ATHEROSCLEROSIS, HYPERTENSION AND DIABETES

PROGRESS IN EXPERIMENTAL CARDIOLOGY

Edited by Naranjan S. Dhalla, Ph.D., M.D. (Hon.), D. Sc. (Hon.)

1. S. Mochizuki, N. Takeda, M. Nagano, N.S. Dhalla (eds.): *The Ischemic Heart.* 1998. ISBN 0-7923-8105-X
2. N.S. Dhalla, P. Zahradka, I. Dixon, R. Beamish (eds.): *Angiotension II Receptor Blockade: Physiological and Clinical Implications.* 1998. ISBN 0-7923-8147-5
3. N. Takeda, M. Nagano, N.S. Dhalla (eds.): *The Hypertrophied Heart,* 2000. ISBN 0-7923-7714-9
4. B. Ostadal, M. Nagano, N.S. Dhalla (eds.): *Cardiac Development,* 2002. ISBN 1-4020-7052-7
5. P. Singal, I. Dixon, L. Kirshenbaum, N.S. Dhalla (eds.): *Cardiac Remodeling and Failure,* 2003. ISBN 1-4020-7177-9
6. N.S. Dhalla, N. Takeda, M. Singh, A. Lukas (eds.): *Myocardial Ischemia and Preconditioning,* 2003. ISBN 1-4020-7195-7
7. N.S. Dhalla, L. Hryshko, E. Kardami, P. Singal (eds.): *Signal Transduction and Cardiac Hypertrophy,* 2003. ISBN 1-4020-7218-X
8. G. Pierce, M. Nagano, P. Zahradka, N.S. Dhalla (eds.): *Atherosclerosis, Hypertension and Diabetes,* 2003. ISBN 1-4020-7311-9

ATHEROSCLEROSIS, HYPERTENSION AND DIABETES

Editors
GRANT N. PIERCE, PhD, FACC
Professor & Director
Division of Stroke & Vascular Disease
St. Boniface General Hospital Research Centre
Faculty of Medicine, University of Manitoba
Winnipeg, Canada

MAKOTO NAGANO, MD, PhD
Professor Emeritus
Department of Medicine, Jikei University School of Medicine
Tokyo, Japan

PETER ZAHRADKA, PhD
Associate Professor
Institute of Cardiovascular Sciences
St. Boniface General Hospital Research Centre
Faculty of Medicine, University of Manitoba
Winnipeg, Canada

NARANJAN S. DHALLA, PhD, MD (Hon), DSc (Hon)
Distinguished Professor and Director
Institute of Cardiovascular Sciences
St. Boniface General Hospital Research Centre
Faculty of Medicine, University of Manitoba
Winnipeg, Canada

KLUWER ACADEMIC PUBLISHERS
BOSTON

Distributors for North, Central and South America:
Kluwer Academic Publishers
101 Philip Drive
Assinippi Park
Norwell, Massachusetts 02061 USA
Telephone (781) 871-6600
Fax (781) 681-9045
E-Mail: kluwer@wkap.com

Distributors for all other countries:
Kluwer Academic Publishers Group
Post Office Box 322
3300 AH Dordrecht, THE NETHERLANDS
Telephone 31 786 576 000
Fax 31 786 576 474
E-Mail: services@wkap.nl

Electronic Services <http://www.wkap.nl>

Atherosclerosis, Hypertension and Diabetes/editors, Grant N. Pierce, Makoto Nagano, Peter Zahradka, Naranjan S. Dhalla.
Series: Progress in Experimental Cardiology
ISBN: 1-4020-7311-9

Printed on acid-free paper.

Printed in the United States of America.

CONTENTS

II. HYPERTENSION

III. DIABETES MELLITUS

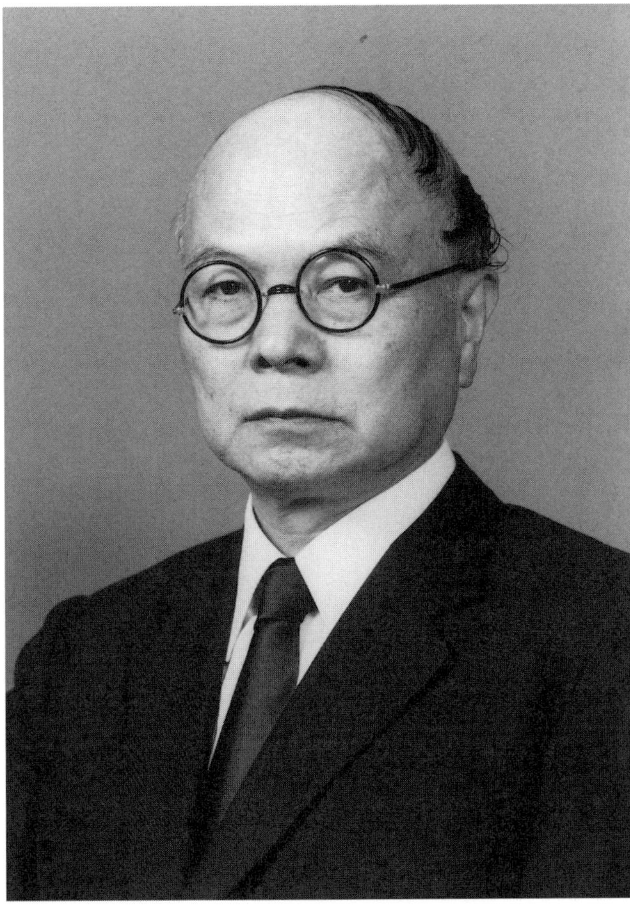

Prof. Setsuro Ebashi, MD, PhD
Okazaki, Japan

A TRIBUTE TO PROFESSOR SETSURO EBASHI, MD, PhD

This book is dedicated to Professor Setsuro Ebashi to recognize his outstanding achievements in the area of Cardiovascular Science and Medicine. Nowadays even students know well that Ca^{2+} plays an important role in cellular activities. However, not many people know that we are greatly indebted to Professor Setsuro Ebashi who made the most important contribution to the establishment of the role of Ca^{2+} as the second messenger first in skeletal muscle.

Deeply impressed by the molecular mechanism of contraction, especially the demonstration of ATP-induced contraction of glycerinated muscle, described in "Chemistry of Muscular Contraction" by A. Szent-Gyorgyi (1949), young Dr. Ebashi determined to work in the field of muscle contraction. The question he first raised was the following. Although ATP induces contractile response of actomyosin system, the removal of ATP does not cause relaxation, which is quite different from acetylcholine-induced contraction of living muscle, where the removal of acetylcholine results in relaxation. He thought that there must be something in living muscle to cause relaxation, which was lost during the preparation of the glycerinated muscle or other actomyosin systems. He started to search for the factor in homogenized muscle and soon found a factor that caused relaxation of glycerinated muscle in the presence of ATP and reported to a meeting of a Japanese muscle physiology group in 1952. Later he realized that Marsh had already reported a similar factor in 1951. However, this was not a disappointment but an encouragement to Dr. Ebashi because it proved that his direction of research was right. Having inquired into the nature of the relaxing factor, he showed in 1955 that the essential component of the relaxing factor was in the particulate fraction, against the general belief at that time that it may be soluble ATP-regenerating enzyme(s).

As for the mechanism of relaxation, Dr. Ebashi conclusively proved in early 1960s that removal of Ca^{2+} from the medium by the relaxing factor is the cause of relaxation. The proof consisted of his several important discoveries: • the relaxing factor strongly takes up Ca^{2+} from the medium into its lumen in the presence of ATP; • chelating agents also cause relaxation and their potency is proportional to their affinity to Ca^{2+} in the ionic condition of the relaxation experiments; • a minute amount of Ca^{2+} is necessary for the contractile reaction of well-washed Ca^{2+}-free natural actomyosin system, and, therefore, the removal of Ca^{2+} from the medium causes the relaxation. (Although physiologists had recognized the contraction-inducing action of Ca^{2+}, it had not been recognized by biochemists before Dr. Ebashi, because Ca^{2+} had been thought to have no effect on the contractile reaction since all the biochemical experiments had been done in the presence of a sufficient amount of Ca^{2+} contamination from reagents and/or exuded from glassware of the day.) Dr. Ebashi further demonstrated that the particulate relaxing factor has a vesicular structure under electron microscopy, indicating that it is fragmented sarcoplasmic reticulum. Since relaxation is the reverse of contraction, these findings led to a clear picture of excitation-contraction coupling: excitation somehow exerts an influence on the sarcoplasmic reticulum to cause a release of Ca^{2+} it accumulated during relaxed state, and the Ca^{2+} released in turn activates the contractile reaction.

In spite of such clear evidence, it took some time for everybody to be convinced of the vital role of Ca^{2+} in contraction, probably because biochemists at that time firmly believed that such an important biological phenomenon as contraction must be managed by some complex organic substance produced by the relaxing factor and not by such a small common inorganic ion Ca^{2+}.

One of the objections against the Ca^{2+} theory was the fact that the effect of Ca^{2+} was sometimes variable depending on the preparation of actomyosin. If it is the important physiological mechanism, the effect of Ca^{2+} should be brought about consistently any time. Dr. Ebashi inquired into this problem and discovered 'the third protein' participating contraction (the first two being myosin and actin), which conferred the Ca^{2+} sensitivity upon the actomyosin system. He further elucidated that • the protein factor is a complex of tropomyosin and a new protein which he named troponin; • tropomyosin and troponin are associated with actin filaments in living muscle; • in the absence of Ca^{2+}, troponin in collaboration with tropomyosin exerts an inhibitory influence on actin to prevent it from interacting with myosin; and • Ca^{2+} is bound to troponin and resulting conformational change of troponin removes the inhibitory influence mentioned above to start contractile reaction. Later it was found that troponin is a heterotrimer consisting of troponin T (the tropomyosin-binding subunit), troponin I (the inhibitory subunit) and troponin C (the Ca^{2+}-binding subunit).

Among the discoveries mentioned above, the fact that a minute amount of Ca^{2+} causes contractile reaction of the actomyosin system was also found independently by Dr. A. Weber, and the fact that the relaxing factor can accumulate Ca^{2+} in the presence of ATP by Drs. W. Hasselbach and M. Makinose, both at about the same time. However, the discovery of troponin, the first Ca^{2+}-receptive protein, and the following elucidation of the molecular mechanism of regulation of contraction and relaxation by Ca^{2+} are Professor Ebashi's unrivaled sphere of activity. Thus, it is no exaggeration to say that Professor Ebashi is the person who opened up the present Ca^{2+} era.

Professor Ebashi was awarded numerous prizes for his great contribution including an Order of Cultural Merits and the Japan Academy Award with an Imperial gift. He is now Professor Emeritus of the University of Tokyo and of National Institute for Physiological Sciences. He is also a member of the Japan Academy, a foreign member of the Royal Society, London, a member of the National Academy of Sciences, USA, and a member of Leopoldina German Academy. He was decorated with the First Order of Merit, the highest rank of decoration in Japan in 1995.

He lives in Okazaki with his wife, Dr. Fumiko Ebashi, who supported him faithfully at home as well as in the laboratory as a coworker and a secretary. Very unfortunately he has been ill for about two years. However, he is mentally still sharp, and everybody who knows him prays earnestly for his recovery and longevity.

Makoto Endo
Moroyama, Japan

PREFACE

This text, as the title states, is a compilation of papers devoted to the study of atherosclerosis, hypertension and diabetes. These three distinct disease entities, although not entirely unrelated, are three of the most important disease conditions in the world today. As such, this volume of research papers is of obvious medical importance. The justification of the energy, time and financial resources directed towards the study of each of these three diseases requires some discussion.

The majority of papers amongst the three diseases that are discussed in this volume are dedicated to the study of atherosclerosis. This is not by accident. Cardiovascular disease is the number one killer today in the world. In the United States almost 61 million Americans have one or more forms of cardiovascular disease. These diseases claimed nearly 1 million lives in 1998 alone. Although approximately 80% of those who die of cardiovascular disease are 65 years of age or older, a significant number of people are killed by cardiovascular disease below the age of 65. Atherosclerotic heart disease in the coronary vasculature caused approximately ½ million deaths in the United States in 1998. At least 12,400,000 people are alive today in the United States with a history of myocardial infarctions or chest pain or both. Clearly, atherosclerotic disease in the heart is a major medical problem. This disease affects both men and women. Although men are more likely to experience a heart attack and are at greater risk for cardiovascular disease, more then ½ of the people alive today with a history of heart attacks or angina are females. As well, women who do have myocardial infarctions are twice as likely to die from the event within a few weeks. Atherosclerotic vascular disease is not limited to just the heart. An atherosclerotic ischemic event is the primary cause of stroke today. Although it is not well appreciated, stroke is the number 3 killer in America today and the leading cause of debilitating neurological damage. Atherosclerotic vascular disease therefore, has a cost in terms of human life, quality of life and financial burden today that no other disease can match. The seriousness of this medical problem demands research attention.

The papers in this volume are directed towards increasing our understanding of novel ways of preventing or treating atherosclerotic disease. We also examine some of the basic mechanisms involved in the atherosclerotic process. For example, nutritional interventions are discussed that may prevent, retard or treat the atherosclerotic process. These include, vitamin therapy (like vitamin D or vitamin B in the treatment of hyperhomocysteinemia), the replacement of hydrogenated fats in the diet because of the influence on cholesterol levels, the use of antioxidants like coenzyme Q10 and other nutritional interventions. Several papers discuss the use of cholesterol lowering agents and their effects both in the control of cholesterol metabolism and atherosclerosis and in the surprising beneficial side-effects that these drugs have in platelet activation. Naturally, lipids themselves are a focus for research intervention. Two papers in our volume address a particular type of lipid, oxidized LDL, as a focus for interventional therapy. The identification of new oxidized LDL receptors and the mechanisms whereby oxy radicals influence cholesterol metabolism may be some of the most important sites for research study in this area that have been identified in the last two decades.

Other sites for research intervention have been identified in this text. The interaction and the use of bone marrow in the study of atherosclerosis is a novel and exciting intervention that has gained enormous popularity in the last few years. Finally, the study of endothelial cell dysfunction and angiotensin and its relationship to atherosclerosis remain exciting avenues to understanding not only how atherosclerosis may block vessels but also how these areas may influence vessel contractile function and the distribution of blood flow through a vascular system.

One of the most novel and intriguing areas of research in the 21st century with regard to cardiovascular disease has been the identified association of infection with atherosclerosis. Although, at first, this seemed to be quite an erratic departure from the dogma of atherogenesis, it is now well recognized that vascular inflammation and the changes in lipid metabolism associated with atherosclerosis may be important stimuli for the development of this disease. Involvement of PPAR-α in the vascular inflammation and a detailed treatise of the use of animals in the study of chlamydia pneumonia as an atherogenic agent are both exciting, new additions in the study of atherosclerotic vascular disease.

Hypertension is often referred to as the silent killer. It is estimated that one in four adults in the United States has hypertension. However, because hypertension has virtually no symptoms, one in three people who have high blood pressure don't even know it. This "silent disease" is deadly. Hypertension killed almost 45,000 Americans in 1998 and contributed to the deaths of 210,000 more. As many as 50 million Americans 6 years of age and older have hypertension. There are racial predispositions for high blood pressure. For example, non-Hispanic blacks and Mexican Americans are more likely to experience high blood pressure than non-Hispanic whites. High blood pressure affects one in three African Americans. Further research into the mechanisms of hypertension is clearly justified. Amazingly, in 90 to 95 percent of cases of people with high blood pressure, the cause is unknown. High blood pressure is the single most important risk factor for strokes. Obviously, the more we understand about how to reduce high blood pressure, the better we can reduce the incidence of stroke, neurological damage, and heart disease.

The papers in this volume dedicated to the study of hypertension focus on factors that may be responsible for high blood pressure. These include examining the genetic predisposition to hypertension as well as how drugs may inhibit the genes involved in vascular hyperplasia and remodeling (two phenomena associated with hypertension). Other papers examine insulin resistance and its involvement in hypertension, and the neurological aspects associated with high blood pressure. These include the involvement of the sympathetic nervous system and hypothalamic peptides in the development of hypertension. An important paper in this volume discusses the cellular function of the endothelium and its relationship to blood pressure. The nutritional basis of hypertension is also examined and discussed. It has long been recognized that kidney dysfunction is involved in the hypertensive condition. One of the papers in this volume examines the effects of leptin on the cardiovascular system and renal function. Although the kidney has long been associated with hypertension as the primary etiological organ, the intriguing involvement of the brain and insulin resistance in the hypertensive condition is identified and discussed in two separate manuscripts. Finally, one paper has advanced novel routes of drug delivery for the treatment of hypertension.

Diabetes is another major disease in the world today. Nearly 60 million Americans have insulin resistance and 25% of these cases will go on to develop diabetes. Diabetes kills 60,000 Americans each year and it is estimated that its complications can contribute to another 190,000 deaths each year. Before the discovery of insulin, most diabetic patients died after lapsing into a coma. Today, with the conventional use of insulin therapy, diabetic patients are living longer but still die sooner than their non-diabetic counterparts. People with diabetes are 2 to 4 times more likely to have stroke or heart disease. If the heart disease does occur, it is more severe in the diabetic and more likely to develop into congestive heart failure than in the non-diabetic population. Diabetes causes lipid abnormalities that are conducive to heart disease. Decreases in high density lipoproteins and increases in low density lipoprotein and triglycerides are common in the diabetic population. Most diabetic patients (approximately 80 to 90 percent) are over weight. The complications of diabetes are not limited to just cardiovascular disease. Diabetes can cause or lead to induction of blindness, kidney disease, nerve disease and limb amputations. Research to discover new methods for the treatment and prevention of diabetes are clearly justified.

The papers in this text on diabetes discuss the risk factors and mechanisms responsible for diabetic vascular and cardiac dysfunction. For example, the involvement of cholesterol and cardiovascular disease in diabetes is discussed. Another paper extends this to a treatise detailing the alterations in the lipid profiles found in diabetic patients and the changes in fibrinolysis. Diabetic vascular disease is discussed as is the role of the endothelium in cardiovascular disease in diabetics. In view of the association of diabetes with excessive body weight, one of the papers examines the mechanisms of adipogenesis and sheds light on the factors involved in this important process. Several papers in this text discuss diabetic heart disease. They describe the mechanisms underlying Type I and Type II diabetic cardiomyopathy, the current research on Type II diabetic heart disease, energy metabolism in the diabetic heart, and a variety of molecular mechanisms responsible for diabetic heart disease. Another interesting paper discusses the use of vanadate as an alternative therapy to insulin in the treatment of diabetes mellitus. New ideas are presented for the mechanism involved in insulin resistance. Finally, one of the significant papers in this manuscript examines how neurotransmitters (like 5 HT) may function as targets for the prevention of cardiovascular disease and diabetes.

This volume brings together nearly 40 papers to discuss the 3 diseases covered by this text; atherosclerosis, hypertension and diabetes. These manuscripts were invited from scientists who presented state of the art lectures at the XVII World Congress of the International Society for Heart Research that was held in Winnipeg, Canada in July, 2001. This Congress, which attracted approximately 2,000 participants, not only served as a venue for scientific interaction and networking but, as evidenced by this volume itself, also resulted in the generation of new science and new thought processes as they pertain to these 3 significant pathological conditions. We certainly hope that you enjoy reading these manuscripts. We believe that they lead to new insights into the management and treatment of atherosclerosis, diabetes and hypertension.

Grant N. Pierce, Winnipeg, Canada
Makoto Nagano, Tokyo, Japan
Peter Zahradka, Winnipeg, Canada
Naranjan S. Dhalla, Winnipeg, Canada

ACKNOWLEDGMENTS

We are grateful to the following corporations and granting agencies for their generous donations in support of the XVII World Heart Congress of the International Society for Heart Research, the first Public Heart Health Forum as well as publication of this book:

PATRONS:
Government of Canada (Dept. of Western Diversification)
Government of Manitoba (Depts. of Industry Trade and Mines; Health; Post-Secondary Education; Culture Heritage and Tourism)
Merck Frosst Canada, Ltd.
Mitsubishi-Tokyo Pharmaceuticals Inc.

PARTNERS:
American Section of the International Society for Heart Research
AstraZeneca
Aventis Pharmaceuticals Inc.
Bayer Canada, Inc.
City of Winnipeg
International Academy of Cardiovascular Sciences
International Society for Heart Research (Kaito Fund, Bayer Yakuhin Fund and Canon Fund)
Kowa Pharmaceuticals
Pfizer Canada
St. Boniface General Hospital Research Foundation

COLLABORATORS:
CanWest Global Foundation
CIHR Institute of Circulatory and Respiratory Health
Eli Lilly
Great West Life and London Life
Manitoba Liquor Control Commission
Mars Incorporated
Medicure, Inc.
Myles Robinson Memorial Heart Fund

Safeway Food and Drug
University of Manitoba (Faculty of Medicine; Departments of Physiology and Human Anatomy & Cell Science)

BENEFACTORS:
ATL Canada
Beckman Coulter Canada Inc.
Canadian Cardiovascular Society
Canadian Institutes of Health Research
Cardiovascular Solutions, Inc.
Dairy Farmers of Canada
De Fehr Foundation
Faculty of Health Sciences, University of Western Ontario
Heart and Stroke Foundation of Manitoba
Institute of Biodiagnostics, National Research Council of Canada
Japanese Working Group on Cardiac Structure and Metabolism
Manitoba Hydro
Merck KGaA (Germany)
Pulsus Group Inc.
St. Boniface General Hospital Research Centre
Wawanesa Mutual Insurance Company
World Heart Corporation

The collaboration of Ms. Eva Little, Ms. Janet Labarre, Ms. Diane Stowe, Ms. Florence Willerton and Ms. Susan Zettler in coordinating diverse editorial activities associated with this book is gratefully acknowledged. Special thanks are due to Mr. Zachary Rolnik, Ms. Mimi T. Breed, Ms. Melissa Ramondetta and their editorial staff at Kluwer Academic Publishers for their patience, interest and hard work in assembling this volume.

ATHEROSCLEROSIS, HYPERTENSION AND DIABETES

I. ATHEROSCLEROSIS AND CARDIOVASCULAR DISEASE

G.N. Pierce, M. Nagano, P. Zahradka, and N.S. Dhalla (eds.).
ATHEROSCLEROSIS, HYPERTENSION AND DIABETES. Copyright © 2003.
Kluwer Academic Publishers. Boston.

PPAR-ALPHA IN LIPID AND LIPOPROTEIN METABOLISM, VASCULAR INFLAMMATION AND ATHEROSCLEROSIS

JEAN-CHARLES FRUCHART, BART STAELS, and PATRICK DURIEZ

Unité de Recherche sur les Lipoprotéines et l'Athérosclérose—Inserm U545—Institut Pasteur et Université de Lille 2—Faculté de Pharmacie—Lille, France

Summary. Peroxisome proliferator-activated receptors (PPARs) are ligand-activated transcription factors belonging to the nuclear receptor superfamily, PPAR-alpha is highly expressed in liver, skeletal muscle, kidney, heart and the vascular wall. PPARs are activated by fatty-acid derivatives and pharmacological agents such as fibrates for PPAR-alpha. PPAR-alpha controls intra- and extracellular lipid metabolisms. Fibric acids decrease triglyceride concentrations by increasing the expression of lipoprotein lipase and decreasing apo C-III concentration. Furthermore, they increase HDL-cholesterol by increasing the expression of apo A-I and apo A-II. In addition, PPARs also modulate the inflammatory response. PPAR activators have been shown to exert anti-inflammatory activities in various cell types by inhibiting the expression of proinflammatory genes such as cytokines, metalloproteases and acute-phase proteins. PPARs negatively regulate the transcription of inflammatory response genes by antagonizing the AP-1, nuclear factor-κB (NF-κB), signal transducer and activator of transcription (STAT) and nuclear factor of activated T-cells (NFAT) signalling pathways and by stimulating the catabolism of proinflammatory eicosanoids. PPAR-alpha activators (gemfibrozil) decrease the risk of coronary heart disease in patients with normal LDL-cholesterol and low HDL-cholesterol (VA-HIT) and they slow the progression of premature coronary atherosclerosis (BECAIT) (bezafibrate), particularly in patients with type 2 diabetes (DAIS) (fenofibrate).

Key words: PPAR-alpha, Lipoproteins, Inflammation, Atherosclerosis

Corresponding Author: Prof. Jean-Charles Fruchart, Département d'Athérosclérose, Inserm U545, Institut Pasteur de Lille, 1 rue du Prof. Calmette, BP 245, 59019 Lille cedex—France. Tel: 33 3 20 87 77 52; Fax: 33 3 20 87 73 60; e-mail: Jean-Charles.Fruchart@pasteur-lille.fr

INTRODUCTION

Epidemiological and intervention studies have now confirmed that dyslipidemias are major risk factors for atherosclerosis and coronary artery disease (CAD). Primary [1] and secondary [2] intervention trials with HMG-CoA reductase inhibitors have undoubtedly proved that a drastic reduction in LDL-cholesterol levels reduces the cardiovascular risk in hyper-LDL-cholesterolaemic patients and even in patients considered as normo-LDL-cholesterolaemics [3]. Nevertheless, other dyslipidaemias, such as hypoalphalipoproteinaemia (low plasma HDL) associated, or not, with concomitant hypertriglyceridemia, may be the cause of a substantial number of cases of CAD [4–5].

In the clinic, PPAR-alpha activators are chemically related to fibric acids (clofibrate, gemfibrozil, fenofibrate, bezafibrate and ciprofibrate).

Fibrates are used in the treatment of hypertriglyceridaemia with or without hypoalphalipoproteinaemia [3,4] and, recently, the VA-HIT (Veterans Affairs-High Density Lipoprotein Cholesterol Intervention Trial) study with a median follow-up of 5.1 years [6] clearly demonstrated that raising HDL-cholesterol and lowering triglycerides, without lowering LDL-cholesterol with gemfibrozil, in men with documented CAD and low HDL-cholesterol reduced the incidence of death from CAD and of non-fatal myocardial infarction by 22% without reducing total mortality.

Nevertheless, although fibrates have been used in clinical practice for over 3 decades now, in depth knowledge of the molecular mechanism of their normolipidaemic effects remained a mystery.

Recently, a direct relationship was evoked between PPAR-alpha activation by fibrates and alteration in lipoprotein metabolism. Furthermore in vivo experiments in animals and in vitro studies suggest that, in humans, fibrates might not only reduce atherosclerosis development through their normolipidaemic properties but also by reducing inflammation at the level of the vascular wall and thrombosis. In this article we review the current knowledge on the role of PPAR-alpha in metabolic diseases and in atherosclerosis.

PEROXISOME PROLIFERATOR-ACTIVATED RECEPTORS (PPARs)

PPAR(s) belong to the family of hormonal activated nuclear receptors. Activated PPAR(s) heterodimerize with activated Rexinoid-X-Receptor (RXR) and bind to the specific so-called "Peroxisome Proliferator Response Elements" (PPREs) which are localized in the promoter of target genes. PPRE(s) are constituted of direct repeat (DR) hexameric sequences which are separated by one or two nucleotides (DR1, DR2). The binding of PPAR to the PPRE induces the expression of the target gene.

To day, 3 different sub-types of PPAR(s) have been reported (alpha, delta, gamma); each specific PPAR sub-type is encoded by one specific gene.

PPAR-alpha is highly expressed in liver, heart, kidney and in brown adipose tissue and moderately in bowel, skeletal muscle, thymus and testis [7].

PPAR-ALPHA ACTIVATORS

PPAR-alpha activators have been synthetized. They include fibric acid derivations (fibrates) and they all induce liver peroxisome proliferation, hepatomegaly and liver cancer in rodents [8].

FIBRIC ACIDS

Wy-14643 and fibric acids (clofibrate, ciprofibrate, bezafibrate, fenofibrate, gemfibrozil . . .) were developed as hypolipidaemic agents in rodents. Clofibric acid and fenofibric acid activate both PPAR-alpha and PPAR-gamma with a 10-fold selectivity for PPAR-alpha. Some fibric acids such as bezafibrate have no specificity for any of the 3 sub-types of PPARs. One common outstanding pharmacological property of clinically used fibric acids is their low affinity for PPAR-alpha (EC50 (μM)) and the resulting required oral high doses (300–1200 mg/day) to achieve clinical efficiency. Newly synthesized PPAR-alpha activators with more than 1000-fold affinity for PPAR-alpha might be promising new drugs for the treatment of dyslipoproteinaemia [9].

EFFECTS OF FIBRIC ACIDS ON PLASMA LIPIDS

Fibric acids are first-line drugs in the treatment of primary hypertriglyceridaemia and are very useful in the treatment of combined hyperlipidaemia, type III dyslipoproteinaemia and secondary lipid abnormalities observed in Non Insulin Dependant Diabetes Mellitus (NIDDM) and obese individuals.

PPAR-alpha activation by fibrates leads to:

- decreased hypertriglyceridaemia by increasing LPL expression [10] and decreasing apo C-III expression [11];
- increased HDL-cholesterol, apo A-I and apo A-II levels [12–14] in human plasma at least partly by increasing apo A-I and apo A-II expression [13,14].
- reduced LDL-cholesterol in combined hyperlipidaemia [15] by decreasing the levels of atherogenic dense LDL, which have poor affinity to the LDL receptor, while increasing buoyant LDL which displays high affinity to this receptor. In primary hypercholesterolaemia, fibrates reduce dense LDL, but not light LDL fractions [16]. In hypercholesterolaemic patients, Caslake M.J. et al. [17] observed that fenofibrate significantly decreased LDL-cholesterol (30%) without decreasing LDL apo B production by shifting LDL from a slowly catabolized pool towards a rapidly catabolized one. Furthermore, the rate of apo B-LDL degradation by the receptor route rose 43% on the drug, whereas the amount cleared by the receptor-independent pathway did not change.

It is generally acknowledged that therapeutic concentrations of fibrates do not inhibit HMG-CoA reductase activity [18].

EFFECT OF FIBRATES ON LIPOPROTEIN METABOLISM

Recent studies have shown that the effects of fibrates on lipoprotein metabolism are due to an increase in cellular FFA catabolism and the resulting inhibition of hepatic VLDL triglyceride secretion, as well as to alterations in genes governing the intravascular hydrolysis of triglycerides and those governing HDL production.

Effects of fibrates on FFA metabolism

PPARα is highly expressed in tissues with elevated rates of FA catabolism, where it regulates genes involved in FA uptake, activation into acyl-CoA esters, degradation via the peroxisomal and mitochondrial beta-oxidation pathways and ketone body synthesis [19].

Fibrate treatment is known to activate PPAR-alpha induced FATP mRNA levels in rat liver and intestine and ACS mRNA levels in the liver and kidney.

PPAR-alpha regulates the entry of FAs into the mitochondria, which is a crucial step in their metabolism, especially in tissues like heart, skeletal muscle and brown adipose tissue in which FAs are a major source of energy.

Three distinct uncoupling protein isoforms, UCP-1, UCP-2 and UCP-3 have been identified and implicated as mediators of thermogenesis. Kelly L.J. et al. [20] reported that the treatment of rats or db/db mice with WY-14,643 (PPAR-alpha ligand) did not affect the expression of UCP-1, 2 or 3 in brown adipose tissue. Nevertheless, hepatic UCP-2 mRNA was increased (x 4 over the control level) in db/db and lean mice, although this effect was not observed in rats. This data shows that PPAR-alpha activators may also regulate UCP proteins, which may be an end-step in the FA catabolic actions of these drugs.

This data as a whole shows that PPAR-alpha activators stimulate different steps in FA oxidative metabolism in different organs and particularly in the liver where they reduce the quantity of FA available for VLDL synthesis and secretion.

Effects of fibrates on genes involved in lipoprotein metabolism

Triglyceride-rich lipoprotein metabolism

One of the major effects of PPAR-alpha activators on plasma lipid metabolism is to reduce triglyceride levels. Kesaniemi Y.A. et al. [21] showed that gemfibrozil decreased the production of VLDL triglyceride by an average of 28%.

Nevertheless, as shown by Kesaniemi Y.A. et al. [21], inhibition of VLDL triglyceride synthesis is not the unique hypotriglyceridaemic effect of fibrates. In this study, gemfibrozil reduced VLDL triglyceride synthesis by only 28% but increased the fractional catabolic rate of VLDL triglyceride by 92%. This suggests that PPAR-alpha activators decrease plasma triglyceride concentrations by increasing VLDL- and chylomicron-triglyceride hydrolysis.

In fact, fibrates increase post-heparin plasma LPL activity.

Schoonjans K. et al. [22] demonstrated that inducibility of the LPL gene by PPAR-alpha correlated with the tissue distribution of this nuclear receptor in rat.

A sequence element was identified as a PPRE in the human LPL promoter that mediates the functional responsiveness to PPAR-alpha activators. The main effect of fibrates is, therefore, on LPL production in rat liver.

Apo C-III acts by delaying the catabolism of triglyceride-rich particles by inhibiting their binding to the endothelial surface and lipolysis by LPL, as well, by interfering with apo E-mediated receptor clearance of remnant particles from plasma [23–28].

Using PPAR-alpha deficient mice, Peters et al. [29] demonstrated an obligatory role for PPAR-alpha in the repression of apo C-III gene expression by fibrates. The regulation of apo C-III gene transcription is complex, being governed by an ensemble of transcription factor binding sites within 1 Kb upstream of the transcription initiation site. Among these sites is the C3P (also called CIIIB) site, to which a number of nuclear receptors such as HNF-4, ARP-1, Ear/COUP-TF [30], RXR and PPAR-alpha bind [31]. Whereas HNF-4, RXR and PPAR-alpha [31] can activate apo C-III gene transcription via this site, ARP-1 and Ear3/COUP-TF act as repressors [30]. Further studies are required to determine whether apo C-III transcriptional repression by PPAR-alpha activators involves any or all of these nuclear factors.

In severe primary hypercholesterolaemia, fenofibrate therapy decreased apo C-III and lipoprotein particles containing both apo C-III and apo B [32]. Staels B. et al. [11] demonstrated that fibrates down-regulate apo C-III expression independently of any induction of peroxisomal acyl CoA oxidase.

These studies show that PPAR-alpha activators decrease human and rat liver apo C-III expression, but the molecular mechanism of this down-regulation has not yet been fully elucidated.

HDL metabolism

Fibric acid therapy increases HDL-cholesterol plasma levels ($\simeq$ 10–15%) in hypertriglyceridaemia [33], combined hyperlipidaemia [34,35] and hypercholesterolaemia [35,36]. These increases in HDL-cholesterol levels are associated with significant increases in levels of apo A-I and apo A-II. Malmendier et al. [12] showed that fenofibrate increased apo A-I in hypercholesterolaemic patients by increasing its synthetic rate much more than its catabolic rate.

Recent studies have demonstrated, in humans, that fibric acids increase plasma HDL concentrations, at least in part, through the induction of the expression of the human apo A-I and apo A-II genes [13,14,37].

Vu-Dac et al. [13] showed that the transcription rate of the human apo A-I gene is induced by PPAR-alpha which interacts with a positive PPRE located in the A site of the human apo A-I gene promoter liver specific enhancer.

In 1995, Vu Dac N. et al. [14] reported that fibric acids induced apo A-II mRNA in primary cultures of human hepatocytes and in human hepatoblastoma cells resulting in increased apo A-II secretion in both cell culture systems. These authors identified a DR1-type PPRE in the J-site of the human apo A-II promoter and demonstrated that fibric acids increase apo A-II plasma levels by stimulating transcription of its gene through the interaction of activated PPAR-alpha with the apo AII-PPRE.

Recently, it has been reported that fibrates increase HDL-receptor activity in human macrophages by stimulating the expression of SR-BI/CLA-1 [38] and ABCA1 [39]. These 2 receptors have been shown to be capable of binding HDL to plasma membrane and of inducing free cholesterol efflux from foam cells derived from human macrophages. This cellular cholesterol efflux corresponds to the first step in the so-called "reverse cholesterol transport" which is responsible for returning excess peripherical cholesterol to the liver to eliminate it in biliary secretion. Therefore, fibrates would not only increase reverse cholesterol transport through increasing the number of cholesterol carriers (HDL) but they would also increase the cellular expression of the HDL receptors whose task is to ensure the binding of these carriers to cell membrane and to induce the efflux of excess cellular cholesterol.

PPAR-ALPHA IN INFLAMMATION

The first evidence indicating a potential role for PPARs in the inflammatory response was the demonstration that leukotriene B4 (LTB4), a proinflammatory eicosanoid, binds to PPAR-alpha and induces the transcription of genes involved in omega- and beta-oxydation which leads to the induction of its own catabolism [40]. Using the mouse ear-swelling test, these authors showed that the duration of the inflammatory response is prolonged in PPAR-alpha deficient mice in response to LTB4 [40]. Several recent studies have been aimed at delineating the cellular and molecular mechanisms explaining the control of the inflammatory response by PPAR-alpha. In primary aortic smooth muscle cells which express substantial amounts of PPAR-alpha, it was demonstrated that PPAR-alpha ligands inhibit interleukin (IL)-1beta-induced IL-6 secretion as well as 6-keto-prostaglandin (PG) F_{1alpha} production. In addition, PPAR-alpha agonists have been reported to decrease cytokine-induced genes, such as expression of vascular cell adhesion molecule-1 and tissue factor in endothelial cells and monocytes respectively [41,42]. Subsequently, it was shown that PPAR-alpha acts by down-regulating the transcription of these genes [43,44]. In vivo evidence for an anti-inflammatory action of PPAR-alpha in the vascular wall came with the demonstration that aortas from PPAR-alpha deficient mice displayed an exacerbated inflammatory response to lipopolysaccharide stimulation [44]. Furthermore, fibrates did not affect LPS-induced IL-6 transcription in PPAR-alpha deficient mice, demonstrating that the anti-inflammatory activities of these agonists require PPAR-alpha expression in vivo. In addition, Poynter and Daynes [45] reported that PPAR-alpha deficient splenocytes produced, in response to lipopolysaccharide (LPS) stimulation, two to three times more IL-6 and IL-12 than splenocytes from wild-type mice. Finally, fibrates were shown to repress the expression of a number of acute-phase proteins in liver, such as fibrinogen, in a PPAR-alpha dependent manner [46]. Taken together, these observations provide evidence that PPAR-alpha plays a role in the inflammatory response at the vascular, splenic and hepatic level.

Studies addressing the molecular mechanisms of this anti-inflammatory action demonstrated that PPAR-alpha negatively interferes with the inflammatory response by antagonizing the nuclear factor-κB (NF-κB) signalling pathway [41,43,44,45]. In fact, a bidirectional antagonism between the PPAR-alpha and NF-κB signalling pathways exists [44]. PPAR-alpha overexpression inhibits NF-κB-driven gene transcription and co-transfection of increasing amounts of p65 led to a dose-dependent inhibition of a PPAR response element (PPRE)-driven promoter construct. Glutathion-S-transferase (GST) pull-down assays revealed that PPAR-alpha physically interacts with p65 via its Rel homology domain which mediates homo- and heterodimerization and interaction with inhibitor of NF-κB (IκB) [44]. Since PPAR-alpha mediated inhibition of NF-κB-driven gene transcription becomes more and more important upon longer exposure to PPAR-alpha ligands, we speculated that a complementary mechanism might exist. NF-κB activity is tightly controlled by the degradation of IκB-alpha which sequesters inactive NF-κB dimers in the cytoplasm. Interestingly, PPAR-alpha activators were found to induce IκB-alpha mRNA and protein expression in primary smooth muscle cells and hepatocytes [47]. IκB-alpha induction by fibrates again requires PPAR-alpha expression. Surprisingly, IκB-alpha induction did not affect p65 nuclear translocation but was associated with reduced NF-κB DNA-binding activity [47]. Western blot analysis revealed that IκB-alpha protein induction occurs mainly in the nucleus which may provide an explanation for the reduced NF-κB binding activity [47]. The induction of IκB-alpha by fibrates in cytokine-activated cells should therefore result in an acceleration of NF-κB nuclear deactivation. In line with this observation, the increase of IκB-alpha protein after treatment with PPAR-alpha activators would lead to a halt in p65-mediated gene activation, thereby reducing the duration of the inflammatory response. This is consistent with a previous report in which PPAR-alpha ligands were shown to affect the duration of the inflammatory response in a PPAR-alpha dependent manner [40]. In view of these results, we propose a model in which PPAR-alpha negatively interferes with NF-κB transcription activity by forming inactive complexes with p65 and by inducing IκB-alpha, the major inhibitor of NF-κB signalling. Chromatin immunoprecipitation experiments revealed that the glucocorticoid receptor antagonizes NF-κB transcription activity by interfering with phosphorylation of the serine-2 of the carboxy-terminal domain of the RNA polymerase II without affecting NF-κB DNA-binding activities, although the glucocorticoid receptor strongly interacts with p65 [48]. It would be of interest to determine whether such a mechanism is also operative for PPAR-alpha using the same technical approach. However, we cannot exclude the existence of additional mechanisms. For instance, PPAR-alpha was reported to play a major role in the control of the cellular redox status [45]. Moreover, Klucis et al. [49] reported that administration of PPAR-alpha activators results in a drastic increase of the activity of catalase, an antioxidant enzyme. Finally, catalase activity and expression were found to be increased in endothelial cells upon fibrate treatment (C. Furman, E. Teissier, B. Staels, P. Duriez, unpublished observations—Data not shown).

A potential involvement of catalase in the control of NF-κB driven transcription by PPAR-alpha activators is under investigation in our laboratory.

Promoter analysis revealed that PPAR-alpha controls IL-6 transcription by negatively interfering not only with NF-κB but also with AP-1 transcriptional activities [44]. GST pull-down experiments as well as electrophoretic mobility shift assays demonstrated that PPAR-alpha activators reduce AP-1 DNA-binding activity by physically interacting with the amino-terminal domain of c-Jun [44,50]. Since most of the proinflammatory genes are under the control of the AP-1 and NF-κB signalling pathways, it is likely that PPAR-alpha agonists regulate a wide spectrum of genes involved in inflammatory disorders.

One of the most relevant indications regarding a role of PPAR-alpha agonists in inflammation control comes from clinical trials. The influence of PPAR-alpha activators on plasma cytokine levels as well as on acute-phase proteins was determined in patients with angiographically established atherosclerosis [43]. Fibrate treatment for 4 weeks (200 mg daily) reduced IL-6, C-reactive protein and fibrinogen levels in patients with coronary artery disease [43]. Another group reported independently that fenofibrate treatment for 1 month resulted in a significant reduction of plasma interferon-gamma (IFNgamma) and tumour necrosis factor-alpha (TNF-alpha) levels in patients with hyperlipoproteinaemia type IIb [51]. These two reports demonstrate that PPAR-alpha activators decrease inflammation in patients, thus indicating a potential use of PPAR-alpha agonists in the treatment of chronic inflammatory diseases.

EFFECTS OF PPAR-ALPHA ACTIVATORS IN THE TREATMENT OF DYSLIPOPROTEINAEMIAS AND IN THE PREVENTION OF ATHEROSCLEROSIS

Reduction of triglyceride and/or increase in HDL-cholesterol plasma levels

In order to stress on the primary targets of fibrates (high triglycerides and low HDL-cholesterol plasma levels) we will present recent clinical data with fibrates that induce strong reduction of triglyceride plasma levels (gemfibrozil, bezafibrate).

Gemfibrozil

In 1997, data of the LOCAT's study (Lipid Coronary Angiography Trial) [52] showed that gemfibrozil therapy retarded the progression of coronary atherosclerosis and the formation of bypass-graft lesions after coronary bypass surgery in men with low HDL cholesterol as their main lipid abnormality.

Syvänne M et al. [53] have studied which lipoproteins, separated by preparative ultracentrifugation, predict angiographic progression in this population. Analysis of the lipoprotein compositions clearly showed that all lipoprotein classes were significantly depleted of triglycerides by gemfibrozil. VLDL were both decreased in number and depleted of lipid, but there was no suggestion of any reduction of IDL or increase of HDL2 particle numbers. Total serum cholesterol and both triglyceride and cholesterol in the IDL and LDL fractions were positively and significantly associated with the risk of global angiographic progression and HDL cholesterol concentration was not associated with protection against progression.

This study adds to the growing evidence of the atherogenecity of triglyceride-rich lipoproteins, especially IDL, and the antiatherogenic influence of HDL3 and suggest that reductions of triglyceride levels that are commonly considered normal seem to provide protection against progressive CAD.

The objective of the Veterans Affairs-High Density Lipoprotein Cholesterol Intervention Trial (VA-HIT) [6] was to test if gemfibrozil decreases CAD death and non-fatal myocardial infarctions in men with documented CAD and HDL-cholesterol ≤40 mg/dl, LDL-cholesterol ≤140 mg/dl and triglycerides ≤300 mg/dl. 2531 patients enrolled into the study and the median follow-up was 5.1 years.

Gemfibrozil (1200 mg/day) decreased total cholesterol by 2.8% and triglycerides by 24.5% but had no effect on LDL-cholesterol and increased HDL-cholesterol by 7.5%.

Gemfibrozil treatment reduced coronary heart death [by 22% ($p = 0.006$)] and non myocardial infarction (274 (21.6%) and 219 (17.3%) in the placebo and gemfibrozil group, respectively). Furthermore, stroke was less frequent in the gemfibrozil group but there was no difference in the rates of coronary revascularisation, or hospitalisation due to unstable angina between the two groups, as there was no difference in the total mortability between the two groups nor in the frequency of new malignancies.

Therefore VA-HIT provides direct clinical evidence of a beneficial effect of reducing triglycerides and increasing HDL-cholesterol without affecting LDL-cholesterol in secondary prevention in patients with low HDL-cholesterol and low-cholesterol.

Bezafibrate

The Bezafibrate Coronary Atherosclerosis Intervention Trial (BECAIT) was initiated to determine whether bezafibrate retards the progression or facilitates regression of premature coronary atherosclerosis [54–56]. The angiographic findings over the 5 years of study indicated that the median change in minimum lumen diameter (MLD) at final assessment was on average 0.13 mm less in the bezafibrate group than in the placebo group ($p < 0.049$).

In 1998, Ruotolo et al [57] examined if there was a relationship between the progression of coronary lesions in the BECAIT and lipoproteins and lipoproteins subfractions. In addition to the decrease in VLDL-cholesterol (−53%) and triglyceride (−46%), bezafibrate treatment resulted in a significant increase in HDL3-cholesterol (+9%) and a shift in the LDL subclass distribution toward larger particle species without any effect on LDL-cholesterol levels. Decreases in small dense LDL and/or VLDL lipid concentrations were unrelated to disease progression. These data suggest that the effect of bezafibrate on progression of focal coronary atherosclerosis could, at least partly, be attributed to a rise in HDL3-cholesterol and a decrease in the total number of apo B-containing lipoproteins.

The goal of the bezafibrate Infarction Prevention (BIP) [58] was to test the benefit of a therapy that increases serum HDL-cholesterol concentrations and lowers triglyceride concentrations on the reduced incidence of myocardial infarctions and mortality among CAD patients.

Bezafibrate treatment significantly reduced serum triglycerides (22%) but not serum total cholesterol (4%) nor LDL-cholesterol (5%), and significantly increased HDL-cholesterol (12%).

Bezafibrate treatment induced 0.13mm less progression in coronary MLD [59], but did not significantly reduced the primary end point (fatal or non-fatal myocardial infarction plus sudden death) (−9%, p = 0.27) with a median fellow-up of 7 years [60] and did no modify total mortality (p = 0.64) [28,31]. Nevertheless, subgroup analysis suggested that bezafibrate had only a beneficial effect in patients with serum triglycerides above 2.3mmol/l (200mg/dl) (p = 0.03) where it significantly decreased primary end-point (p = 0.03).

Fenofibrate

The incidence of CAD is greatly increased in those diabetes mellitus. The Diabetes Atherosclerosis Intervention Study (DAIS) [61] is the first intervention trial designed to examine directly whether correcting dyslipoproteinaemia in men and women with non-insulin-dependent diabetes will reduce their CAD. The DAIS is a multinational angiographic study using the 200mg micronized form of fenofibrate in a double-blind, placebo-controlled protocol. Preliminary oral reports have indicated that fenofibrate reduced coronary stenosis progression in type 2 diabetes.

MIXED DYSLIPOPROTEINEMIA

It is clearly demonstrated that the convenient treatments for pure hypercholesterolaemia and pure hypertriglyceridaemia are statins and fibrates respectively. However, the most appropriate therapy of combined hyperlipidaemia remains to be determined. Zambon et al. [34] compared in a randomized crossover study the effects of gemfibrozil versus lovastatin in familial combined hyperlipidaemia and the additive effects of combination treatment on lipid regulation. Gemfibrozil (1,200mg/day) had no effect on LDL-cholesterol levels but favourably influenced triglyceride levels and apo B-containing lipoprotein composition that are related to hypertriglyceridaemia (reduction of both the number and size ofVLDL particles). Conversely, lovastatin markedly decreased LDL-cholesterol (reduction of the number of LDL particles) but had little effect on triglyceride-rich lipoproteins. Combined treatment was safe and had additive effects on lipids, causing significant reduction in total cholesterol, triglycerides, LDL-cholesterol and an increase in HDL-cholesterol. In this condition, target LDL-cholesterol levels (<130mg/dl) (3.4mmol/l) were achieved in 71% of patients with established CAD. The overall result of combination gemfibrozil-lovastatin was a normalization of the lipid profile in 68% of the patients: LDL-cholesterol <150mg/dl (3.9mmol/l) in all cases, triglycerides <200mg/dl (2.3mmol/l) in 96% of the patients, and HDL-cholesterol >35mg/dl in 68% of the patients.

REFERENCES

1. Shepherd J, Cobbe SM, Ford I, Isles CG, Lorimer AR, MacFarlane PW, McKillop JH, Packard CJ. 1995. Prevention of coronary heart disease with pravastatin in men with hypercholesterolemia. West of Scotland Coronary Prevention Study Group. N Engl J Med 333:1301–1307.

2. 1994 Randomised trial of cholesterol lowering in 4,444 patients with coronary heart disease: the Scandinavian Simvastatin Survival Study (4S). Lancet 344:1383–1389.
3. Sacks FM, Moye LA, Davis BR, Cole TG, Rouleau JL, Nash DT, Pfeffer MA, Braunwald E. 1998. Relationship between plasma LDL concentrations during treatment with pravastatin and recurrent coronary events in the Cholesterol and Recurrent Events trial. Circulation 97:1446–1452.
4. Sprecher DL. 1998. Triglycerides as a risk factor for coronary artery disease. Am J Cardiol 82:49U–56U.
5. Saku K, Zhang B, Ohta T, Arakawa K. 1999. Quantity and function of high density lipoprotein as an indicator of coronary atherosclerosis. J Am Coll Cardiol 33:436–443.
6. Rubins HB, Robins SJ, Collins D, Fye CL, Anderson JW, Elam MB, Faas FH, Linares E, Schaefer EJ, Schectman G, Wilt TJ, Wittes J. 1999. Gemfibrozil for the secondary prevention of coronary heart disease in men with low levels of high-density lipoprotein cholesterol. Veterans Affairs High-Density Lipoprotein Cholesterol Intervention Trial Study Group. N Engl J Med 341:410–418.
7. Braissant O, Foufelle F, Scotto C, Dauca M, Wahli W. 1996. Differential expression of peroxisome proliferator-activated receptors (PPARs): tissue distribution of PPAR-alpha, -beta, and -gamma in the adult rat. Endocrinology 137:354–366.
8. Issemann I, Green S. 1990. Activation of a member of the steroid hormone receptor superfamily by peroxisome proliferators. Nature 347:645–650.
9. Willson TM, Brown PJ, Sternbach DD, Henke BR. 2000. The PPARs: from orphan receptors to drug discovery. J Med Chem 43:527–550.
10. Heller F, Harvengt C. 1983. Effects of clofibrate, bezafibrate, fenofibrate and probucol on plasma lipolytic enzymes in normolipaemic subjects. Eur J Clin Pharmacol 25:57–63.
11. Staels B, Vu-Dac N, Kosykh VA, Saladin R, Fruchart JC, Dallongeville J, Auwerx J. 1995. Fibrates downregulate apolipoprotein C-III expression independent of induction of peroxisomal acyl coenzyme A oxidase. A potential mechanism for the hypolipidemic action of fibrates. J Clin Invest 95:705–712.
12. Malmendier CL, Delcroix C. 1985. Effects of fenofibrate on high and low density lipoprotein metabolism in heterozygous familial hypercholesterolemia. Atherosclerosis 55:161–169.
13. Vu-Dac N, Schoonjans K, Laine B, Fruchart JC, Auwerx J, Staels B. 1994. Negative regulation of the human apolipoprotein A-I promoter by fibrates can be attenuated by the interaction of the peroxisome proliferator-activated receptor with its response element. J Biol Chem 269:31012–31018.
14. Vu-Dac N, Schoonjans K, Kosykh V, Dallongeville J, Fruchart JC, Staels B, Auwerx J. 1995. Fibrates increase human apolipoprotein A-II expression through activation of the peroxisome proliferator-activated receptor. J Clin Invest 96:741–750.
15. Cattin L, Da Col PG, Feruglio FS, Finazzo L, Rimondi S, Descovich G, Manzato E, Zambon S, Crepaldi G, Siepi D. 1990. Efficacy of ciprofibrate in primary type II and IV hyperlipidemia: the Italian multicenter study. Clin Ther 12:482–488.
16. Tilly-Kiesi M, Tikkanen MJ. 1991. Low density lipoprotein density and composition in hypercholesterolaemic men treated with HMG CoA reductase inhibitors and gemfibrozil. J Intern Med 229:427–434.
17. Caslake MJ, Packard CJ, Gaw A, Murray E, Griffin BA, Vallance BD, Shepherd J. 1993. Fenofibrate and LDL metabolic heterogeneity in hypercholesterolemia. Arterioscler Thromb 13:702–711.
18. Stange EF, Fruhholz M, Osenbrugge M, Reimann F, Ditschuneit H. 1991. Bezafibrate fails to directly modulate HMG-CoA reductase or LDL catabolism in human mononuclear cells. Eur J Clin Pharmacol 40 Suppl 1:S37–S40.
19. Schoonjans K, Staels B, Auwerx J. 1996. The peroxisome proliferator activated receptors (PPARS) and their effects on lipid metabolism and adipocyte differentiation. Biochim Biophys Acta 1302:93–109.
20. Kelly LJ, Vicario PP, Thompson GM, Candelore MR, Doebber TW, Ventre J, Wu MS, Meurer R, Forrest MJ, Conner MW, Cascieri MA, Moller DE. 1998. Peroxisome proliferator-activated receptors gamma and alpha mediate in vivo regulation of uncoupling protein (UCP-1, UCP-2, UCP-3) gene expression. Endocrinology 139:4920–4927.
21. Kesaniemi YA, Grundy SM. 1984. Influence of gemfibrozil and clofibrate on metabolism of cholesterol and plasma triglycerides in man. JAMA 251:2241–2246.
22. Schoonjans K, Peinado-Onsurbe J, Lefebvre AM, Heyman RA, Briggs M, Deeb S, Staels B, Auwerx J. 1996. PPARalpha and PPARgamma activators direct a distinct tissue-specific transcriptional response via a PPRE in the lipoprotein lipase gene. EMBO J 15:5336–5348.
23. Quarfordt SH, Michalopoulos G, Schirmer B. 1982. The effect of human C apolipoproteins on the in vitro hepatic metabolism of triglyceride emulsions in the rat. J Biol Chem 257:14642–14647.

24. Windler E, Chao Y, Havel RJ. 1980. Regulation of the hepatic uptake of triglyceride-rich lipoproteins in the rat. Opposing effects of homologous apolipoprotein E and individual C apoproteins. J Biol Chem 255:8303–8307.
25. Clavey V, Lestavel-Delattre S, Copin C, Bard JM, Fruchart JC. 1995. Modulation of lipoprotein B binding to the LDL receptor by exogenous lipids and apolipoproteins CI, CII, CIII, and E. Arterioscler Thromb Vasc Biol 15:963–971.
26. Aalto-Setala K, Fisher EA, Chen X, Chajek-Shaul T, Hayek T, Zechner R, Walsh A, Ramakrishnan R, Ginsberg HN, Breslow JL. 1992. Mechanism of hypertriglyceridemia in human apolipoprotein (apo) CIII transgenic mice. Diminished very low density lipoprotein fractional catabolic rate associated with increased apo CIII and reduced apo E on the particles. J Clin Invest 90:1889–1900.
27. Aalto-Setala K, Weinstock PH, Bisgaier CL, Wu L, Smith JD, Breslow JL. 1996. Further characterization of the metabolic properties of triglyceride- rich lipoproteins from human and mouse apoC-III transgenic mice. J Lipid Res 37:1802–1811.
28. Ebara T, Ramakrishnan R, Steiner G, Shachter NS. 1997. Chylomicronemia due to apolipoprotein CIII overexpression in apolipoprotein E-null mice. Apolipoprotein CIII-induced hypertriglyceridemia is not mediated by effects on apolipoprotein E. J Clin Invest 99:2672–2681.
29. Peters JM, Hennuyer N, Staels B, Fruchart JC, Fievet C, Gonzalez FJ, Auwerx J. 1997. Alterations in lipoprotein metabolism in peroxisome proliferator- activated receptor alpha-deficient mice. J Biol Chem 272:27307–27312.
30. Ladias JA, Hadzopoulou-Cladaras M, Kardassis D, Cardot P, Cheng J, Zannis V, Cladaras C. 1992. Transcriptional regulation of human apolipoprotein genes ApoB, ApoCIII, and ApoAII by members of the steroid hormone receptor superfamily HNF-4, ARP-1, EAR-2, and EAR-3. J Biol Chem 267:15849–15860.
31. Vu-Dac N, Gervois P, Pineda Torra IP, Fruchart JC, Kosykh V, Kooistra T, Princen HM, Dallongeville J, Staels B. 1998. Retinoids increase human apo C-III expression at the transcriptional level via the retinoid X receptor. Contribution to the hypertriglyceridemic action of retinoids. J Clin Invest 102:625–632.
32. Bard JM, Parra HJ, Camare R, Luc G, Ziegler O, Dachet C, Bruckert E, Douste-Blazy P, Drouin P, Jacotot B. 1992. A multicenter comparison of the effects of simvastatin and fenofibrate therapy in severe primary hypercholesterolemia, with particular emphasis on lipoproteins defined by their apolipoprotein composition. Metabolism 41:498–503.
33. Kahri J, Sane T, Van Tol A, Taskinen MR. 1995. Effect of gemfibrozil on the regulation of HDL subfractions in hypertriglyceridaemic patients. J Intern Med 238:429–436.
34. Zambon D, Ros E, Rodriguez-Villar C, Laguna JC, Vazquez M, Sanllehy C, Casals E, Sol JM, Hernandez G. 1999. Randomized crossover study of gemfibrozil versus lovastatin in familial combined hyperlipidemia: additive effects of combination treatment on lipid regulation. Metabolism 48:47–54.
35. Steinmetz A, Schwartz T, Hehnke U, Kaffarnik H. 1996. Multicenter comparison of micronized fenofibrate and simvastatin in patients with primary type IIA or IIB hyperlipoproteinemia. J Cardiovasc Pharmacol 27:563–570.
36. Schaefer EJ, Lamon-Fava S, Cole T, Sprecher DL, Cilla DDJ, Balagtas CC, Rowan JP, Black DM. 1996. Effects of regular and extended-release gemfibrozil on plasma lipoproteins and apolipoproteins in hypercholesterolemic patients with decreased HDL cholesterol levels. Atherosclerosis 127:113–122.
37. Berthou L, Duverger N, Emmanuel F, Langouet S, Auwerx J, Guillouzo A, Fruchart JC, Rubin E, Denefle P, Staels B, Branellec D. 1996. Opposite regulation of human versus mouse apolipoprotein A-I by fibrates in human apolipoprotein A-I transgenic mice. J Clin Invest 97:2408–2416.
38. Chinetti G, Gbaguidi FG, Griglio S, Mallat Z, Antonucci M, Poulain P, Chapman J, Fruchart JC, Tedgui A, Najib-Fruchart J, Staels B. 2000. CLA-1/SR-BI is expressed in atherosclerotic lesion macrophages and regulated by activators of peroxisome proliferator-activated receptors. Circulation 101:2411–2417.
39. Chinetti G, Lestavel S, Bocher V, Remaley AT, Neve B, Torra IP, Teissier E, Minnich A, Jaye M, Duverger N, Brewer HB, Fruchart JC, Clavey V, Staels B. 2001. PPAR-alpha and PPAR-gamma activators induce cholesterol removal from human macrophage foam cells through stimulation of the ABCA1 pathway. Nat Med 7:53–58.
40. Devchand PR, Keller H, Peters JM, Vazquez M, Gonzalez FJ, Wahli W. 1996. The PPARα-leukotriene B4 pathway to inflammation control. Nature 384:39–43.

41. Marx N, Sukhova GK, Collins T, Libby P, Plutzky J. 1999. PPARalpha activators inhibit cytokine-induced vascular cell adhesion molecule-1 expression in human endothelial cells. Circulation 99:3125–3131.
42. Neve BP, Corseaux D, Chinetti G, Zawadzki C, Fruchart JC, Duriez P, Staels B, Jude B. 2001. PPA-Ralpha agonists inhibit tissue factor expression in human monocytes and macrophages. Circulation 103:207–212.
43. Staels B, Koenig W, Habib A, Merval R, Lebret M, Torra IP, Delerive P, Fadel A, Chinetti G, Fruchart JC, Najib J, Maclouf J, Tedgui A. 1998. Activation of human aortic smooth-muscle cells is inhibited by PPARα but not by PPARγ activators. Nature 393:790–793.
44. Delerive P, De Bosscher K, Besnard S, Vanden Berghe W, Peters JM, Gonzalez FJ, Fruchart JC, Tedgui A, Haegeman G, Staels B. 1999. Peroxisome proliferator-activated receptor alpha negatively regulates the vascular inflammatory gene response by negative cross-talk with transcription factors NF-kappaB and AP-1. J Biol Chem 274:32048–32054.
45. Poynter ME, Daynes RA. 1998. Peroxisome proliferator-activated receptor alpha activation modulates cellular redox status, represses nuclear factor-kappaB signaling, and reduces inflammatory cytokine production in aging. J Biol Chem 273:32833–32841.
46. Kockx M, Gervois P, Poulain P, Derudas B, Peters JM, Gonzales FJ, Princen HM, Kooistra T, Staels B. 1999. Fibrates suppress fibrinogen gene expression in rodents via activation of the peroxisome proliferator-activated receptor-alpha. Blood 93:2991–2998.
47. Delerive P, Gervois P, Fruchart JC, Staels B. 2000. Induction of IkappaBalpha expression as a mechanism contributing to the anti-inflammatory activities of peroxisome proliferator-activated receptor-alpha activators. J Biol Chem 275:36703–36707.
48. Nissen RM, Yamamoto KR. 2000. The glucocorticoid receptor inhibits NFkappaB by interfering with serine-2 phosphorylation of the RNA polymerase II carboxy-terminal domain. Genes Dev 14:2314–2329.
49. Klucis E, Crane D, Masters C. 1984. Sequential alterations in the micro-localization of catalase in mouse liver after treatment with hypolipidemic drugs. Mol Cell Biochem 65:73–82.
50. Delerive P, Martin-Nizard F, Chinetti G, Trottein F, Fruchart JC, Najib J, Duriez P, Staels B. 1999. Peroxisome proliferator-activated receptor activators inhibit thrombin-induced endothelin-1 production in human vascular endothelial cells by inhibiting the activator protein-1 signaling pathway. Circ Res 85:394–402.
51. Madej A, Okopien B, Kowalski J, Zielinski M, Wysocki J, Szygula B, Kalina Z, Herman ZS. 1998. Effects of fenofibrate on plasma cytokine concentrations in patients with atherosclerosis and hyperlipoproteinemia IIb. Int J Clin Pharmacol Ther 36:345–349.
52. Frick MH, Syvanne M, Nieminen MS, Kauma H, Majahalme S, Virtanen V, Kesaniemi YA, Pasternack A, Taskinen MR. 1997. Prevention of the angiographic progression of coronary and vein-graft atherosclerosis by gemfibrozil after coronary bypass surgery in men with low levels of HDL cholesterol. Lopid Coronary Angiography Trial (LOCAT) Study Group. Circulation 96:2137–2143.
53. Syvanne M, Nieminen MS, Frick MH, Kauma H, Majahalme S, Virtanen V, Kesaniemi YA, Pasternack A, Ehnholm C, Taskinen MR. 1998. Associations between lipoproteins and the progression of coronary and vein-graft atherosclerosis in a controlled trial with gemfibrozil in men with low baseline levels of HDL cholesterol. Circulation 98:1993–1999.
54. de Faire U, Ericsson CG, Hamsten A, Nilsson J. 1995. Design features of a five-year Bezafibrate Coronary Atherosclerosis Intervention Trial (BECAIT). Drugs Exp Clin Res 21:105–124.
55. de Faire U, Ericsson CG, Grip L, Nilsson J, Svane B, Hamsten A. 1996. Secondary preventive potential of lipid-lowering drugs. The Bezafibrate Coronary Atherosclerosis Intervention Trial (BECAIT). Eur Heart J 17 Suppl F:37–42.
56. Ericsson CG, Nilsson J, Grip L, Svane B, Hamsten A. 1997. Effect of bezafibrate treatment over five years on coronary plaques causing 20% to 50% diameter narrowing (The Bezafibrate Coronary Atherosclerosis Intervention Trial [BECAIT]). Am J Cardiol 80:1125–1129.
57. Ruotolo G, Ericsson CG, Tettamanti C, Karpe F, Grip L, Svane B, Nilsson J, de Faire U, Hamsten A. 1998. Treatment effects on serum lipoprotein lipids, apolipoproteins and low density lipoprotein particle size and relationships of lipoprotein variables to progression of coronary artery disease in the Bezafibrate Coronary Atherosclerosis Intervention Trial (BECAIT). J Am Coll. Cardiol 32:1648–1656.
58. Goldbourt U, Brunner D, Behar S, Reicher-Reiss H. 1998. Baseline characteristics of patients participating in the Bezafibrate Infarction Prevention (BIP) Study. Eur Heart J 19 Suppl H:H42-7.

59. Ericsson CG, Hamsten A, Nilsson J, Grip L, Svane B, de Faire U. 1996. Angiographic assessment of effects of bezafibrate on progression of coronary artery disease in young male postinfarction patients. Lancet 347:849–853.
60. Kaplinsky E, Brunner D. 1998. The bezafibrate infarction prevention (BIP) study results. XXth Congress of the European Society of Cardiology Vienne, August 22–August 26.
61. Steiner G. 1996. The Diabetes Atherosclerosis Intervention Study (DAIS): a study conducted in cooperation with the World Health Organization. The DAIS Project Group. Diabetologia 39:1655–1661.

G.N. Pierce, M. Nagano, P. Zahradka, and N.S. Dhalla (eds.).
ATHEROSCLEROSIS, HYPERTENSION AND DIABETES. Copyright © 2003.
Kluwer Academic Publishers. Boston.

THE CHOICE OF AN APPROPRIATE ANIMAL SPECIES IN THE STUDY OF CHLAMYDIA PNEUMONIAE AS AN ATHEROGENIC AGENT

SATORU HIRONO, MD, PHD and
GRANT N. PIERCE, PHD, FACC, FAHA

Division of Stroke and Vascular Disease, St. Boniface General Hospital Research Centre and Department of Physiology, Faculty of Medicine, University of Manitoba, Winnipeg, Canada

Summary. Different animal models have been used to increase our understanding of the mechanisms responsible for atherosclerosis. We have used the same animal models to study the relationship of atherosclerosis to infection. The data generated from these studies have yielded valuable insights into the mechanisms whereby an infectious agent like *Chlamydia pneumoniae* augments the atherosclerotic process. The appropriate choice of the optimal animal species in which to study these interactions is critical. This review discusses some of the choices facing the researcher in this field and some of the interesting data that has been generated using the different animal species.

***Key words*:** Atherosclerosis, Infection, Inflammation, Cholesterol, Virus, Bacteria, Atherogenesis

INTRODUCTION

Coronary artery disease and stroke are vascular lesions that result in more deaths, debilitating injury and at a greater economic cost than any other diseases today. Coronary artery disease and stroke achieve these devastating effects through an ischemic event induced by an atherosclerotic blockage. Knowledge of the mechanisms responsible for atherogenesis, therefore, represents some of the most important medical information that we could obtain today.

Correspondence to: Dr. Grant N. Pierce, Director, Division of Stroke and Vascular Disease, St. Boniface General Hospital Research Centre, 351 Tache Avenue, Winnipeg, Manitoba, Canada, R2H 2A6. Phone: (204) 235-3414; Fax: (204) 235-1151; e-mail: gpierce@sbrc.ca

Atherosclerosis is now regarded as a chronic inflammatory disease. Recent data suggest that infection may be a novel cardiovascular risk factor [1]. *C. pneumoniae* is one infectious agent that has received particular attention as a potent atherogenic agent [2,3]. Despite the growing evidence for a link between *C. pneumoniae* infection and atherosclerosis, a precise causative role of the organism in coronary artery disease has not yet been proven [4,5]. Several large, long-term secondary prevention clinical trials with antibiotic treatment [6–8] are now under way to address the causative role of *C. pneumoniae* in coronary artery disease. The best way, however, to determine causality is still through animal investigations where direct interventions can unequivocally identify cause-and-effect relationships.

Atherosclerotic disease in animals is modulated by the animal species in which it is investigated. Some species accurately represent the disease to the human condition and others are inappropriate in which to study its pathogenesis. The most extreme example is rodents. Rats are completely resistant to atherosclerotic disease (except in unusual cases or if the rat has undergone some manner of gene manipulation) and are not a good model in which to study atherosclerotic disease. This dilemma is further complicated when an investigator wishes to study the effects of an infectious agent upon atherogenesis. The infection characteristics are another variable that will influence the applicability of the animal data to the human condition. The choice, therefore, of an appropriate animal model in which to study the effects of an infectious agent on atherogenic disease is a critical decision. Several animal models have been used to study a possible causal relationship between *C. pneumoniae* infection and atherosclerosis [9]. This manuscript discusses data obtained to date concerning the use of different infectious agents in a variety of animals in order to provide some guidance for choosing the best animal model in which to study the effects of an infectious agent like *C. pneumoniae* on atherosclerotic disease.

THE MOUSE MODEL OF *CHLAMYDIA PNEUMONIA* INFECTION AND ATHEROSCLEROSIS

i) General introduction

Several mouse models have been used for the study of *C. pneumoniae* as an atherogenic agent. The most popular of these are the atherosclerosis-susceptible inbred strain C57BL/6J mice [10], and genetically modified low-density lipoprotein receptor deficient (LDLR–/–) mice [11] and apolipoprotein E-deficient (apoE–/–) mice [12–14]. Both of the former strains of mice develop hypercholesterolemia and atherosclerotic lesions only on a cholesterol-enriched diet, whereas the latter spontaneously develops hypercholesterolemia and atherosclerotic lesions even on a normal chow diet. Each strains of mouse has its own unique advantages and disadvantages with regards to how closely they mimic atherosclerosis in humans. These characteristics are reviewed in detail elsewhere [15,16]. To summarize, it is fair to conclude that these mice models of atherosclerosis are among the best representations of the human atherosclerotic condition [15,16].

Mouse models have been used to study the respiratory pathology of *C. pneumoniae* infection [17,18]. Intranasal inoculation of mice with *C. pneumoniae* results in systemic dissemination of the organism from the respiratory tract to other organs like the vasculature [19–21]. The infection with *C. pneumoniae* in the respiratory tract appears to be transferred to alveolar macrophages that subsequently enter the vascular circulation [22]. Strong evidence exists that the atherosclerotic coronary and carotid arteries and aorta are frequently infected with *C. pneumoniae* [23–26]. One would suspect, therefore, that other vascular beds that have not been investigated to date (e.g. renal arteries) might also be susceptible to this infection and the subsequent atherogenic lesions.

ii) The apoE deletion mouse

The genetically modified apoE−/− mice have been used to study the effects of infection on atherosclerosis in a number of laboratories. Moazed and colleagues [27] evaluated the effects of chronic *C. pneumoniae* infection on the development of atheromatous lesions in the apoE−/− mice. Eight-week-old male apoE−/− mice were inoculated intranasally with 3×10^7 inclusion forming unit (IFU) of *C. pneumoniae* AR-39 strain 3 times at 1-week intervals. After inoculations, the areas of fatty streaks and early atheromatous lesions of the aortic arch were significantly larger (2.4- and 1.6-fold greater at 8 and 12 weeks after the first inoculation, respectively) in infected than in non-infected mice. These results indicate that respiratory infection with *C. pneumoniae* results in dissemination of the organism to the aorta of the apoE−/− mice, leading to the aggravation of atherosclerotic lesions induced by hypercholesterolemia.

The age of the apoE−/− mouse or the stage of its pre-existing atherosclerotic lesion development may also influence the capacity of *C. pneumoniae* to successfully infect the vasculature. When apoE−/− mice received a single inoculation at 16 weeks of age, *C. pneumoniae* DNA was detected by PCR in the aorta in 100% (8/8) of the inoculated mice through 8 weeks after inoculation in comparison to 50% (8/16) of mice infected at 8 weeks of age [20]. In another study [28], the mice inoculated with *C. pneumoniae* (A-03 strain [29], at 5×10^6 IFU) twice at 12–14 weeks of age were more susceptible to the atherogenic effect of *C. pneumoniae* than the mice inoculated at 10–12 weeks of age. In apoE−/− mice, fatty streak lesions begin to appear at 10–12 weeks of age and intermediate lesions containing foam cells and spindle-shaped smooth muscle cells develop at 15 weeks [15,28]. Therefore, pre-existing atherosclerotic lesions may sensitize the vessel to the atherogenic effects of *C. pneumoniae.* These data suggest that an atheromatous lesion, even if it is at a relatively early stage, must precede the infection in order to allow the infection to further stimulate the atherogenic process. This hypothesis is a critical one that deserves further study but is in agreement with conclusions obtained elsewhere using another mouse model of atherosclerosis [21].

The animal strain itself may be an important factor to consider when examining the effects of *C. pneumoniae.* For example, the ability of *C. pneumoniae* to infect and reside in the aortic tissue in C57BL/6J mice was compared to apoE−/− mice [20]. Whereas aortic samples from apoE−/− mice were successfully infected with *C. pneumoniae* for extended time periods, *C. pneumoniae* DNA was detected in the aorta of C57BL/6J mice only up to 14 days after a single inoculation of the organism. These data demonstrated the variability of the host animal strain to accommodate the infection and emphasizes the importance of careful selection of an appropriate animal model for study. In unpublished work from our labs (G. Zhong and G.N. Pierce), we also detected a resistance in the apoE−/− mouse to the atherogenic effect of *C. pneumoniae* using the same chlamydia strain that was atherogenic in the LDLR−/− mouse [21]. This would suggest that the mouse model itself was a variable of importance to control.

Some investigators have generated results that may question the use of the apoE−/− mouse as an appropriate model for the study of infection/atherosclerosis interactions. Two laboratories have recently reported an inability to either detect evidence of successful dissemination of *C. pneumoniae* to the vessels or an atherogenic effect in the apoE−/− mice. Caligiuri et al. [30] inoculated 6- to 8-week-old female apoE−/− mice intranasally with 1×10^6 IFU of *C. pneumoniae* strain Kajaani 7 (Finnish epidemic strain [31]) once or twice at 18-week intervals and atherosclerotic lesions were evaluated 22 weeks after primary infection. Aalto-Setala et al. [32] inoculated 8-week-old male apoE−/− mice on an atherosclerosis-resistant background, FVB, 3 times at 1-week intervals with 3×10^6 IFU of the same *C. pneumoniae* strain Kajaani 7. Atherosclerotic lesions were measured in the aortic root at 10 weeks after primary infection. In another set of experiments, 8-week-old apoE−/− mice on male FVB or both male and female C57BL/6J backgrounds were inoculated with 1×10^6 IFU of *C. pneumoniae* and re-infected 3 times with 1×10^5 IFU at 3- to 4-weeks intervals. Atherosclerotic lesions were measured 18 weeks later. In both studies, no statistically significant difference was found in the size of the atherosclerotic lesion between *C. pneumoniae* infected and non-infected control mice, despite serological evidence of a successful infection. Aalto-Setala and co-workers could not demonstrate *C. pneumoniae* DNA in aortic tissue by PCR [32], and Caligiuri and colleagues found only rare, occasional *C. pneumoniae* antigen positive macrophages in arterial lesions by immunohistochemical staining [30]. The lack of dissemination of the organism from lung to arterial tissue may be a result of the different *C. pneumoniae* strain used or some differences in the experimental protocols from those used by Moazed and colleagues [27].

It should be noted that the sex of the mouse may also influence the atherogenic effect of *C. pneumoniae.* Differences in atherosclerotic lesion development between male and female mice have previously been demonstrated [33]. Burnett and coworkers [34] inoculated both male and female apoE−/− mice with *C. pneumoniae* at 6 and 8 weeks of age, and the atherosclerotic lesions were evaluated at 8 weeks after the final inoculation. Infection with the organism increased lesion size by 70% in males, whereas no significant increase was found in infected females compared to uninfected controls. However, because uninfected female apoE−/− mice had greater (~2-fold lesion area) baseline atherosclerotic lesions than did male mice [33], the authors speculated that this high background level of atherosclerosis in female apoE–/– mice may explain the lack of additive effect of *C. pneumoniae* infection. Thus, caution should be taken in selecting the appropriate animal sex with which to study the atherogenic effect of an infectious agent.

In summary, the apoE–/– mouse is an excellent model of atherosclerosis. The plaques found in this mouse are representative of the human atheromatous lesion and the plaques develop in a relatively short period of time. However, its use as a model to test the effects of infection on atherosclerosis has met with mixed success. Unfortunately, it is not entirely clear what factors have led to the negative results. This may result in a less enthusiastic endorsement of this mouse model in the future for the study of *C. pneumoniae* and its involvement in atherosclerosis.

iii) The LDL receptor deletion mouse

Another genetically manipulated mouse has been identified as an excellent model of atherosclerosis. The LDLR–/– mouse [14] is an excellent model of atherosclerotic disease that closely mimics this condition in humans [15,16]. This mouse will develop hypercholesterolemia and atherosclerotic lesions only on a cholesterol-enriched diet [14].

Recently, Hu et al. [21] have developed a mouse model of *C. pneumoniae* infection and atherosclerosis using these LDLR–/– mice. The LDLR–/– mice were fed with a regular mouse chow or a 2% cholesterol-enriched diet, and inoculated intranasally with the *C. pneumoniae* AR-39 strain at 0.5–1 × 10^7 IFU once monthly for 9 months. The atherosclerotic lesions were evaluated at 20 to 25 days after the final inoculation. The chlamydial LPS antigen was detected in the aorta from mice infected with the *C. pneumoniae.* The *C. pneumoniae* AR39 infection also significantly enhanced the development of atherosclerotic lesions induced by a cholesterol-enriched diet. Interestingly, regardless of chlamydial infection, neither the chlamydial antigen nor measurable atherosclerotic lesions was detected in the aorta from LDL–/– mice fed a regular chow. Infection with a different chlamydial strain, *C. trachomatis* MoPn strain, had very different effects. MoPn is a mouse pneumonitis strain of *C. trachomatis* that causes mouse pneumonia [35] and has, therefore, been used to study the respiratory pathology induced by chlamydial infection in mice. *C. trachomatis* inoculation at 0.5–1 × 10^4 IFU once monthly for 9 months produced no significant effects on atherosclerotic development in the mice fed a cholesterol-enriched diet, despite evidence of dissemination to the aorta [21]. These results implied that the *C. pneumoniae* species (or AR39 strain) may possess a unique property that contributes to its role in atherogenesis [36], and that the initial lesion induced by hypercholesterolemia may be necessary for *C. pneumoniae* to successfully infect, reside persistently in the aortic tissues and, ultimately stimulate the atherogenic process. It would be worth investigating what is responsible for the species-specific difference of atherogenic property between *C. pneumoniae* and *C. trachomatis.*

The important observation that a cholesterol-enriched environment is critical for the atherogenic effects of an infectious agent is in agreement with the previous findings that *C. pneumoniae* can disseminate to, but cannot persist in the aorta following a single intranasal inoculation of normocholesterolemic C57BL/6J mice [20]. The same group has reported that repeated inoculations of C57BL/6J mice on a normal chow diet resulted in a more persistent infection of *C. pneumoniae* and inflammatory changes in the aorta [37] but did not initiate any measurable atherosclerotic lesions in the mice [38]. These authors recently demonstrated that *C. pneumoniae* infection accelerated atherosclerotic lesion formation in C57BL/6J mice on a high fat, high cholesterol diet [39]. These results suggest that persistent infection with *C. pneumoniae* alone may be insufficient for the induction of atherosclerotic lesions in mice but must be accompanied by a cholesterol-enriched diet.

The LDLR−/− mouse can be used effectively in the study of the causal relationship of infection with atherosclerosis by taking advantage of its unique gene expression to answer complex biochemical questions. For example, *C. pneumoniae* increased DiI-LDL uptake and induced foam cell formation in macrophages isolated from LDL receptor (ApoB/E receptor)-deficient mice [40]. This suggested that *C. pneumoniae* increases LDL uptake by macrophages through a mechanism independent of the native LDL receptors [40]. The authors subsequently identified the component of *C. pneumoniae* that induces macrophage foam cell formation as chlamydial lipopolysaccharide (LPS) [41]. In support of this conclusion, LPS extracted from *E. coli* has been shown to induce macrophage lipid accumulation and foam cell formation [42,43].

Thus, the LDLR−/− mouse is an excellent animal model in which to study the effects of *C. pneumoniae* infection on atherosclerotic disease. It mimics the human condition well. It can be infected relatively easily through the intranasal route with *C. pneumoniae* and this will disseminate successfully to the aorta. This results in successful inflammatory responses and a significant stimulation of atherosclerotic plaque formation. Because the animal is small, relatively small amounts of *C. pneumoniae* are required for inoculations. This is a distinct advantage when it is recognized that *C. pneumoniae* is a notoriously difficult compound with which to work, grow and culture. A decided disadvantage of using the LDLR−/− mouse for this kind of study is the length of time required to generate a significant atherogenic effect. The model requires 6 [44] to 9 months [21] of dietary intervention and infection in order to induce a significant effect. Shorter periods of study (3 months) do not demonstrate any effects of the *C. pneumoniae* on atherogenesis [12]. Finally, the genetic make-up of knock-out mouse models allows the researcher to answer mechanistic questions in a definitive manner that simply could not be accomplished in other animal or human experimental conditions.

THE RABBIT MODEL OF *CHLAMYDIA PNEUMONIAE* INFECTION AND ATHEROSCLEROSIS

The rabbit has long been used as a convenient model for diet induced atherosclerosis. It is probably the most frequently used animal model for the study of atherosclerosis. Unfortunately, it is now recognized as less than ideal as a representative model for human atherosclerotic disease [16]. The cellular and compositional characteristics of the atheromatous plaque, as well as the differences in the LDL particle itself are amongst the main problems that limit the application of these data to the human disease state. However, despite these concerns, the rabbit has been used quite successfully as a model system in which to test the role of infection in atherosclerosis.

Laitinen et al. [45] demonstrated that intranasal inoculation of New Zealand White rabbits with the *C. pneumoniae* strain Kajaani 7 (1×10^7 IFU, twice at 3-week interval) resulted in inflammatory changes in the aorta 2 to 4 weeks after reinfection. Fong et al. [46] inoculated New Zealand White rabbits with $1–5 \times 10^7$ IFU of *C. pneumoniae* (ATCC strain VR1310). Two of the six infected animals showed fatty streaks in the aortic arch and spindle cell proliferation of vascular smooth muscle cells (intermediate lesion) as early as 7 and 14 days after the single inoculation, respectively. The authors extended these observations to further assess the role of *C. pneumoniae* in atherogenesis, using two separate strains of *C. pneumoniae*, the ATCC strain VR1310 and the TWAR strain AR39. Three months after a single inoculation of *C. pneumoniae* ($1.0–2.6 \times 10^7$ IFU), six of 23 (26.1%) rabbits showed microscopic changes of atherosclerosis of the aorta. When the rabbits were inoculated 3 times within 6 weeks, eight of 23 (34.8%) animals developed more advanced atheromatous lesions at 12 weeks after the first inoculation [47]. These results indicate that in rabbits, a species that is more prone to atherosclerosis, *C. pneumoniae* infection of the arterial wall can initiate development of atherosclerotic lesions even in the absence of hypercholesterolemia.

This animal model has been used successfully to study preventative therapy. Muhlestein and colleagues [48] studied the effect of azithromycin on atherosclerotic lesions of infected animals. A 7-week course of azithromycin after multiple inoculations successfully prevented the intimal thickening of the aorta in infected rabbits with a 0.25% cholesterol diet. These data provide important information regarding treatment strategies that can be used against *C. pneumoniae* as well as to clarify a causal role for *C. pneumoniae* in atherogenesis.

In summary, rabbits remain an effective and useful animal model in which to study the effects of infection on atherogenesis. The time course of the atherogenesis is conducive to obtaining rapid answers to experimental questions. The size of the animal is both an advantage and a disadvantage. It is advantageous because of the relatively large amount of tissue sample that can be obtained. This will allow more detailed biochemical and histochemical characterization of the effects of the experimental interventions. The greater body mass will also, however, create a need for larger quantities of *C. pneumoniae* to induce a successful infection.

CONCLUSIONS

In summary, in vivo animal models are extremely useful in order to learn more about the cause-and-effect relationship of infection with atherosclerosis. They are now beginning to inform us about potentially useful therapeutic strategies that can be implemented in human trials. Specifically, we can conclude that animal studies to date have furthered our understanding of the role of *C. pneumoniae* infection in atherogenesis in the following ways: 1) respiratory tract infection of animals with *C. pneumoniae* results in systemic dissemination to other organs including vascular tissue; 2) repeated infection of animals with *C. pneumoniae* may cause longer persistence of the organism in aortic tissue, leading to more advanced lesions; 3) *C. pneumoniae* appears to augment atheromatous lesions induced by hypercholesterolemia; 4) the *C. pneumoniae* species may possess a unique property leading to atherogenesis. Each animal species has its own unique advantages and disadvantages. There is no ideal, perfect model. In our judgement, the LDLR−/− mouse is probably the best overall model in which to study *C. pneumoniae* and its role in atherosclerosis. Despite the lack of available tissue to complete detailed biochemical analyses and the length of time needed to generate appreciable atherosclerotic plaques, the animals show consistent dissemination of the infection, significant and clear stimulatory effects on atherogenesis and the unique genetic composition can be used to answer cellular questions about LDL metabolism as it relates to infection. The use of animal models remains an important option for researchers in which to study the fundamental pathologic question of the relationship of *C. pneumoniae* infection to atherosclerotic vascular disease.

ACKNOWLEDGEMENTS

This work was supported by a grant from the Canadian Institutes for Health Research and by a grant-in-aid from the Tsukada Medical Foundation (Japan). GN Pierce is a CIHR Senior Scientist. S. Hirono is a Postdoctoral Fellow of the Faculty of Medicine at the University of Manitoba.

REFERENCES

1. Danesh J, Collins R, Peto R. 1997. Chronic infections and coronary heart disease: is there a link? Lancet 350:430–436.
2. Grayston JT. 2000. Background and current knowledge of *Chlamydia pneumoniae* and atherosclerosis. J Infect Dis 181(Suppl 3):S402–410.
3. Gaydos CA and Quinn TC. 2000. The role of *Chlamydia pneumoniae* in cardiovascular disease. Advances in Internal Medicine 45:139–173.
4. Muhlestein JB, Anderson JL, Carlquist JF, Salunkhe K, Horne BD, Pearson RR, Bunch TJ, Allen A, Trehan S, Nielson C. 2000. Randomized secondary prevention trial of azithromycin in patients with coronary artery disease—primary clinical results of the ACADEMIC study. Circulation 102:1755–1760.
5. Gurfinkel E, Bozovich G, Beck E, Testa E, Livellara B, Mautner B. 1999. Treatment with the antibiotic roxithromycin in patients with acute non-Q-wave coronary syndromes: the final report of the ROXIS study. Eur Heart J 20:121–127.
6. Dunne M. 1999. WIZARD and the design of trials for secondary prevention of atherosclerosis with antibiotics. Am Heart J 138:S542–544.
7. Grayston JT, Jackson LA, Kennedy WJ, Kronmal RA. 1999. Secondary prevention trials for coronary artery disease with antibiotic treatment for *Chlamydia pneumoniae:* design issues. Am Heart J 138:S545–S549.
8. Jackson LA. 2000. Description and status of the azithrimycin and coronary events study (ACES). J Infect Dis 181(Suppl 3):S579–581.
9. Saikku P, Laitinen K, Leinonen M. 1998. Animal model of *Chlamydia pneumoniae* infection. Atherosclerosis 140(Suppl 1):S17–19.

10. Paigen B, Morrow A, Brandon C, Mitchell D, Holmes P. 1985. Variation in susceptibility to atherosclerosis among inbred strains of mice. Atherosclerosis 57:65–73.
11. Ishibashi S, Brown MS, Goldstein JL, Gerard RD, Hammer RE, Herz J. 1993. Hypercholesterolemia in low density lipoprotein receptor knockout mice and its reversal by adenovirus-mediated gene delivery. J Clin Invest 92:883–893.
12. Zhang SH, Reddick RL, Piedrahita JA, Maeda N. 1992. Spontaneous hypercholesterolemia and arterial lesions in mice lacking apolipoprotein E. Science 258:468–471.
13. Plump AS, Smith JD, Hayek T, Aalto-Setala K, Walsh A, Verstuyft JG, Rubin EM, Breslow JL. 1992. Severe hypercholesterolemia and atherosclerosis in apolipoprotein E-deficient mice created by homologous recombination in ES cells. Cell 71:343–53.
14. Nakashima Y, Plump AS, Raines EW, Breslow JL, Ross R. 1994. ApoE-deficient mice develop lesions of all phases of atherosclerosis throughout the arterial tree. Arterioscler Thromb 14:133–140.
15. Breslow JL. 1996. Mouse models of atherosclerosis. Science 272:685–688.
16. Moghadasian MH, Frohlich JJ, McManus BM. 2001. Advances in experimental dyslipidemia and atherosclerosis. Lab Invest 81:1173–1183.
17. Yang ZP, Kuo CC, Grayston JT. 1993. A mouse model of *Chlamydia pneumoniae* strain TWAR pneumonitis. Infect Immun 61:2037–2040.
18. Kaukoranta-Tolvanen SSE, Laurila AL, Saikku P, Leinonen M, Liesirova L, Laitinen K. 1993. Experimental infection of *Chlamydia pneumoniae* in mice. Microb Pathog 15:293–302.
19. Yang ZP, Kuo CC, Grayston JT. 1995. Systemic dissemination of *Chlamydia pneumoniae* following intranasal inoculation in mice. J Infect Dis 171:736–738.
20. Moazed TC, Kuo CC, Grayston JT, Campbell LA. 1997. Murine models of *Chlamydia pneumoniae* infection and atherosclerosis. J Infect Dis 175:883–890.
21. Hu H, Pierce GN, Zhong G. 1999. The atherogenic effects of chlamydia are dependent on serum cholesterol and specific to *Chlamydia pneumoniae*. J Clin Invest 103:747–753.
22. Moazed TC, Kuo CC, Grayston JT, Campbell LA. 1998. Evidence of systemic dissemination of *Chlamydia pneumoniae* via macrophages in the mouse. J Infect Dis 177:1322–1325.
23. Kuo CC, Grayston JT, Campbell LA, Goo YA, Wissler RW, Benditt EP. 1995. *Chlamydia pneumoniae* (TWAR) in coronary arteries of young adults (15–34 years old). Proc Natl Acad Sci USA 92:6911–6914.
24. Jackson LA, Campbell LA, Schmidt RA, Kuo CC, Cappuccio AL, Lee MJ, Grayston JT. 1997. Specificity of detection of *Chlamydia pneumoniae* in cardiovascular atheroma—evaluation of the innocent bystander hypothesis. Am J Pathol 150:1785–1790.
25. Yamashita K, Ouchi K, Shirai M, Gondo T, Nakazawa T, Ito H. 1998. Distribution of *Chlamydia pneumoniae* infection in the atherosclerotic carotid artery. Stroke 29:773–778.
26. Taylor-Robinson D. 1998. *Chlamydia pneumoniae* in vascular tissue. Atherosclerosis 140(Suppl 1): S21–S24.
27. Moazed TC, Campbell LA, Rosenfeld ME, Grayston JT, Kuo CC. 1999. *Chlamydia pneumoniae* infection accelerates the progression of atherosclerosis in apolipoprotein E-deficient mice. J Infect Dis 180;238–241.
28. Rothstein NM, Quinn TC, Madico G, Gaydos CA, Lowenstein CJ. 2001. Effect of azithromycin on murine arteriosclerosis exacerbated by *Chlamydia pneumoniae*. J Infect Dis 183:232–238.
29. Ramirez JA. 1996. Isolation of *Chlamydia pneumoniae* from coronary artery of a patients with coronary atherosclerosis. *Chlamydia pneumoniae*/Atherosclerosis Study Group. Ann Intern Med 125:979–982.
30. Caligiuri G, Rottenberg M, Nicoletti A, Wigzell H, Hansson GK. 2001. *Chlamydia pneumoniae* infection does not induce or modify atherosclerosis in mice. Circulation 103:2834–2838
31. Ekman MR, Grayston JT, Visakorpi R, Kleemola M, Kuo CC, Saikku P. 1993. An epidemic of infection due to *Chlamydiae pneumonia* in military conscripts. Clin Infect Dis 17:420–425.
32. Aalto-Setala K, Laitinen K, Erkkila L, Leinonen M, Jauhiainen M, Ehnholm C, Tamminen M, Puolakkainen M, Penttila I, Saikku P. 2001. *Chlamydia pneumoniae* does not increase atherosclerosis in the aortic root of apolipoprotein E-deficient mice. Arterioscler Thromb Vasc Biol 21:578–584.
33. Paigen B, Holmes PA, Mitchell D, Albee D. 1987. Comparison of atherosclerotic lesions and HDL-lipid levels in male, female, and testosterone-treated female mice from strains C57BL/6, BALB/c, and C3H. Atherosclerosis 64:215–221.
34. Burnett MS, Gaydos CA, Madico GE, Glad SM, Paigen B, Quinn TC, Epstein SE. 2001. Atherosclerosis in apo E knockout mice infected with multiple pathogens. J Infect Dis 183:226–231.

35. Nigg C and Eaton MD. 1944. Isolation from normal mice of a pneumotropic virus which forms elementary bodies. J Exp Med 79:497–510.
36. Blessing E, Nagano S, Campbell LA, Rosenfeld ME, Kuo CC. 2000. Effect of *Chlamydia trachomatis* infection on atherosclerosis in apolopoprotein E-deficient mice. Infect Immun 68:7195–7197.
37. Campbell LA, Blessing E, Rosenfeld M, Lin TM, Kuo CC. 2000. Mouse models of *C. pneumoniae* infection and Atherosclerosis. J Infect Dis 181(suppl 3);S508–513.
38. Blessing E, Lin T, Campbell LA, Rosenfeld ME, Lloyd D, Kuo CC. 2000. *Chlamydia pneumoniae* induces inflammatory changes in the heart and aorta of normocholesterolemic C57BL/6J mice. Infect Immun 68:4765–4768.
39. Blessing E, Campbell LA, Rosenfeld ME, Chough N, Kuo CC. 2001. *Chlamydia pneumoniae* infection accelerates hyperlipidemia induced atherosclerotic lesion development in C57BL/6J mice. Atherosclerosis 158:13–17.
40. Kalayoglu MV, Miranpuri GS, Golenbock DT, Byrne GI. 1999. Characterization of low-density lipoprotein uptake by murine macrophages exposed to *Chlamydia pneumoniae*. Microb Infect 1:409–418.
41. Kalayoglu MV and Byrne GI. 1998. A *Chlamydia pneumoniae* component that induces macrophage foam cell formation is chlamydial lipopolysaccharide. Infect Immun 66:5067–5072.
42. Lopes-Virella M, Klein R, Stevenson H. 1987. Low density lipoprotein metabolism in human macrophages stimulated with microbial or microbial-related products. Arteriosclerosis 7:176–184.
43. Funk J, Feingold K, Moser A, Grunfeld C. 1993. Lipopolysaccaride stimulation of RAW 264.7 macrophages induces lipid accumulation and foam cell formation. Atherosclerosis 98:67–82.
44. Liu L, Hu H, Ji H, Murdin AD, Pierce GN, Zhong G. 2000. *Chlamydia pneumoniae* infection significantly exacerbates aortic atherosclerosis in an LDLR−/− mouse model within six months. Mol Cell Biochem 215:123–128.
45. Laitinen K, Laurila A, Pyhala L, Leinonen M, Saikku P. 1997. *Chlamydia pneumoniae* infection induces inflammatory changes in the aortas of rabbits. Infect Immun 65:4832–4835.
46. Fong IW, Chiu B, Viira E, Fong MW, Jang D, Mahony J. 1997. Rabbit model for *Chlamydia pneumoniae* infection. J Clin Microbiol 35:48–52.
47. Fong IW, Chiu B, Viira E, Jang D, Mahony JB. 1999. De novo induction of atherosclerosis by *Chlamydia pneumoniae* in a rabbit model. Infect Immun 67:6048–6055.
48. Muhlestein JB, Anderson JL, Hammond EH, Zhao L, Trehan S, Schwobe EP, Carlquist JF. 1998. Infection with *Chlamydia pneumoniae* accelerates the development of atherosclerosis and treatment with azithromycin prevents it in a rabbit model. Circulation 97:633–636.

G.N. Pierce, M. Nagano, P. Zahradka, and N.S. Dhalla (eds.).
ATHEROSCLEROSIS, HYPERTENSION AND DIABETES.
Kluwer Academic Publishers. Boston.

ENDOTHELIAL CELL DYSFUNCTION— A KEY FACTOR IN ATHEROGENESIS AND ITS REVERSAL (LABORATORY AND CLINICAL STUDY)

GURMUKH S. SAINANI, MANISHA SAWHNEY BHATIA, and RAJESH SAINANI

Department of Medicine, Jaslok Hospital and Research Centre, Peddar Road, Mumbai 400 026, India

Summary. In macrophage cell cultures and DNA studies, we recorded morphological changes and DNA damage caused by hydrogen peroxide exposure. In another experiment, interaction of altered macrophages and OX-LDL resulted in foam cells. In another experiment native LDL was converted to oxidised LDL by exposure to cigarette smoke extract. However pre-treatment with anti-oxidants-superoxide dismutase (SOD), nitric oxide (NO), glutathione peroxidase (GPx), vitamins A, E, C, β-carotene in all above experiments reversed partially/completely oxidative damage of macrophages, DNA, LDL and prevented foam fell formation. Clinical study included 100 documented cases of coronary artery disease (CAD), (50-angiographically proved, 50 acute myocardial infarction patients and 100 healthy controls (angiographically negative). We estimated oxidative stress (thiobarbituric acid reactive substances and conjugated diene levels) and antioxidant levels (SOD, NO, GPx, vitamins A, E, C, β-carotene, selenium) in all. Oxidative stress was significantly increased and anti-oxidant levels were significantly low in CAD group. Low NO levels in CAD reflect endothelial cell dysfunction (ECD). Coronary artery lesions improved with treatment.

We conclude that ECD is the key factor in CAD and with timely treatment, ECD and coronary artery blocks can be reversed to variable extent.

***Key words*:** Endothelial cell dysfunction, Atherogenesis, Oxidative Stress, Anti-oxidants

Correspondence: Dr. G.S. Sainani, 201, Buena vista, Gen. Jagannath Bhosle Road, Mumbai 400 021, India. Tel: (Res) 22024139, 22846363; Clinic 23868292, 23872131; Fax No. 91-22-24959598; e-mail: drsainani@vsnl.com

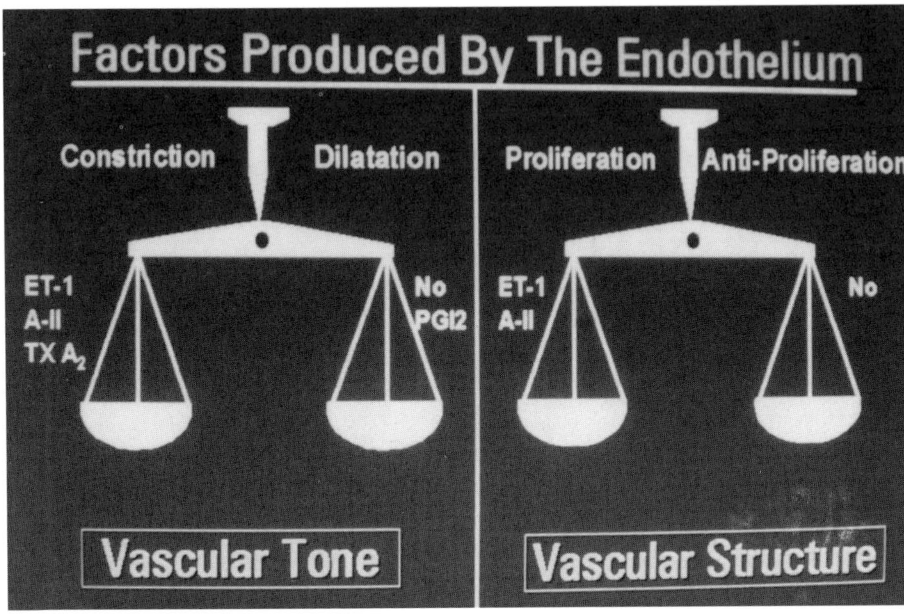

Figure 1. Factors produced by the endothelium, balancing in healthy state.

INTRODUCTION

Over last 10 years, endothelium has assumed a vital role. Earlier endothelium was thought to be a smooth, intact non-thrombogenic lining of the arterial wall. But now it is clear that endothelium produces several vasoactive substances which regulate vascular tone and structure. As a matter of fact, with its total mass of approximate five normal hearts weighing about 1,800 gms, the endothelium is considered as the largest endocrine organ. Total vascular surface area is equivalent to six tennis courts in an adult weighing 70 kg. The vascular endothelium that lines the luminal surface of the coronary arteries is a physiologically active organ that plays an important role in the regulation of coronary artery vasomotion as well as in the prevention of platelet, neutrophil and monocyte activation and adhesion to the lumen surface [1]. The endothelial factors that help to regulate vasomotion are divided into two groups—Endothelial derived relaxing factors (EDRF) and Endothelial derived constricting factors (EDCF). Endothelial derived relaxing factors include nitric oxide (NO) and prostacyclin (PG2) and Endothelial derived constricting factors include endothelin 1 (ET1) and thromboxane A2 (TxA2). These factors balance the effects of vascular tone and vascular structure as shown in Fig. 1. All work together in the normal coronary vascular endothelium to regulate vasomotion and to preserve a smooth non-thrombotic luminal surface (Fig. 2). The alterations in these factors, if allowed to become chronic, are responsible for changes in

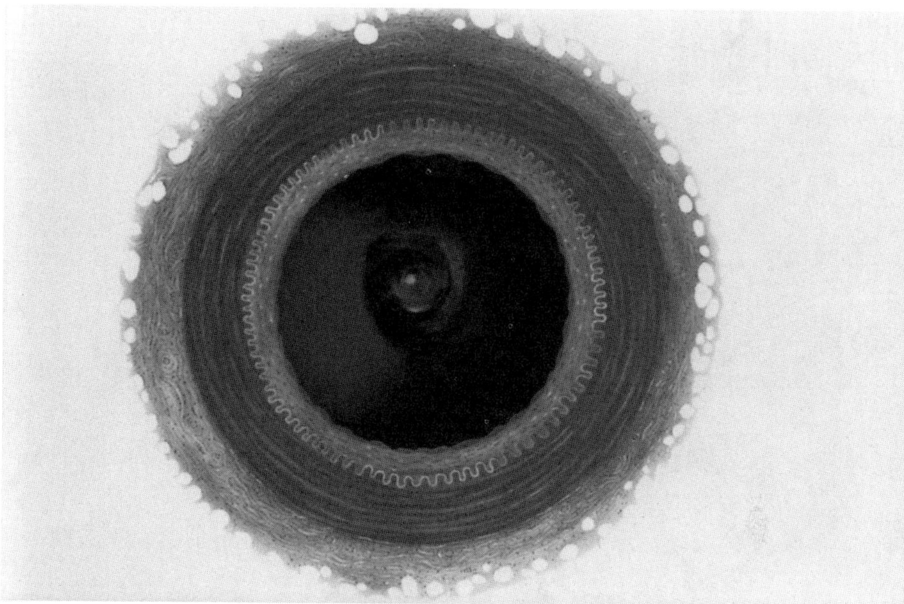

Figure 2. Normal vascular endothelium-with a smooth non thrombotic luminal surface.

vascular structure and growth and adhesivity to platelets and leukocytes leading to atherosclerosis [2,3].

Our aim should be to maintain smooth endothelial lining by proper diet and life-style. That will ensure the integrity of vascular structure of our body (Fig. 3). The most important vasculature are coronary, cerebral and peripheral blood vessels.

The functions of endothelium are **(1)** Maintenance of normal vascular tone and growth by a balanced secretion of vasoconstrictor growth promoting (endothelin-1, thromboxane A2) as well as vasorelaxant/antiproliferative (nitric oxide, prostacyclin) factors. **(2)** Regulate transport of macromolecules from the blood stream into the vessel wall. **(3)** Prevent circulating blood cells (monocytes, platelets) from adhering to the vessel wall.

Nitric oxide (NO) has been the most important molecule of the last decade. It has multifaceted role in the vessel wall (Fig. 4). It inhibits platelet aggregation, inhibits neutrophil adhesion, inhibits adhesion cell molecules, causes vasodilatation and it prevents smooth muscle proliferation. Thus NO is very vital agent as it protects against vasoconstriction and atherosclerosis [4–6].

Endothelin-1 is the most potent endogenous vasoconstrictor and growth promoting factor. It stimulates the release of oxygen free radicals from leukocytes. Oxygen free radicals cause destruction of cell membrane and stimulate atherosclerosis. In healthy individuals, very small amount of ET-1 are released and the effects of NO and ET-1 are well balanced. But NO release is impaired in case of endothe-

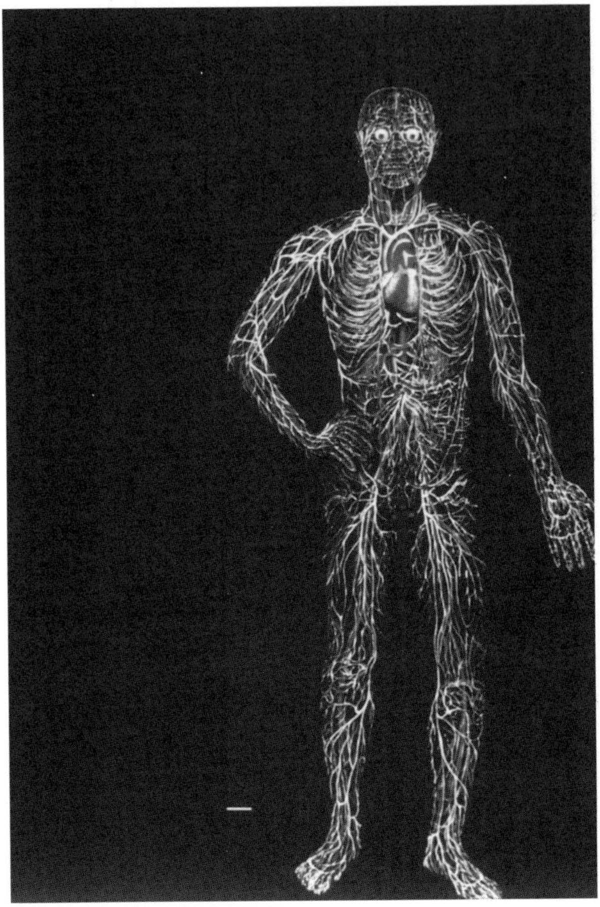

Figure 3. Vasculature of human body.

lial dysfunction, the predominant action of ET-1 leads to vasoconstriction and atherosclerosis [7].

One may surmise that a healthy endothelium is not leaky, not sticky and able to mediate relaxation through NO release. Endothelial cell dysfunction is triggered by risk factors such as hypertension, hyperlipidemia, hyperglycemia, smoking. This results in reduction of NO activity, increase in E-1 activity, increase in endothelial cell permeability. Macromolecules such as LDL as well as monocytes penetrate into the vessel wall and get converted into oxidized LDL and macrophages secrete adhesion cell molecules. Monocytes and platelets stick to the endothelium. Monocytes penetrate in the vessel wall and change into macrophages which pick up oxidized-

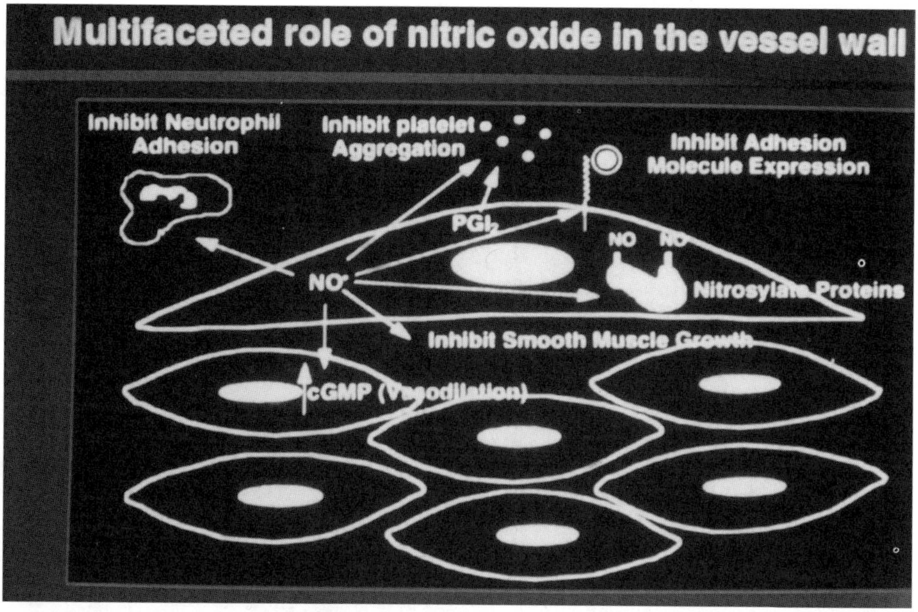

Figure 4. Multifaceted role of nitric oxide in the vessel wall.

LDL (OX-LDL) and get transformed into foam cells leading to formation of fatty streak. At the same time, thrombogenic factors such as platelets, factors VII, fibrinogen come into play and lead to formation of atheromatous plaque [8]. Amongst the atheromatous plaques, it is the vulnerable (unstable) plaque which has tendency to rupture resulting in acute coronary syndromes such as unstable angina, acute myocardial infarction and sudden cardiac death. The vulnerable plaque (Fig. 5) consists of central lipid core which is covered by smooth muscle cells and thin collagen cap and at the periphery of the plaque, there are plenty of cells (macrophages and neutrophils). Interplay between plaque vulnerability and haemodynamic stresses determines the moment and point of rupture resulting in acute coronary syndromes [5,6].

Endothelin 1 (ET-1), Angiotensin II (AII) and Thromboxane (TB-A2) cause vasoconstriction where as nitric oxide (NO) and prostacyclin (PG2) cause vasodilation. Endothelin-I and angiotensin II cause proliferation of smooth muscle whereas nitric oxide has anti-proliferative action.

Endothelial cells regulate the homeostasis of arterial wall. Healthy endothelium is not leaky, not sticky and is able to relax (Fig. 6). Risk factors such as hypertension, diabetes mellitus, smoking and hyperlipidemia cause endothelial cell dysfunction and induce vascular remodelling. Damaged endothelium is leaky, sticky and unable to relax [9] (Fig. 7).

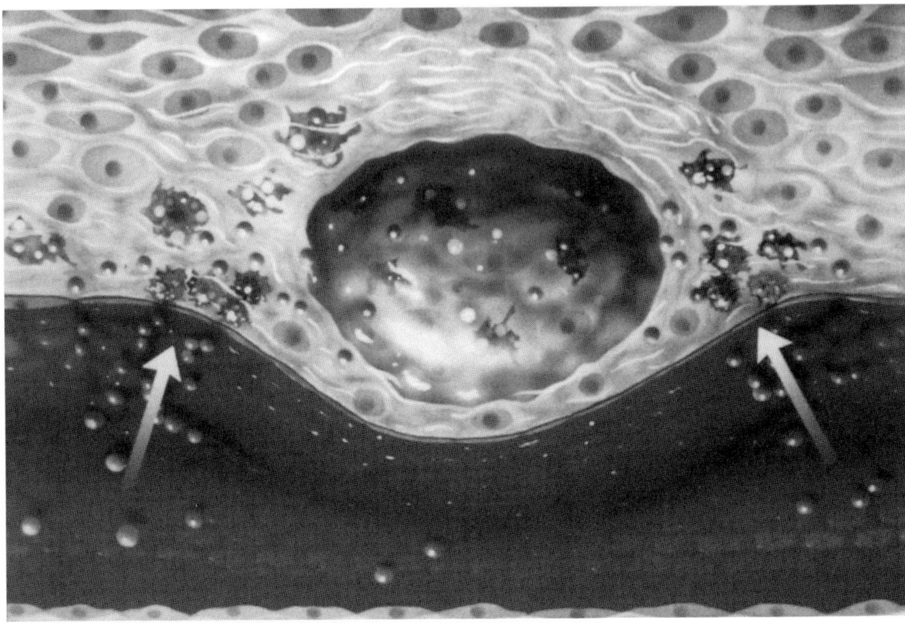

Figure 5. The vulnerable plaque-consisting of lipid core covered by smooth muscle cells and thin collagen cap and plenty of macrophages, neutrophils at the periphery.

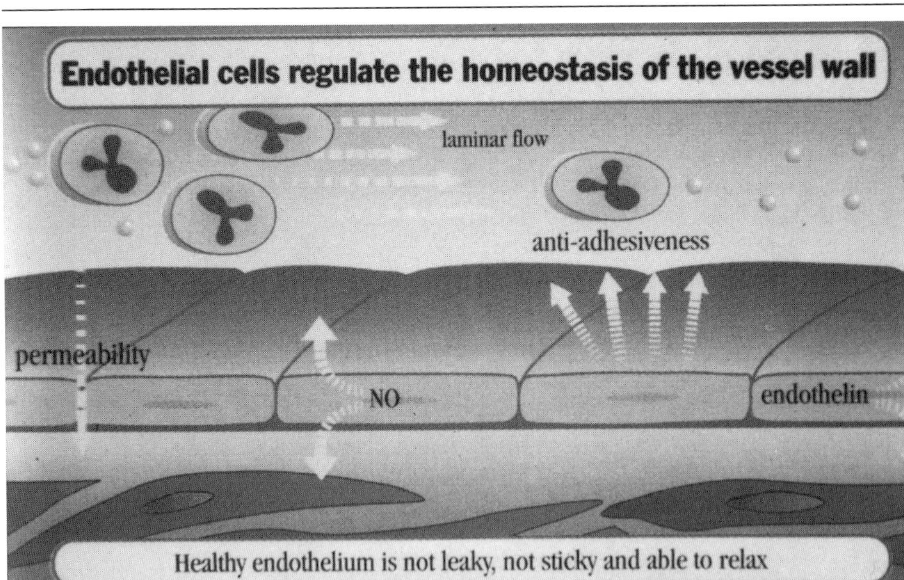

Figure 6. Healthy endothelium-is not leaky, not sticky and able to relax. Regulation of homeostasis of the vessel wall regulated by the endothelial cells.

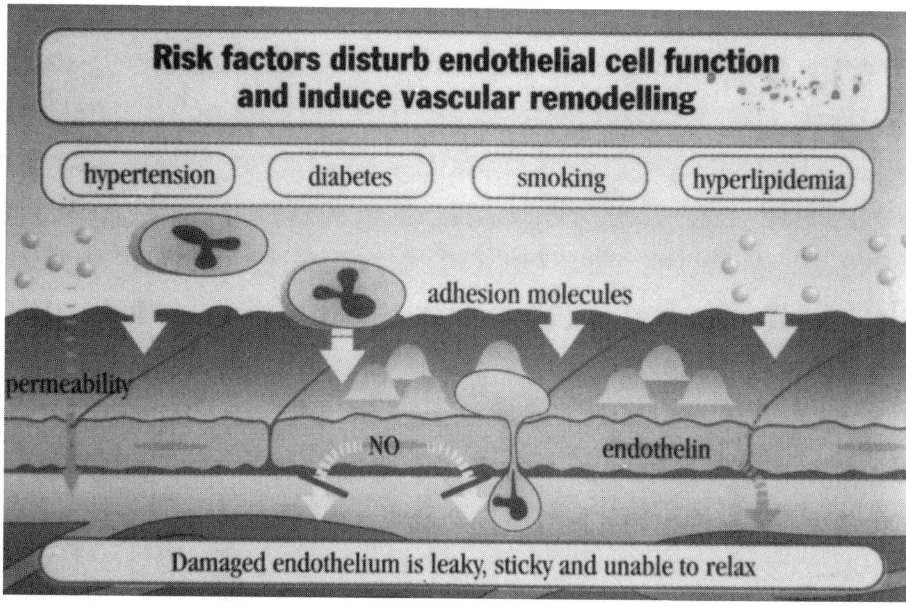

Figure 7. Damaged endothelium due to various risk factors is leaky, sticky and unable to relax.

MATERIAL AND METHODS

I Laboratory experiments

1 Effects of H_2O_2 on human macrophages

Human macrophages were cultured from blood and were treated with 0.1 nmol/l of hydrogen peroxide (H_2O_2). Cell viability and morphology were studied under phase contrast microscope and serial photographs were taken.

2 Conversion of native LDL to OX-LDL

Macrophages were cultured with native LDL first and then culture plate was exposed to H_2O_2 for a variable period to convert native LDL to minimally modified LDL and oxidized LDL and microphotographs were taken to see the entry of LDL particles in macrophages. Finally the culture plates were challenged with various antioxidants (SOD, GPx, NO, vitamins A, C and E) to see the effect.

3 Cigarette smoke extract and LDL oxidation

Smoke from two lit cigarettes was consecutively bubbled through 1 ml phosphate buffer saline (PBS) at room temperature. For controls, PBS was bubbled with plain air. Both preparations were filtered separately through 0.2 μm Micron filters. LDL (0.2 mgm) was incubated with CSE and control preparation (filtrates) at 37°C for 6 hours in a total incubation volume of 0.5 ml. Various anti-oxidants (SOD, GPx, NO, vitamins, A, C, E) were also added separately to the CSE filtrate to evaluate their capacity to prevent LDL oxidation. The observations were made on electrophoresis.

4 Experiments on DNA

We also carried out experiments showing oxidative damage to DNA. Human macrophages were cultured in minimal essential medium with 20% foetal calf serum. Subcultured macrophages were treated with H_2O_2. DNA from pre-treated macrophages were isolated. Agarose electrophoresis was carried out for 2–3 hours. Migration was seen on transillumination, oxidative damage to DNA was induced by exposure of isolated macrophage cell cultures to H_2O_2. The electrophoretic mobility of DNA was altered by oxidative damage as seen in agarose gel electrophoresis. Anti-oxidants (SOD, GPx, NO, vitamin A,C,E) were added to cell culture along with H_2O_2 to study their protective effect.

II Clinical study

Documented cases of ischaemic heart disease (IHD) were compared with age and sex matched healthy controls. One hundred cases of IHD (50 cases of documented AMI and 50 cases of IHD confirmed by coronary angiography) were compared with 100 age and sex matched healthy controls (non-diabetic, non-hypertensive, negative stress test and normal coronary angiography) All subjects underwent a detailed history for coronary risk factors, detailed physical examination, X-Ray chest, ECG, stress test in normal controls and suspected IHD cases, coronary angiography, blood examination for blood sugar, lipid profile. The healthy controls had normal blood sugar, normal lipid profile, negative stress test and/or normal coronary angiograms. All 50 cases of acute myocardial infarction were diagnosed on strict criteria of abnormal ECGs and elevated cardiac enzymes. 50 cases of IHD were confirmed on coronary angiography. Oxidative stress was estimated by measuring Thiobarbituric acid reactive substances (TBARS) and diene conjugate levels. Anti-oxidant status was evaluated by estimating SOD, NO, GPx, selenium, vitamins A, C, E. Also total anti-oxidant status was estimated in patients of IHD and normal healthy controls.

METHODOLOGY

I Oxidant panel

Parameters	**Methods**
	Yagi's Fluorometric Method [10]
Thiobarbituric acid Reactive substance (TBARS)	LDL is mixed with Thiobarbituric acid reagent On heating TBARS measured Fluorometrically
Conjugated dienes	Measured spectrophotometrically from the diene vs time profile [11]

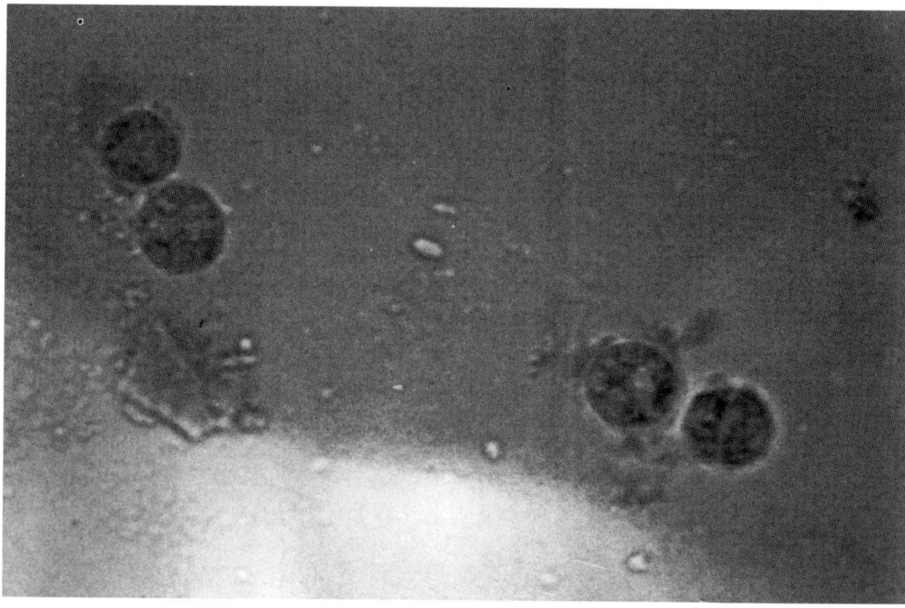

Figure 8. Effect of H_2O_2 on human macrophages. After 2 hours exposure of macrophages to H_2O_2 shows no significant changes in cell morphology.

II Anti-oxidant panel

Parameters	**Methods**
Superoxide dismutase (SOD)	Estimated using Ransod Kit [12]
Nitrite	Estimated colorimetrically by Griess Reagent [13]
Glutathione Peroxidase (GPx) and selenium	Estimated using Ransod Kit [14]
Vitamin A, β-carotene	Estimated using trifluoroacetic acid [15]
Vitamin C	Estimated by 26-Dichlorophenol-Indophenol [15]
Vitamin E	Colorimetrically [15]
Total anti-oxidant status	Estimated using Randox Total Anti-oxidant status kit [16]

RESULTS

1 Effect of H_2O_2 on human macrophages

After 2 hours exposure of macrophages to H_2O_2 (Fig. 8) there was no significant change in cell morphology. But after 8 hours incubation with H_2O_2 (oxidant), cells retract, cytoplasm retracts from cell membrane (Fig. 9). After 24 hours incubation with H_2O_2, macrophage cells get distorted and there is loss of viability (Fig. 10). Cytoplasm and nucleus cannot be differentiated. Altered morphology of

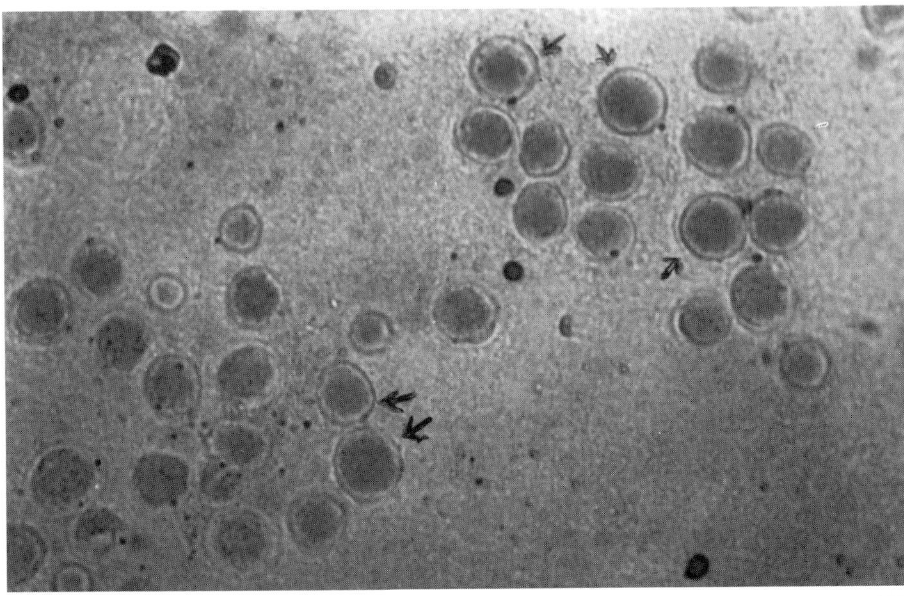

Figure 9. Effect of H_2O_2 on human macrophages. After 8 hours exposure of macrophages to H_2O_2 shows cell retraction cytoplasm retract from cell membrane shown by arrows.

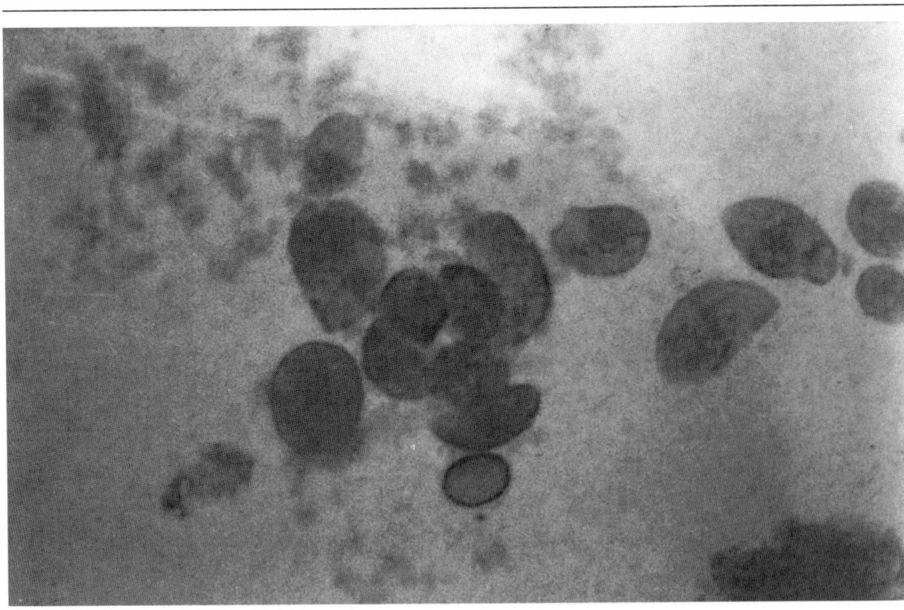

Figure 10. Effect of H_2O_2 on human macrophages. After 24 hours exposure of macrophages to H_2O_2 shows macrophage cells are distorted and there is loss of viability.

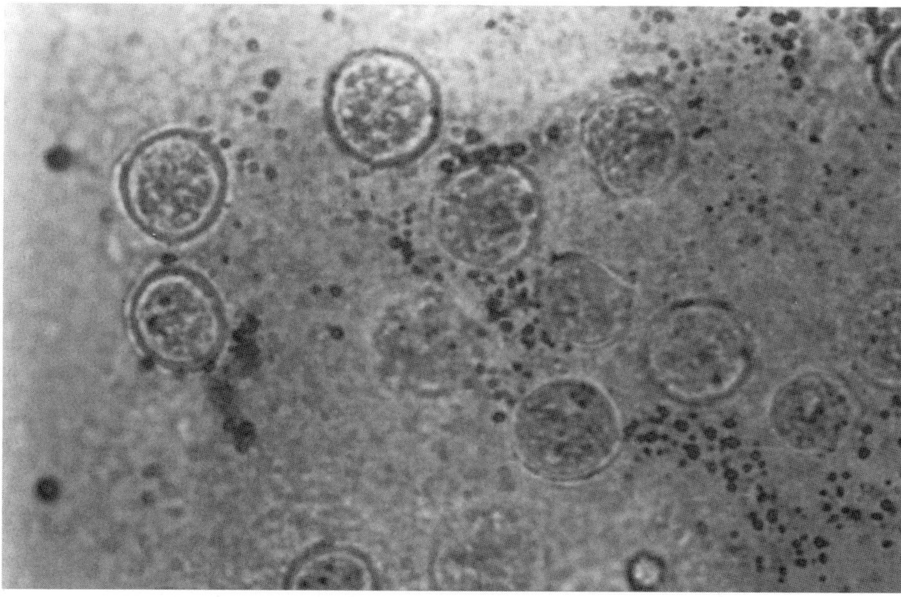

Figure 11. Macrophages cultured with native LDL-No uptake of LDL by macrophages.

macrophages leads to altered surface markers which leads to increased uptake of oxidized LDL leading to atherosclerosis.

2 Conversion of native LDL to OX-LDL

Macrophages were cultured with native LDL, there was no uptake of LDL by macrophages (Fig. 11). When exposed to oxidants, native LDL was converted to minimally modified LDL (MM/LDL) and the morphology of macrophages was slightly altered with the result that few lipid particles (stained by oil 'O' Red) were seen in macrophage cells (Fig. 12). Further exposure to oxidants led to copper oxidised LDL (ox-LDL). There was distinct uptake of ox-LDL (stained dark orange and there was disruption of cell membrane resembling foam cells (Fig. 13). Hence foam cells were formed in laboratory experiments. We then challenged the cultured macrophages with ox-LDL with different antioxidants eg. superoxide dismutase (SOD), Glutathione peroxidase (GPx), Nitric oxide (NO). It was observed that lipid particles (ox-LDL) were extruded from the cells (Fig. 14). Hence from these experiments, one can conclude that it is the ox-LDL which enters the modified macrophages to form foam cells. Addition of different anti-oxidants in culture medium showed extrusion of lipid particles from cells after 12 hours. Hence our experimental study confirms importance of oxidative stress in initiating atherosclerosis and protective function of anti-oxidants. Our experiments have also confirmed

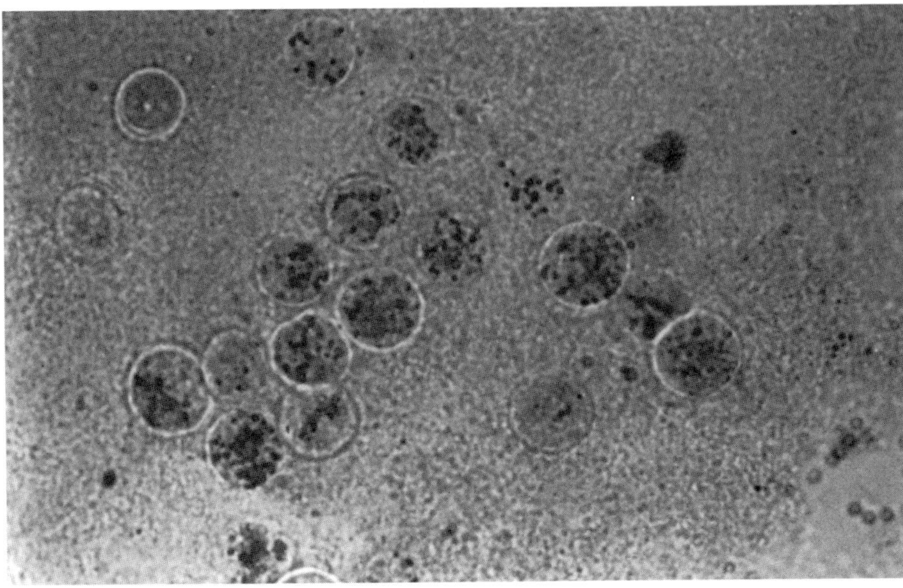

Figure 12. Cultured macrophages and native LDL when exposed to H_2O_2 leads to change in morphology of macrophages and minimally modified LDL with the result that few lipid particles (stained by oil "O" Red) are seen in macrophages.

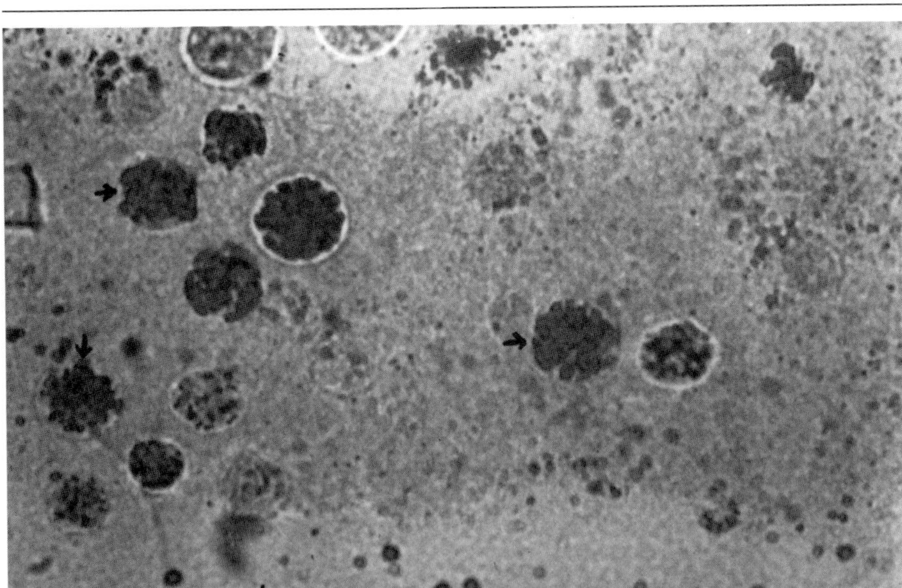

Figure 13. More exposure to H_2O_2 leads to copper oxidised LDL (ox-LDL) and there is distinct uptake of ox-LDL (stained dark orange) and there is disruption of cell membrane resembling foam cells.

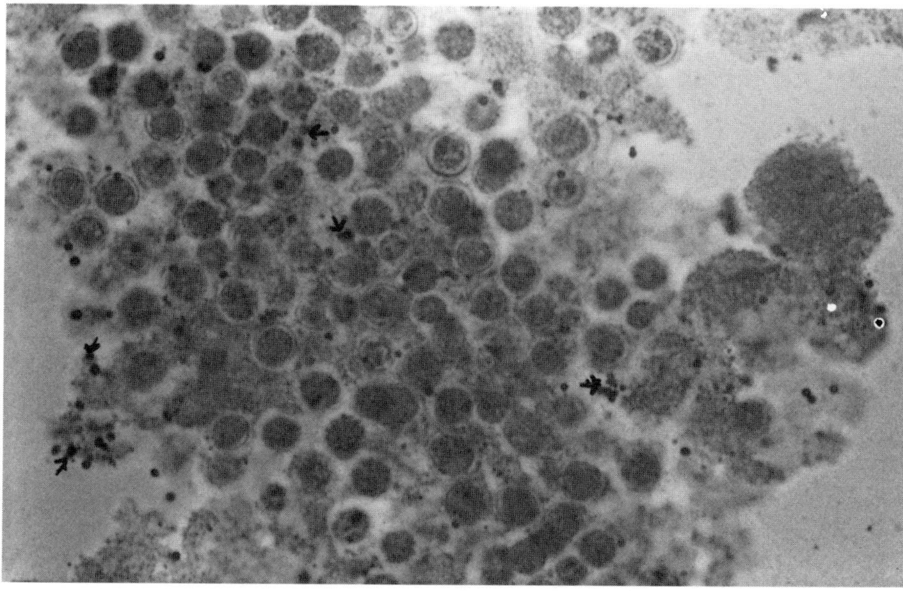

Figure 14. Cultured macrophages with ox-LDL when challenged with anti-oxidants showed that lipid particles (shown by arrows) are excluded from the cells.

that morphological changes in macrophages and oxidation of LDL by oxidants is the important requirement for entry of ox-LDL to form foam cells which leads to formation of fatty streak. Our experimental results discussed above are shown schematically in Fig. 15.

3 Cigarette smoke extract and LDL oxidation

On electrophoresis, 8 columns were observed and recorded (Fig. 16). Number 1 column is the control where the native LDL is at baseline. Number 2 column represents LDL incubated with CSE which has migrated further towards the anode as it is oxidised by CSE. Whereas SOD (No. 3) Nitric oxide (No. 5) and vitamin E (No. 6) prevented completely, the oxidation of LDL; Vit. C (No. 4), Vit. A (No. 5) and GPx (No. 8) prevented partially the LDL oxidation. One can therefore conclude that cigarette smoking is an important risk factor for cardiovascular disease. Also one may infer that anti-oxidants (fresh fruits, green vegetables and sprouts or supplements of vitamins A, C, E) can protect to some extent the smokers. Smokers should therefore take more natural antioxidants in form of fruits, vegetables sprouts.

4 Experiments on DNA

On Gel electrophoresis, pure preparations of DNA were seen as distinct single band (Figs 17, 18, column 1) and damaged DNA band was smeared (Figs 17, 18 columns

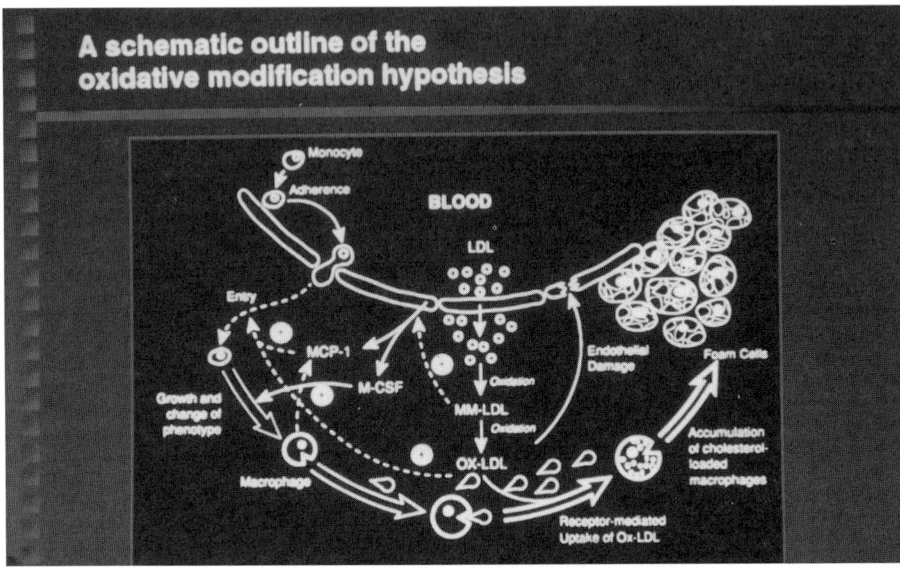

Figure 15. Schematic outline of oxidative modification hypothesis.

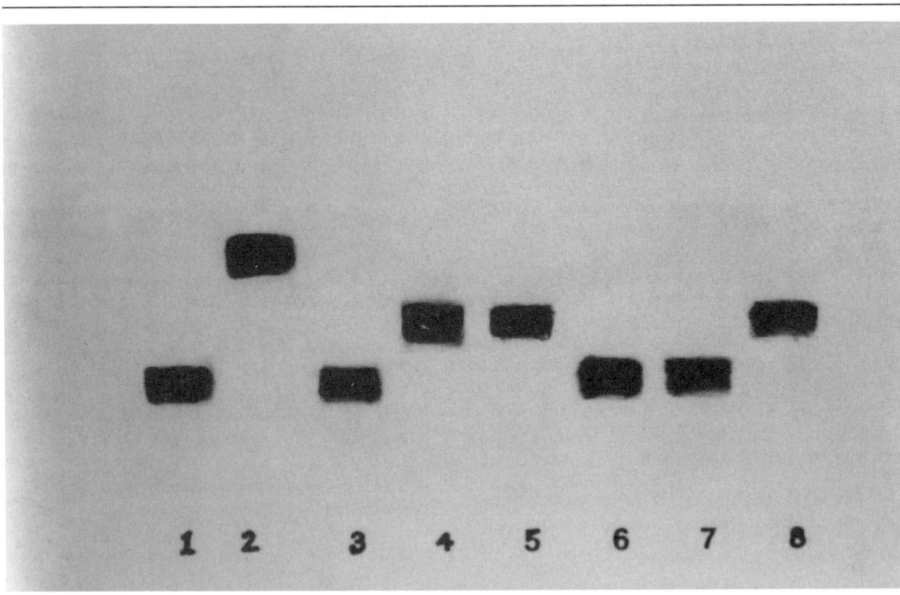

Figure 16. Exposure of CSE with ox-LDL. Column 1 control + native LDL, column 2 LDL incubated with CSE has migrated towards anode, column 3 CSE + ox-LDL + SOD, column 4 CSE + ox-LDL + vitamin C, column 5 CSE + ox-LDL + vitamin A, Column 6 CSE + ox-LDL + vitamin E, Column 7 CSE + ox-LDL + vitamin nitric oxide and column 8 CSE + ox-LDL + vitamin Gpx. Limited mobility in columns with CSE + Ox-LDL and various anti oxidants.

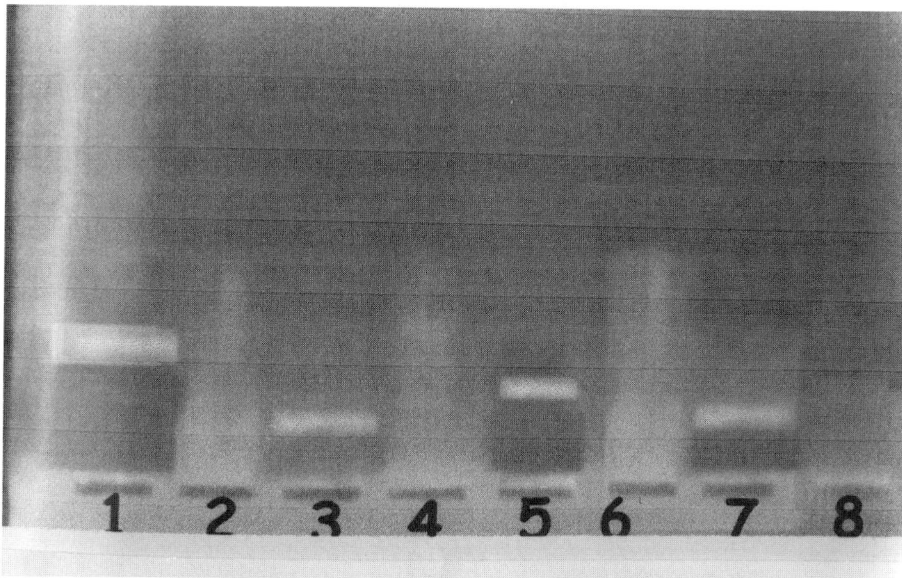

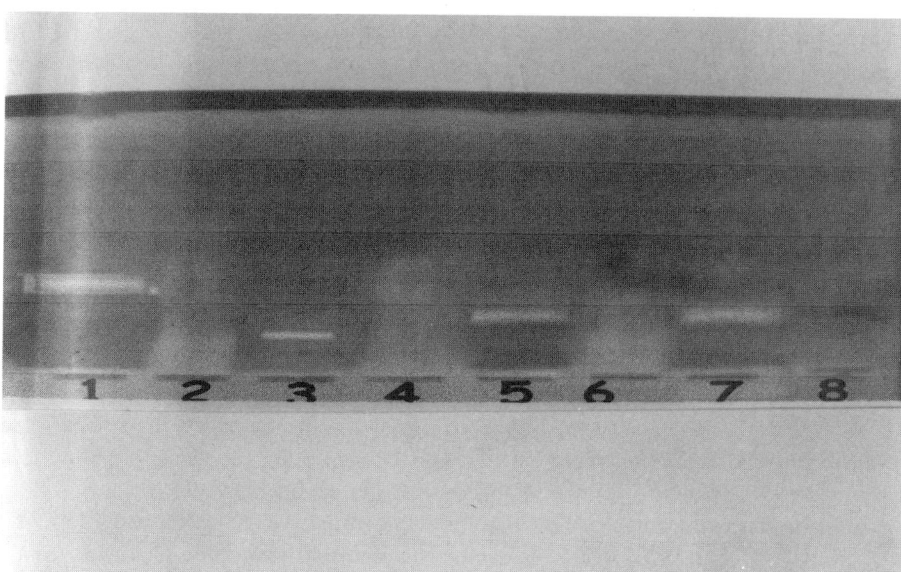

Figure 17 & 18. Oxidative damage to DNA with free ox-LDL. On gel electrophoresis pure preparation of DNA are seen as distinct bands and damage DNA bands are smeared columns 2, 4, 6 and 8. **Protective action of anti-oxidants to DNA treated with ox-LDL.** Limited mobility but distinct bands are observed in columns 3(SOD) 5, (nitric oxide) 7, (GPx) of Fig 17 and columns 3, (Vitamin A) 5, (vitamin C) 7 (vitamin E) of Fig. 18.

Table 1. Showing comparative values for oxidative stress in IHD patients and controls

Oxidative Stress parameters	IHD	Controls
Thiobarbituric Acid Reactive Substances (TBARS) μmol/l	5.8	3.45
Diene Conjugate Level (O.D. Units)	46.0	27.5

There is significant increase in TBARS and Diene Conjugate levels in IHD patients compared to the healthy controls.

Table 2. Showing anti-oxidant values in cases of IHD and health controls

Anti-Oxidant Parameters	IHD	Controls
SOD (Ug/Hb)	450	1,030
Nitrite (u/L)	1.4	2.0
GPx (Ug/Hb)	30	45
Selenium (ug/Hb)	0.5	0.7

There is a significant decrease in various anti-oxidant parameters in IHD patients.

Table 3. Showing antioxidant values in cases of IHD and controls

Anti-oxidant Parameters	IHD	CONTROLS
Vitamin-A [mg/L]	20	47
β-Carotene [mg/L]	0.1	0.5
Vitamin-C [mg/L]	16	30
Vitamin-E [mg/L]	13	30
Total Anti-oxidant status [mmol/lL plasma]	1.28	1.85

There is a significant decrease in various anti-oxidants parameters in IHD patients compared to healthy controls.

2, 4, 6). Antioxidants were able to limit the damage. The bands were distinct but mobility was limited (Fig. 17 column 3-SOD; column 5 NO, column 7 GPx—Fig. 18, column 3 vitamin A, column 5 Vitamin C, column 7 Vitamin E.).

CLINICAL STUDY

It was found that oxidative stress (TBARS and Diene conjugates) were significantly increased in IHD patients compared to controls (Table 1).

As regards anti-oxidants, SOD, NO, GPx, Selenium were significantly low in IHD patients (Table 2). Also anti-oxidants vitamin A, β-Carotene, C, E and total anti-oxidant status were significantly low in IHD patients compared to controls (Table 3).

DISCUSSION

Our laboratory experiments on macrophages confirm that human macrophages when exposed to hydrogen peroxide (H_2O_2) are altered. The cell morphology and viability is changed. After exposure for 2 hours, there is very little alteration, but after 8 hours incubation with H_2O_2 (oxidant), cells retract, cytoplasm retracts from cell membrane. After 24 hours incubation with H_2O_2, the cells are distorted and there is loss of viability. Cytoplasm and nucleus cannot be differentiated. Our experimental results are in conformity with those of Bono and Yang [17]. Further photomicrographs after 48 hours and 72 hours revealed totally unviable macrophages. Altered morphology of macrophages results in altered surface makers which leads to increased uptake of oxidized LDL forming foam cells which then results in formation of fatty streak. These results of morphological studies of macrophages are consistent with those of endothelial cell studies [17;18].

Thorne et al. [19] and Ester Bauer et al. [20] have described 3 forms of LDL i.e. native LDL, minimally modified LDL (mm-LDL) and oxidised LDL (ox-LDL), Both the oxidized forms of LDL have been shown to selectively induce monocyte chemotaxis, adhesion to and transmigration across the arterial wall into the intima and macrophage proliferation within the atherosclerotic plaque.

We have demonstrated in our experiments the selective uptake of mm-LDL and ox-LDL as compared to native LDL. Macrophages when cultured with native LDL, did not pick up LDL. However when this culture plate was exposed to oxidants (hydrogen peroxide), native LDL was initially converted to minimally modified LDL (MMLDL) and the morphology of macrophages was also altered as seen in first experiments, with the result that few lipid particles (stained by oil "O" Red) were seen in macrophage cells. Further exposure to H_2O_2 resulted in copper oxidized LDL (ox-LDL) and further alteration of macrophage morphology. This led to distinct uptake of ox-LDL (stained dark orange) and there was disruption of cell membrane and the cell resembled foam cells. We then challenged the cultured macrophages with ox-LDL with different anti-oxidants eg. Superoxide dismutase (SOD), nitric oxide (NO) and glutathione peroxide (GPx) and it was observed that after 12 hours of challenge, the lipid particles were extruded from the cells. Hence these experiments confirm that it is the ox-LDL which enters the modified macrophages to form foam cells. Addition of different anti-oxidants in culture medium showed extrusion of lipid particles from cells after 12 hours. Our experiments have also confirmed that morphological changes in macrophages and oxidation of LDL by oxidants is the important requirement for entry of ox-LDL to form foam cells which leads to formation of fatty streak.

A number of studies have implicated free radicals in cigarette smoke to be involved in the progression of coronary heart disease. Prya and Stone [21] have reported that gas-phase cigarette smoke contains approximately 1×10^{15} radicals per puff, which are primarily of the alkyl, alkoxyl, peroxyl type. Carbon monoxide, an active constituent of gas-phase cigarette smoke could be involved in atherogenesis by causing hypoxia and vascular injury [22]. Free radicals in cigarette smoke can deplete anti-oxidants and initiate peroxidation of unsaturated lipids [23]. Our experiments on cigarette smoke extract revealed that cigarette smoke acts as an oxidant converting native LDL to ox-LDL. LDL was incubated with CSE and control preparation for 6 hours. Various anti-oxidants (SOD, GPx, NO, Vitamins A, C, E) when added separately to the CSE filtrate, prevented to a variable extent oxidation of LDL. Whereas SOD, NO and vitamin E prevented completely, the others (GPx, vitamins A & C) prevented partially oxidation of LDL. We know that it is the ox-LDL which is atherogenic. Hence our experiments confirm that cigarette smoking is an important risk factor for coronary artery disease. Also one may infer that anti-oxidants (vitamins A, C, E) present in fresh fruits, green vegetables, tomatoes and sprouts, can protect to some extent the smokers. Therefore smokers from low socio-economic group who cannot afford to take plenty of fruits, vegetables are more at risk from smoking than those who can afford to take anti-oxidant vitamins and minerals in natural form.

We carried out experiments to demonstrate DNA damage by oxidative stress and the protective action of different anti-oxidants. Nuclear DNA is readily oxidized by toxic free radicals. Hydrogen peroxide causes DNA strand breaks after conversion to the hydroxyl radical via the Fenton reaction [24,25], although calcium responsive nucleases and the action of lipid peroxides have also been implicated in its genotoxicity [26]. We carried out experiments on DNA which were isolated from pre-treated macrophages and they were treated with H_2O_2. The electrophoretic mobility of DNA was altered by oxidative damage by H_2O_2 as seen in agarose gel electrophoresis. Anti-oxidants (SOD, GPx, NO, vitamins A, C, E) were added to cell culture along with H_2O_2 to study their protective effect. It was observed that anti-oxidants were able to limit the damage.

Role of oxidative stress and anti-oxidants in coronary artery disease is important. Evidence that low intake of anti-oxidants are relevant to the development of CAD comes from four sources, epidemiological data, case control studies, observational surveys of the effects of supplementation in selected populations and prospective controlled trials. In India, the work by Singh et al. [27], Singhal et al. [28], Nand et al. [29] and animal studies by Subramanyam et al. [30] have emphasized the beneficial role of anti-oxidants in the progression of CHD.

OXIDATIVE STRESS IN CORONARY ARTERY DISEASE

One major target of vascular oxidative stress is LDL, the oxidative modification of which is an event that is central to the contemporary hypothesis of atherogenesis and the progression to atherosclerosis. Lipid peroxides (formed by the peroxidation of unsaturated fatty acids by free radicals) are important in the pathogenesis of atherosclerosis. Measurement of lipid peroxides involve use of specific and expensive procedure. However we wanted to establish simple laboratory procedure to assess oxidative stress. Estimation of plasma lipid peroxides by the thiobarbituric acid reaction (TBARS) is well established, sensitive method which measures the amount malonyldialdehyde formed as a breakdown product of lipoperoxide. Raised TBARS levels in plasma of 48 symptomatic CAD patients as compared to the 92 controls were reported by Chiu et al. [31]. Sandersen et al. [32] reported elevated plasma lipid peroxide levels measured as TBARS in patients with peripheral vascular disease and smokers. The potential role of lipoperoxides in atherogenesis is supported by the increase in serum and aortic lipid peroxide concentration (as measured by TBARS) in animals maintained with atherogenic diets. Goto et al. [33], Heinle et al. [34].

As in above studies, oxidative stress in our study was measured. The level of TBARS was significantly raised in our CAD subjects (5.862 ± 0.3 μmol/l) as compared to normal controls (3.23 ± 0.23 μmol/l). This raised level of TBARS signifies the increased susceptibility of LDL oxidation in our CAD patients. The oxidized LDL causes endothelial cell injury, uncontrolled uptake by macrophages, reduced endothelial prostacyclin synthesis, thrombogenesis, all of these characterising the pathogenesis of atherosclerosis. Thus, as seen from our study and the various above mentioned studies, the estimation of lipid peroxides by TBARS may be useful laboratory index of the severity of atherosclerosis.

Conjugated dienes are intermediates, formed in the oxidative attack on PUFA's resulting from the abstraction of hydrogen. They are formed when there is no longer any protection from anti-oxidants and can be conveniently quantified by continuous measurement of their ultraviolet light absorption of 234 nm. Mehemeticik et al. [11] found raised conjugated diene levels in hypercholesterolemic patients (n = 50) as compared to the normolipidemics (n = 44).

We have measured conjugated diene levels as the propagation rate, expressed in μmol diene/min per mgm LDL, which is the maximal rate of LDL oxidation detection in the kinetic curve. We found elevated levels of conjugated diene (145.86 ± μmol diene/min/mgm LDL) in our CAD patients as compared to the normal controls (127.54 ± 12.06 μmol diene/min/mgm LDL). Hence the raised conjugated diene levels in our study and other reported studies confirm raised oxidative stress in the CAD patients. Therefore one may infer that elevated TBARS and diene conjugates in our CAD patients reflect LDL oxidation which is a key factor in atherogenesis.

ANTI-OXIDANTS AND CORONARY HEART DISEASE

Basic research results reveal that several vitamins may decrease risk of cardiovascular disease. Vitamin E inhibits LDL-c oxidation, while β-carotene prevents endothelial damage in inhibiting LDL oxidation within the tissue. Thus different anti-oxidants have different modes of action [35–37].

In epidemiological studies, some carried out in Europe [38,39] and USA [40,41] showed that large intake of dietary vitamins have lower risk of C.V. disease. Besides dietary studies, there are reports that establish a relation between the anti-oxidant status and CHD. The MONICA study [42,43] examined the plasma concentrations of vitamins E, C, A and β-carotene in 16 European regions with about 100 males (40–59 years age). This study showed that the incidence of CHD is inversely related to the anti-oxidant status. The Basel Prospective Study [39] involved 2000 Swiss males (mean age 62 years). An inverse relation between plasma β-carotene, vitamin C and the risk for ischaemic heart disease and stroke was observed. An inverse relationship between plasma β-carotene and risk of myocardial infarction was obtained in the prospective study, by Morris et al. in the Lipid Research Clinics Coronary Primary Prevention Trial (LRCCPPT) [44]. In the present study, we have estimated levels of enzymatic and non-enzymatic anti-oxidants in relation with oxidative stress in angiographically proved CAD patients (n = 50) and 50 patients of AMI. The protein enzymatic and non-enzymatic anti-oxidants studied by us were superoxide dismutase (SOD), NO, glutathione peroxidase (GPx), selenium and albumin. We found an inverse relation between levels of SOD and CHD. SOD levels in CHD patients (n = 50) was 452.06 ± 60.28 μ/gm Hb and in AMI patients (n = 50) was 441.00 ± 60.28 μ/gm Hb and in controls (n = 100) was 1,040.5 ± 98.13 μ/gm Hb. Burton et al. [45] have experimentally shown a reduction in infarct size by IV administration of SOD. The low levels of SOD with raised oxidative stress in our IHD patients are consistent with observations of other workers.

We found significant decline in the GPx levels of CAD (30.18 + 2.33 μg/Hb) and AMI patients (30.54 ± 2.33 μg/Hb) as compared to the normal controls (47.11 ± 11.82 μg/Hb) observed in our study. Reduced levels in our CAD patients and in AMI subjects implied reduced anti-oxidant status in these patients. Araujo et al. [46] have reported low levels of glutathione peroxidase in hyperlipidemics as compared to normolipidemics.

The antioxidant properties of selenium, a constituent of glutathione peroxidase have been studied by Rotruck et al. [47]. In Finland, a low selenium region, persons with selenium levels less than 45 μg/l had an increased risk of CV death and AMI [48]. In our study, selenium was 0.523 ± 0.18 μg/Hb in IHD patients, 0.505 ± 0.16 μg/Hb in AMI patients versus 0.754 ± 0.298 μg/Hb in healthy controls. Our results showed an inverse relationship between selenium concentration and risk of CHD. Deficiency of selenium reduces the peroxidation capacity of GPx thus increasing accumulation of lipid peroxide leading to endothelial injury.

LOW MOLECULAR WEIGHT ANTI-OXIDANTS AND CHD

The low molecular weight anti-oxidants studied were vitamins A, β-carotene, C and E. The results of various studies have been variable. The MONICA vitamin sub-study [42,43] did not reveal a protective association between β-carotene and risk of IHD. Inverse relationship between β-carotene and risk of CHD was confirmed by Health Professional [49] and the Nurses Health Study. [40]. The Lipid Research Clinics Coronary Primary Prevention Trial (LRCCPPT) [44], a 13 year follow up study of 1899 hyperlipidemic men revealed that CV disease events were significantly lower in persons with higher carotenoid concentrations. In US Physicians Health Study [49], the therapeutic effect of β-carotene supplements (50 mgm/day) on 330 patients of CHD was examined. The 5 year follow up revealed a significant reduction in cases of MI and stroke. In our study, β-carotene levels were significantly reduced in IHD and AMI subjects as compared to the controls. The mean levels of β-carotene were 0.099 ± 0,025 μm in CAD patients, 0.104 ± 0.026 μm in AMI patients and 0.497 ± 0.03 μm in controls. Our results are consistent with most other studies [50–52].

Ascorbic acid (vitamin C) has been shown to efficiently scavenge superoxide, hydrogen peroxide, hydroxyl, peroxyl radical and singlet oxygen. Frie et al. [53] stressed that the antioxidant mode of action of vitamin C is due to their ability to trap peroxyl radicals in the aqueous phase before they initiate lipid peroxidation. Ascorbic acid also protects membranes against peroxidation by enhancing the activity of α-tocopherol, the chief chain breaking anti-oxidants (Golumbic and Mattil) [54]. Vollset and Bjelke [38] found an inverse relationship between vitamin C intake as judged by diet questionnaires and risk of CV disease. This was a 11 year follow up study of 16,713 men/women (Finland) of which 438 cases had fatal C.V. disease. Similar results are reported by Enstram et al. [41] in their 10 year follow up study of 11,349 middle aged men/women. However the Health Professional follow up study [49]; (total n = 4667, MI = 106, non-MI = 201 and revascularization = 360) showed no relation between vitamin C intake and risk of CV diseases. Similarly no significant relation between vitamin C levels and risk for CHD was reported by Nurses Health Study [40].

In our study, we found levels of vitamin C significantly low in our CAD and AMI patients compared to controls. Thus an inverse relationship between levels of ascorbic acid and CHD is seen in our study and is in echo with other studies [39, 50, 55].

In models involving normal animal fed with a high cholesterol diet, significant inhibition of atherosclerosis with vitamin-E treatment has been shown in rabbits [56], squail and monkeys [57]. Various vitamin E dietary supplementation studies reveal that oral intake of α-tocopherol leads to a significant increase of the tocopherol content of the LDL particles. Amongst epidemiological studies, Nurses Health Study [40], based on detailed questionnaire comprising 116 items from food and supplements revealed a significant inverse relationship between vitamin-E intake and risk of CAD. Similarly Health Professional follow up study (HPFS) [49] involved 39,910 male medical professionals. This 4 year follow up study showed a significant inverse relationship between vitamin-E intake and risk of CHD. In our study, the mean vitamin E levels were 13.16 ± 2.9 mg/l in IHD patients, 12.66 ± 2.54 mg/dl/l in AMI patients as compared to 30.98 ± 3.76 mg/L in controls. Thus an inverse relationship between plasma vitamin E levels and CHD is established. Our findings are in echo with other reports [29,58–60].

NITRIC OXIDE AND CORONARY HEART DISEASE

The biologic link between endothelial damage and atherosclerosis may be related to decreased arterial bioavailability of NO, which may predispose to leucoctye and platelet adhesion, vasoconstriction and smooth muscle cell proliferation.

Supplementation with oral L-arginine the physiologic substrate for NO production has profound anti-atherogenic effects in cholesterol fed animals (Cooke et al.) [61]. Owing to short life of NO and its unstability, it is difficult to do direct measurement of NO in vitro and in vivo. Hence we measured plasma concentrations of nitrite/nitrate, the stable metabolic products of NO by Greiss reagent. In our study the mean nitrate levels were 12.22 ± 1.83 μm/ml in IHD patients, 11.00 ± 1.34 μm/ml in AMI patients and 20.0 ± 3.18 μm/ml in our controls. Green et al. [13] and Jilma et al. [62] have also reported same nitrate levels as ours in their normal controls.

Our results confirm the importance of nitric oxide as an important anti-oxidant as we found low levels of nitric oxide estimated as nitrate levels in our IHD and AMI patients compared to healthy controls.

TOTAL ANTI-OXIDANT STATUS AND CORONARY HEART DISEASE

All anti-oxidants do not contribute to the total anti-oxidant capacity in an analogous manner, since all anti-oxidants in vivo do not have the same reaction kinetics and they may interact with one another. It is more meaningful to measure the total anti-oxidant status as the anti-oxidant system is composed of a number of elements which exert anti-oxidant activity in different way [63,64].

The total anti-oxidant status in our IHD and AMI patients was significantly reduced as compared to controls ($P < 0.001$). Hence in these patients, the overall anti-oxidant protection (including estimated anti-oxidants plus other unidentified anti-oxidants) was reduced.

OXIDATIVE STRESS, ANTI-OXIDANTS AND SEVERITY OF CAD

Since atherosclerosis and its progression are associated with increased vascular oxidative stress, it is postulated that anti-oxidant therapy may improve vascular function limiting further complications [49,65,66].

In our study, oxidative stress (as determined by TBARS and conjugated diene) was directly related to severity of CAD. Both these parameters were significantly raised in the triple vessel disease group as compared to the single vessel group. Similarly anti-oxidant parameters had relations with severity of CAD. Anti-oxidant levels in single vessel disease were > double vessel disease group > triple vessel disease group. Hence our study shows that severity of coronary artery stenosis is related to rising oxidative stress and declining anti-oxidant levels.

REGRESSION OF ATHEROMATOUS PLAQUES

An attempt was made to follow up patients of documented coronary artery disease after advising them strict diet, life style modifications, strict lipemic control with statins, long acting nifedipine (20 mgm BD), ramipril (10 mgm daily) and supplementation with vitamin C (500 mgm daily), vitamin E (400 mgm daily). Patients showed improvement as frequency of ischemic events was considerably reduced and in 10 patients in whom repeat coronary angiography was possible, there was regression in plaque size.

ACKNOWLEDGEMENT

We are most grateful to the trustees of Jaslok Hospital, for the research grant and to Lt. Gen. Dr. P K Chakrabarty (Chief Executive Director) and Dr. MP Lekhi

(Medical Director), Jaslok Hospital and Research Centre for the facilities provided for carrying out the research study. We also thank all the physicians/cardiologists who provided us the clinical cases for this study.

REFERENCES

1. Kaiser L, Sparks HV. 1987. Endothelial cells: not just a cellophane wrapper. Arch Intern Medicine 147:569–573.
2. Petty PG, Pearson JD. 1989. Endothelium the axis of vascular health and disease. Jr Royal Coll Physicians 23:92–101.
3. Celermajor DS. 1997. Endothelial dysfunction: Does it matter? Is it reversible?. Am Col of Cardiology 30:325–333.
4. Kelly RA, Smith IW. 1996. Nitric oxides and nitrovasodilators—Similarities, differences and interactions and interactions. Amer Journ of Cardiol 2C–7C.
5. Dinerman JL, Mehta JL. 1990. Endothelial platelet and leukocyte interactions in ischaemic heart disease in sights into potential mechanism and their clinical relevance, Journ Am Coll Cardiology 16:207–222.
6. Shah PK. 1997. New insights into the pathogenesis and prevention of acute coronary syndromes Am. Journ. Cardiol 79(12B):17–23.
7. Masaki T. 1989. The discovery, the present state and the future prospects of endothelin. Journ Cardio vas. Pharmacology, 1989, 13, suppl 5: S1–S4.
8. Awiram M, Dankner G, Brook JG. 1990. Platelet secretory products increases LDL oxidation, enhance its uptake by macrophages and reduces its fluidity. Arteriosclerosis 10:559–563.
9. Shah PK. 1996. Pathophysiology of plaque rupture and concept of plaque stabilisation. Cardiol Clin 14:17–29.
10. Yagi K. 1984. Increased serum lipid peroxides initiate atherogeneses. Bioassays 1:58–60.
11. Mehmetcik GT, Uysal M. 1997. Endogenous and Copper-induced lipid peroxidation and antioxidant activity of serum in hypercholesterolemic subject. Hormone Metabolism Research 29: 63–65.
12. Mc Cord JM, Crapo JD, Fidovich I. 1997. Superoxided ismutase assays. A review of methodology. In: superoxide and superoxide dismutases, Ed. AM Michelson, JM McCord, I Fidovich, 11–17, London, UK Academic.
13. Green LC, Wagner DA, Glogoswski J, Skipper PL, Wishnok JS, Tannendaum SR. 1982. Analysis of nitrate, nitrate and (^{5}N) nitrate in biological fluids. Analytical Biochem 126:131–138.
14. Buczynski A, Wachowicz B, Kedziora—Kornatowaska K, Tkaczewski W, Kedziora J. 1993. Changes in antioxidant enzyme activities, aggregrability and malonyldialdehyde concentrations in blood, platelets from patients with CHD, Atherosclerosis 100(2):223–228.
15. Gey KF, Puska P. 1989. Plasma vitamin E and A inversely correlated to mortality from ischaemic heart disease in cross-cultural epidemiology, Ann New York Acad Sci 57:254–282.
16. Lantos J, Roth E, Czopf L, Nemes J, Gal I. 1997. Monitoring of plasma total antioxidant status in different diseases, Acta Chirurgica Hungarica 36(1–4):188–189.
17. de Bono DP, Yang WD. 1995. Exposure to low concentrations of H_2O_2 causes delayed endothelial cell death and inhibits proliferations of surviving cells. Atherosclerosis 114:235–245.
18. Whorton AR, Montgomery ME, Kent RS. 1985. Effects of hydrogen peroxide on prostaglandins production and cellular integrity in cultured porcine endothelial cells, Journ Clinical Investigations 76:295–296.
19. Tharng SA, Abbot SE, Winward PG, Blake DR, Mills PG. 1996. Extent of oxidative modification of LDL, determines the degree of cytotoxicity to human coronary artery cells, Heart 75:11–16.
20. Esterbauer H, Dicher-Rothencder M, Wagg G, Streiyel G, Jurgens G. 1990. Biochemical structural and functional properties of oxidised LDL, Chem Res Toxicol 3:77–92.
21. Prya WA, Stone K. 1993. Oxidants in cigarette smoke, Radicals hydrogen peroxide peroxynitrate and peroxynitrite. Ann New York Acad Sci 686:12–27.
22. Wald NS, Howard PG, Smith, Kjeldsen K. 1973. Association between atherosclerosis diseases and carboxy-haemoglobin levels in tobacco smokers. British Med Journ 1:761–765.
23. Frie B, Forte TM, Ames BM, Cross CE. 1991. Gas phase oxidants of cigarette smoke induce lipid perioxidant and changes in lipoprotein properties in human blood plasma Protective effects of ascorbic acid, Biochem Journ 117:133–138.

24. Mello AC, Hoftmann ME, Menghini R. 1984. Cell Killing and DNA damage by hydrogen peroxide are mediated by intracellular iron, Biochem Journ 218:273–275.
25. Schranf S, Hyslop PA, Jackson H, Cochrane LG. 1988. Oxidant included DNA damage of target cells, Journ Clin Invest 82:1040–1050.
26. Cantoni O, Sestili P, Cattabeni F B, Bellomo G, Pou S, Cohen M, Cerutti P. 1989. Calcium chelator Quin 2 prevents hydrogen peroxide induced DNA breakage and cytotoxicity, Eur Journ Biochem 182:209–212.
27. Singh RB, Niaz MA. 1993. CHD in Indians, Pakistanis and Bangladeshis; aetiology and possibilities for prevention (letter) British Heart Journ 69:572.
28. Singhal S, Gupta P, Mathur B, Banda S, Dandia R, Gupta R. 1998. Educational status and dietary fat and antioxidant intake in urban subjects. JAPI 46/8:684–688.
29. Nand N, Budhiraja N, Singh GP, Sharma M, Aggarwal HK. 1997. Lipid peroxidation and vitamin-E in IHD, JAPI 45/11:839–841.
30. Subramanyam G. 1998. Role of trace elements and antioxidants in cardiovascular diseases. Cardiology Today II/1:59–64.
31. Chin HC, Jeng JR, Shiel SM. 1994. Increased oxidizability of plasma LDL from patients with CAD, Biochem Biophys, Acta 1225:200–208.
32. Sanderson KJ, Vanrij AM, Wade CR, Sutherland HF. 1995. Lipid peroxidation of circulating LDL with age, smoking and in peripheral vascular disease, Atherosclerosis 118:45–51.
33. Goto Y. 1982. Lipid peroxides as a cause of vascular disease. In: Lipid peroxides in biology and medicine. Edn Yogi K 295:303-NY Academic Press Inc.
34. Heinle H, Liebich H. 1980. The influence of diet—induced hypercholesterolemia with the degree of oxidation of glutathione in rabbit aorta. Atherosclerosis 37:637–640.
35. Sies H. 1993. Strategies on antioxidant defense. Eur, J Biochem 215:213–219.
36. Steinberg D, Parthasarathy T, Carew J. 1989. Beyond cholesterol-Modification of LDL that increases its atherogenicity. New England of Medicine 320(14):915–924.
37. Goldstein S, Czapski G. 1984. Mannitol as an OH scavenger in aqueous solutions and in biological systems, Int. Journ. Radiation Biology 46:725–729.
38. Vollset SE, Bjelke E. 1983. Does consumption of fruits and vegetables protect against stroke, Lancet 2:742 (letter).
39. Gey KF, Stahelin HB, Eichhdzer M. 1993. Poor plasma status of carotene and Vitamin C is associated with higher mortality from IHD and stroke. Prospective Basel Study. Clinical Invest 7:3–6.
40. Stampfer MJ, Hennekns CH, Mansan JF, Colditz GA, Rosner B, Willett WC. 1993. Vitamin E consumption and the risk of coronary disease in women. New England Journ of Med 328:1444–1449.
41. Enstram JE, Kanim LE, Klein MA. 1992. Vitamin C intake and mortality among a sample of the United States population. Epidemiology 3:194–202.
42. Gey KF. 1993. Vitamin E and other essential antioxidant regarding CHD: Risk assessment studies. In Vitamin E in health and disease, edn. L-Packer and J Fuchs, 589–633, New York, Dekkes.
43. Gey KF, Puska P, Jordan P, Meser UK. 1991. Inverse correlation between plasma Vitamin-E and mortality from IHD in cross epidemiology. Am Journ, Clin Nutr 53:326S–334S.
44. Morris Dl, Kritchevksy SB, Davis CE. 1994. Serum carotenoids and coronary heart disease, the lipid research clinics coronary primary prevention trial and follow-up stud., Jr. Am Med. Assoc 272:1439–1441.
45. Burton KP. 1985. SOD enhances recovery following myocardial ischaemia. American Journal of Physiology 248:4637–4643.
46. Araujo FB, Barbosa DS, Hsin CY, Maranhao RC, Abadalla DS. 1995. Evaluation of oxidative stress in patients with hyperlipidemia. Atherosclerosis 117:61–71.
47. Rotruck JT, Pope AL, Ganther HE, Swanson AB, Hafeman DG, Hoekstra WG. 1973. Selenium biochemical role as a component of glutathione peroxidase, Science 179:585–590.
48. Salonen JT, Alfthan GH, Hunthuenen JK, Pikkarainen J, Puska P. 1982. Association between cardiovascular death and myocardial infarction and serum selenium in a matched pair longitudinal study. Lancet 2:175–179.
49. Rimm EB, Stampfer MJ, Ascherio A, Giovannucci E, Colditz GA, Willet WC. 1993. Vitamin E consumption and the risk of coronary heart disease in men. New England Journ of Med 328: 1450–1456.
50. Singh RB, Nizam MA, Bishnoi I, Sharma JP, Gupta S, Rastogi SS, Singh R, Begum R, Chibo H, Shoumin Z 1994. Diet, antioxidant vitamins, oxidative stress and the risk of CAD, The Peerzada prospective study. Acta Cardiologica XLIX:453–467.

51. Singh RB, Rastogi S, Ghosh S, Nizam MA, Singh NK. 1993. The diet and moderate exercise trial (DAMET) results after 24 weeks. Acta Cardiologica 48:543–547.
52. The alpha tocopherol, Beta-carotene, cancer prevention study group (ATBC-group) 1994. The effect of vitamin E and beta carotene on the incidence of lung cancer and other cancers in male smokers. New England Journ Of Medicine 330:1029–1035.
53. Frei B, England L, Ames BN. 1998. Ascorbate is an outstanding antioxidant in human blood plasma, Proc Natl Acad Sci USA 86:6377–6381.
54. Golumbic C, Mattil HA. 1941. Antioxidants and the antioxidants of fats XIII The antioxygenic action of ascorbic acid in association with tocopherols hydroquinoes and related compounds, Journ Am Chem Soc 63:1279–1280.
55. Riemersma RA, Wood DA, Macintyre CH, Elton RA, Gey KP, Oliver MF. 1991. Risk of angina pectoris and plasma concentrations of vitamins A, C, E and carotene. Lancet 337:1–5.
56. Prasad K, Kalra J. 1993. Oxygen free radicals and hypercholesterolemic atheroclerosis, effect of vitamin E, American Heart Journ 25:958–973.
57. Verlangieri AJ, Bush MJ. 1992. Effects of d α-tocopherol supplementation on experimentally induced primate atherosclerosis, Journ Am Coll. Nutrition 11:131–138.
58. Gupta V, Chandra M, Johri AK, Mishra R, Kumar A, Gujrati V, Shanker K. 1994. Effect of oral vitamin E on oxy free radicals in AMI, Indian Heart Journal 46:222–224.
59. Daga MK, Madhuchhanda, Mishra TK, Mohan A. 1997. Lipid peroxide, beta carotene and alpha tocopherol in ischaemic stroke and effect of exogenous vitamin E supplementation on outcome, JAPI 45/11:843–846.
60. Singh RB, Niaz M, Rastogi SS. 1996. Usefulness of antioxidant vitamins in suspected AMI (The Indian Experiment of Infarct survival-3) Am Journ of Cardiology 77:232–236.
61. Cooke JP, Singer AH, Tsao P, Zera P, Rowan RA, Billinghem OF, Eichler HG. 1992. Antiatherogenic effects of L arginine in the hypercholesterolemic rabbit. Journ Clin Invest 90:1168–1172.
62. Jilma B, Kastner J, Mensik C, Vondrovec B, Mildebrandt J, Krejcy K, Wagneri ••. 1996. Sex differences in concentrations of exhaled NO and plasma nitrate, Life Science 58:469–476.
63. Jacob RA. 1995. The integrated antioxidant system, Nutrition Research 15:755–756.
64. Halliwell B, Gutteridge JMC. 1990. The antioxidant of human extracellular fluids, Arch Biochem Biophys 289:1–8.
65. Gaziano JM, Mansen JE, Branch LG, Colditz GA, Willett WC, Buring JE. 1992. Dietary beta-carotene and decreased cardiovascular mortality in an elderly cohort, Journ, Am Coll Cardiology 19:377 (abstract).
66. Gage JE, Hess OM, Murakami T, Ritter M, Grimm J, Krayenbuchl HP. 1986. Vasoconstriction of stenotic coronary arteries during dynamic exercise in patients with classic angina pectoris. Reversibility by nitroglycerin. Circulation 73:865–876.

G.N. Pierce, M. Nagano, P. Zahradka, and N.S. Dhalla (eds.).
ATHEROSCLEROSIS, HYPERTENSION AND DIABETES. Copyright © 2003.
Kluwer Academic Publishers. Boston.

BIOCHEMICAL MECHANISMS OF HYPERHOMOCYSTEINEMIA IN ATHEROSCLEROSIS: ROLE OF CHEMOKINE EXPRESSION

KARMIN O, MB, PHD and YAW L. SIOW, PHD

Department of Pharmacology, Faculty of Medicine, University of Hong Kong, Hong Kong, People's Republic of China

Summary. Abundant epidemiological evidence has demonstrated that hyperhomocysteinemia is a common and independent risk factor for cardiovascular disorders due to atherosclerosis. Monocyte infiltration into the subendothelial space in the arterial wall and later differentiation into macrophages are important initial steps in the development of atherosclerotic lesions. Macrophages can then take up large amount of lipids to form foam cells in the lesion. The findings that macrophages and foam cells accumulate in the atherosclerotic lesions of hyperhomocysteinemic patients suggest that the recruitment of monocytes is enhanced during atherogenesis. Monocyte chemoattractant protein-1 (MCP-1) is a potent chemokine that stimulates migration of monocytes into the intima of arterial walls. The level of MCP-1 is increased in atherosclerotic lesions in both human and experimental animals. MCP-1 exerts its action mainly through the interaction with C-C chemokine receptor (CCR2) on the surface of monocytes. In this article, we reviewed recent studies on the homocysteine-induced MCP-1 and its receptor CCR2 expression in vascular cells as well as the involvement of oxidative stress and nuclear factor kappa B (NF-κB) activation. Homocysteine-stimulated CCR2 expression in monocytes together with increased MCP-1 expression in vascular cells may represent a mechanism for homocysteine-enhanced monocyte infiltration into the arterial wall during atherogenesis.

***Key words*:** Hyperhomocysteinemia, Atherosclerosis, Chemokines, Oxidative stress, Nuclear factor kappa B

Address for Correspondence: Dr. Karmin O, MB, PhD, Department of Pharmacology, Faculty of Medicine, The University of Hong Kong, 2/F. Laboratory Block, New Medical Complex, 21 Sassoon Road, Hong Kong, People's Republic of China. Tel: (852) 2819-2861; Fax: (852) 2817-0859; e-mail: okarmin@hkucc.hku.hk

INTRODUCTION

Hyperhomocysteinemia, a condition of elevated serum levels of homocysteine, is one of the important risk factors for atherosclerosis [1–4]. Atherosclerosis is the principal contributor to the pathogenesis of myocardial and cerebral infarction, which are the leading causes of mortality and morbidity in many countries [3]. Abnormal elevations of homocysteine (a thiol containing amino acid) levels up to 0.1–0.25 mM in blood have been reported in patients with hyperhomocysteinemia [3,5]. Many factors may regulate plasma levels of homocysteine. For example, severe hyperhomocysteinemia seen in children is usually the result of rare homozygous deficiency of enzymes necessary for homocysteine catabolism [3,4]. Moderate increases in blood homocysteine levels occur more frequently and are often found in patients with heterozygous enzyme deficiency, folate or pyridoxine (vitamin B_6) deficiency, impaired renal function as well as in elderly people and postmenopausal women [3–5].

HYPERHOMOCYSTEINEMIA AND ATHEROSCLEROSIS

Epidemiological studies have revealed that hyperhomocysteinemia is associated with an increased risk of atherosclerosis [1–4]. Elevated homocysteine levels have been observed in a significant proportion of patients with coronary artery disease (up to 30–40%) [5–9]. Several plausible mechanisms for homocysteine-induced atherosclerosis have been proposed. These include endothelial dysfunction [10,11], increased proliferation of smooth muscle cells [12,13], enhanced coagulability [13,14], and increased cholesterol synthesis in hepatocytes [15,16]. Although the precise molecular mechanisms responsible for the pathogenicity of hyperhomocysteinemia remain uncertain, endothelial injury and dysfunction are considered to be one of the leading mechanisms contributing to atherogenesis [2–4,11,17–19]. It has been proposed that homocysteine-caused endothelial injury may be due to oxidative stress, attenuation of nitric oxide-mediated vasodilatation and disturbances in the antithrombotic activities of the endothelium [17–20]. Upon injury, endothelial cells are capable of producing various cytokines and growth factors that in turn participate in the development of atherosclerotic lesions. We recently reported that homocysteine stimulated the expression of monocyte chemoattractant protein-1 (MCP-1) in endothelial cells [21], vascular smooth muscle cells [22] and monocyte-derived macrophages [23] leading to enhanced monocyte chemotaxis and adhesion to endothelial cells. Several animal models with hyperhomocysteinemia have been developed in monkeys [24], in apoE-null mice [25] as well as in cystathionine β-synthase (CBS) deficient mice [18]. In the vessels of diet-induced moderate hyperhomocysteinemic monkeys, Lentz et al. reported increased platelet-mediated vasoconstriction, impaired endothelium-dependent vasodilation, and decreased thrombomodulin-dependent activation of protein C when compared to that of monkeys fed a normal diet [24]. In the apoE-null mice with dietary-induced hyperhomocysteinemia, Hoffman et al. reported a 2-fold increase in the aortic root lesion size [25]. These mice also had significantly elevated levels of vascular cell adhesion molecule-1 (VCAM-1) and tumor necrosis factor-α (TNF-α). An impaired endothelium-dependent vasodilator function, likely due to diminished nitric oxide bioactivity was observed in the CBS-deficient mice (which had impaired homocysteine metabolism) [18]. These studies indicate that homocysteine may enhance vascular inflammation and endothelial dysfunction in animals that are prone to the development of atherosclerosis.

EFFECT OF HOMOCYSTEINE ON CHEMOKINE EXPRESSION

MCP-1 expression

One of the earliest detectable cellular responses in the formation of atherosclerotic lesions is the local recruitment of monocytes by the endothelium [26,27]. Such localized accumulation of monocytes is mediated by endothelial expression of specific adhesion/chemoattractant molecules [28]. MCP-1 is a potent chemokine that stimulates the migration of monocytes into the intima of arterial walls [29–32]. The amount of this chemokine appears to be increased in atherosclerotic lesions in both human and experimental animals [29,33,34]. Several in vitro studies have demonstrated that the expression of MCP-1 mRNA was upregulated in macrophages treated with oxidized LDL and oxidized VLDL [35], in human vascular endothelial cells and in smooth muscle cells treated with modified lipoproteins [36,37]. During the development of atherosclerosis, the origin of inflammatory signals including MCP-1 is thought to be the vessel wall itself [38]. Our laboratory demonstrated that the secretion of MCP-1 protein was significantly increased (195% as compared to the control) in human umbilical cord vein endothelial cells (HUVEC) treated with homocysteine (0.02–0.1 mM) [21]. Further analysis revealed that such effect was accompanied by an increased expression of MCP-1 mRNA (176% as compared to the control) in endothelial cells which resulted in enhanced monocyte chemotaxis. Homocysteine-induced MCP-1 expression and subsequent monocyte chemotaxis were blocked by a p38 MAP kinase inhibitor (SB203580) suggesting that the p38 MAP kinase pathway might be involved in homocysteine-induced MCP-1 expression in endothelial cells [21]. Indeed, p38 MAP kinase as well as other members of the p38 MAP kinase pathway, including MKK3, MKK6, ATF-2 and Elk-1, were activated in homocysteine-treated cells [21]. In contrast, staurosporine, a protein kinase C (PKC) inhibitor, had no effect on homocysteine-induced MCP-1 expression. However, an increase in MCP-1 expression in human aortic vascular smooth muscle cells (VSMCs) was associated with the activation of PKC [22]. Homocysteine treatment (0.05–0.2 mM) significantly increased the expression of MCP-1 mRNA (up to 2.7 fold) and protein (up to 3.3 fold) in VSMCs [22]. Similar effect was observed in human monocyte-derived macrophage [23]. Homocysteine (0.05–0.2 mM) was shown to significantly enhance the expression of MCP-1 mRNA (up to 2.6 fold) and protein (up to 4.8 fold) in human peripheral blood monocyte-derived macrophage or THP-1-derived macrophage. Homocysteine-induced MCP-1 expression resulted in an increased monocyte chemotaxis and adhesion to endothelial cells. It is well known that upon infiltration into the arterial wall, monocytes differentiate into macrophages that are able to take up large amount of lipids to become foam cells [26,27]. We observed that homocysteine-treated monocytes/macrophages as well as endothelial cells were able to take up oxidized LDL (Fig. 1). Following 6-h incubation with 0.1 mM homocysteine, endothelial cells were treated with THP-1 monocytes (0.1×10^5) for an additional hour. At the end of the incubation period, non-adhered THP-1 cells were washed off. The attached THP-1 cells and endothelial cells were incubated for 24 h in the absence or presence of oxidized LDL (ox-LDL). Cells were then stained with Oil Red O and counter-stained with Harris Hematoxylin to identify cellular lipid droplets. Figure 1 showed that monocytes/macrophages and endothelial cells accumulated large amount of lipid droplets to form foam cell-like cells in the presence of ox-LDL. Addition of anti-MCP-1 antibodies to the culture medium abolished monocyte adhesion to endothelial cells. These results suggest that homocysteine-induced MCP-1 production may play an important role in mediating monocyte adhesion to endothelial cells. In the presence of oxidized lipoproteins, attached monocytes as well as endothelial cells are capable of taking up large amount of lipids to form foam cells.

Other investigators also reported that homocysteine stimulated the interaction between leukocytes (predominantly neutrophils) and endothelial cells in vitro causing endothelial cell damage [39]. Such increased adhesion of leukocytes to the mesenteric wall in rats was not due to an increase in the expression of endothelial surface adhesion molecules (ICAM-1, E-selectin, VACAM-1 and P-selectin) but involved surface changes in neutrophils [39]. A transendothelial leukocyte migration into the perivascular tissues was also reported [39].

It is generally believed that endothelial expression of MCP-1 initiates the migration of monocytes into the arterial wall. Based on results obtained from our laboratory (21–23) as well as others, we speculate that homocysteine-induced endothelial MCP-1 expression may be associated with early stages of atherosclerosis by stimulating monocyte transmigration to the subendothelial space and differentiation into macrophages. On the other hand, MCP-1 produced in smooth muscle cells as well as in macrophages may facilitate the recruitment of additional monocytes into the lesion at later stages of atherosclerosis in patients with hyperhomocysteinemia.

Oxidative stress and nuclear factor kappa B activation

Nuclear factor kappa B (NF-κB), a transcription factor, plays an important role in up-regulating the expression of MCP-1 and other inflammatory factors in atherosclerotic lesions [40–42]. The promoter region of the MCP-1 gene consists of several putative binding sites for transcription factors including two binding sites for NF-κB [43]. NF-κB is normally present in the cytoplasm in an inactive form that is associated with an inhibitory protein, named IκB [44–46]. Upon dissociation from IκB, the active NF-κB is translocated into the nucleus where it binds to the κB binding motifs in the promoters or enhancers of the genes encoding cytokines. The active dimeric forms of NF-κB are frequently composed of several DNA binding subunit such as p50, p65 and/or c-rel. Activated NF-κB (found in the nucleus) has

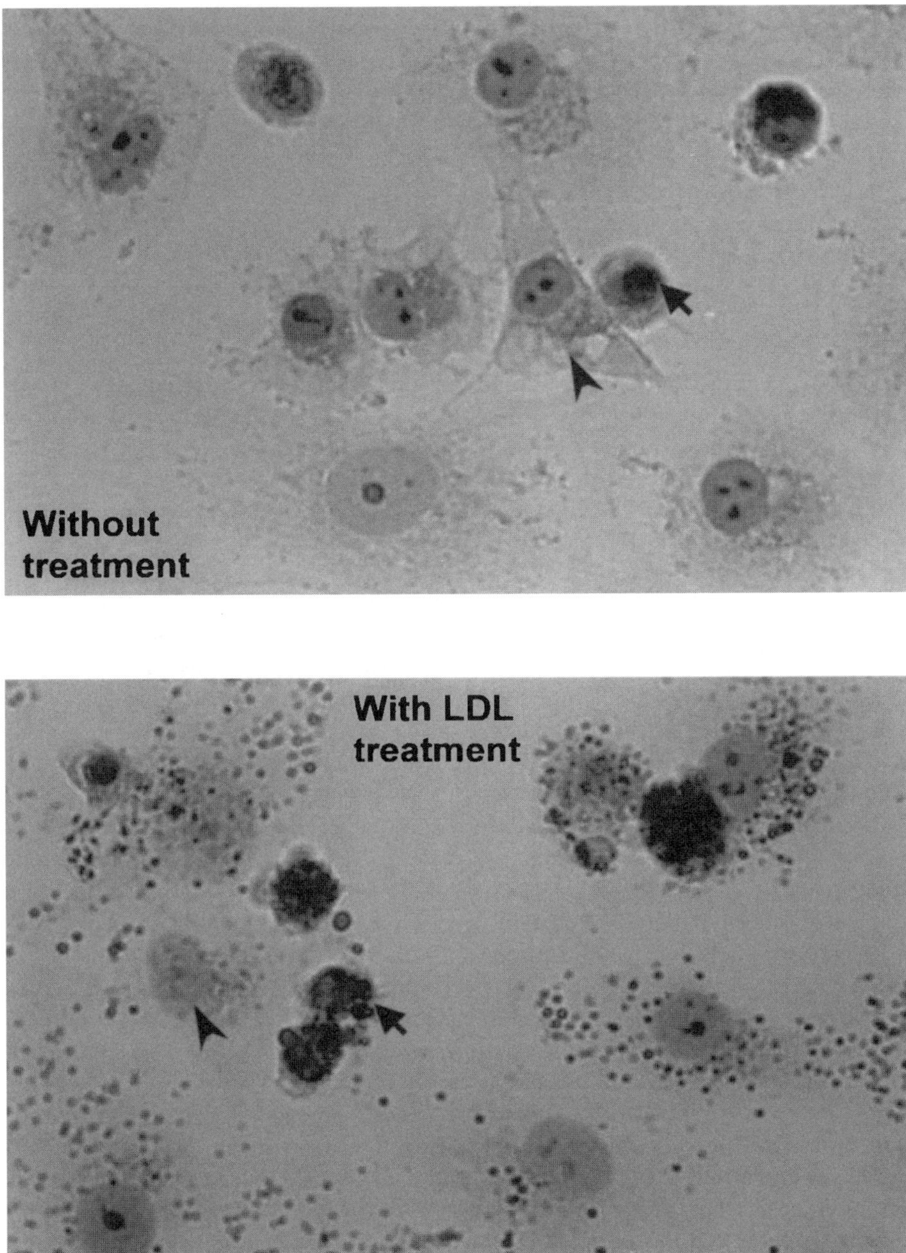

Figure 1. Uptake of lipoproteins by monocytes and endothelial cells. Endothelial cells (HUVEC purchased from ATCC) were incubated with homocysteine (0.1 mM) in F-12K nutrient medium containing endothelial cell growth supplement for 6 h. THP-1 monocytes (0.5×10^5) were then added to the culture dish containing endothelial cells and the incubation was continued for another 24 h in the absence or presence of oxidized LDL (50 µg/mL). At the end of the incubation, cells were washed with PBS and stained with Oil Red O (ORO) and counter-stained with Harris Hematoxylin. Arrows indicate foam cells from THP1- derived macrophages and arrowheads point to endothelial cells.

been detected in macrophages, endothelial cells and vascular smooth muscle cells in human atherosclerotic lesions [40,41]. In contrast, little or no activation of NF-κB is found in normal aorta or arteries. Results from our in vitro studies suggest that NF-κB activation may play an important role in homocysteine-induced MCP-1 expression [22,23]. In VSMCs and in macrophages, the increase in MCP-1 expression was associated with activation of NF-κB due to increased phosphorylation of IκB-α as well as reduced expression of IκB-α mRNA in homocysteine-treated cells. Our results also suggest that oxidative stress is involved in homocysteine-induced NF-κB activation and subsequent MCP-1 expression [22,23].

CCR2 expression

MCP-1 exerts its action mainly through the interaction with the chemokine receptor (CCR2) on the surface of monocytes [38,47,48]. An increased expression of CCR2 gene was reported in patients with hypercholesterolemia [49]. The importance of MCP-1 and its receptor CCR2 in the development of atherosclerosis was further revealed in CCR2 deficient mice [50]. Boring et al. reported a dramatic reduction in atherosclerotic lesion formation in apo E null mice (genetically modified to develop atherosclerosis) that also lacked CCR2 [50]. We investigated the effect of homocysteine on CCR2 expression in human THP-1 monocytic cells as well as in human peripheral blood monocytes [51]. Homocysteine treatment (0.05–0.2 mM) significantly enhanced the expression of CCR2 mRNA (129–209% of the control) and CCR2 protein (up to 183% of control) in monocytes after 24 h of incubation [51]. Such stimulation on CCR2 expression was associated with a parallel increase in the binding activity of CCR2 (129–191% of control) to MCP-1 as well as enhanced chemotactic response of homocysteine-treated monocytes. Further investigation revealed that the levels of superoxide were significantly elevated in cells incubated with homocysteine for 12–48 h. Addition of superoxide dismutase, a superoxide scavenger, to the culture medium completely abolished the stimulatory effect of homocysteine on CCR2 expression as well as on the binding activity of CCR2 to MCP-1. A recent study revealed that H_2O_2 and the GSH-depleting drug buthionine sulphoximine stimulated CCR2 expression in human monocytes [52]. Furthermore, treatment with antioxidants such as pyrrolidine dithiocarbamate could decrease the expression of CCR2 and other chemokine receptors in monocytes, indicating a positive effect of oxidative stress on CCR2 expression [52]. Results obtained from the in vitro study [51] suggest that homocysteine-induced superoxide formation may serve as one of the underlying mechanisms for enhanced CCR2 expression in monocytes. Although results from several studies indicate that superoxide dismutase might have a role in homocysteine-induced vascular cell dysfunction [53,54], the causative effect of homocysteine on the activity of this enzyme remains to be further verified experimentally.

On the basis of the results obtained from our studies [21–23,51], we propose the following mechanisms by which homocysteine stimulates the expression of MCP-1 in endothelial cells, vascular smooth muscle cells and macrophages as well

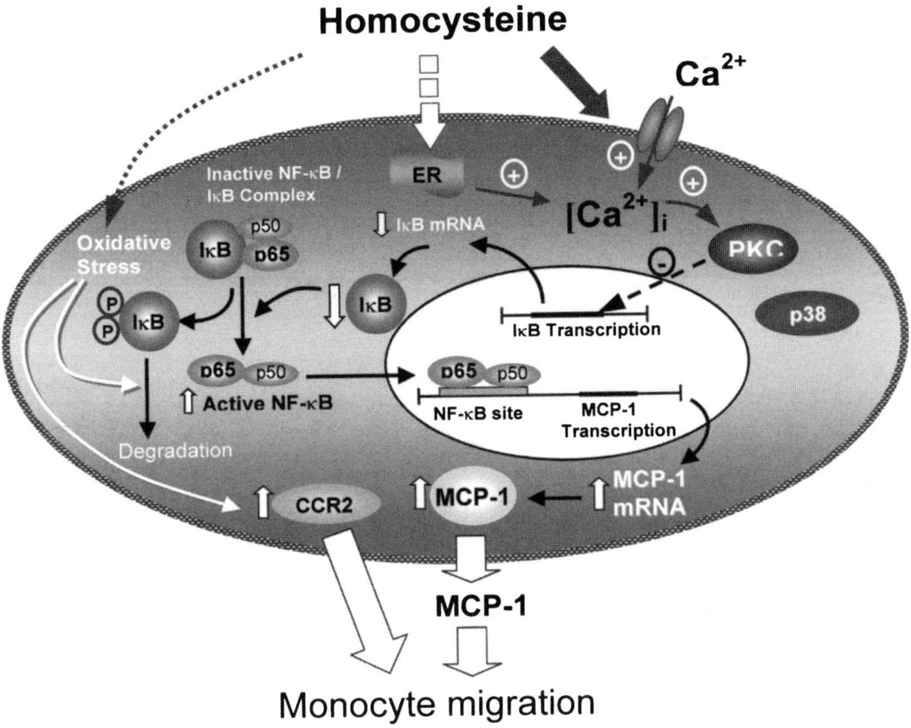

Figure 2. Proposed mechanisms of homocysteine-induced expression of MCP-1 and CCR2 leading to atherosclerosis.

as induces the expression CCR2 in monocytes leading to enhanced monocyte binding to endothelial cells (Fig. 2). In an early event following homocysteine treatment, the phosphorylation and subsequent degradation of IκBα protein might be responsible for the activation of NF-κB. At a later stage, the reduced IκBα mRNA expression due to increased oxidative stress and changes in activities of protein kinases might contribute to NF-κB activation. Independently, homocysteine-induced oxidative stress may also lead to increased expression of CCR2 in monocytes. Together, homocysteine-stimulated CCR2 expression in monocytes and increased MCP-1 expression in vascular cells may represent the underlying mechanism of homocysteine-enhanced monocyte infiltration into the arterial wall during atherogenesis.

CONCLUDING REMARKS

Our results have clearly demonstrated that homocysteine stimulates MCP-1 mRNA expression in endothelial cells, vascular smooth muscle cells and macrophages as well as CCR2 expression in monocytes. We are currently exploring the underlying mechanisms of enhanced monocyte binding to the vascular endothelial in an animal model with hyperhomocysteinemia. It remains to be investigated whether homocysteine displays similar effect on the expression of chemokines and/chemokine receptors in patients with hyperhomocysteinemia.

ACKNOWLEDGEMENT

The work presented in this article was supported, in part, by a grant from the Research Grant Council of Hong Kong SAR.

REFERENCES

1. Clarke R, Daly L, Robinson K, Naughten E, Cahalane S, Fowler B, Graham I. 1991. Hyperhomocysteinemia: an independent risk factor for vascular disease. N Engl J Med 324:1149–1155.
2. McCully KS. 1996. Homocysteine and vascular disease. Nat Med (NY) 2:386–389.
3. Duell PB, Malinow MR. 1997. Homocyst(e)ine: an important risk factor for atherosclerotic vascular disease. Curr Opin Lipidol 8:28–34.
4. Refsum H, Ueland PM, Nygard O, Vollset SE. 1998. Homocysteine and Cardiovascular Disease. Annu Rev Medicine 49:31–62.
5. Mudd SH, Levy HL, Skovby F. 1995. Disorders of transsulfuration. In: The Metabolic Basis of Inherited Disease. Ed. CR Scriver, AL Beaudet, WS Sly, D Valle, 1279–1327. New York: McGraw-Hill.
6. Nygard O, Nordrehaug JE, Refsum H, Ueland PM, Farstad M, Vollset SE. 1997. Plasma homocysteine levels and mortality in patients with coronary artery disease. N Engl J Med 337:230–236.
7. Genest JJ Jr, McNamara JR, Upson B, Salem DN, Ordovas JM, Schaefer EJ, Malinow MR. 1991. Prevalence of familial hyperhomocyst(e)inemia in men with premature coronary artery disease. Arterioscler Thromb 11:1129–1136.
8. Gallagher PM, Meleady R, Shields DC, Tan KS, McMaster D, Rozen R, Evans A, Graham IM, Whitehead AS. 1996. Homocysteine and risk of premature coronary heart disease. Evidence for a common gene mutation. Circulation 94:2154–2158.
9. Boushey CJ, Beresford SA, Omenn GS, Motulsky AG. 1995. A quantitative assessment of plasma homocysteine as a risk factor for vascular disease. Probable benefits of increasing folic acid intakes. JAMA 274:1049–1057.
10. Harker LA, Ross R, Slichter SJ, Scott CR. 1976. Homocysteine-induced arteriosclerosis. The role of endothelial cell injury and platelet response in its genesis. J Clin Invest 58:731–741.
11. Weiss N, Heydrick S, Zhang YY, Bierl C, Cap A, Loscalzo J. 2002. Cellular redox state and endothelial dysfunction in mildly hyperhomocysteinemic cystathionine beta-synthase-deficient mice. Arterioscler Thromb Vasc Biol 22:34–41.
12. Tsai JC, Perrella MA, Yoshizumi M, Hsieh CM, Haber E, Schlegel R, Lee ME. 1994. Promotion of vascular smooth muscle cell growth by homocysteine: a link to atherosclerosis. Proc Natl Acad Sci USA 91:6369–6373.
13. Chen C, Halkos ME, Surowiec SM, Conklin BS, Lin PH, Lumsden AB. 2000. Effects of homocysteine on smooth muscle cell proliferation in both cell culture and artery perfusion culture models. J Surg Res 88:26–33.
14. Durand P, Lussier-Cacan S, Blache D. 1997. Acute methionine load-induced hyperhomocysteinemia enhances platelet aggregation, thromboxane biosynthesis, and macrophage-derived tissue factor activity in rats. FASEB J 11:1157–1168.
15. O K, Lynn EG, Chung YH, Siow YL, Man RYK, Choy PC. 1998. Homocysteine stimulates the production and secretion of cholesterol in hepatic cells. Biochim Biophys Acta 1393:317–324.
16. Werstuck GH, Lentz SR, Dayal S, Hossain GS, Sood SK, Shi YY, Zhou J, Maeda N, Krisans SK, Malinow MR, Austin RC. 2001. Homocysteine-induced endoplasmic reticulum stress causes dysregulation of the cholesterol and triglyceride biosynthetic pathways. J Clin Invest 107:1263–1273.
17. Schlaich MP, John S, Jacobi J, Lackner KJ, Schmieder RE. 2000. Mildly elevated homocysteine concentrations impair endothelium dependent vasodilation in hypercholesterolemic patients. Atherosclerosis 153:383–389.

18. Eberhardt RT, Forgione MA, Cap A, Leopold JA, Rudd MA, Trolliet M, Heydrick S, Stark R, Klings ES, Moldovan NI, Yaghoubi M, Goldschmidt-Clermont PJ, Farber HW, Cohen R, Loscalzo J. 2000. Endothelial dysfunction in a murine model of mild hyperhomocyst(e)inemia. J Clin Invest 106:483–491.
19. Morita H, Kurihara H, Yoshida S, Saito Y, Shindo T, Oh-Hashi Y, Kurihara Y, Yazaki Y, Nagai R. 2001. Diet-induced hyperhomocysteinemia exacerbates neointima formation in rat carotid arteries after balloon injury. Circulation 103:133–139.
20. Mujumdar VS, Aru GM, Tyagi SC. 2001. Induction of oxidative stress by homocyst(e)ine impairs endothelial function. J Cell Biochem 82:491–500.
21. Sung FL, Siow YL, Wang G, Lynn EG, O K. 2001. Homocysteine stimulates the expression of monocyte chemoattractant protein-1 in endothelial cells leading to enhanced monocyte chemotaxis. Mol Cell Biochem 216:121–128.
22. Wang G, Siow YL, O K. 2000. Homocysteine stimulates nuclear factor kappa B activity and monocyte chemoattractant protein-1 expression in vascular smooth muscle cells: a possible role for protein kinase C. Biochem J 352:817–826.
23. Wang G, Siow YL, O K. 2001 Homocysteine induces monocyte chemoattractant protein-1 expression by activating NF-kappa B in THP-1 macrophage. Am J Physiol Heart Cir Physiol 280: H2840–2847.
24. Lentz SR, Sobey CG, Piegors DJ, Bhopatkar MY, Faraci FM, Malinow MR, Heistad DD. 1996. Vascular dysfunction in monkeys with diet-induced hyperhomocyst(e)inemia. J Clin Invest 98:24–29.
25. Hofmann MA, Lalla E, Lu Y, Gleason MR, Wolf BM, Tanji N, Ferran LJ Jr, Kohl B, Rao V, Kisiel W, Stern DM, Schmidt AM. 2001. Hyperhomocysteinemia enhances vascular inflammation and accelerates atherosclerosis in a murine model. J Clin Invest 107:675–683.
26. Gerrity RG. 1981. The role of the monocyte in atherogenesis: I. Transition of blood-borne monocytes into foam cells in fatty lesions. Am J Pathol 103:181–190.
27. Ross R. 1993. The pathogenesis of atherosclerosis: a perspective for the 1990s. Nature 362:801–809.
28. Rollins BJ, Yoshimura T, Leonard EJ, Pober JS. 1990. Cytokine-activated human endothelial cells synthesize and secrete a monocyte chemoattractant, MCP-1/JE. Am J Pathol 136:1229–1233.
29. Nelken NA, Coughlin SR, Gordon D, Wilcox JN. 1991. Monocyte chemoattractant protein-1 in human atheromatous plaques. J Clin Invest 88:1121–1127.
30. Valente AJ, Rozek MM, Sprague EA, Schwartz CJ. 1992. Mechanisms in intimal monocyte-macrophage recruitment. A special role for monocyte chemotactic protein-1. Circulation 86: III20–III25.
31. Li YS, Shyy YJ, Wright JG, Valente AJ, Cornhill JF, Kolattukudy PE. 1993. The expression of monocyte chemotactic protein (MCP-1) in human vascular endothelium in vitro and in vivo. Mol Cell Biochem 126:61–68.
32. Brown Z, Gerritsen ME, Carley WW, Strieter RM, Kunkel SL, Westwick J. 1994. Chemokine gene expression and secretion by cytokine-activated human microvascular endothelial cells. Differential regulation of monocyte chemoattractant protein-1 and interleukin-8 in response to interferon-gamma. Am J Pathol 145:913–921.
33. Takeya M, Yoshimura T, Leonard EJ, Takahashi K. 1993. Detection of monocyte chemoattractant protein-1 in human atherosclerotic lesions by an anti-monocyte chemoattractant protein-1 monoclonal antibody. Hum Pathol 24:534–539.
34. Ylä-Herttuala S, Lipton BA, Rosenfeld ME, Särkioja T, Yoshimura T, Leonard EJ, Witztum JL, Steinberg D. 1991. Expression of monocyte chemoattractant protein 1 in macrophage-rich areas of human and rabbit atherosclerotic lesions. Proc Natl Acad Sci USA 88:5252–5256.
35. Wang GP, Deng ZD, Ni J, Qu ZL. 1997. Oxidized low density lipoprotein and very low density lipoprotein enhance expression of monocyte chemoattractant protein-1 in rabbit peritoneal exudate macrophages. Atherosclerosis 133:31–36.
36. Shi W, Haberland ME, Jien ML, Shih DM, Lusis AJ. 2000. Endothelial responses to oxidized lipoproteins determine genetic susceptibility to atherosclerosis in mice. Circulation 102:75–81.
37. Cushing SD, Berliner JA, Valente AJ, Territo MC, Navab M, Parhami F, Gerrity R, Schwartz CJ, Fogelman AM. 1990. Minimally modified low density lipoprotein induces monocyte chemotactic protein 1 in human endothelial cells and smooth muscle cells. Proc Natl Acad Sci USA 87:5134–5138.
38. Reape TJ, Groot PH. 1999. Chemokines and atherosclerosis. Atherosclerosis 147:213–225.
39. Dudman NP, Temple SE, Guo XW, Fu W, Perry MA. 1999. Homocysteine enhances neutrophil-endothelial interactions in both cultured human cells and rats in vivo. Circ Res 84:409–416.

40. Brand K, Page S, Rogler G, Bartsch A, Brandl R, Knuechel R, Page M, Kaltschmidt C, Baeuerle PA, Neumeier D. 1996. Activated transcription factor nuclear factor-kappa B is present in the atherosclerotic lesion. J Clin Invest 97:1715–1722.
41. Brand K, Page S, Walli AK, Neumeier D, Baeuerle PA. 1997. Role of nuclear factor-kappa B in atherogenesis. Exp Physiol 82:297–304.
42. Marumo T, Schini-Kerth VB, Fisslthaler B, Busse R. 1997. Platelet-derived growth factor-stimulated superoxide anion production modulates activation of transcription factor NF-kappaB and expression of monocyte chemoattractant protein 1 in human aortic smooth muscle cells. Circulation 96:2361–2367.
43. Ueda A, Ishigatsubos Y, Okubo T, Yoshimura T. 1997. Transcriptional regulation of the human monocyte chemoattractant protein-1 gene. Cooperation of two NF-kappaB sites and NF-kappaB/Rel subunit specificity. J Biol Chem 272:31092–31099.
44. Baldwin AS Jr. 1996. The NF-kappa B and I kappa B proteins: new discoveries and insights. Annu Rev Immunol 14:649–683.
45. Thurberg BL, Collins T. 1998. The nuclear factor-kappa B/inhibitor of kappa B autoregulatory system and atherosclerosis. Curr Opin Lipidol 9:387–396.
46. Simeonidis S, Stauber D, Chen G, Hendrickson WA, Thanos D. 1999. Mechanisms by which IkappaB proteins control NF-kappaB activity. Proc Natl Acad Sci USA 96:49–54.
47. Charo IF. 1999. CCR2: from cloning to the creation of knockout mice. Chem Immunol 72:20–41.
48. Charo IF, Myers SJ, Herman A, Franci C, Connolly AJ, Coughlin SR. 1994. Molecular cloning and functional expression of two monocyte chemoattractant protein 1 receptors reveals alternative splicing of the carboxyl-terminal tails. Proc Natl Acad Sci USA 91:2752–2756.
49. Han KH, Tangirala RK, Green SR, Quehenberger O. 1998. Chemokine receptor CCR2 expression and monocyte chemoattractant protein-1-mediated chemotaxis in human monocytes A regulatory role for plasma LDL. Arterioscler Thromb Vasc Biol 18:1983–1991.
50. Boring L, Gosling J, Cleary M, Charo IF. 1998. Decreased lesion formation in $CCR2^{-/-}$ mice reveals a role for chemokines in initiation of atherosclerosis. Nature 394:894–897.
51. Wang G, O K. 2001. Homocysteine stimulates monocyte chemoattractant protein-1 receptor CCR2 expression in human monocytes: involvement of oxygen free radicals. Biochem J 357:233–240.
52. Saccani A, Saccani S, Orlando S, Siron M, Bernasconi, S, Ghezz P, Mantovan A, Sica A. 2000. Redox regulation of chemokine receptor expression. Proc Natl Acad Sci USA 97:2761–2766.
53. Wilcken DEL, Wang XL, Adachi T, Hara H, Duarte N, Green K, Wilcken B. 2000. Relationship between homocysteine and superoxide dismutase in homocystinuria Possible relevance to cardiovascular risk. Arterioscler Thromb Vasc Biol 20:1199–1202.
54. Upchurch GR Jr, Welch GN, Fabian AJ, Freedman JE, Johnson JL, Keaney JF Jr, Loscalzo J. 1997. Homocyst(e)ine decreases bioavailable nitric oxide by a mechanism involving glutathione peroxidase. J Biol Chem 272:17012–17017.

G.N. Pierce, M. Nagano, P. Zahradka, and N.S. Dhalla (eds.).
ATHEROSCLEROSIS, HYPERTENSION AND DIABETES. Copyright © 2003.
Kluwer Academic Publishers. Boston.

OXYRADICALS AND HYPERCHOLESTEROLEMIC ATHEROSCLEROSIS

PAUL LEE and KAILASH PRASAD

Department of Physiology, College of Medicine, University of Saskatchewan, Saskatoon, Saskatchewan, Canada

Summary. The data presented in this short review suggest that the oxidative stress is elevated in hypercholesterolemia and that the oxidative stress induces the development of atherosclerosis. The data also suggest that protective effect of various antioxidants is due to a decrease in the oxidative stress. The review supports the hypothesis that hypercholesterolemic atherosclerosis is mediated through oxidative stress.

***Key words*:** Oxidative stress, Antioxidants, Free radicals

INTRODUCTION

Hypercholesterolemia is a major risk factor for coronary artery disease and stroke [1–5]. Atherosclerosis is a disease resulting from cascades of complex interaction among the endogenous cellular and non-cellular elements of the arterial wall; blood components including plasma lipoproteins, mononuclear leukocytes and platelets; environmental factors; hemodynamic factors; and genetic factors. Endothelial cell injury is the basic mechanism for initiation and maintenance of atherosclerosis [6–8]. Hypercholesterolemia is known to produce endothelial cell injury [6,9,10]. Oxygen radicals produce endothelial cell injury [11–13]. It is possible that hypercholesterolemia-induced atherosclerosis is mediated through elevated levels of

Address for Correspondence: K. Prasad, MD, PhD, Department of Physiology, College of Medicine, University of Saskatchewan, 107 Wiggins Road, Saskatoon, Saskatchewan, S7N 5E5 Canada. Phone: (306) 966-6539; Fax No: (306) 966-6532; e-mail: prasadk@sask.usask.ca

oxyradicals. This review provides evidence that hypercholesterolemic atherosclerosis is due to increased levels of oxyradicals.

Hypercholesterolemia and oxyradicals

Hypercholesterolemia increases the cholesterol content of various cells in the body [14–16]. Cholesterol-rich platelets release substances such as thrombin, histamine, and adenosine diphosphate (ADP) [17]. Histamine and ADP activate phospholipase A_2 (PLA_2) activity [18]. Increase in PLA_2 activity may also arise from increases in intracellular Ca^{++} [19] which accompany hypercholesterolemia [20]. Synthesis and release of platelet-activating factor (PAF) are dependent upon thrombin and intracellular Ca^{++} [21–23]. Activation of PLA_2 would ultimately lead to increased synthesis and release of prostaglandins and leukotrienes. Increased production of thromboxane A_2 and prostacyclin in aorta of experimental atherosclerosis has been reported [24]. Oxygen radicals are generated during synthesis of prostaglandins [25] and leukotrienes [26]. Hypercholesterolemia activates complements C_3 and C_5 [27,28]. Hypercholesterolemia through PAF would increase the synthesis and release of interleukin-1 (IL-1) [29] and tumor necrosis factor (TNF) [30]. PAF [31], IL-1 [32] and TNF [33] are known to stimulate polymorphonuclear leukocytes (PMNLs) and monocytes to produce oxyradicals. These data suggest that oxyradicals could be elevated in hypercholesterolemia.

Hypercholesterolemic atherosclerosis and oxyradicals

The studies in rabbits show that high cholesterol diet produces increases in the serum levels of total cholesterol (TC), and low-density lipoprotein-cholesterol (LDL-C) [33–40]. Hypercholesterolemia was associated with development of atherosclerosis in aorta [34–41] and in coronary artery [35,36]. Atherosclerotic plaques were assessed by staining the aorta with Herxheimer's solution containing Sudan IV that stains lipids [42]. The surface area of the atheromatous plaques was measured from a photograph of the aorta and expressed as a percentage of total aortic intimal surface area. Extent of atherosclerosis was related to the dose and duration of cholesterol consumption [34–37,39].

The parameters of oxidative stress measured in these studies were a) malondialdehyde (MDA), lipid peroxidation production, a measure of levels of oxyradicals; b) oxygen free radical producing activity of PMNLs (PMNL-CL) using luminometer; c) antioxidant reserve of aortae [Aortic-chemiluminescence (Aortic-CL)] using luminometer. An increase in aortic-CL indicates a decrease in the antioxidant reserve and vice-versa; and d) antioxidant enzymes [superoxide dismutase (SOD), catalase and glutathione peroxidase (GSH-Px)] in the blood and aorta. The methods of measurement of MDA in aorta and blood [34], PMNL-CL [34,39], antioxidant reserve [35,43], and antioxidant enzymes [44] are detailed elsewhere.

Hypercholesterolemic atherosclerosis is associated with increases in the serum [34] and aortic MDA [34–37,41], PMNL-CL [34,39] and decreases in the antioxidant reserve in the aortae [35–37,41]. There is a decrease in the activity of SOD and

GSH-Px and an increase in the activity of catalase in hypercholesterolemia [44]. There is a consistent increase in activities of catalase and GSH-Px in atherosclerotic aortae [36,37,44,45]. The activity of SOD in aorta is reported to increase [44,45] and to remain unchanged [36,37]. An increase in the SOD and GSH-Px and a decrease in catalase activity in aortic tissue of cholesterol-fed rabbits have also been reported [46]. The increase in the activities of antioxidant enzymes could be due to oxidative stress. Elevation of GSH-Px activity is commonly associated with a small increase in oxidative stress [47,48]. Induction of SOD, catalase and GSH-Px activity with different forms of oxidative stress has been shown [49]. Differential effect of hypercholesterolemia on SOD activity in aorta is not clearly understood. It could be due to the extent and duration of atherosclerotic lesions.

Hypercholesterolemic atherosclerosis is asso ciated with an increase in the presence of oxidized-LDL in the plasma of both patients and New Zealand white rabbits [50]. Oxidized-LDL is present in the blood and atherosclerotic plaques [51–55]. Not only LDL but also very low-density lipoprotein (VLDL) and high-density lipoprotein (HDL) are oxidatively modified in vivo in rabbits fed on high cholesterol diet [56].

Hypercholesterolemic atherosclerosis and antioxidants

Several studies have investigated the ability of various antioxidants in the prevention of atherosclerosis in animals. Vitamin E treatment did not affect the serum TC, LDL-C, HDL-C and VLDL-C in high cholesterol-fed rabbits [34]. It, however, prevented the development of atherosclerosis by approximately 75%. Protective effect of vitamin E against hypercholesterolemic atherosclerosis is associated with a decrease in the blood and aortic tissue MDA. It, however, did not reduce the PMNL-CL. Hypercholesterolemia in rabbits decreases the activity of both SOD and GSH-Px and increases the activity of catalase [44]. Vitamin E treatment in hypercholesterolemic rabbit prevents the decrease in SOD and GSH-Px activity of blood but did not affect the changes in the catalase activity. Vitamin E prevents the cholesterol-induced rise in the catalase and GSH-Px activity in aorta but does not prevent the rise in SOD activity [44]. Probucol, a lipid soluble cholesterol-lowering drug with potent antioxidant properties [57] inhibited the formation of atherosclerotic lesions independent of its cholesterol lowering properties [58]. Probucol reduces the formation of atherosclerotic lesions in cholesterol fed monkeys [59]. Probucol in 0.5% cholesterol fed rabbits did not affect serum TC and LDL-C but decreased HDL-C [35]. It reduced the development of atherosclerosis which was associated with a decrease in the aortic MDA. Probucol was ineffective in lowering TC, LDL-C, and reducing atherosclerosis in aorta and coronary arteries in 1% cholesterol-fed rabbits [35]. This ineffectiveness was associated with its inability to reduce aortic tissue MDA and to increase the antioxidant reserve. Probucol in general was ineffective in hypercholesterolemia-induced changes in SOD, and catalase activity except GSH-Px activity of aorta which increased in 0.5% cholesterol-fed rabbits [45].

Purpurogallin, an antioxidant [60], reduced the development of atherosclerosis in aorta and coronary arteries without lowering the serum TC and LDL-C in high cholesterol-fed rabbits [36]. The protective effect of purpurogallin was associated with an increase in the antioxidant reserve and reversal of the increase in the hypercholesterolemia-induced rise in activity of SOD, catalase and GSH-Px in aorta [36].

Garlic which has antioxidant activity [61], prevented the development of atherosclerosis in high cholesterol-fed rabbits without significantly affecting serum TC, LDL-C, and HDL-C [37]. The protective effect of garlic was associated with a decrease in MDA, and an increase in the antioxidant reserve of aorta [37]. Garlic produced a decrease in the activity of catalase in aortae of hypercholesterolemic rabbits but did not affect the activity of SOD and GSH-Px.

In a recent study with secoisolariciresinol diglucoside (SDG) an antioxidant [62] in high cholesterol-fed rabbits it has been shown that it reduces the development of atherosclerosis [41]. The protective effect of SDG was associated with a decrease in the serum lipids (TC and LDL-C), and aortic MDA; and an increase in the antioxidant reserve of the aortae [40].

Comments

The studies to-date suggest that hypercholesterolemic atherosclerosis is associated with an increase in a) the production of oxyradicals by PMNLs, b) serum lipid peroxidation product malondialdehyde; c) aortic tissue malondialdehyde, and d) the presence of oxidized LDL in the plasma. It is also associated with a decrease in the antioxidant reserve of aorta. SOD and GSH-Px activity of blood is depressed while activity of catalase is elevated. However, the activity of antioxidant enzymes are elevated in the aortic tissue of hypercholesterolemic rabbit.

Endothelial cell damage is prerequisite for development of atherosclerosis according to response to injury hypothesis [63]. Oxidative stress produced by hypercholesterolemia could damage the endothelial cell and hence initiate the development of atherosclerosis. Oxyradicals are known to produce damage of endothelial cells [11–13]. Oxidized-LDL (OX-LDL) has also been implicated in the development of atherosclerosis [64–66]. Oxidized-LDL can also produce endothelial cell damage [67]. Besides endothelial cell damage, OX-LDL induces local vascular cells to produce monocyte chemotactic protein 1 (MCP-1) and granulocyte and macrophage colony stimulating factor which stimulate monocyte recruitment and differentiation to macrophages in the arterial wall [68]. Oxidized LDL is recognized by scavenger receptors on macrophages and is interlized to form foam cells. In addition, OX-LDL has direct chemotactic effect on monocyte migration [69].

Antioxidants prevented the development of atherosclerosis without lowering serum cholesterol. The protection was associated with decrease in the oxidative stress.

These results suggest the role of oxygen radicals in the pathogenesis of hypercholesterolemic atherosclerosis.

ACKNOWLEDGMENT

This work was supported by the Heart and Stroke Foundation of Saskatchewan and the CIHR—Regional Partnership of Saskatchewan.

REFERENCES

1. Kannel WB, Castelli WP, Gordon T, McNamara PM. 1971. Serum cholesterol, lipoproteins, and the risk of coronary heart disease. The Framingham Study. Ann Intern Med 74:1–12.
2. Castelli WP. 1988. Cholesterol and lipids in the risk of coronary artery disease. The Framingham Heart Study. Can J Cardiol 4:5A–10A.
3. Castelli WP, Garrison RJ, Wilson PWF, Abbot RD, Kalousdian S, Kannel WB. 1986. Incidence of coronary artery disease and lipoprotein cholesterol levels. JAMA 256:2835–2838.
4. Gotto AM, Gorry GA, Thompson JR, Cole JS, Trost R, Yeshurn D, DeBakry MR. 1977. Relationship between plasma lipid concentration and coronary artery disease in 496 patients. Circulation 56:875–883.
5. Goldstein JL, Schrott HG, Hazzard WR, Bierman EL, Motulsky AG. 1973. Hyperlipidemia in coronary artery disease II. Genetic analysis of lipid levels in 176 families and delineation of a new inherited disorder, combined hyperlipidemia. J Clin Invest 52:1544–1568.
6. Ross R, Harker L. 1976. Hyperlipidemia and atherosclerosis: chronic hyperlipidemia initiates and maintains lesions by endothelial cell desquamation and lipid accumulation. Science 193:1094–1100.
7. Ross R. 1986. The pathogenesis of atherosclerosis—an update. N Engl J Med 314:488–500.
8. French JE. 1966. Atherosclerosis in relation to the structure and function of the arterial intima, with special reference to the endothelium. Int Rev Exp Pathol 5:253–353.
9. Nelson E, Gertz SD, Forbes MS, Rennels MI, Heald FP, Kahn MA, Farber TM, Miller E, Husain MM, Earl FL. 1976. Endothelial lesions in the aorta of egg yolk-fed miniature swine: a study by scanning and transmission electron microscopy. Exp Mol Pathol 25:208–220.
10. Thomas WA, Florentin R, Nam SC, Kim DN, Jones RM, Lee KT. 1968. Preproliferative phase of atherosclerosis in swine fed cholesterol. Arch Pathol 86:621–643.
11. Ram JI, Hiebert LM. 2001. Marked variation in free radical injury between bovine and porcine endothelial cells cultured in different medium. In Vitro & Molecular Toxicology 14:209–217.
12. Hiebert LM, Liu J. 1994. Dextran sulphates protect porcine arterial endothelial cells from free radical injury. Human & Experimental Toxicology 13:223–239.
13. Hiebert LM, Liu J. 1990. Heparin protects cultured arterial endothelial cells from damage by toxic oxygen metabolities. Atherosclerosis 83:47–51.
14. Prisco D, Rogasi PG, Matucci M, Pannicia R, Abbate R, Gensini GF, Serneri GG. 1986. Age related changes in platelet lipid composition. Thromb Res 44:427–437.
15. Stuart MJ, Gerrard JM, White JG. 1980. Effect of cholesterol on production of thromboxane B_2 by platelets in vitro. N Engl J Med 302:6–10.
16. Görg P, Kakkar VV. 1987. Increased uptake of monocyte-treated low density lipoproteins by aortic endothelium in vivo. Atherosclerosis 65:99–107.
17. Shattil SJ, Anaya-Galindo R, Bennet J, Colman RW, Cooper RA. 1975. Platelet hypersensitivity induced by cholesterol incorporation. J Clin Invest 55:636–643.
18. Ruzicka T, Printz MP. 1984. Arachidonic acid metabolism in skin: a review. Rev Physiol Biochem Pharmacol 100:121–160.
19. Van den Bosch H. 1980. Intracellular phospholipases A. Biochim Biophys Acta 604:191–246.
20. Quan-sang KHL, Levenson J, Simon A, Meyer P, Devynck MA. 1987. Platelet cytosolic free Ca^{++} concentration and plasma cholesterol in untreated hypertensives. J Hypertension 5 (suppl 5): S251–S254.
21. Whatley RE, Nelson P, Zimmerman GA, Stevens DL, Parker CT, McIntyre TM, Prescott SM. 1989. The regulation of platelet-activating factor production in endothelial cells. The role of calcium and protein kinase C. J Biol Chem 264:6325–6333.
22. Heller R, Bussolino F, Ghigo D, Garbarino G, Schroder H, Pescarmona G, Till U, Bosia A. 1991. Protein kinase C and cyclic AMP modulate thrombin-induced platelet activating factor synthesis in human endothelial cells. Biochim Biophys Acta 1093:55–64.
23. Bussolino F, Camussi G. 1995. Platelet-activating factor produced by endothelial cells. A molecule with autocrine and paracrine properties. Eur J Biochem 229:327–337.
24. Henriksson P, Stamberger M, Diezfalusy U. 1987. Increased aortic thromboxane production in experimental atherosclerosis. Prostaglandins Leukot Med 29:71–77.
25. Panganamala RV, Sharma HM, Heikkila JC, Geer JC, Cornwell DG. 1976. Role of hydroxyl radical scavengers, dimethyl sulfoxide, alcohol and methanol in the inhibition of prostaglandin biosynthesis. Prostaglandins 11:599–607.
26. Murota S, Morita I, Suda N. 1990. The control of vascular endothelial cell injury. Ann NY Acad Sci 598:182–187.

27. Vogt W, Von Zabern I, Damerau B, Hesse D, Lühmann B, Nalte R. 1985. Mechanisms of complement activation by crystalline cholesterol. Mol Immunol 22:101–106.
28. Seifert PS, Kazatchkine MD. 1987. Generation of complement anaphylatoxins C_{5b-9} by crystalline cholesterol oxidation derivatives depends on hydroxyl group number and position. Mol Immunol 24:1303–1308.
29. Pignol B, Henane S, Mencia-Huerta JM, Rola-Pleszczynski M, Braquet P. 1987. Effect of platelet-activating factor (PAF-acether) and its specific receptor antagonist, BN 52021, on interleukin 1 (IL1) release and synthesis by rat spleen adherent monocytes. Prostaglandins 33:931–939.
30. Bonavida B, Mencia-Huerta JM, Braquet P. 1989. Effect of platelet-activating factor on monocyte activation and production of tumor necrosis factor. Int Arch Allergy Appl Immunol 88:157–160.
31. Rouis M, Nigon F, Chapman MJ. 1998. Platelet-activating factor is a potent stimulant of the production of active oxygen species by human monocyte-derived macrophages. Biochem Biophys Res Commun 156:1293–1301.
32. Braquet P, Hosfard D, Braquet M, Bourgain R, Bussolino F. 1989. Rose of cytokines and platelet-activating factor in microvascular immune injury. Int Arch Allergy Appl Immunol 88:88–100.
33. Paubert-Braquet M, Lonchampt MO, Koltz P, Guilbaud J. 1988. Tumor necrosis factor (TNF) primes human neutrophil (PMN) platelet-activating factor (PAF)-induced superoxide generation. Consequences in promoting PMN-mediated endothelial cell (EC) damages (abstract). Prostaglandins 35:803.
34. Prasad K, Kalra J. 1993. Oxygen free radicals and hypercholesterolemic atherosclerosis; effect of vitamin E. Am J Heart 125:958–973.
35. Prasad K, Kalra J, Lee P. 1994. Oxygen free radicals as a mechanism of hypercholesterolemic atherosclerosis: effects of probucol. Intl J Angiol 3:100–112.
36. Prasad K, Mantha SV, Kalra J, Kapoor R, Kamalarajan BRC. 1997. Purpurogallin in the prevention of hypercholesterolemic atherosclerosis. Intl J Angiol 6:157–166.
37. Prasad K, Mantha SV, Kalra J, Lee P. 1997. Prevention of hypercholesterolemic atherosclerosis by garlic, an antioxidant. J Cardiovasc Pharmacol Therapeut 2:309–320.
38. Pearson TA, Malmros H, Dillman J, Sternby N, Heptinstall RH. 1987. Atherosclerosis in the hypercholesterolemic hare. Comparison of coronary artery lesions induced by dietary cholesterol in the hare and rabbit. Atherosclerosis 63:125–135.
39. Prasad K. 1997. Dietary flax seed in the prevention of hypercholesterolemic atherosclerosis. Atherosclerosis 132:69–76.
40. Prasad K, Mantha SV, Muir AD, Westcott ND. 1998. Reduction of hypercholesterolemic atherosclerosis by CDC-flaxseed with very low alpha-linolenic acid. Atherosclerosis 136:367–375.
41. Prasad K. 1999. Reduction of serum cholesterol and hypercholesterolemic atherosclerosis in rabbits by secoisolariciresinol diglucoside isolated from flaxseed. Circulation 99:1355–1362.
42. Holman RS, McGill HC Jr, Strong JP, Greer JC. 1958. Technics for studying atherosclerotic lesions. Lab Invest 7:42–47.
43. Prasad K, Lee P, Mantha SV, Kalra J, Prasad M, Gupta JB. 1992. Detection of ischemia-reperfusion injury by cardiac muscle chemiluminescence. Mol Cell Biochem 115:49–58.
44. Mantha SV, Prasad M, Kalra J, Prasad K. 1993. Antioxidant enzymes in hypercholesterolemia and effects of vitamin E in rabbits. Atherosclerosis 101:135–144.
45. Mantha SV, Kalra J, Prasad K. 1996. Effects of probucol on hypercholesterolemia-induced changes in antioxidant enzymes. Life Sci 58:503–509.
46. Del Boccio G, Lapenna D, Porreca E, Pennelli A, Savini F, Feliciani P, Ricci G, Cuccurullo F. 1990. Aortic antioxidant defence mechanisms: time related changes in cholesterol-fed rabbits. Atherosclerosis 81:127–135.
47. Frank L, Messaro D. 1980. Oxygen toxicity. Am J Med 69:117–126.
48. Oei HH, Stroo WE, Burton KP, Schaffer SW. 1982. A possible role of xanthine oxidase in producing oxidative stress in the heart of chronically ethanol-treated rats. Res Commun Chem Pathol Pharmacol 38:453–461.
49. Shull S, Heintz NH, Periasamy M, Manohar M, Jansen YM, Marsh JP, Mossman BT. 1991. Differential regulation of antioxidant enzymes in response to antioxidant. J Biol Chem 266:24398–24403.
50. Palinski W, Rosenfeld ME, Yla-Herttuala S, Gurtner GC, Socher SS, Butler SW, Parthasarathy S, Carew TE, Steinberg D, Witztum JL. 1989. Low density lipoprotein undergoes oxidative modification in vivo. Proc Natl Acad Sci USA 86:1372–1376.

51. Demuth K, Myara I, Chappey B, Vedie B, Pech-Amsellem MA, Haberland ME, Moatti N. 1996. A cytotoxic electronegative LDL subfraction is present in human plasma. Arterioscler Thromb Vasc Biol 16:773–783.
52. Sevanian A, Hwang J, Hodis H, Cazzolato G, Avogaro P, Bittolo-Bon G. 1996. Contribution of an in vivo oxidized LDL to LDL oxidation and its association with dense LDL subpopulations. Arterioscler Thromb Vasc Biol 16:784–793.
53. Juul K, Nielsen, LB, Munkoholm K, Stender S, Nordestgaard BG. 1996. Oxidation of plasma low-density lipoprotein accelerates its accumulation and degradation in the arterial wall in vivo. Circulation 94:1698–1704.
54. Inoue T, Hayashi M, Takayanagi K, Morooka S. 2002. Lipid lowering therapy with fluvastatin inhibits oxidative modification of low density lipoprotein and improves vascular endothelium function in hypercholesterolemic patients. Atherosclerosis 160:369–376.
55. Sasaki S, Kuwahara N, Kunitomo K, Harada S, Yamada T, Azuma A, Takeda K, Nakagawa M. 2002. Effects of atorvastatin on oxidized low-density lipoprotein, low-density lipoprotein subfraction distribution, and remnant lipoprotein in patients with mixed hyperlipoproteinemia. Am J Cardiol 89:386–389.
56. Jiang Y, Liu B, Fu M. 1997. Oxidative modification of serum LDL, VLDL and HDL induced by fed on high cholesterol diet in vivo in rabbits. Hua Xi Yi Ke Da Xue Xue Bao 28:1–5.
57. Reaven PD, Parthasarathy S, Beltz WF, Witztum JL. 1992. Effect of probucol on plasma lipid and lipoprotein levels and on protection of low density lipoprotein against in vitro oxidation in humans. Arterioscler Thromb 12:318–324.
58. Carew TE, Schwenke DC, Steinberg D. 1987. Antiatherogenic effect of probucol unrelated to its hypocholesterolemic effect: evidence that antioxidants in vivo can selectively inhibit low density lipoprotein degradation in macrophage-rich fatty streaks and slow the progression of atherosclerosis in Watanabe heritable hyperlipidemic rabbit. Proc Natl Acad Sci USA 84:7725–7729.
59. Sasahara M, Raines EW, Chait A. 1994. Inhibition of hypercholesterolemia-induced atherosclerosis in the non-human primate by probucol. I. Is the extent of atherosclerosis related to resistance of LDL to oxidation? J Clin Invest 94:155–164.
60. Prasad K, Kapoor R, Lee P. 1994. Purpurogallin, a scavenger of polymorphonuclear leukocyte-derived oxyradicals. Mol Cell Biochem 139:27–32.
61. Prasad K, Laxdal VA, Yu M, Raney BL. 1996. Evaluation of hydroxyl radical scavenging property of garlic. Mol Cell Biochem 154:55–63.
62. Prasad K. 1997. Hydroxyl radical scavenging property of secoisolariciresinol diglucoside (SDG) isolated from flaxseed. Mol Cell Biochem 168:117–123.
63. Ross R. 1986. The pathogenesis of atherosclerosis—an update. N Engl J Med 314:488–500.
64. Steinberg D, Parthasarathy S, Carew TE, Khoo JC, Witztum JL. 1989. Beyond cholesterol: modifications of low density lipoprotein that increase its atherogenicity. N Engl J Med 320:915–924.
65. Steinberg D. 1991. Antioxidants and atherosclerosis. A current assessment. Circulation 84:1420–1425.
66. Parthasarathy S, Steinberg D, Witztum JL. The role of oxidized low-density lipoproteins in the pathogenesis of atherosclerosis. Annu Rev Med 43:219–225.
67. Schwartz CJ, Valente AJ, Sprague EA, Kelley JL, Nerem RM. 1991. The pathogenesis of atherosclerosis: an overview. Clin Cardiol 14 (suppl I):I1–I16.
68. Parhami F, Fang ZT, Fogelman AM, Andalibi A, Territo MC, Berliner JA. 1993. Minimally modified low density lipoprotein-induced inflammatory responses in endothelial cells are mediated by cyclic adenosine monophosphate. J Clin Invest 92:471–478.
69. Quinn MT, Parthasarathy S, Steinberg D. 1988. Lysophosphatidylcholine: a chemotactic factor for human monocytes and its potential role in atherosclerosis. Proc Natl Acad Sci USA 85:2805–2809.

G.N. Pierce, M. Nagano, P. Zahradka, and N.S. Dhalla (eds.).
ATHEROSCLEROSIS, HYPERTENSION AND DIABETES. Copyright © 2003.
Kluwer Academic Publishers. Boston.

IDENTIFICATION, REGULATION AND FUNCTION OF LOX-1, A NOVEL RECEPTOR FOR OX-LDL

JACOB JOSEPH, MD, DAYUAN LI, MD, PHD, HONGJIANG CHEN, MD, and JAWAHAR L. MEHTA, MD, PHD, FACC

Division of Cardiovascular Medicine, Department of Internal Medicine, University of Arkansas for Medical Sciences and the Central Arkansas Veterans Healthcare System, Little Rock, AR USA
Supported by a Merit Review Award from the VA Central Office, Washington, DC; a contract with the Department of Defense, Washington, DC; and a Scientist Development Grant from the American Heart Association, Dallas, Texas

Summary. Oxidatively modified low-density lipoprotein (ox-LDL) causes endothelial activation, dysfunction and injury, which are considered primary steps in atherogenesis. Recently, a novel lectin-like receptor for ox-LDL (LOX-1) has been identified, primarily in endothelial cells. This receptor mediates uptake of ox-LDL into the endothelial cells and activates a variety of signal transduction mechanisms that lead to endothelial cell activation and expression of adhesion molecules. LOX-1 receptor is transcriptionally upregulated by various stimuli accompanying pathogenic states, including TNF-α, angiotensin II, shear stress and ox-LDL itself. LOX-1 receptor expression has been demonstrated in animal models and humans with hypertension, diabetes mellitus and atherosclerosis. Expression of this receptor may also be pathogenically involved in arterial thrombosis and myocardial ischemia-reperfusion injury. Understanding the regulation and signal transduction pathways of this receptor may lead to new therapies in prevention and treatment of atherosclerosis, and its complications.

Key words: Atherosclerosis, Diabetes mellitus, Hypertension, Oxidized-low-density lipoprotein, Renin-angiotensin-system

INTRODUCTION

Oxidized LDL (ox-LDL) is a key molecule in the pathogenesis of atherosclerosis. Many of its effects are thought to be due to uptake by monocyte/macrophages and smooth muscle cells with resultant pro-atherogenic effects. This uptake is mediated

Address Correspondence to: J. L. Mehta, MD, PhD, University of Arkansas for Medical Sciences, 4301 W. Markham St., Slot 532, Little Rock, AR 72205. Tel: (501) 296-1401; Fax: (501) 686-6180; e-mail: mehtajl@uams.edu

by a variety of scavenger receptors, such as SR-AI/II, CD36, SR-BI, macrosialin/CD68 [1,2]. Ox-LDL also leads to functional and structural changes in endothelium, which are early steps in atherogenesis. Endothelial activation by ox-LDL can lead to expression of vasoactive and pro-atherogenic genes such as endothelin, tissue factor, cyclo-oxygenase, nitric oxide synthase, growth factors and monocyte chemoattractant protein-1 (MCP-1). Activated endothelial cells also express adhesion molecules, which initiate a cascade of events including inflammatory cell attachment, cell rolling, and subendothelial migration of inflammatory cells [3–8]. In addition, ox-LDL causes endothelial injury, including apoptosis [9].

The precise mechanism of ox-LDL uptake by endothelial cells has been a subject of debate, since the traditional scavenger receptors are absent or present in very small amounts on endothelial cells [10]. It has been suggested that endothelial cells internalize and degrade modified forms of LDL, including ox-LDL, utilizing cell surface receptors [11–13]. The identification of a novel lectin-like receptor for ox-LDL, termed LOX-1, in bovine aortic endothelial cells by Sawamura and colleagues [14] opened a new avenue of investigation. Subsequently, these findings were confirmed by independent groups of investigators. Understanding the function, regulation and pathogenic role of this receptor should allow development of therapeutic interventions directed at steps in atherogenesis. In this review, we will attempt to describe the current knowledge about LOX-1 receptor function, regulation and alteration in selected pathologic states.

LOX-1: identification and binding characteristics

LOX-1 spans the cell membrane and is a ~50 kDa type II membrane protein with a C-type lectin-like extracellular domain and a short cytoplasmic tail. LOX-1 has been identified in the endothelium of human coronary arteries, rabbit and rat aorta, and bovine endothelial cells [14–18]. In addition, LOX-1 has also been identified in macrophages, platelets and smooth muscle cells, albeit in small amounts [19–21].

Human coronary artery endothelial cells possess a single class of ox-LDL receptors with a B_{max} of approximately 30 ng/mg protein and K_D of 1.7×10^{-8} M (determined by radioligand-binding studies) [16,17]. The binding characteristics are specific for ox-LDL, but not native or acetylated LDL (Ac-LDL) [22]. Delipidation does not decrease ox-LDL binding or degradation in LOX-1 expressing cells (LOX-1-CHO). Fucoidin and maleylated BSA, which inhibit ox-LDL binding to class A scavenger receptors, do not inhibit ox-LDL binding or degradation in LOX-1-CHO [16]. However, polyinosinic acid and carrageenan significantly reduce ox-LDL binding to LOX-1-CHO. These observations show the specificity of LOX-1 for ox-LDL compared to that for native- or Ac-LDL. LOX-1 recognizes specific protein moieties of ox-LDL, with a different ligand specificity compared to other receptors for ox-LDL, including class A and B scavenger receptors [22]. At this time, it is unclear whether oxidized phospholipids and minimally oxidized LDL also bind to LOX-1.

Sawamura and coworkers [23] have recently demonstrated that the lectin-like domain of LOX-1 is crucial for ligand binding, while the neck domain is not essential. More specifically, a large loop between the third and fourth cysteine residues of the lectin-like domain appears to play a critical role in ox-LDL binding. Directed mutagenesis of the basic amino acid residues around this region showed that all basic residues in this region are involved in ox-LDL binding, since simultaneous mutations of these basic residues almost abolished the ox-LDL-binding activity of LOX-1. It is thought that the electrostatic interaction between basic residues in the lectin-like domain of LOX-1 and negatively charged ox-LDL is critical for the binding of ox-LDL to LOX-1.

Endothelial activation or dysfunction elicited by ox-LDL and its lipid constituents has been shown to play a crucial role in the pathogenesis of atherosclerosis. LOX-1 was identified as the major receptor for ox-LDL in endothelial cells. This receptor can support binding, internalization and proteolytic degradation of ox-LDL, but not of significant amounts of acetylated LDL, which is a well-known high-affinity ligand for class A scavenger receptors and scavenger receptor expressed by endothelial cells (SR-EC) [14,16].

Regulation of LOX-1 receptor function

Expression and function of the LOX-1 receptor is altered in several pathologic states. A number of molecules, including ligands, have been shown to alter the function of LOX-1.

Lipids

Ox-LDL increases the expression of LOX-1 mRNA in cultured endothelial cells. Mehta and Li [16] and Aoyama et al. [24] have shown this phenomenon to be time-dependent peaking at 12–24 hours in vitro. The effect of increasing ox-LDL concentrations on LOX-1 expression is biphasic with an increase in expression from 10–40 μg/ml, and a decline in expression at higher concentrations (80–100 μg/ml), probably secondary to toxicity at higher concentrations [9]. Native-LDL, as expected, does not alter LOX-1 expression in vitro. Lysophosphotidylcholine (LPC), another lipid moiety thought to play a role in atherogenesis also increases transcription of LOX-1 mRNA [24].

Inflammatory cytokines

TNF-α, a pro-inflammatory cytokine, is expressed in atherosclerotic lesions and has been implicated in plaque vulnerability [25–27]. Kume and coworkers [28] demonstrated that TNF-α increases cell surface expression of LOX-1 in a concentration-dependent manner with a peak effect at 8–12 hrs, whereas interferon-γ, does not increase the expression of LOX-1. TNF-α can also induce the expression of class A scavenger receptors in cultured vascular smooth muscle cells [29,30], but has a suppressive effect in macrophages [31].

Shear Stress

Shear stress modulates endothelial cell gene expression and effects endothelial function. Physiologic shear stress (1–15 dynes/cm^2) was shown by Murase and coworkers [32] to increase LOX-1 transcription and translation in a time-dependent fashion. This effect is probably mediated through Ca^{++} dependent mechanisms, since shear-stress-induced LOX-1 mRNA expression was reduced by chelation of intra-cellular Ca^{++}, while ionomycine, a Ca^{++} ionophore enhanced the effect of shear stress. Obviously, shear stress-induced upregulation of endothelial LOX-1 expression could have important implications for atherogenesis.

Angiotensin II

The renin-angiotensin system (RAS) and its effector molecule angiotensin II (Ang II) have been postulated to play a critical role in atherogenesis. RAS inhibition by angiotensin converting enzyme inhibition has been shown to be effective in limiting progression of atherosclerosis [33] and decreasing atherosclerotic cardiovascular morbidity [34]. These effects are thought to be predominantly mediated through the angiotensin II type I (AT1) receptor. Ang II has direct effects on atherogenic molecular processes like endothelial apoptosis, nitric oxide synthase inhibition, reactive oxygen species (ROS) formation and expression of endothelial adhesion molecule expression [35–38], which are similar to the effects of ox-LDL. Hence great potential exists for synergism between RAS and ox-LDL.

Ang II markedly increases LOX-1 mRNA and protein expression in a concentration-dependent fashion [17]. This is accompanied by increase in I^{125}-ox-LDL uptake by endothelial cells. Ang II also potentiates the pathogenic effects of ox-LDL on endothelial cell viability and function. These interactions between the two systems are mediated via the AT1 receptor, since they were blocked by specific AT1 receptor blocker losartan, but not the AT2 receptor blocker PD123 319 blocked Ang II-mediated LOX-1 upregulation. Ox-LDL itself upregulates Ang II AT1 receptor expression, thereby augmenting the interaction between the two systems [39]. Angiotensin converting enzyme inhibitors also markedly decrease LOX-1 gene expression [40]. Several studies show that hyperlipidemia increases AT1 receptor expression, indicating the potential clinical importance of this interaction [41,42]. This cross-talk between the RAS and dyslipidemia may have great implications in the pathogenesis of atherosclerosis.

Downregulation of LOX-1 expression

Recently, oligonucleotide based therapy was shown to decrease LOX-1 expression by our group. A specific antisense phosphorothioate oligodeoxynucleotide directed at 5′-coding sequence of human LOX-1 mRNA blocked ox-LDL induced upregulation of LOX-1 [43,44]. In addition, antibodies to the ox-LDL receptor have also been developed [15].

MOLECULAR MECHANISMS OF ATHEROGENESIS AND LOX-1

Endothelial dysfunction is an important determinant of atherogenesis, and ox-LDL induces endothelial activation, dysfunction and injury [3,9,45,46]. Ox-LDL also causes apoptosis in human coronary artery endothelial cells, associated with FAS (pro-apoptotic) upregulation and Bcl2 (anti-apoptotic) downregulation [9]. This effect of ox-LDL is accompanied by LOX-1 upregulation, and is inhibited by chemical inhibitors of LOX-1 and specific antisense to LOX-1 mRNA [43].

We have investigated the role of LOX-1 activation in mediating endothelial responses to ox-LDL, especially in its effect on the expression of endothelial constitutive nitric oxide synthase (eNOS) and the adhesion molecules E- and P-selectins, ICAM-1 and VCAM-1 [47,48]. Specific antisense to LOX-1 reduced the effect of ox-LDL on the expression of eNOS and adhesion molecules, indicating the importance of LOX-1 in the effects of ox-LDL on markers of endothelial dysfunction.

Ox-LDL plays a role in monocyte chemotaxis, an early step in atherogenesis [3]. Upregulation of MCP-1 results from ox-LDL induced activation of protein kinase C and mitogen-activated protein kinases (MAPK) [49–51]. We have found similar results in HCAECs upon exposure to ox-LDL [44], with MAPK phosphorylation, MCP-1 expression (protein and mRNA) and monocyte adhesion to the endothelial cells resulting from activation of LOX-1. These effects were blocked by an antisense to LOX-1 mRNA.

The intracellular pathways mediating endothelial injury secondary to ox-LDL include intracellular generation of ROS, activation of protein kinases and transcription factors [51–55]. NF-κB activation and intracellular ROS formation was shown by Cominacini and coworkers to result from ox-LDL binding to LOX-1[51]. These effects were blocked by a monoclonal antibody to LOX-1. We have recently shown that LOX-1 expression leads to inactivation of protein kinase B (PKB) pathway [56]. PKB is important in signal transduction downstream of phosphatidylinositide (PI) 3-kinase [57] and appears to be critically important in the expression of eNOS.

LOX-1 IN PATHOLOGIC STATES

Atherosclerosis

Ox-LDL has been identified in the atherosclerotic plaque, particularly the rupture-prone plaque [58]. Elevated plasma levels of ox-LDL accompany acute manifestations of atherosclerosis [58]. As discussed above, significant cross-talk has been demonstrated between the RAS and ox-LDL, which could potentiate their atherogenic effects.

Animal models of atherosclerosis have shown increased LOX-1 expression. Chen et al. [15], in their studies in Watanabe heritable hyperlipidemic rabbit model, showed increased LOX-1 protein and mRNA expression in 8-week old aortas. Early stages of atherosclerosis in this model was correlated with augmented expression of LOX-1 in the arterial intima, with endothelial cells showing the most prominent staining; however, endothelium in non-lesion areas also demonstrated LOX-1 expression. This indicates that LOX-1 expression may be a very early event in atherogenesis. In New Zealand White rabbits fed 10 weeks of high-cholesterol diet, we observed an upregulation of LOX-1 expression in the aortas from hypercholesterolemic rabbits, but not controls [59]. The neointima was the primary site of expression. The treatment of rabbits with the Ang II AT1 receptor blocker losartan decreased the extent of atherosclerosis and LOX-1 expression (RT-PCR and immunostaining). This model of atherosclerosis is associated with over-expression of AT1 receptors [42]. This study provides another evidence for the cross-talk between RAS and LOX-1.

In a study of human carotid endarterectomy specimens, Kataoka et al. [60] showed LOX-1 expression in early atherosclerotic lesions, with greater expression in early compared to advanced lesions. Endothelial cells, macrophages and smooth muscle cells in the intima of advanced atherosclerotic plaques were seen to express LOX-1. We have identified LOX-1 expression in the intima of advanced human atherosclerotic lesions. Interestingly, double immunostaining revealed co-localization of LOX-1 in cells undergoing apoptosis (endothelial cells, smooth muscle cells and macrophages). Oka and coworkers [61] have corroborated these findings and shown that LOX-1 mediates phagocytosis of aged and apoptotic cells. These observations confirm the results of in vitro studies [9], and suggest that LOX-1 expression in the initial stages of atherosclerosis may facilitate uptake of ox-LDL, activation of endothelial cells, and adhesion of inflammatory cells. With progression of atherosclerosis, LOX-1 is expressed in the smooth muscle cells and monocytes/macrophages where LOX-1 may serve to induce apoptosis and phagocytosis.

Hypertension

Nagase et al. [62] studied LOX-1 expression in animal models of hypertension. Northern analysis showed minimal expression of LOX-1 mRNA in aorta and vein of control Wistar-Kyoto rats, while expression was markedly increased in spontaneously hypertensive rats. Wistar-Kyoto rats, Dahl salt-sensitive and salt-resistant rats were fed., but markedly upregulated in spontaneously hypertensive rats. LOX-1 expression was lower in the aorta of Dahl salt-resistant rats on salt-loaded or control diet, but elevated in salt-loaded Dahl salt-sensitive rats. It may be speculated that a dynamic regulation of LOX-1 expression resulting in increased ox-LDL uptake in endothelial cells and diminished endothelium-dependent vasorelaxation may contribute to the pathogenesis of hypertension [63].

Thrombosis

Thrombosis leads to the major acute complications of atherosclerosis, and is initiated by platelet attachment at the site of endothelial dysorption [64]. Ox-LDL is internalized by platelets with consequent decrease in type 3 NOS (eNOS) activity and enhanced platelet aggregation [65]. Recently, LOX-1 expression has been demonstrated in platelets [19]. Preliminary studies by Kakatani et al. [66] indicate the ability of LOX-1 antibody to decrease arterial thrombus formation in the rat. Hence we can speculate that LOX-1 expression in platelets may play an important role in atherosclerotic complications.

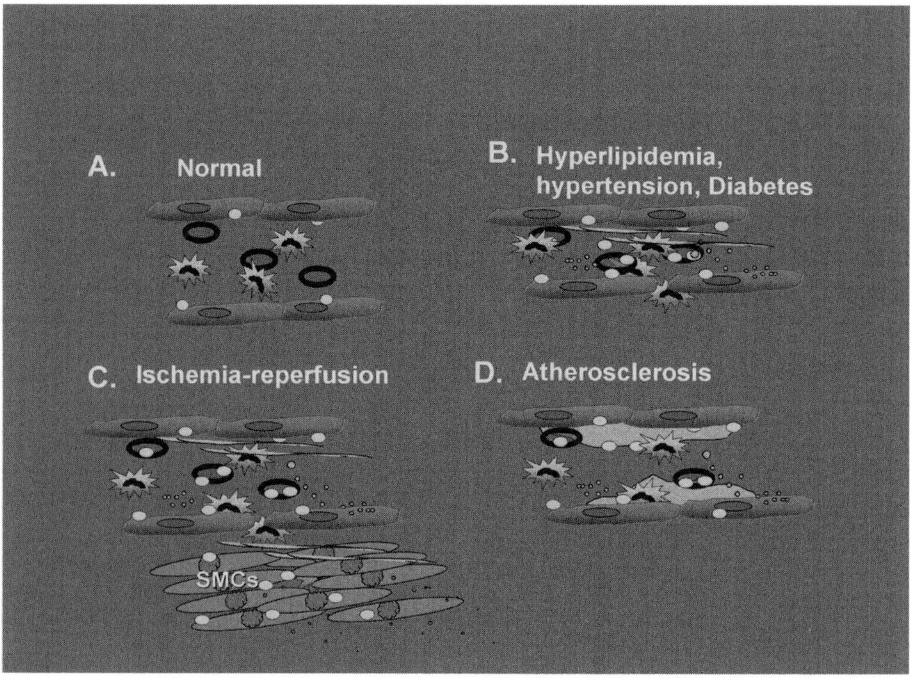

Figure 1. This figure shows LOX-1 (yellow dots) expression in normal and pathologic states. A. In physiologic state, there is very little LOX-1 expression. B. In dyslipidemia, hypertension (sate of increased shear stress), and diabetes mellitus, there is increased LOX-1 expression in endothelial cells and platelets, which may relate to endothelial activation, dysfunction and injury, and platelet activation. Endothelial activation and separation allows inflammatory cell adhesion and migration to sub-endothelial layers. C. During ischemia-reperfusion, there is intense expression of LOX-1 in endothelial cells, platelets and cardiac smooth muscle cells. LOX-1 activation may lead to reperfusion injury. D. Atherosclerotic regions show intense upregulation of LOX-1.

Myocardial Ischemia

Coronary thrombosis is most often the proximate cause of acute coronary syndromes [64]. As stated earlier, ox-LDL accumulates in the rupture-prone segments of atherosclerotic tissues, and myocardial ischemia is accompanied by oxidative stress that facilitates oxidation of native-LDL [58]. Further, perfusion with ox-LDL of the isolated rat heart significantly decreases myocardial contraction [67]. We examined LOX-1 expression in the myocardium of rats undergoing total coronary occlusion for one hour followed by reperfusion for one hour. We observed extensive LOX-1 expression in the ischemic-reperfused myocardium, but not in the hearts of rats subjected to sham surgery. Ischemia alone did not upregulate LOX-1 expression. To examine the relation of LOX-1 expression with infarct size and cardiac function, a group of rats were treated with LOX-1 antibody before initiation of ischemia. We observed a marked decrease in myocardial LOX-1 expression in rats given the antibody. More importantly, there was a 48% reduction in infarct size with preservation of left ventricular function after ischemia-reperfusion in rats given the LOX-1 antibody [68,69].

These studies imply an important role of LOX-1 expression during myocardial ischemia on cardiac function and infarct size.

Diabetes mellitus

Diabetes mellitus creates a powerful pro-atherogenic mileu, characterized by a state of oxidative stress, endothelial dysfunction and upregulated expression of adhesion molecules for inflammatory cells. In the streptozotocin-induced diabetic rat model, LOX-1 expression was found to be increased in diabetic rat aorta compared with that in the non-diabetic rat [70]. Immunohistochemistry revealed that endothelial cells were the major cell type expressing LOX-1, especially at the aortic bifurcation. In vitro studies have corroborated these findings. In cultured aortic endothelial cells, LOX-1 expression was induced by diabetic rat serum and advanced glycation end-products, but not by control rat serum with high glucose. Further, competitive inhibition assay revealed that LOX-1 ligand activity in the diabetic rat serum, mainly in the VLDL/LDL fractions.

CONCLUSIONS

Identification of LOX-1 and definition of its biological role provides new information regarding the uptake of ox-LDL into endothelial cells, smooth muscle cells and macrophages. Internalization of ox-LDL leads to a cascade of events including endothelial dysfunction, activation and injury; hence LOX-1 could play a major role in atherogenic effects of hyperlipidemia. Alteration of endothelial cell function by ox-LDL via the LOX-1 receptor may be a key event in hypertension, diabetes mellitus and dyslipidemia, the most important risk factors for atherosclerosis. Cross-talk between the RAS and dyslipidemia may serve to enhance tissue injury.

REFERENCES

1. Freeman MW. 1997. Scavenger receptors in atherosclerosis. Curr Opin Hematol 4:41–47.
2. Steinbrecher UP. 1999. Receptors for oxidized low density lipoprotein. Biochem Biophys Acta 1436:279–298.
3. Ross R. 1993. The pathogenesis of atherosclerosis: a perspective for the 1990's. Nature 362:801–809.
4. Kume N, Cybulsky MI, Gimbrone MA Jr. 1992. Lysophosphatidylcholine, a component of atherogenic lipoproteins, induces mononuclear leukocyte adhesion molecules in cultured human and rabbit arterial endothelial cells. J Clin Invest 90:1138–1144.
5. Kume N, Gimbrone MA Jr. 1994. Lysophosphatidylcholine transcriptionally induces growth factor gene expression in cultured human endothelial cells. J Clin Invest 93:907–911.
6. Zembowicz A, Tang JL, Wu KK. 1995. Transcriptional induction of endothelial nitric oxide synthase type III by lysophosphatidylcholine. J Biol Chem 270:17006–17010.
7. Hirata K, Miki N, Kuroda Y, Sakoda T, Kawashima S, Yokoyama M. 1995. Low concentration of oxidized low-density lipoprotein and lysophosphatidylcholine upregulate constitutive nitric oxide synthase mRNA expression in bovine aortic endothelial cells. Circ Res 76:958–962.
8. Zembowicz A, Jones SL, Wu KK. 1995. Induction of cyclooxygenase-2 in human umbilical vein endothelial cells by lysophosphatidylcholine. J Clin Invest 96:1688–1692.

9. Li DY, Yang BC, Mehta JL. 1998. Ox-LDL enhances anoxia-reoxygenation-mediated apoptosis in human coronary endothelial cells: Role of PKC, PTK, Bcl-2 and Fas. Am J Physiol 275:H568–H576.
10. Bickel PE, Freeman M. 1992. Rabbit aortic smooth muscle cells express inducible macrophage scavenger receptor messenger RNA that is absent from endothelial cells. J Clin Invest 90:1450–1457.
11. Kume N, Arai H, Kawai C, Kita T. 1991. Receptors for modified low-density lipoproteins in human endothelials cells: different recognition for acetylated low-density lipoprotein and oxidized low-density lipoprotein. Biochem Biophys Acta 1091:63–67.
12. van Berkel TJC, De Rijke YB, Kruijt JK. 1991. Different fate in vivo of oxidatively modified low density lipoprotein and acetylated low density lipoprotein in rats. J Biol Chem 266:2282–2289.
13. De Rijke YB, van Berkel TJC. 1994. Rat liver Kupffer and endothelial cells express different binding proteins for modified low density lipoproteins. J Biol Chem 269:824–827.
14. Sawamura T, Kume N, Aoyama T, Moriwaki H, Hoshikawa H, Aiba Y, Tanaka T, Miwa S, Katsura Y, Kita T, Masaki T. 1997. An endothelial receptor for oxidized low-density lipoprotein. Nature 386:73–77.
15. Chen M, Kakutani M, Minami M, Kataoka H, Kume N, Narumiya S, Kita T, Masaki T, Sawamura T. 2000. Increased expression of lectin-like oxidized low density lipoprotein receptor-1 in initial atherosclerotic lesions of Watanabe heritable hyperlipidemic rabbits. Arterioscler Thromb Vasc Biol 20:1107–1115.
16. Mehta JL, Li DY. 1998. Identification and autoregulation of receptor for OX-LDL in cultured human coronary artery endothelial cells. Biochem Biophys Res Commun 248:511–514.
17. Li DY, Zhang YC, Philips MI, Sawamura T, Mehta JL. 1999. Upregulation of endothelial receptor for oxidized low-density lipoprotein (LOX-1) in cultured human coronary artery endothelial cells by angiotensin II type 1 receptor activation. Circ Res 84:1043–1049.
18. Nagase M, Hirose S, Sawamura T, Masaki T, Fujita T. 1997. Enhanced expression of endothelial oxidized low-density lipoprotein receptor (LOX-1) in hypertensive rats. Biochem Biophys Res Commun 237:496–498.
19. Chen M, Kakutani M, Naruko T, Ueda M, Narumiya S, Masaki T, Sawamura T. 2001. Activation-dependent surface expression of LOX-1 in human platelets. Biochem Biophys Res Commun Mar 23;282:153–158
20. Kataoka H, Kume N, Miyamoto S, Minami M, Morimoto M, Hayashida K, Hashimoto N, Kita T. 2001. Oxidized LDL modulates Bax/Bcl-2 through the lectin-like Ox-LDL receptor-1 in vascular smooth muscle cells. Arterioscler Thromb Vasc Biol 21:955–960
21. Yoshida H, Kondratenko N, Green S, Steinberg D, Quehenberger O. 1998. Identification of the lectin-like receptor of oxidized low-density lipoprotein in human macrophages and its potential role as a scavenger receptor. Biochem J 334:9–13.
22. Moriwaki H, Kume N, Sawamura T, Aoyama T, Hoshikawa H, Ochi H, Nishi E, Masaki T, Kita T. 1998. Ligand specificity of LOX-1, a novel endothelial receptor for oxidized low density lipoprotein. Arterioscler Thromb Vasc Biol 18:1541–1547.
23. Chen M, Inoue K, Narumiya S, Masaki T, Sawamura T. 2001. Requirements of basic amino acid residues within the lectin-like domain of LOX-1 for the binding of oxidized low-density lipoprotein. FEBS Lett 499:215–219.
24. Aoyama T, Fujiwara H, Masaki T, Sawamura T. 1999. Induction of lectin-like oxidized LDL receptor by oxidized LDL and lysophosphatidylcholine in cultured endothelial cells. J Mol Cell Cardiol 31:2101–2114.
25. Tipping PG, Hancock WW. 1993. Production of tumor necrosis factor and interleukin-1 by macrophages from human atheromatous plaques. Am J Pathol 142:1721–1728.
26. Barath P, Fishbein MC, Cao J, Berenson J, Helfant RH, Forrester JS. 1990. Tumor necrosis factor gene expression in human vascular intimal smooth muscle cells detected by in situ hybridization. Am J Pathol 137:503–509.
27. Lee RT, Libby P. 1997. The unstable atheroma. Arterioscler Thromb Vasc Biol 17:1859–1867.
28. Kume N, Murase T, Moriwaki H, Aoyama T, Sawamura T, Masaki T, Kita T. 1998. Inducible expression of lectin-like oxidized LDL receptor-1 in vascular endothelial cells. Circ Res 83:322–327.
29. Pitas RE. 1990. Expression of the acetylated low density lipoprotein receptor by rabbit fibroblasts and smooth muscle cells: up-regulation by phorbol esters. J Biol Chem 265:12722–12727.
30. Li H, Freeman MW, Libby P. 1995. Regulation of smooth muscle scavenger receptor expression in vivo by atherogenic diets and in vitro by cytokines. J Clin Invest 95:122–133.
31. Hsu HY, Nicholson AC, Hajjar DP. 1996. Inhibition of macrophage scavenger activity by tumor necrosis factor-α is transcriptionally an post-transcriptionally regulated. J Biol Chem 271:7767–7773.

32. Murase T, Kume N, Korenaga R, Ando J, Sawamura T, Masaki T, Kita T. 1998. Fluid shear stress transcriptionally induces lectin-like oxidized LDL receptor-1 in vascular endothelial cells. Circ Res 83:328–333.
33. Chobanian AV, Hauderschild CC, Nickerson C, Hope S. 1992. Trandolapril inhibits atherosclerosis in the Watanabe heritable hyperlipidemic rabbit. Hypertension 20:473–477.
34. Pitt B. 1994. Angiotensin-converting enzyme inhibitors in patients with coronary atherosclerosis. Am Heart J 128:1328–1332.
35. Li DY, Yang BC, Phillips MI, Mehta JL. 1999. Proapoptotic effects of Ang II in human coronary artery endothelial cells: role of AT_1 receptor and PKC activation. Am J Physiol 276:H786–H792.
36. Raij L. 2001. Hypertension and cardiovascular risk factors: role of the angiotensin II-nitric oxide interaction. Hypertension 37:767–773.
37. Lassegue B, Sorescu D, Szocs K, Yin Q, Akers M, Zhang Y, Grant SL, Lambeth JD, Griendling KK. 2001. Novel gp91(phox) homologues in vascular smooth muscle cells : nox1 mediates angiotensin II-induced superoxide formation and redox-sensitive signaling pathways. Circ Res 88:888–894.
38. Dzau VJ. 2001. Tissue angiotensin and pathobiology of vascular disease: a unifying hypothesis. Hypertension 37:1047–1052.
39. Li D, Saldeen T, Romeo F, Mehta JL. 2000. Oxidized LDL upregulates angiotensin II type 1 receptor expression in cultured human coronary artery endothelial cells: the potential role of transcription factor NF-kappaB. Circulation 102:1970–1976.
40. Morawietz H, Rueckschloss U, Niemann B, Duerrschmidt N, Galle J, Hakim K, Zerkowski HR, Sawamura T, Holtz J. 1999. Angiotensin II induces LOX-1, the human endothelial receptor for oxidized low-density lipoprotein. Circulation 100:899–902.
41. Strehlow K, Wassmann S, Bohm M, Nickenig G. 2000. Angiotensin AT1 receptor over-expression in hypercholesterolaemia. Ann Med 32:386–389.
42. Yang BC, Phillips MI, Mohuczy D, Meng H, Shen L, Mehta P, Mehta JL. 1998. Increased angiotensin II type 1 receptor expression in hypercholesterolemic atherosclerosis in rabbits. Arterioscler Thromb Vasc Biol 18:1433–1439.
43. Li D, Mehta JL. 2000. Upregulation of endothelial receptor for oxidized LDL (LOX-1) by oxidized LDL and implications in apoptosis of human coronary artery endothelial cells: evidence from use of antisense LOX-1 mRNA and chemical inhibitors. Arterioscler Thromb Vasc Biol 20:1116–1122.
44. Li D, Mehta JL. 2000. Antisense to LOX-1 inhibits oxidized LDL-mediated upregulation of monocyte chemoattractant protein-1 and monocyte adhesion to human coronary artery endothelial cells. Circulation 101:2889–2895.
45. Walsh K, Isner JM. 2000. Apoptosis in inflammatory-fibroproliferative disorders of the vessel wall. Cardiovasc Res 45:756–765.
46. Sam F, Sawyer DB, Chang DL, Eberli FR, Ngoy S, Jain M, Amin J, Apstein CS, Colucci WS. 2000. Progressive left ventricular remodeling and apoptosis late after myocardial infarction in mouse heart. Am J Physiol Heart Circ Physiol 279:H422–428.
47. Li D, Chen H, Mhatre A, Romeo F, Saldeen T, Mehta JL. 2000. Statins inhibit ox-LDL-induced expression of adhesion molecules and monocyte adhesion to human coronary endothelial cells: Role of mitogen-activated protein kinase and NF-κB. Circulation 102:1229
48. Mehta JL, Li DY, Chen HJ, Joseph J, Romeo F. 2001. Inhibition of LOX-1 by statins may relate to upregulation of eNOS. Biochemical Biophysical Research Communications 289:857–861.
49. Voraberger G, Schafer R, Strotowa C. 1991. Cloning of the human gene for intercellular adhesion molecule 1 and analysis of its 5′-regulatory region. Induction by cytokines and phorbol ester. J Immunol 147:2777–2786.
50. Iademarco MF, McQuillan JJ, Rosen GD, Dean DC. 1992. Characterization of the promoter for vascular cell adhesion molecule-1 (VCAM-1). J Biol Chem 267:16323–16329.
51. Cominacini L, Pasini AF, Garbin U, Davoli A, Tosetti ML, Campagnola M, Rigoni A, Pastorino AM, Lo Cascio V, Sawamura T. 2000. Oxidized low density lipoprotein (ox-LDL) binding to ox-LDL receptor-1 in endothelial cells induces the activation of NF-κB through an increased production of intracellular reactive oxygen species. J Biol Chem 275:12633–12638.
52. Cominacini L, Rigoni A, Pasini AF, Garbin U, Davoli A, Campagnola M, Pastorino AM, Lo Cascio V, Sawamura T. 2001. The binding of oxidized low density lipoprotein (ox-LDL) to ox-LDL receptor-1 reduces the intracellular concentration of nitric oxide in endothelial cells through an increased production of superoxide. J Biol Chem 276:13750–13755.
53. Kusuhara M, Chait A, Cader A, Berk BC. 1997. Oxidized LDL stimulates mitogen-activated protein kinases in smooth muscle cells and macrophages. Arterioscler Thromb Vasc Biol 17:141–148.

54. Han KH, Tangirala RK, Green SR, Quehenberger O. 1998. Chemokine receptor CCR2 expression and monocyte chemoattractant protein-1-mediated chemotaxis in human monocytes: a regulatory role for plasma LDL. Arterioscler Thromb Vasc Biol 18:1983–1991.
55. Wang GP, Deng ZD, Ni J, Qu ZL. 1997. Oxidized low density lipoprotein and very low density lipoprotein enhance expression of monocyte chemoattractant protein-1 in rabbit peritoneal exudates macrophages. Atherosclerosis 133:31–36.
56. Li DY, Chen HJ, Mehta JL. 2001. Statins inhibit oxidized-LDL-mediated LOX-1 expression, uptake of ox-LDL and reduction in PKB phosphorylation. Cardiovasc Res, 52:130–135
57. Tang X, Downes CP, Whetton AD, Owen-Lynch PJ. 2000. Role of phosphatidylinositol 3-kinase and specific protein kinase B isoforms in the suppression of apoptosis mediated by the Abelson protein-tyrosine kinase. J Biol Chem 275:3142–3148.
58. Ehara S, Ueda M, Naruko T, Haze K, Itoh A, Otsuka M, Komatsu R, Matsuo T, Itabe H, Takano T, Tsukamoto Y, Yoshiyama M, Takeuchi K, Yoshikawa J, Becker AE. 2001. Elevated levels of oxidized low density lipoprotein show a positive relationship with the severity of acute coronary syndromes. Circulation 103:1955–1960.
59. Chen H, Li D, Sawamura T, Inoue K, Mehta JL. 2000. Upregulation of LOX-1 expression in aorta of hypercholesterolemic rabbits: modulation by losartan. Biochem Biophys Res Commun 276:1100–1104.
60. Kataoka H, Kume N, Miyamoto S, Minami M, Moriwaki H, Murase T, Sawamura T, Masaki T, Hashimoto N, Kita T. 1999. Expression of lectinlike oxidized low-density lipoprotein receptor-1 in human atherosclerotic lesions. Circulation 99:3110–3117.
61. Oka K, Sawamura T, Kikuta K, Itokawa S, Kume N, Kita T, Masaki T. 1998. Lectin-like oxidized low-density lipoprotein receptor 1 mediates phagocytosis of aged/apoptotic cells in endothelial cells. Proc Natl Acad Sci USA 95:9535–9540.
62. Nagase M, Hirose S, Sawamura T, Masaki T, Fujita. 1997. Enhanced expression of endothelial oxidized low-density lipoprotein receptor (LOX-1) in hypertensive rats. Biochem Biophys Res Commun 237:496–498.
63. Panza JA, Quyyumi AA, Brush JE Jr, Epstein SE. 1990. Abnormal endothelium-dependent vascular relaxation in patients with essential hypertension. N Engl J Med 323:22–27.
64. Conti CR, Mehta JL. 1987. Acute myocardial ischemia: Role of atherosclerosis, in situ thrombosis, platelet activation, coronary vasospasm, and altered arachidonic acid metabolism. Circulation 75:V84–V95.
65. Chen LY, Mehta P, Mehta JL. 1996. Oxidized LDL decreases L-arginine uptake and nitric oxide synthase protein expression in human platelets: relevance of the effect of oxidized LDL on platelet function. Circulation 93:1740–1746.
66. Kakatani M, Sawamura T, Chen M. 2000. Role of Lox-1 in thrombosis. Circulation 102:II-191.
67. Harrison GJ, Jordan LR, Selley ML, Willis RJ. 1995. Low-density lipoproteins inhibit histamine and $NaNO_2$ relaxation of the coronary vasculature and reduce contractile function in isolated rat hears. Heart Vessels 10:249–257.
68. Dayuan Li, MD, PhD, Victor Williams, MD, Ling Liu, MD, Hongjiang Chen, MD, Tatsuya Sawamura, MD, PhD, Francesco Romeo, MD, Jawahar L. Mehta, MD, PhD. 2001. Expression of LOX-1 during ischemia-reperfusion and its role in determination of apoptosis and left ventricular dysfunction in rats. Circulation 104:II-11.
69. Williams V, Li DY, Liu L, Chen HJ, Sawamura T, Antakli T, Mehta JL. 2001. The role of LOX-1, an oxidized LDL Receptor, in myocardial ischemia-reperfusion injury in rats. Circulation 104:II-92.
70. Kita T, Kume N, Yokode M, Ishii K, Arai H, Horiuchi H, Moriwaki H, Minami M, Kataoka H, Wakatsuki Y. 1999. Oxidized LDL and expression of monocyte adhesion molecules. Diabetes Res Clin Pract 45:123–126.

G.N. Pierce, M. Nagano, P. Zahradka, and N.S. Dhalla (eds.).
ATHEROSCLEROSIS, HYPERTENSION AND DIABETES.
Kluwer Academic Publishers. Boston.

ATHEROSCLEROSIS AND ANGIOTENSIN II IN HYPERCHOLESTEROLEMIA AND DIABETES. A ROLE FOR AT_1 RECEPTORS BEYOND HYPERTENSION

WILLIAM B. STRAWN, DVM, PHD, RICHARD H. DEAN, MD, and CARLOS M. FERRARIO, MD

Hypertension and Vascular Disease Center, Wake Forest University School of Medicine, Winston-Salem, North Carolina 27157, USA

Summary. The pathophysiological continuum that presumably begins with endothelial injury and dysfunction and ends with the fibronecrotic plaque, occlusive coronary artery disease, and diabetes-related nephropathy is potentially influenced by an association between hyperglycemia, hypercholesterolemia and activation of the renin-angiotensin system. It is known that the resultant proliferative and progressive responses of the arterial wall in atherosclerosis and glomerulosclerosis are the culmination of the effects of a variety of mitogenic and inhibitory hormonal and trophic factors exerting their actions at stages that may be far removed both spatially and temporally from the initial injurious event. These processes are likely also at work in the diabetic kidney, but are not as well investigated. Regardless of the initiating mechanism, the vascular endothelium, inflammatory cell infiltration and the resultant tissue response have become the focus of attention in the pathogenesis of both atherosclerosis and diabetic nephropathy. A vast array of effects of angiotensin II likely to be mediated through both type 1 and type 2 angiotensin receptors are now described in the literature. Current data indicates that the role of angiotensin II in vascular remodeling and renal injury may originate from a local tissue source rather than the circulation. Regardless of its origin, angiotensin peptides and angiotensin receptors may contribute in significant ways to the atherogenic processes. While the stages of atherosclerosis and renal diabetic nephropathy in humans and animals are well defined morphologically, the mechanisms within vascular and renal tissues that contribute to these pathologies represent a spectrum of events

Corresponding Author: Carlos M. Ferrario, MD, The Hypertension and Vascular Disease Center, Wake Forest University School of Medicine, Winston-Salem, North Carolina 27157. Phone: 336-716-5819; Fax: 336-716-6644 e-mail: cferrari@wfubmc.edu

occurring in different microenvironments over prolonged periods. This review describes well-established and novel aspects of angiotensin II-mediated actions as they relate to hypercholesterolemia-induced atherogenesis and diabetic nephropathy, and suggests potential pathways where angiotensin II might be substantially involved through the AT_1 receptor in these processes, and thus may be blocked by AT_1 receptor antagonists.

***Key words*:** Angiotensin II, Atherosclerosis, Diabetes mellitus, Hypercholesterolemia AT1 receptor, AT2 receptor

INTRODUCTION

Diabetes and hypercholesterolemia are major risk factors for coronary artery and renal vascular and functional abnormalities, and are commonly present in combination in the clinical setting. The coexistence of dyslipidemia and hyperglycemia greatly increases the incidence of cardiovascular morbidity and mortality secondary to atherosclerosis and likely exacerbates the deterioration of diabetic renal function. The public health burden of type 2 diabetes mellitus and of hypercholesterolemia is significant and rapidly increasing. The potent effects of angiotensin II (Ang II) type I (AT_1) receptor blockers (ARBs) to decrease proteinuria in both experimental and human diabetic nephropathy and to improve survival of individuals with coronary artery disease suggest that RAS activation is responsible for many of these deleterious effects [1]. Ang II may exert its most important pathophysiologic actions through the remodeling of coronary artery and renovascular tissue by inducing pro-inflammatory and pro-oxidative responses [2]. Hypercholesterolemia-induced and diabetic atherosclerosis as well as renal glomerulosclerosis and interstitial fibrosis involve changes that are consistent with the inflammatory actions of angiotensin II. Emerging evidence suggests that an intravascular and intrarenal RAS may be activated in the presence of hypercholesterolemia and hyperglycemia, leading to production of local tissue Ang II production. Once formed, Ang II exerts most of its well-characterized effects through binding to AT_1 receptors that are abundantly present in the cells of the coronary arteries and glomeruli, tubules, and the renal vasculature and interstitium. Adult coronary arteries and kidney also express angiotensin II type 2 (AT_2) receptors whose balance with AT_1 receptors may regulate the outcome of increased Ang II generation. Stimulation of AT_2 receptors, associated with increased nitric oxide (NO) production, inhibition of cell growth and matrix synthesis, in effect tends to oppose those of AT_1 receptors. Upregulation of both AT_1 and AT_2 receptors in atherosclerotic coronary arteries and the reduction in kidney AT_1 receptor expression in diabetic nephropathy suggests that the balance between AT_1 and AT_2 receptor-mediated cell-signaling events may be a determinant of the progression rate of these processes. This review briefly examines the role of the RAS in the increased risk for coronary artery disease and nephropathy in diabetic patients, and the potential impact of AT_1 receptor blockade on the development of clinical outcomes in these patients.

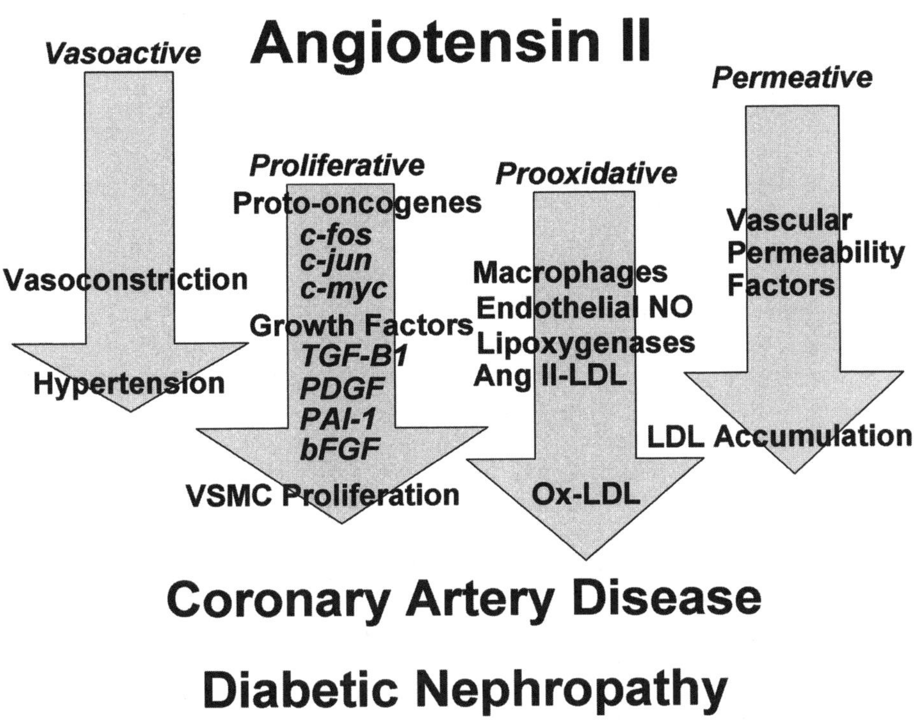

Figure 1. Cellular effects of angiotensin II (Ang II) contributing to the pathological effects on the heart and kidneys.

EVIDENCE FOR ANGIOTENSIN II AT_1 RECEPTOR-MEDIATED ATHEROSCLEROSIS AND GLOMERULOSCLEROSIS

Experimental evidence derived mainly from animal and in vitro studies associates Ang II with arterial lipid deposition, reactive oxygen species (ROS) production, activation of monocytes, increasing adhesion of monocytes to endothelial cells, direct modification of low density lipoprotein (LDL) molecules, and increased oxidized LDL uptake into monocytes. Figure 1 illustrates the well-described vasoactive and proliferative aspects of Ang II actions; newly described pro-oxidative and permeative effects that are associated with inflammatory responses in early coronary artery disease and diabetic nephropathy are indicated as potential pathways in these disease processes. Vascular angiotensin converting enzyme (ACE) and vascular smooth muscle cell (VSMC) AT_1 receptor expression are up regulated in atherosclerotic lesions, potentially serving as a source for local production of angiotensin II and sites for its actions, respectively [3]. Furthermore, the inhibitory effect of ARBs on the progression of atherogenic changes in rabbits and nonhuman primates fed a cholesterol-containing diet and in apolipoprotein E–deficient mice suggest that angiotensin II plays a key role in the initiation and progression of atherosclerosis [4]. Since all components of the RAS including Ang II and its receptors are detected in arteries with atherosclerotic plaque and in diabetic kidneys, it is likely that Ang II is influential at this stage of athero- and glomerulosclerosis [5–9]. Human VSMCs respond to Ang II AT_1 receptor stimulation by secreting types I and III collagen which may extend extracellular matrix (ECM) formation in the plaque. Conversely, matrix metalloproteinases (MMP) produced by resident macrophages disrupt ECM and may increase the probability of plaque rupture. ARBs inhibit MMP-1 and MMP-2 activity suggesting that Ang II exacerbates the tendency for plaque rupture through AT_1-mediated macrophage MMP production. These findings indicate that the atheroma is a microenvironment where Ang II-producing and -sensitive macrophages, VSMCs and ECM are in close proximity to a microvasculature capable of synthesizing and delivering Ang II. Whether reduction of the influence of Ang II in the advanced, vascularized plaque by ACE inhibition or AT_1 receptor blockade might result in lesion regression in humans is not yet known.

Adhesion of monocytes to human aortic endothelial cells induced by Ang II is dose-dependent, saturable, and sensitive to AT_1 receptor blockade. Monocyte migration into rat type-I mesenteric arteries is enhanced by Ang-II infusion independently of its pressor effects. Elevated plasma low density lipoprotein (LDL) concentrations correlate in vitro and in vivo with enhanced vascular ACE and Ang II production, AT_1 receptor gene expression and receptor density that leads to enhanced biological effects of Ang II. Ang II stimulates the deposition of oxidized LDL contributing to increased intracellular adhesion molecule (ICAM)-1 and vascular cell adhesion molecule (VCAM)-1 expression, and Ang II-modified LDL is taken up by macrophages via the scavenger receptor at an enhanced rate. Endothelial cell (EC) expression of VCAM-1 precedes the subendothelial accumulation of monocytes and is increased by Ang II through the AT_1 receptor suggesting a role for Ang II in the early stages of vascular activation. Production of monocyte chemoattractant protein (MCP)-1, expressed by monocytes, ECs and VSMCs, is stimulated by AT_1 receptor-mediated activation of nuclear factor (NF)-κB. E-selectin mRNA and protein increased in human coronary endothelial cells in response to Ang II stimulation of AT_1 receptors. These findings suggest that Ang II may be a significant stimulus for both the recruitment and subendothelial infiltration of monocytes and their transformation into macrophage foam cells in early atherosclerosis as well as glomerulosclerosis.

The earliest fatty streak lesions in atherogenesis are composed of primarily lipid-laden macrophage foam cells. Figures 2 and 3 illustrate typical fatty streak formation in the early atherogenesis associated with diet-induced hypercholesterolemia in the cynomolgus monkeys model of atherosclerosis. The efficacy of ARBs to reduce the extent of fatty streak in animal models of diet-induced and genetic hypercholesterolemia is well-established. Several recent studies indicate that the RAS plays a role in the development of fatty streak in cynomolgus monkeys. Fatty streak formation induced by hypercholesterolemia was associated with increased ACE activity, Ang II concentration, and AT_1 receptor expression. We showed a direct effect

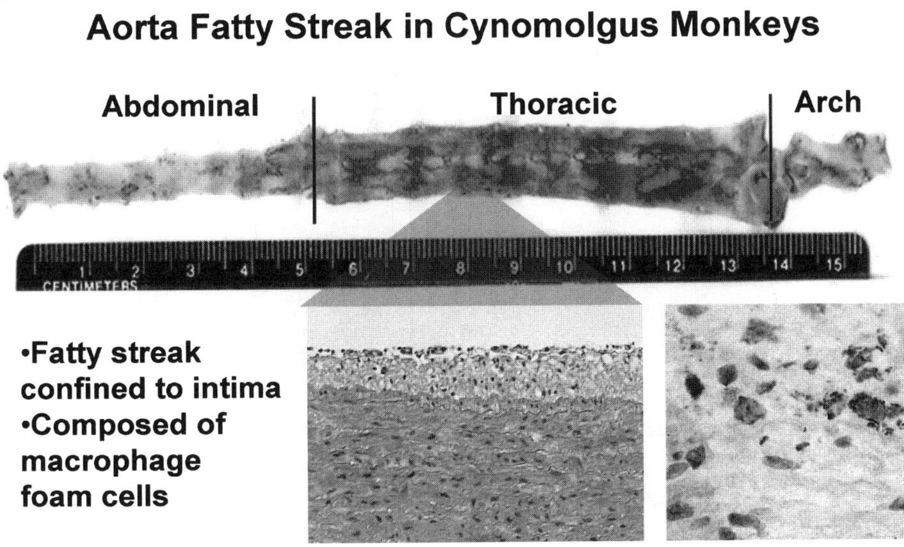

Figure 2. Morphological characteristics of the early stages of plaque development in non-human primates.

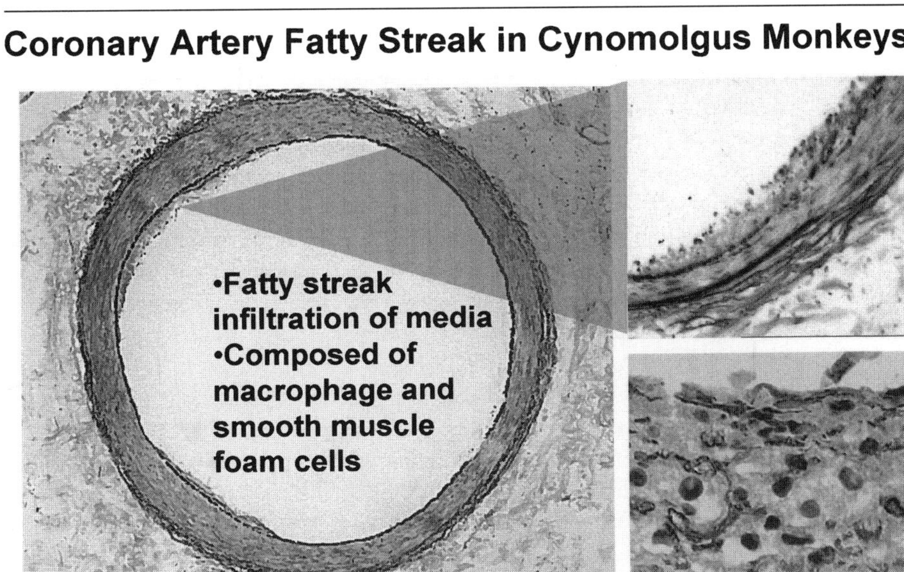

Figure 3. Infiltration of monocytes which mature into lipid-laden macrophages denote the characteristic early fatty streak lesion that progresses to the stable plaque.

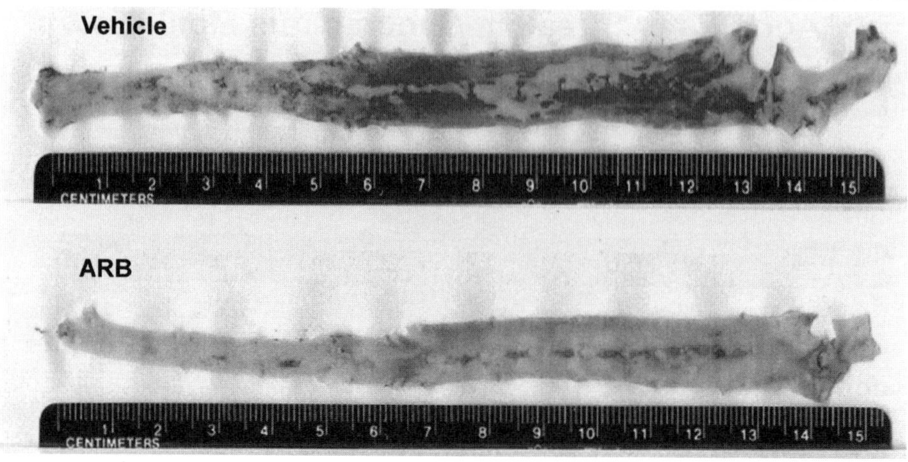

Figure 4. In the cholesterol-fed cynomolgus monkeys, six-weeks of continuous administration of losartan (ARB) was associated with a robust prevention of fatty streak deposition in the abdominal and thoracic aorta. (Reprinted by permission from reference 4).

of AT_1 receptor blockade on inhibition of fatty streak formation that could not be explained by changes in blood pressure or the atherogenic profile of plasma lipoproteins [4]. Our study was the first to show that AT_1 receptor blockade inhibits diet-induced atherogenesis in nonhuman primates at vascular sites corresponding to atherosclerosis-prone sites in humans. Figures 4 and 5 illustrate the robust inhibitory effect in cynomolgus monkeys of short-term Ang II AT_1 receptor blockade on fatty streak in the aorta and left anterior descending coronary artery, respectively.

Lipid abnormalities mediated by Ang II AT_1 receptors may be important in the pathogenesis of glomerulosclerosis just as in atherosclerosis [10] Proposed mechanisms include lipid interactions with glomerular macrophages, alterations in vascular and mesangial functions, changes in production of mediator substances, or alterations in membrane fluidity. Among many risk factors for the development of lipid-mediated diabetic nephropathy, recent interest has been focused on a possible involvement of oxidative modification of LDL since numerous lines of evidence indicate that diabetes mellitus is associated with increased oxidative stress. In fact, several reports showed increased circulating levels of oxidized LDL in the plasma of diabetic patients. In addition, it has also been shown that LDL isolated from patients with poorly controlled diabetes mellitus has an enhanced susceptibility to oxidation. Nephrotoxicity from elevated circulating lipids occurs in experimental and clinical situations. Experimental evidence linking hyperlipidemias to renal injury and progression of renal fibrogenesis indicates that renal accumulation of fatty acids and cholesteryl esters occurs concurrently with progression of tubulointerstitial fibrosis and glomerulosclerosis. It is not clear how diet-induced hypercholesterolemia may

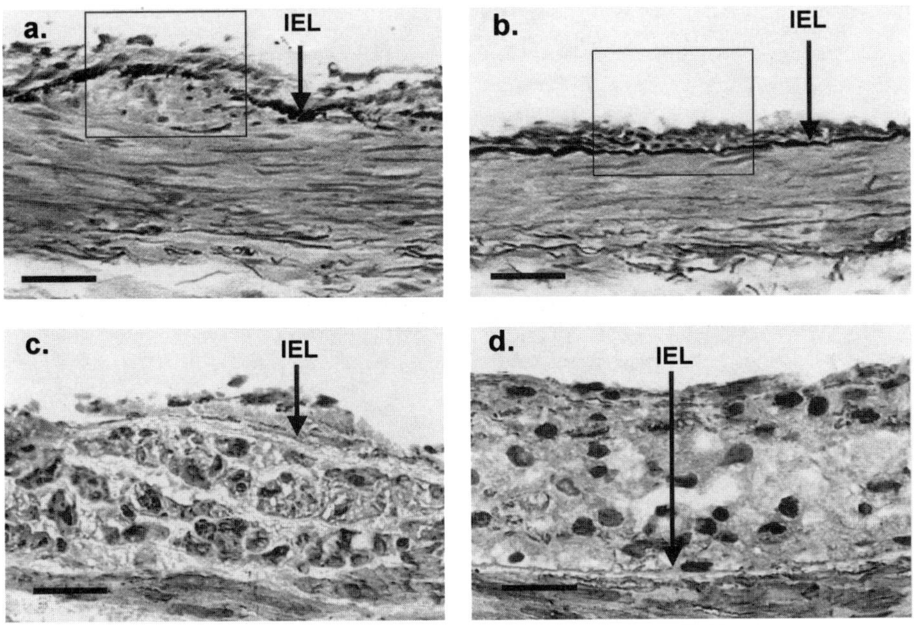

Figure 5. Histological characteristic of fatty streak lesions in cynomolgus monkeys given either vehicle (panels a and c) or losartan (panels b and d) for six weeks document the prevention of early atherogenesis with reduction in lipid accumulation, no fragmentation of the internal elastic laminae (IEL), and reduced thickening of the vascular intima. (Reprinted by permission from reference 4).

evoke renal toxicity, although it is suspected that the injury process is mediated in part by oxidized LDL.

The concept that hyperlipidemia, hyperglycemia and the RAS may interact to initiate diabetic nephropathy is a hypothesis based, in part, on their experimentally established interactions within the vascular wall during atherogenesis and clinical evidence for the benefit of RAS suppression on coronary artery disease. Modification of the vascular microenvironment toward increased oxidant production leads to the generation of oxidized lipid moieties that are thought to play a role in early fatty streak formation in coronary arteries. Disruption of endothelial function by oxidized LDL is presumed to evoke both activation of the local vascular RAS and diminished expression of endothelial NO synthase. The enhanced expression of vascular ACE, AT_1 receptors and angiotensin II production observed in nonhuman models of hyperlipoproteinemia effectively increases the bioavailability and biological effect of plasma and tissue Ang II. The pressor-independent pro-oxidative and pro-inflammatory actions of Ang II that precipitate endothelial dysfunction, monocyte binding to endothelial cells, ECM proliferation and oxidative changes may exacerbate the actions of lipids in early atherogenesis as well as lipid-associated nephropathies. Ang II-mediated accumulation of cells in atherosclerotic arteries is

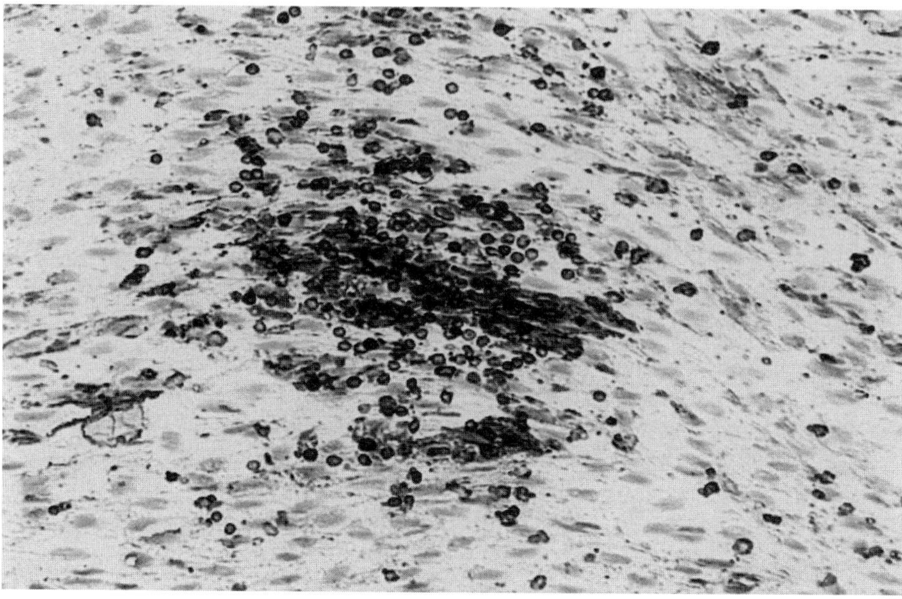

Figure 6. Apposition of monocytes to vascular endothelium in the thoracic aorta of a transgenic rat model of hypertension within areas in which the vascular endothelium is injured as a consequence of the hypertensive process. (Adapted from reference 30).

associated with a variety of adhesion and adhesion-related molecules, including selectins [11], integrins and chemokines that are also stimulated by hyperlipidemia [12,13,14]. Ang II may be a significant stimulus for both the recruitment and sub-endothelial infiltration of monocytes and their transformation into macrophage foam cells in early atherosclerosis. Figures 6 and 7 illustrate Ang II AT_1 receptor-mediated inflammatory responses in the transgenic m(ren2)27 rat, a model with an inherently activated vascular RAS. Whether hyperlipidemia- and hyperglycemia-induced monocyte recruitment mechanisms are directly related to RAS activation in the diabetic kidney is not known, though evidence for interactions between LDL and Ang II in coronary arteries suggests this possibility. Deposition of oxidized LDL within the vascular wall thought to initiate fatty streak lesions is stimulated by Ang II [15,16], and Ang II-modified LDL is taken up by macrophage scavenger receptors at an enhanced rate compared to native LDL. Ang II increases macrophage lipoxygenase activity via AT_1 receptor-mediated mechanisms, which increases the ability of these cells to generate oxidized LDL [17]. The up-regulation of oxidized LDL endothelial receptor (LOX-1) gene expression and increased uptake of oxidized LDL by AT_1 receptor activation in human coronary artery endothelial cells are the likely pathways involved in Ang II- and oxidized LDL-mediated decreased NO generation and increased lipid peroxidation by these cells [18,19,20]. These findings illustrate the interplay between pro-atherogenic lipoproteins and Ang II AT_1

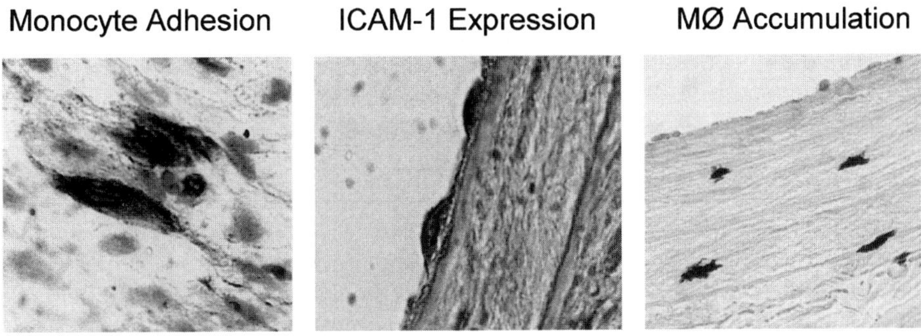

Figure 7. Immunohistochemical demonstration in hypertensive (mRen2)27 transgenic rat aorta of Angiotensin II (Ang II), AT1 receptor mediated monocyte adhesion to endothelium (small, round cell adherent to endothelial cell, left panel), endothelial cell ICAM-1 expression (dark—staining cells adjacent to lumen, middle panel), and macrophage accumulation within media (dark—staining cells, right panel) suggests vascular renin-angiotensin system mediated inflammation (adapted from reference 30 and unpublished data from the same authors).

receptor-mediated pro-inflammatory pathways within the vascular wall and suggest that commonalities to early diabetic nephropathy may employ the same or similar mechanisms.

ANGIOTENSIN II IN THE DIABETIC KIDNEY

Accumulating evidence suggests that components of the intrarenal RAS are selectively activated in the diabetic kidney as they are in the coronary circulation [21]. Increased intrarenal angiotensinogen expression, and redistribution of ACE protein has been shown in both rats and humans. Activation of a local RAS in the diabetic kidney could lead to increased concentrations of Ang II in the region of the glomerulus and/or proximal tubule. Activation of mesangial cell AT_1 receptors induces a contractile response and enhanced expression of glomerular MCP-1. Mesangial cell protein synthesis is also stimulated by AT_1 receptors, with enhanced production of ECM and elaboration of tumor growth factor (TGF)-β1. In addition, mesangial cell production of such autocrine growth factors as endothelin, interleukin-6, and platelet-derived growth factor is stimulated by Ang II, which may contribute to a proliferative response. In human mesangial cells, AT_1 receptors were linked to vascular permeability factor/vascular endothelial growth factor production, suggesting a mechanism by which Ang II might contribute to increased capillary permeability and proteinuria in glomerular diseases. Activation of mesangial cell AT_1 receptors is also associated with decreased degradation of matrix through the inhibition of tissue metalloproteinases and enhanced production of plasminogen activator inhibitor. AT_1 receptors have also been detected on cells of the macula densa and in both the cortical collecting duct and inner medullary collecting duct. These effects could therefore be involved in mediating progressive fibrosis diabetic nephropathy.

Glucose-induced activation of the intrarenal RAS may in part explain some of the impact of hyperglycemia on the initiation and progression of diabetic nephropathy. While the diabetic kidney showed marked decreases in AT_1 receptor density, the intrarenal response to Ang II was reported to increase in diabetic rats. This enhanced responsiveness is in agreement with the Ang II-mediated accumulation of ECM in the diabetic kidney. This apparent contradiction may be explained by considering the nature of the renal RAS and the morphological changes that occur in early untreated diabetes. First, AT_1 receptors are present at various densities throughout the nephron as well as in the glomerular mesangial cells. It is therefore quite possible that differential regulation occurs within the kidneys, although the overall changes show up as a downregulation in radioreceptor assays of membranes from whole kidney. The intrarenal RAS and the production of Ang II may be stimulated in the diabetic rat resulting in greater activity, in spite of lower receptor density. It is known that the greatest sensitivity to the vascular effects of Ang II is found in the kidney, and that infusion of low doses of Ang II that do not affect systemic blood pressure can induce a substantial constriction of renal vessels resulting in a decline in renal blood flow, and an anti-natriuresis. Hyperglycemia tends to blunt these responses, resulting in less impressive, although still significant, changes from baseline. This observation is also consistent with a glucose-mediated increase in intrarenal RAS activity in that higher intrarenal Ang II levels may be expected to cause refractoriness to exogenous Ang II by down regulating angiotensin receptors. The mechanism whereby increased glucose can activate the RAS is unknown, though recent studies suggest that hyperglycemia can modulate expression of the renal angiotensinogen gene in vivo. It is therefore possible that hyperglycemia can activate the renal RAS through molecular rather than hemodynamic or physiologic mechanisms.

Because there is now convincing evidence for adult kidney AT_2 receptor expression and these receptors are linked to increased intrarenal NO production, it is possible to speculate that some of the beneficial effects of AT_1-receptor antagonism in diabetic nephropathy may relate to unopposed activation of intrarenal AT_2 receptors [22]. Despite the possibility of increased local production of Ang II, several studies have determined suppression of AT_1-receptor mRNA or protein expression in the diabetic kidney. A number of studies have demonstrated a downregulation of glomerular and tubular AT_1 receptors in early diabetes. Nonetheless, the importance of AT_1 receptor activation in mediating progressive diabetic glomerulosclerosis is suggested by studies in experimental diabetes in which AT_1 receptor blockade significantly reduced proteinuria and inhibited development of glomerulosclerosis. In glomerular endothelial cells, AT_2 receptors stimulate expression of the chemokine regulated on activation of normal T cells expressed and secreted (RANTES), which may contribute to recruitment of monocytes and macrophages in glomerular inflammation. The effects of glucose and Ang II on mesangial matrix metabolism may be mediated by TGF-β1 since exposure of mesangial cells to glucose or Ang II increases TGF-beta expression and secretion. Their effects on matrix metabolism were blocked by anti-TGF-beta antibody or ARBs, which also prevents the glucose-induced increment in TGF-beta secretion. Taken together, these findings support the hypothesis that the high-glucose milieu of diabetes increases Ang II production by renal, and especially, mesangial cells, which results in stimulation of TGF-β1 secretion, leading to increased synthesis and decreased degradation of matrix proteins, thus producing matrix accumulation. This may be an important mechanism linking hyperglycemia and Ang II in the pathogenesis of diabetic nephropathy.

CLINICAL APPLICABILITY OF ARBS IN DIABETIC NEPHROPATHY

Diabetic nephropathy is responsible for over 40% of all patients requiring renal replacement therapy in the U.S. and is the second most common cause of renal failure in Europe, carrying with it considerable excess cardiovascular mortality. There is clinical evidence that ARBs might convey protection against diabetic nephropathy since treatment by ACE inhibition in type 1 diabetic patients with advanced nephropathy reduced the risk of end-stage renal failure or death by 50% over a 3 year period. These effects are thought to be due to an ACE inhibitor-specific renoprotective action, which appears, at least in part, to be independent of blood pressure control. ACE inhibitors also reduced the risk of progression from microalbuminuria to overt nephropathy in type 1 diabetic patients, an effect that was also partly independent of BP reduction. A recent study in hypertensive type 1 diabetic patients with diabetic nephropathy showed that AT_1 receptor blockade was associated with decreased proteinuria presumably related to reduce glomerular capillary filtration pressure [1]. The same investigators further showed that serum levels of VCAM-1 and E-selectin were reduced compared to placebo-treated controls, suggesting that ARBs may provide additional protection against the inflammatory response related to Ang II production in diabetic kidneys [23]. Although the majority of studies indicate a downregulation of intrarenal AT_1 receptors, a concurrent reduction in AT_2 receptor expression might result in a net augmentation of AT_1 mediated signal transduction. It is conceivable that in diabetic nephropathy, the balance between AT_1 and AT_2 receptor signaling pathways determines the rate of disease progression. This hypothesis will require validation in both in vitro models involving renal cells in culture and in vivo studies of experimental animals using AT_1 and AT_2 antagonists. In addition, it will be of interest to determine the effect of selective activation of AT_2 receptors with specific agonists on the progression of diabetic nephropathy.

SUMMARY

It is increasingly evident that dyslipidemia evoke human coronary atherosclerosis through the oxidative, inflammatory and proliferative actions of Ang II (Fig. 8). Studies in vitro and in models of dietary and genetic hypercholesteremia demonstrated that angiotensin II modifies atherogenesis at multiple points beginning as early as fatty streak formation. Evidence indicates that angiotensin II contributes to atherogenesis at both transcriptional and translational levels by up regulating adhesion molecule mRNA and protein synthesis. Measurements of components of the

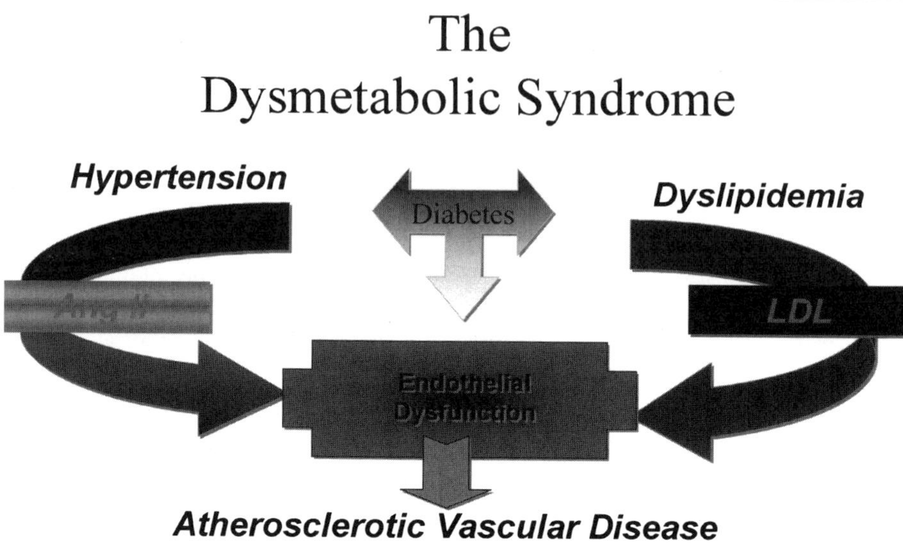

Figure 8. Diagrammatic view of the interaction between angiotensin II (Ang II), oxidize LDL (LDL) and hyperglycemia as the mechanisms which impinging on vascular endothelium begin the process of atherosclerotic vascular disease.

RAS in plasma have suggested suppression of this system in diabetes mellitus, though there is increasing evidence for activation of local RAS in the kidney. In the proximal tubule, there is evidence for upregulation of renin and angiotensinogen expression. Within the glomerulus, an increase in ACE level was reported in diabetes, as have direct effects of high extracellular glucose levels on mesangial cell expression of RAS components. Despite the possibility of increased local production of Ang II, several studies showed suppressed AT_1 receptor mRNA or protein expression in the diabetic kidney. Because AT_1 receptor blockade exerts beneficial effects on the progression of diabetic nephropathy, this indicates that cellular signaling pathways for kidney AT_1 receptors may be amplified. The recent demonstration of Ang II AT_2 receptors in the adult kidney and their potential to oppose the vasoconstrictive, anti-natriuretic, and pro-fibrotic properties of AT_1 receptors suggests that the balance of intrarenal AT_1 and AT_2 receptors may be important in determining the cellular responses to Ang II in diabetic nephropathy.

The coexistence of hypercholesterolemia and diabetes dramatically and synergistically increases the risk of microvascular and macrovascular complications. Perhaps most important among these is the increased risk of cardiovascular events in this patient population. Whereas the complications of type 1 diabetes mellitus are mostly microvascular, patients with type 2 diabetes mellitus are more susceptible to acceleration of atherosclerosis; the most important macrovascular complication, coronary artery disease, is responsible for about half of the deaths in these patients. While the classic risk factors of high cholesterol levels and hyperglycemia are important in the pathogenesis of coronary artery disease their mechanisms of action are not fully explained. The coexistence of type 2 diabetes mellitus and hypercholesterolemia may be related to endothelial dysfunction, which has been demonstrated in patients who have these conditions. Endothelial dysfunction and injury begin a cascade of events leading to the formation of fatty streaks, atherosclerotic plaque, and glomerulosclerosis. While the base of information regarding ARBs in high-risk patients with diabetes and hypercholesterolemia is lacking, preclinical and pilot trial data suggest that the ARBs should be reno- and vasculo-protective in these patients.

A single unifying mechanism of increased production of ROS by Ang II may serve as a causal link between hyperglycemia and hypercholesterolemia and many of the major pathways responsible for atherogenic and diabetic pathologies. Several lines of evidence suggest a crucial role for Ang II-mediated oxidative stress and in the pathogenesis of hyperglycemia- and hypercholesterolemia-associated endothelial dysfunction. Endothelial dysfunction in these scenarios may be due to impaired NO synthesis and/or inactivation of endothelium-derived NO by ROS [24]. That Ang II plays an important role in the development of atherosclerosis and glomerulosclerosis is supported by numerous studies indicating that ARBs retard the progression of these pathologies in both experimental animal models and humans [7,25–28]. Results of these studies suggest that hypercholesterolemia and hyperglycemia can induce a proinflammatory response within coronary arteries and the kidney glomerulus, involving production of well-described macrophage chemotactic and adhesion molecules, which results in macrophage recruitment and the development of acute and chronic injury. Glomerular macrophage recruitment in experimental diabetes was via Ang II-stimulated MCP-1 expression, suggesting that the RAS is an important regulator of local MCP-1 expression, and strongly implicating macrophage recruitment and activation in the pathogenesis of early diabetic glomerular injury. Diabetes-associated vascular complications may involve an activation of the NF-κB by hyperglycemia. NF-κB activation is also related to AT_1 receptor-mediated pathways, and is believed to be dependent on activation of the Rho family of GTPases [29]. Preincubation of VSMC with insulin doubled NF-κB transactivation by Ang II and hyperglycemia, suggesting a potential mechanism for crosstalk between the RAS and hyperglycemia. Taken together, these data suggest that activation of the RAS is a mechanism for the initiation and progression of inflammatory cell infiltration found in early changes common to both hypercholesterolemia and hyperglycemia. Therapeutic blockade of Ang II AT_1 receptors in diabetic and hypercholesterolemic humans by ARBs, with concomitant elevation in plasma and tissue Ang II levels, may provide vascular and renal protection not only by reducing AT_1 receptor-mediated pro-oxidative effects, but also by unopposed AT2 receptor stimulation.

REFERENCES

1. Andersen S, Tarnow L, Rossing P, Hansen BV, Parving H-H. 2000. Renoprotective effects of angiotensin II receptor blockade in type 1 diabetic patients with diabetic nephropathy. Kidney International 57:601–606.

2. Dzau VJ. 2001. Tissue angiotensin and pathobiology of vascular disease: a unifying hypothesis. Hypertension 37:1047–1052.
3. Strawn WB, Dean RH, Ferrario CM. 2000. Novel mechanisms linking angiotensin II and early atherogenesis. J. Renin-Angiotensin-Aldosterone System 1:11–17.
4. Strawn WB, Chappell MC, Dean RH, Kivlighn S, Ferrario CM. 2000. Inhibition of early atherogenesis by losartan in monkeys with diet-induced hypercholesterolemia. Circulation 101:1586–1593.
5. de Las H, Aragoncillo P, Maeso R, Vazquez-Perez S, Navarro-Cid J, DeGasparo M, Mann J, Ruilope LM, Cachofeiro V, Lahera V. 1999. AT(1) receptor antagonism reduces endothelial dysfunction and intimal thickening in atherosclerotic rabbits. Hypertension 34:969–975.
6. Ferrario CM, Deitch JS, Dean RH, Strawn WB. 1996. Hypertension and atherosclerosis: a mechanistic understanding of disease progression. Cardiovasc Risk Factors 6:1–12.
7. Fukuhara M, Geary RL, Diz DI, Gallagher PE, Wilson JA, Glazier SS, Dean RH, Ferrario CM. 2000. Angiotensin-converting enzyme expression in human carotid artery atherosclerosis. Hypertension 35:353–359.
8. Hilgers KF, Mann JFE. 1997. Role of angiotensin II in glomerular injury—lessons from experimental and clinical studies. Kidney &. Blood Pressure Research 19:254–262.
9. Kim S, Iwao H. 2000.—Molecular and cellular mechanisms of angiotensin II-mediated cardiovascular and renal diseases. Pharmacological Reviews 52:11–34.
10. Dominguez JH, Tang N, Xu W, Evan AP, Siakotos AN, Agarwal R, Walsh J, Deeg M, Pratt JH, March KL, Monnier VM, Weiss MF, Baynes JW, Peterson R. 1999. Studies of renal injury III: lipid-induced nephropathy in type II diabetes. Kidney International 57:92–104.
11. Grafe M, Auch-Schwelk W, Zakrzewicz A, Regitz-Zagrosek V, Bartsch P, Graf K, Loebe M, Gaehtgens P, Fleck E. 1997.—Angiotensin II-induced leukocyte adhesion on human coronary endothelial cells is mediated by E-selectin. Circ Res 81:804–811.
12. Devaraj S, Jialal I. 2000.—Low-density lipoprotein postsecretory modification, monocyte function, and circulating adhesion molecules in type 2 diabetic patients with and without macrovascular complications: the effect of alpha-tocopherol supplementation. Circulation Jul 11;102(2):191–196.
13. Frostegard J, Wu R, Haegerstrand A, Patarroyo M, Lefvert AK, Nilsson J. 1993.—Mononuclear leukocytes exposed to oxidized low density lipoprotein secrete a factor that stimulates endothelial cells to express adhesion molecules. Atherosclerosis 103:213–219.
14. Fuhrman B, Judith O, Keidar S, Ben-Yaish L, Kaplan M, Aviram M. 1997.—Increased uptake of LDL by oxidized macrophages is the result of an initial enhanced LDL receptor activity and of a further progressive oxidation of LDL. Free Radical Biology & Medicine 23:34–46.
15. Keidar S, Attias J, Heinrich R, Coleman R, Aviram M. 1999.—Angiotensin II atherogenicity in apolipoprotein E deficient mice is associated with increased cellular cholesterol biosynthesis. Atherosclerosis 146:249–257.
16. Keidar S, Attias J, Smith J, Breslow J, Hayek T. 1997. The angiotensin-II receptor antagonist, losartan, inhibits LDL lipid peroxidation and atherosclerosis in apolipoprotein E-deficient mice. Biochem Biophys Res Comm 236:622–625.
17. Wen Y, Scott Y, Liu Y, Gonzales N, Nadler J. 1997. Evidence that angiotensin II and lipoxygenase products activate c-Jun NH_2-terminal kinase. Circ Res 81:651–655.
18. Nickenig G, Sachindis A, Michaelsen F, Böhm M, Seewald S, Vetter H. 1997. Upregulation of vascular angiotensin II receptor gene expression by low-density lipoprotein in vascular smooth muscle cells. Circulation 95:473–478.
19. Nickenig G, Jung O, Strehlow K, Zolk O, Linz W, Schölkens BA, Böhm M. 1997. Hypercholesterolemia is associated with enhanced angiotensin AT_1-receptor expression. Am J Physiol 272:H2701–H2707.
20. Li D, Saldeen T, Romeo F, Mehta JL. 2000. Oxidized LDL upregulates angiotensin II type 1 receptor expression in cultures human coronary artery endothelial cells. Circulation 102:1970.
21. Burns, KD. 2000. Angiotensin II and its receptors in the diabetic kidney. American Journal of Kidney Diseases 36:449–467.
22. Wehbi GJ, Zimpelmann J, Carey RM, Levine DZ, Burns KD. 2001. Early streptozotocon-diabetes mellitus downregulates rat kidney AT2 receptors. Am J of Renal Physiol 280:F254–F265.
23. Andersen S, Schalkwijk CG, Stehouwer CDA, Parving H-H. 2000. Angiotensin II blockade is associated with decreased plasma leukocyte adhesion molecule levels in diabetic nephropathy. Diabetes Care 23:1031–1032.
24. Harrison DG. 1994. Endothelial dysfunction in atherosclerosis. Basic Res Cardiol 89:87–102.
25. Aberg G, Ferrer P. 1990. Effects of captopril on atherosclerosis in cynomolgus monkeys. J Cardiovasc Pharmacol 15:S65l–S72.

26. Beisiegel U, St. Clair R. 1996. An emerging understanding of the interactions of plasma lipoproteins with the arterial wall that leads to the development of atherosclerosis. Curr Op Lipid 7:265–268.
27. Cheng JWM, Ngo MN. 1997. Current perspective on the use of angiotensin-converting enzyme inhibitors in the management of coronary (atherosclerotic) artery disease. Ann Pharmacotherapy 31:1499–1506.
28. Fennessy PA, Campbell JH, Mendelsohn FAO, Campbell GR. 1996. Angiotensin-converting enzyme inhibitors and atherosclerosis: Relevance of animal models to human disease. Clin Exp Pharmacol Physiol 23:S30–S32.
29. Thurberg BL, Collins T. 1998. The nuclear factor-kB/inhibitor of kappa B autoregulatory system and atherosclerosis. Curr Op Lipid 9:387–396.
30. Strawn WB, Gallagher PE, Tallant EA, Ganten D, Ferrario CM. 1999. Angiotensin II A_1-receptor blockade inhibits monocyte activation and adherence in transgenic (mRen2)27 rats. J Cardio Pharma 33:341–351.

G.N. Pierce, M. Nagano, P. Zahradka, and N.S. Dhalla (eds.).
ATHEROSCLEROSIS, HYPERTENSION AND DIABETES. Copyright © 2003.
Kluwer Academic Publishers. Boston.

BASIC AND CLINICAL RESULTS OF NEW STATIN: PITAVASTATIN

PROF. YASUSHI SAITO

Department of Clinical Cell Biology Graduate School of Medicine, Chiba University, 1-8-1 Inohana Chuoku Chiba 260-8670 Japan

Summary. Pitavastatin ((+)-monocalcium bis [(3R, 5S, 6E)-7-[2-cyclopropyl-4-(4-fluorophenyl)-3-quinolyl]-3,5-dihydroxy-6-heptenoate] is a new potent HMG-CoA reductase inhibitor. It has been suggested that this agent decreases plasma cholesterol by strongly enhancing the expression of hepatic low density lipoprotein (LDL) receptor and decreases plasma triglycerides (TG) by suppressing the secretion of very low density lipoprotein (VLDL)-TG from the liver. Furthermore, pitavastatin inhibited the accumulation of lipids into macrophages and the intimal thickening. In the Japanese long-term clinical study, its efficacy and safety have been confirmed.

These results suggested that pitavastatin possesses a great potential to suppress atherosclerosis with its potent lipid-lowering effect and additional extrahepatic actions. In addition, pitavastatin was scarcely metabolized with CYP2C9 and CYP2C8 of cytochrome P450 drug metabolizing enzymes. The drug interaction might hardly occur as compared to other statins. Furthermore, in the Japanese long-term clinical study, the usefulness of pitavastatin as a lipid lowering agent has been confirmed, and is expected to launch early.

***Key words*:** Pitavastatin, HMG-CoA reductase inhibitor, LDL-cholesterol, Triglyceride, Cytochrome P450

Address Correspondence to: Prof. Yasushi Saito, Department of Clinical Cell Biology Graduate School of Medicine, Chiba University, 1-8-1 Inohana Chuoku Chiba 260-8670 Japan. Tel: +81 (0)43 226 2092; Fax: +81 (0)43 226 2095
To whom correspondence should be addressed: Mr. Yoshitaka Kuwabara, Mr. Shunji Nakagawa, Kowa Company Ltd., 3-4-14 Nihonbashi-Honcho, Chuo-Ku, Tokyo 103-8433, Japan. Tel: +81 (0)3 3279 7296; Fax: +81 (0)3 3242 2270; e-mail: y-kuwabr@kowa.co.jp, s-nakagw@kowa.co.jp

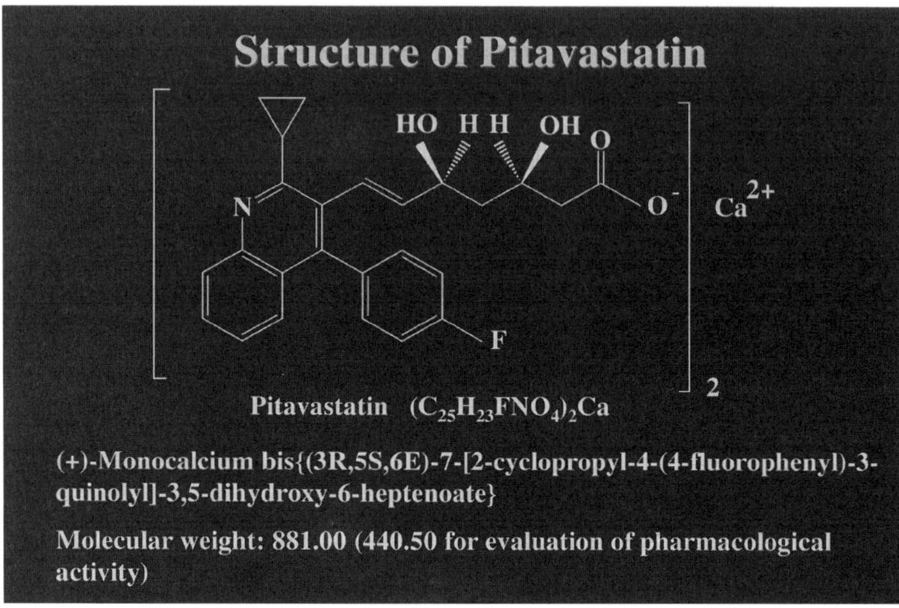

Figure 1. Chemical structure of Pitavastatin.

INTRODUCTION

Low density lipoprotein (LDL)-cholesterol is considered to be the most dangerous factor on the development of coronary heart disease (CHD). Now, the treatment with HMG-CoA reductase inhibitors (statins) is the strong LDL lowering therapy because LDL is dramatically decreased by the inhibition of HMG-CoA reductase, a rate limiting enzyme of the cholesterol biosynthesis pathway. Furthermore, the relationship between the decrease in LDL by statins and the decrease in CHD events has been reported [1,2]. Currently, pravastatin, lovastatin, simvastatin, fluvastatin and atorvastatin are prescribed in the world. However, the patients, whose therapeutic target level of total cholesterol and LDL-cholesterol are not achieved after administration of these drugs alone, remain to be solved. Pitavastatin is being developed as a new "strong statin". In this review, we report the pharmacological and pharmacokinetic characteristics of pitavastatin and the results of Japanese long-term clinical study.

STRUCTURE

Pitavastatin ((+)-monocalcium bis [(3R, 5S, 6E)-7-[2-cyclopropyl-4-(4-fluorophenyl)-3-quinolyl]-3,5-dihydroxy-6-heptenoate] is a new HMG-CoA reductase inhibitor synthesized by Nissan Chemical Industries, Ltd., and is developed by Kowa Company, Ltd. (Fig. 1).

Table 1. Pharmacokinetic properties of Pitavastatin

Absorption	Good (>75%, rat)
T-max	0.5–1.8 h
Plasma $T_{1/2}$	9–12 h
Protein Binding	>99%
Renal Excretion	<2%
Active Metabolites	<2
Cross of BBB	No
CYP Catabolism	Little (2C9, 2C8)

PHARMACOKINETICS

It has been reported that pitavastatin exhibited high bioavailability (BA) in the pharmacokinetic studies in several animals as well as the absorption rate was 75% or more in rats [3] (Table 1). In humans, the time reaching the maximum plasma concentration (Tmax) was within 2 hr after administration, suggesting that the gastrointestinal absorption of pitavastatin was excellent [4].

In addition, the plasma half-life was long in humans (9–12 hr), demonstrating that pitavastatin remained in the body for relatively a long time [4]. It has been reported that pitavastatin was employed to entero-hepatic circulation after it was excreted into bile and reabsorbed in rats and dogs [3,5]. These results supported the relatively long plasma half-life.

The drug tissue distribution studies revealed that pitavastatin was mostly distributed to the liver, but hardly to the other organs [3]. The drug distribution was very little in the brain, suggesting that pitavastatin exhibited no blood brain barrier (BBB) transition. The protein binding ratio of pitavastatin was very high (99% or more). It has also been reported that pitavastatin bound to albumin and acid alpha glycoprotein among plasma proteins [6]. Whereas no mutual interaction in protein binding was found between pitavastatin and various highly protein binding drugs such as warfarin [6].

It has been known that metabolites of atorvastatin are strongly involved in the pharmacological effect. The presence of active metabolites is also reported in pitavastatin, but the generated amount was very low, suggesting less involvement in the pharmacological effect [6]. Although pitavastatin was mildly metabolized by P450 isoforms such as CYP2C9 and CYP2C8, but it has been demonstrated that it was hardly metabolized by cytochrome P450 as compared to other statins [6].

Human urine excretion rate of unchanged pitavastatin was low (less than 2%), and the excretion of metabolites was hardly detected, suggesting that pitavastatin was a drug of fecal excretion type mainly via bile [4].

PHARMACOLOGICAL EFFECTS

Effects on HMG-Co-A reductase

The inhibitory effects of several statins on HMG-Co-A reductase were determined using rat liver microsomes. The results demonstrated that pitavastatin exhibited the

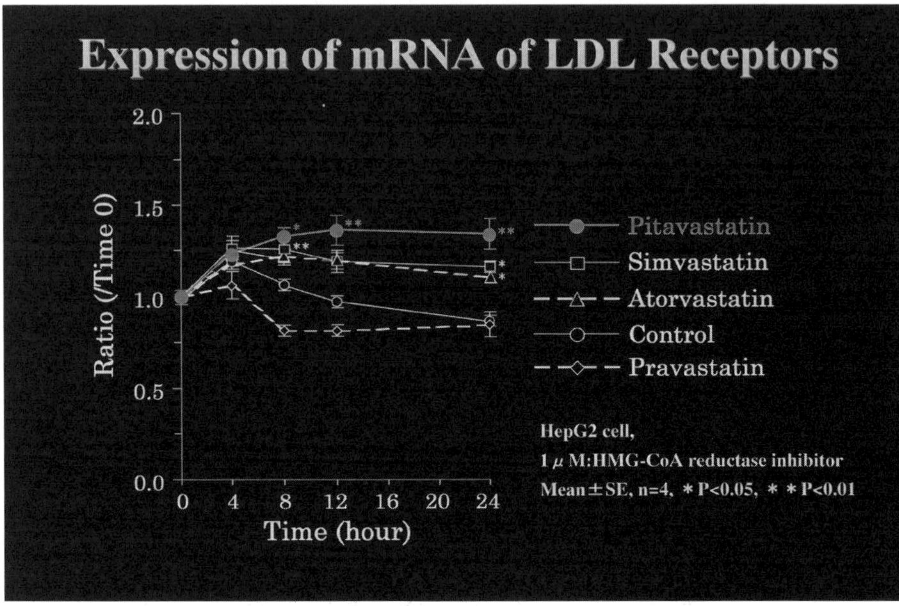

Figure 2. Effect of HMG-CoA reductase inhibitors (1 μM) on the levels of mRNA for LDL receptor in HepG2 cells. Each HMG-CoA reductase inhibitor was added to the medium containing 10% LPDS (Lipid depleted serum), three days after the change into 10% LPDS medium. The induction of mRNA for LDL receptors was measured by RNase protection assay. Results are given as mean ± SE (n = 4). *p < 0.05, **p < 0.01, significantly different.

competitive type inhibition. The IC_{50} value was 1.9 nM. The effect of pitavastatin was 1.8 times, 21 times and 216 times stronger, respectively, than those of atorvastatin, fluvastatin and simvastatin [7].

Effects on LDL receptor

After 1 μM each of pitavastatin or several statins (simvastatin, atorvastatin and fluvastatin) was added to HepG2 cells, LDL receptor mRNA was determined with a ribonuclease protection assay within 24 hr. As a result, the strongest induction of LDL receptor mRNA expression was observed in pitavastatin [8] (Fig. 2). LDL receptor activity was determined by degradation of LDL. HepG2 cells were preincubated with 1 μM each of pitavastatin and several other statins (simvastatin, atorvastatin and fluvastatin) for 24 hr, followed by addition of ^{125}I-LDL. After further incubation, ^{125}I-LDL degradation was measured. LDL degradation was accelerated with all the statins used. However, the acceleration by pitavastatin was the highest, suggesting the strongest enhancement of LDL receptor activity in pitavastatin [8].

LIPID LOWERING EFFECTS

In dogs, pitavastatin dose-dependently decreased blood cholesterol and triglycerides from 0.1 mg/kg. On the other hand, atorvastatin dose-dependently decreased blood

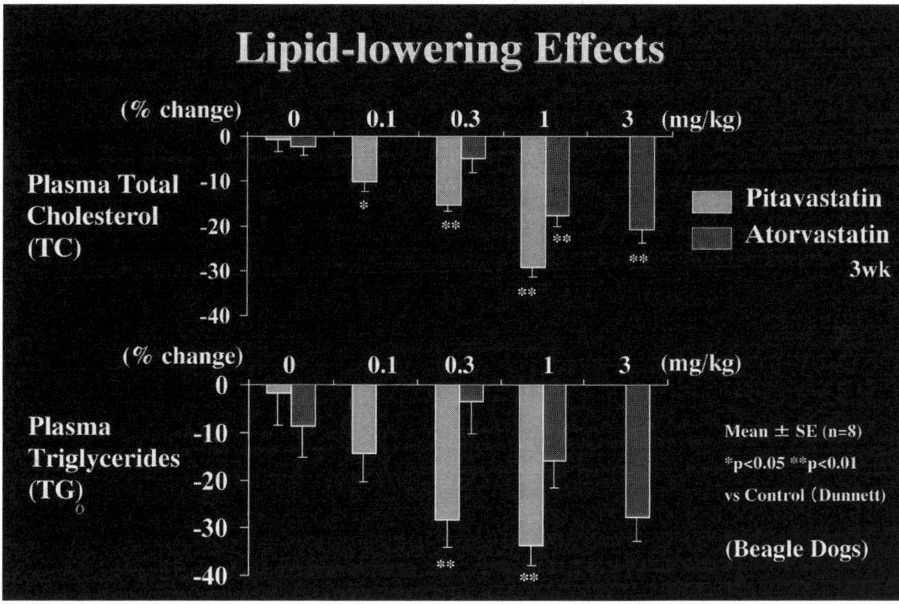

Figure 3. Cholesterol lowering effect of Pitavastatin vs Atorvastatin. Plasma TC and TG were measured after oral administration of pitavastatin or atorvastatin to dogs for 3 weeks. Data represent the mean ± SE (n = 8). *p < 0.05, **p < 0.01, significantly different.

cholesterol and triglycerides from 1 mg/kg (Fig. 3). These results suggested a strong blood lipid lowering effect of pitavastatin, and were considered to be based on the strong enhancement effect on LDL receptor of pitavastatin. In addition, in HepG2 cells, the addition of pitavastatin decreased the intracellular cholesteryl ester content and apo B secretion [9]. Furthermore, in the perfusion system of guinea pig liver after pitavastatin was administered at 3 mg/kg for 2 weeks, the secretion of VLDL-TG and VLDL-apo B was decreased [10] (Fig. 4). These results suggested that the plasma TG lowering effect of pitavastatin was attributed to the suppression ofVLDL-TG secretion.

ANTI-ATHEROSCLEROSIS EFFECT

The accumulation of lipids by pitavastatin was investigated in RAW macrophages treated with oxidized LDL [11]. Pitavastatin dose-dependently inhibited the accumulation of cholesteryl ester. The effect of pitavastatin was 3 times stronger than that of simvastatin and 39 times stronger than that of atorvastatin, when compared with IC_{50} (pitavastatin; 56.3 nM). The effect was eliminated by mevalonic acid, suggesting that it was the effect based on the inhibition of HMG-CoA reductase. In the carotid artery scraping model in rabbits, the carotid artery was scrapped at 8 days after start of administration of pitavastatin, and it was removed at 21 days after administration. The intima/media ratios were compared at 1 mg/kg

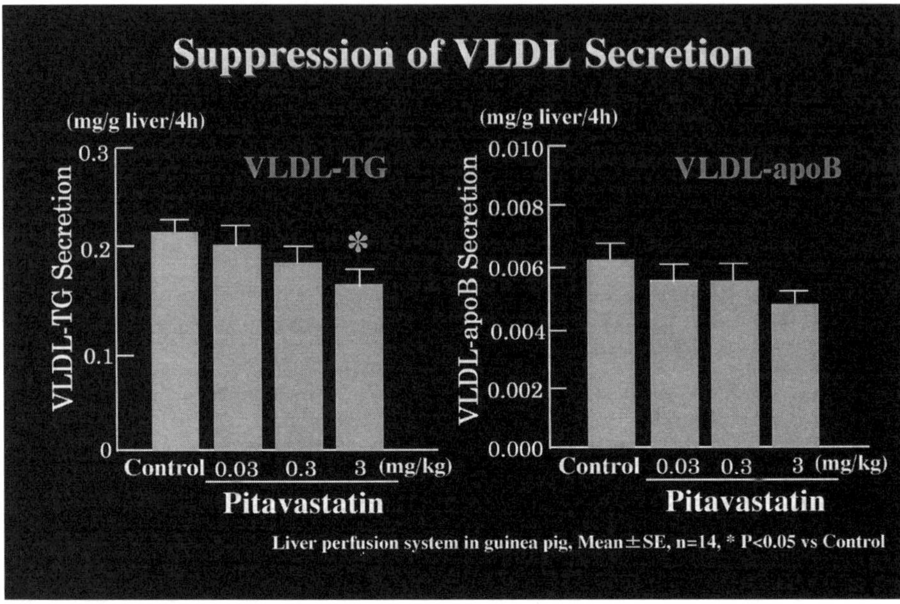

Figure 4. Suppression of VLDL secretion by pitavastatin. The livers were taken for liver perfusion from guinea pigs dosed with pitavastatin 3 mg/kg for 2 weeks. At the end of the liver perfusion, the perfusate was collected and analyzed for VLDL. Data represent the mean ± SE (n = 14). *$p < 0.05$, significantly different.

of pitavastatin, 9.6 mg/kg of pravastatin and 3 mg/kg of simvastatin. As a result, pitavastatin inhibited the accumulation of lipids in macrophages, and inhibited the intimal thickening, suggesting a contribution to the suppression of atherosclerosis [12] (Fig. 5).

CLINICAL STUDY

In order to obtain the information of efficacy and safety after long-term administration of pitavastatin, we conducted a long-term study in Japan for 6 months or longer to 12 months of treatment period.

The subjects were hyperlipemic patients with 220 mg/dl or more of total cholesterol (TC). The administration was started from 2 mg. The doses from 8 weeks were selected from 1, 2 and 4 mg in each patient depending on the TC levels at week 4 (Fig. 6). As a result, the LDL-C levels were significantly decreased from 4 weeks, thereafter continuously and stably changed in the range between −38.7 and −40.9% until 52 weeks.

The triglyceride (TG) levels were significantly decreased in patients with 150 mg/dl or more of TG before administration, thereafter continuously and stably changed in the range between −25.1 and −31.2% until 52 weeks.

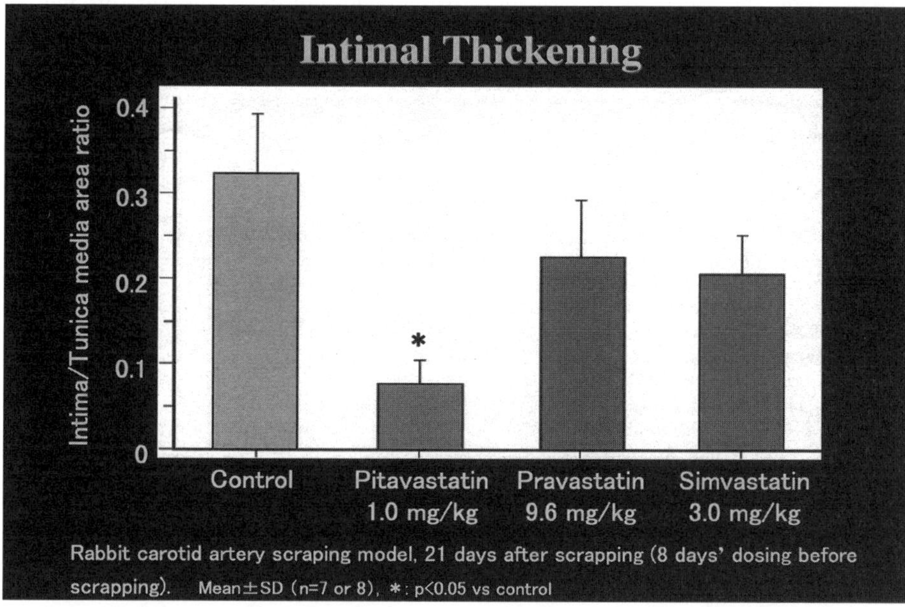

Figure 5. Effect of pitavastatin, pravastatin and simvastatin on the neointimal thickening after balloon injury in rabbits. Data represent the mean ± SD (n = 7 or 8). *p < 0.05, significantly different.

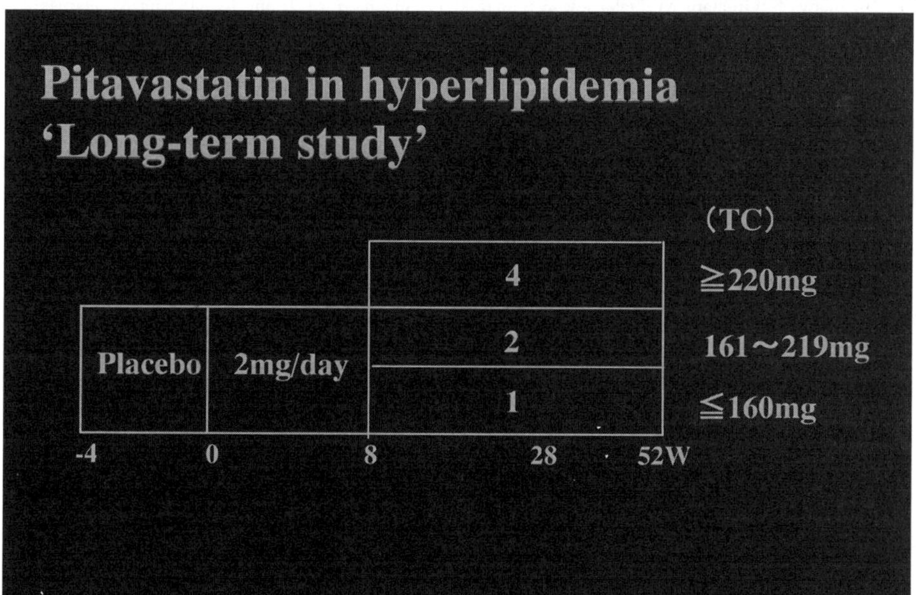

Figure 6. Dosing schedule for long term study. 0–8 W: One 2 mg NK-104 tablet, once a day. After 8 W: Decided based on TC levels at 4 W with reference to the following standards: (1) $161 \leq TC \geq 219$ mg/dL: One 2 mg NK-104 tablet, once a day for maintenance. (2) $TC \geq 220$ mg/dL: Increased to two 2 mg NK-104 tablets, once a day. (3) $TC \leq 160$ mg/dL: Decreased to one 1 mg NK-104 tablet, once a day.

Regarding the safety in 893 Japanese patients administered, the patients with 3 times or more of upper limits of normal ranges of alanine aminotransferase (ALT) and aspartate aminotransferase (AST) were 4 cases (0.4%) and 1 case (0.1%), respectively. The patients with 6 times or more of the upper limit of normal range of creatine kinase (CK) were 3 cases (0.3%).

REFERENCES

1. Shepherd J, Cobbe SM, Ford I, Isles CG, Lorimer AR, MacFarlane PW, Mckillop JH, Packard CJ. 1995. Prevention of coronary heart disease with pravastatin in men with hypercholesteremia. West of Scotland Coronary Prevention Study Group. N Engl J Med 333:1301–1307.
2. Sacks FM, Pfeffer MA, Moye LA, Rouleau JL, Rutherford JD, Cole TG, Brown L, Warnica JW, Arnold JM, Wun CC, Davis BR, Braunwald E. 1996. The effect of pravastatin on coronary events after myocardial infarction in patients with average cholesterol levels. Cholesterol and Recurrent Events Trial Investigators. N Engl J Med 335:1001–1009.
3. Kimata H, Fujino H, Koide T, Yamada Y, Tsunenari Y, Yanagawa Y. 1998. Studies on the metabolic fate of NK-104, a new inhibitor of HMG-CoA Reductase (1): Absorption, distribution, metabolism and excretion in rats. Xenobio Metabol and Dispos 13:484–498.
4. Fujino H, Kojima J, Yamada Y, Kanda H, Kimata H. 1999. Studies on the metabolic fate of NK-104, a new inhibitor of HMG-CoA Reductase (4): Interspecies variation in laboratory animals and humans. Xenobio Metabol and Dispos 14:79–91.
5. Kojima J, Ohshima T, Yoneda M, Sawada H. 2001. Effect of biliary excretion on the pharmacokinetics of pitavastatin (NK-104) in dogs. Xenobio Metabol and Dispos 16:497–502.
6. Fujino H, Yamada I, Kojima J, Hirano M, Matsumoto H, Yoneda M. 1999. Studies on the metabolic fate of NK-104, a new inhibitor of HMG-CoA Reductase (5): In Vitro metabolism and plasma protein binding in animals and human. Xenobio Metabol and Dispos 14:415–424.
7. Aoki T, Nishimura H, Nakagawa S, Kojima J, Suzuki H, Tamaki T, Saito Y. 1997. Pharmacological profile of a novel synthetic inhibitor of 3-hydroxy-3-methylglutaryl-coenzyme A reductase. Arzneim-Forsch/Drug Res 47:904–909.
8. Morikawa S, Umetani M, Nakagawa S, Yamazaki H, Suganami H, Inoue K, Kitahara M, Hamakubo T, Kodama T, Saito Y. 2000. The relative induction of mRNA for HMG-CoA reductase and LDL receptor by five different HMG-CoA reductase inhibitors in cultured human cells. J Atheroscler Thromb 7:138–144.
9. Yanagita T, Hara E, Yotsumoto H, Rahman SM, Han SY, Cha JY, Yamamoto K. 1999. NK-104, a potent new 3-hydroxy-3-methylglutaryl coenzyme A reductase inhibitor, enhances posttranslational catabolism of apolipoprotein B-100 and inhibits secretion of apolipoprotein B-100 and triacylglycerols from HepG2 cells. Cur Ther Res 60:423–434.
10. Suzuki H, Aoki T, Tamaki T, Sato F, Kitahara M, Saito Y. 1999. Hypolipidemic effect of NK-104, a potent HMG-CoA reductase inhibitor, in guinea pigs. Atherosclerosis 146:259–270.
11. Kitahara M, Kanaki T, Tamaki T, Saito Y. 2000. Itavastatin inhibits modified LDL-induced foam cell formation and scavenger pathway, mediated with Rab, Rho and Rac small G-protein, in RAW264.7 macrophages. Atherosclerosis 151:295. Abstract.
12. Kitahara M, Kanaki T, Toyoda K, Miyakoshi C, Tanaka S, Tamaki T, Saito Y. 1998. NK-104, a newly developed HMG-CoA reductase inhibitor, suppresses neointimal thickening by inhibiting smooth muscle cell growth and fibronectin production in balloon-injured rabbit carotid artery. Jpn J Pharmacol 77:117–128.

G.N. Pierce, M. Nagano, P. Zahradka, and N.S. Dhalla (eds.).
ATHEROSCLEROSIS, HYPERTENSION AND DIABETES. Copyright © 2003.
Kluwer Academic Publishers. Boston.

REDUCING CARDIOVASCULAR RISK WITH HMG CoA REDUCTASE INHIBITORS, POTENTIAL CONTRIBUTION FROM PLATELETS

STEPHEN HENRY,[1] PER L. KATZMAN,[2] RATNA BOSE,[1] YVETTE PERRY,[1] SHAUN WALKER,[1] DAVID MYMIN,[1] and PETER BOLLI[3]

[1] *Faculty of Medicine, University of Manitoba, Winnipeg, Canada;* [2] *Department of Medicine, Central Hospital, Helsingborg, Sweden;* [3] *Niagara Clinical Teaching and Research Centre, St. Catharines, Canada*

Summary. Platelets, when activated contribute to the development of atherosclerosis through releasing growth promoting, vasoconstricting, and pro-aggregating substances. The end product is atherosclerotic plaque formation and thrombus formation, an important cause of fatal and morbid cardiac events. HMG CoA reductase inhibitors have been shown to reduce fatal and morbid cardiovascular events significantly. The objective of the present study was to determine whether treatment with the HMG CoA reductase inhibitor simvastatin would reduce the increased state of platelet activation in hyperlipidemic patients and thereby contribute to the beneficial effect of HMG CoA reductase inhibitors.

Fasting blood was drawn from 9 patients with dyslipidemia and 9 age and sex matched normolipidemic control subjects. Platelet activation was determined by measuring the intracellular free calcium concentration ($[Ca^{2+}]_i$) under basal conditions and following stimulation with thrombin. These measurements were done in hyperlipidemic patients before and after treatment with simvastatin. For controls, platelet activation was determined in age and sex matched normolipidemic subjects.

In nine hyperlipidemic patients basal and thrombin stimulated $[Ca^{2+}]_i$ were significantly higher in the platelets of hyperlipidemic patients than in the platelets of nine normolipidemic controls. Following a three months' treatment with simvastatin at the mean dose 18 mg/day, serum total and LDL cholesterol fell significantly but remained significantly above those of the control subjects. Basal and thrombin stimulated $[Ca^{2+}]_i$ decreased significantly following simvastatin treatment. However, compared to the $[Ca^{2+}]_i$ in the platelets of normolipidemic

Correspondence to: Dr. Peter Bolli, Hotel Dieu Health Sciences Hospital, Niagara, Niagara Clinical Teaching and Research Centre, 155 Ontario Street—2C, St. Catharines, Ontario, Canada, L2R 5K3. Telephone: (905) 682-1610 ext. 243; Fax: (905) 641-5218; e-mail: peter.bolli@hdhsc.org

controls, $[Ca^{2+}]_i$ in the treated hyperlipidemic patients decreased significantly below the $[Ca^{2+}]_i$ in the normolipidemic control subjects even though serum total and LDL cholesterol remained above those of the control subjects. There was a direct correlation between the serum LDL/HDL ratio and $[Ca^{2+}]_i$. There was an inverse relationship between serum HDL cholesterol concentration and $[Ca^{2+}]_i$.

Platelets are activated in hyperlipidemic patients, the degree of activation relates directly to the serum LDL concentration and inversely to the serum HDL concentration. Since treatment with simvastatin reduced the degree of platelet activation to below that of normolipidemic controls even though serum total and LDL cholesterol concentrations were still higher than those of the control subjects, indicates that simvastatin reduced platelet activation by mechanisms beyond its' lipid lowering effect. This could contribute to the marked risk reduction for morbid and fatal cardiovascular events observed with HMG CoA reductase inhibitor treatment.

Key words: Hyperlipidemia, Platelets, Simvastatin, Intracellular calcium

INTRODUCTION

Dyslipidemia, in particular abnormally elevated plasma concentrations of low density lipoprotein (LDL) is associated with an increased incidence of cardiovascular events and there is a direct relationship between the plasma level of total and LDL cholesterol and the risk for a cardiovascular event [1]. The pathogenesis of atherosclerosis and the development of the atherosclerotic lesion is now well understood [2]. The initiating factor of the atherosclerotic process is an impairment of the function the endothelial cells caused by the presence of cardiovascular risk factors such as smoking, hypertension, diabetes mellitus and dyslipidemia [2]. In patients with dyslipidemia, endothelial function is impaired [3–5] and lipid lowering treatment has been shown to restore endothelial function [6–9].

There is a close interrelationship between the function of the endothelial cells and platelets [10]. Platelets become activated during the atherosclerotic process and contribute to it by releasing growth promoting and vasoconstrictor substances and by increasing their aggregability, lead to thrombus formation [2,11]. Normally functioning endothelial cells protect against platelet activation in part by their ability to produce nitric oxide [12]. Consequently, impaired endothelial function can lead to platelet activation and eventually aggregation [10]. Thus, enhanced platelet aggregation in patients with hyperlipidemia has been reported [13,14] and plasma lipoproteins were found to influence platelet aggregation in normal healthy subjects [15]. Besides through their interaction with dysfunctional endothelial cells, platelets have been found to be activated by LDL [16–20] particularly in its' oxidized form [21–23]. The mechanism by which platelets could be activated by LDL is through an agonistic effect on the platelet LDL receptor [24,25] which has been suggested to involve the II b/ III a receptor for the binding of oxidized LDL [24] but seems to share it with native LDL. Activation of platelets seems to occur via the phosphatidyl inositol cycle [16].

The purpose of the present study was to examine the state of platelet activation under basal conditions and their reactivity to thrombin in platelets taken from patients with hyperlipidemia before and after lipid lowering therapy and compare the results with platelets from age and sex matched normolipidemic controls. The degree of platelet activation was determined by measuring changes in the $[Ca^{2+}]_i$ in platelets since $[Ca^{2+}]_i$ represents the second messenger for most of the platelet related functions [26].

MATERIAL AND METHODS

Patients and control subjects

Nine hyperlipidemic patients were included. Their fasting total cholesterol was >7 mmol/l and triglycerides <2.8 mmol/l on two separate occasions. All patients had primary Type IIa hyperlipidemia, presumably on a polygenic basis. Secondary causes of dyslipidemia such as diabetes mellitus, hypothyroidism and liver and renal disease were excluded by appropriate laboratory evaluations. Exclusion criteria included hypertension, (diastolic BP >90 mmHg or systolic BP >140 mmHg), familial homozygous hyperlipidemia, clinical evidence of atherosclerotic vascular disease or a history of angina pectoris, myocardial infarction, cerebrovascular accident or intermittent claudication. All patients were non-smokers except for one female who smoked 1–3 cigarettes/day. None of the patients ingested any drugs with known or possible effects on platelet function within 14 days of being studied.

Nine sex matched control subjects of comparable age had a fasting total cholesterol <5.2 mmol/l and triglycerides <2.8 mmol/l. Their blood pressures were <140/90 mmHg measured in the sitting position on 2 separate occasions. They were all non-smokers and did not take any medications that could have a possible effect on platelet function within 14 days of the study. This study was approved by the local Ethics Committee and all patients and controls gave informed consent.

After baseline lipid and platelet studies were done, patients were started on simvastatin 10 mg. given once daily. If after one month's treatment the total cholesterol was not reduced by 10% of its initial value, the dose of simvastatin was increased to 20 mg. once daily. The total treatment time was 3 months following which lipid and platelet studies were repeated.

MEASUREMENT OF LIPID PROFILE

Measurement of total and HDL cholesterol as well as triglycerides were done using routine laboratory techniques at the Department of Clinical Biochemistry, Health Sciences Centre, Winnipeg. Fasting serum LDL cholesterol was calculated according to Friedewald et al. [27]. Body mass index (BMI) was calculated from weight (kg) and height (m) as BMI = kg/m^2.

PLATELET ISOLATION AND MEASUREMENT OF PLATELET INTRACELLULAR FREE CALCIUM CONCENTRATION

After overnight fasting venous blood was drawn into dextrose/citrate tubes (Vacutainer[R]). Platelet-rich plasma (PRP) was obtained after a twenty-minutes centrifugation (120 × g) at 20°C. The PRP was incubated with fura-2/AM (3.85 μM.

30 min. 37°C) and then filtered through a Sepharose 2B-CL column [28,29] equilibrated with elution buffer (145 mMNaCl.5 mM KCl.1 mM Mg SO_4. 0.5 mM NaH_2PO_4. 6 mM glucose and 10 mM HEPES, pH 7.4). Thereafter the platelet suspension was kept a 4°C until measurements were performed [21]. Platelet count was adjusted 4–7 × 10^7 per ml (Coulter Counter). Calcium measurements were determined using a Jasco CA-100 Ca^{2+} analyzer (Jasco Inc., Easton, MD, USA) equipped with a thermostat-controlled cuvette holder (0.5 ml) and a magnetic stirrer (1,000 rpm). Platelet suspension samples (0.5 ml) were placed in the cuvette holder and warmed up to 37°C for 2 min. before $CaCl_2$ was added (final concentration 1 mM). The mixture was then kept at 37°C for a further 3 min. before measurements of $[Ca^{2+}]_i$ were performed. Storage of platelets at 4°C did not influence their reactivity to various agonists when warmed up to 37° prior to the experiments. Previous experiments (unpublished) showed that with platelet storage at 4°C there was a minimal leak of Fura-2 from platelets. Therefore the baseline values were stable and enabled platelet stimulation experiments over a total of 2 h. $[Ca^{2+}]_i$ was calculated using the equation [30]:

$$[Ca^{2+}]_i = K_D \times (R - R_{min}/R_{max} - R) \times \beta,$$

where K_D is the dissociation constant of the Fura-2/Ca^{2+} complex [224 nM at 37°C] [30], R the ratio of fluorescence at excitation wavelengths 340 and 380 nm, with an emission wavelength of 500 nm, R_{max} and R_{min} the ratio of fluorescence at these wavelengths for calcium-saturated and calcium-free fura-2 and β the ratio of fluorescence between calcium-free and calcium-saturated fura-2 at 380 nm. R_{max} was determined using ≥0.5% Triton X-100, and R_{min} by subsequent addition of ≥10 mM EGTA. The intraassay coefficient of variance for basal $[Ca^{2+}]_i$ was 6%. Correction for fura-2 contamination and leak (2.2 ± 0.1% and 0.2 ± 0.3% per hour, respectively) was performed on basal $[Ca^{2+}]_i$ values [31].

Measurements of $[Ca^{2+}]_i$ were performed before and following stimulation with human thrombin, 0.1 u/ml, 0.2 u/ml, 1.0 u/ml (Sigma Chemical Co., St. Louis, MO 2,000 NIH u/mg). Determinations were made in duplicate, and the mean value was used for analysis.

Statistical Analysis

Paired and unpaired student's t tests and linear regression analysis were used when appropriate. A two-tailed p value of <0.05 was considered to indicated statistical significance. All values are expressed as mean ± SEM.

RESULTS

Characteristics of patients and control subjects, effect of simvastatin treatment

Hyperlipidemic patients and control subjects were of comparable age and BMI (Table 1). Pre-treatment total and plasma LDL cholesterol concentrations and LDL/HDL ratio were significantly higher and HDL cholesterol concentration sig-

Table 1. Baseline characteristics and lipid profile of hyperlipidemic patients and normal control subjects. Lipid profile in hyperlipidemic patients before (–simvastatin) and following 3 months' treatment with simvastatin (+simvastatin) (mean dose 18/mg/day)

		Patients	
	Controls	–Simvastatin	+Simvastatin
Sex (M/F)	2/7	2/7	
Age	44.7 ± 4	49.3 ± 5	
BMI	21.2 ± 1.6	25.2 ± 4.7	
Total CHOL	4.7 ± .2	8.3 ± .5★★	6.4 ± .03*#
HDL-CHOL	1.47 ± .1	1.31 ± 0.9★	1.32 ± .09
TRIGLYC	1.5 ± .2	2.0 ± .3	2.0 ± .3
LDL-CHOL	2.5 ± .2	6.0 ± .4★★	4.1 ± .3**##
LDL/HDL	2.0 ± .5	4.8 ± .4★	3.2 ± .3*#

★p < .005 vs. controls.
★★p < .001 vs controls.
*p < .005 vs—simvastatin.
**p < .001 vs—simvastatin.
#p < 0.05 vs controls.
##p < 0.01 vs controls.
Mean values ± SEM.
BMI = body mass index, CHOL = cholesterol, HDL = high density lipoprotein, LDL = low density lipoprotein, TRIGLYC = triglyerides.

nificantly lower in patients compared to controls. Following treatment with simvastatin, mean dose 18 mg./day for three months, there was a significant decrease in total and LDL plasma cholesterol concentrations as well as in the LDL/HDL ratio. However, values following simvastatin treatment remained significantly higher than in the control subjects. Plasma HDL and triglycerides concentrations remained unchanged (Table 1).

Basal and thrombin-stimulated intra-cellular free calcium concentration in platelets

Basal platelet $[Ca^{2+}]_i$ was higher in the untreated hyperlipidemic patients compared to the platelets from normal control subjects (48 ± 5 nM vs. 37 ± 5 nM; $p < 0.01$). Following simvastatin treatment $[Ca^{2+}]_i$ fell to 37 ± 5 nM; $p = 0.11$ (Fig. 1).

Stimulation of platelets with human thrombin at a dose of 0.2 u/ml resulted in a greater rise in $[Ca^{2+}]_i$ in the platelets from untreated patients as compared to control subjects. Treatment with simvastatin reduced thrombin-stimulated $[Ca^{2+}]_i$ in patients significantly and to below the $[Ca^{2+}]_i$ measured in normal controls (Fig. 1). The $[Ca^{2+}]_i$ in response to 0.1 u/ml of thrombin was also higher in untreated hyperlipidemic patients (546 ± 44 nM) than in controls (360 ± 56 nM, $p < 0.005$). Following simvastatin treatment $[Ca^{2+}]_i$ fell to 358 ± 44 nM; $p < 0.02$. Similarly the $[Ca^{2+}]_i$ response to thrombin 1.0 u/ml was greater in the untreated hyperlipidemic patients (1,174 ± 168 nM) than in controls (974 ± 168 nM; $p < 0.1$) and again fell to (759 ± 77 nM; $p < 0.05$) following simvastatin treatment.

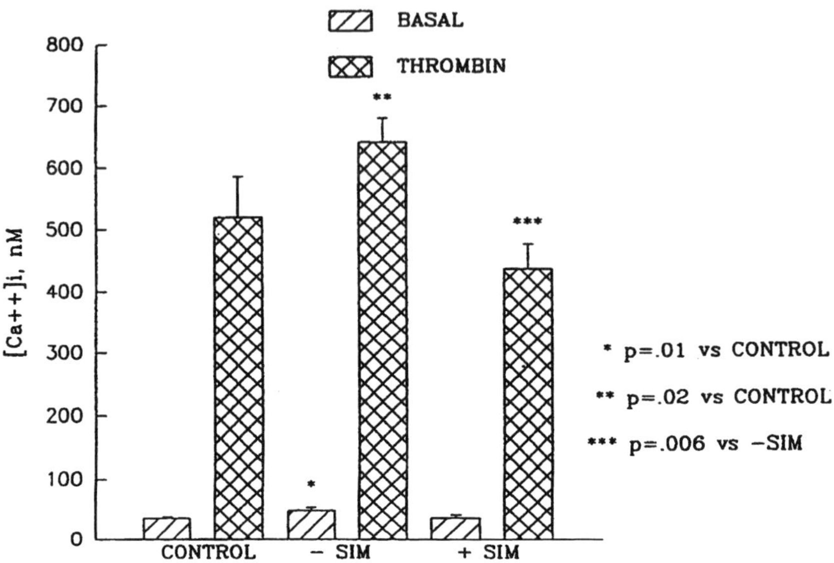

Figure 1. Basal (hatched bars) thrombin-stimulated (0.2 u/ml; (cross hatched bars)) intracellular free calcium concentrations ($[Ca^{2+}]_i$) in platelets from normolipidemic healthy subjects (control) and from hyperlipidemic patients before (–SIM) and after treatment with simvastatin (mean dose 18 mg/day) (+SIM). Mean ± SEM.

Basal as well as the thrombin (0.2 u/ml) stimulated $[Ca^{2+}]$: in platelets of normal control subjects and in the untreated patients correlated directly with the serum LDL/HDL ratio (r = 0.72, r = 0.63, respectively) (Fig. 2) and inversely with the serum HDL concentration (r = 0.59, r = 0.66, respectively) (Fig. 3).

DISCUSSION

The results of the present study show that platelets are in a state of activation and show greater reactivity to an agonist such as thrombin in patients with hyperlipidemia compared to normolipidemic control subjects. This is supported by the direct relationship between serum LDL cholesterol levels (here expressed as LDL/HDL ratio) and the concentration of $[Ca^{2+}]_i$ in platelets. On the other hand, there was an inverse relationship between serum levels of HDL cholesterol and the platelet $[Ca^{2+}]_i$. This parallels the observed effect of elevated serum LDL concentrations and the LDL/HDL ratio on the risk of coronary artery disease and the beneficial effect of a higher serum HDL concentration [1,32]. This also concurs with our findings that the secretion of platelet derived growth factor correlates with $[Ca^{2+}]_i$ [33].

The significant reduction in basal platelet activation and in the reactivity of platelets to thrombin as reflected by a significant decrease in platelet $[Ca^{2+}]_i$ following lipid lowering treatment with simvastatin, also supports the notion that

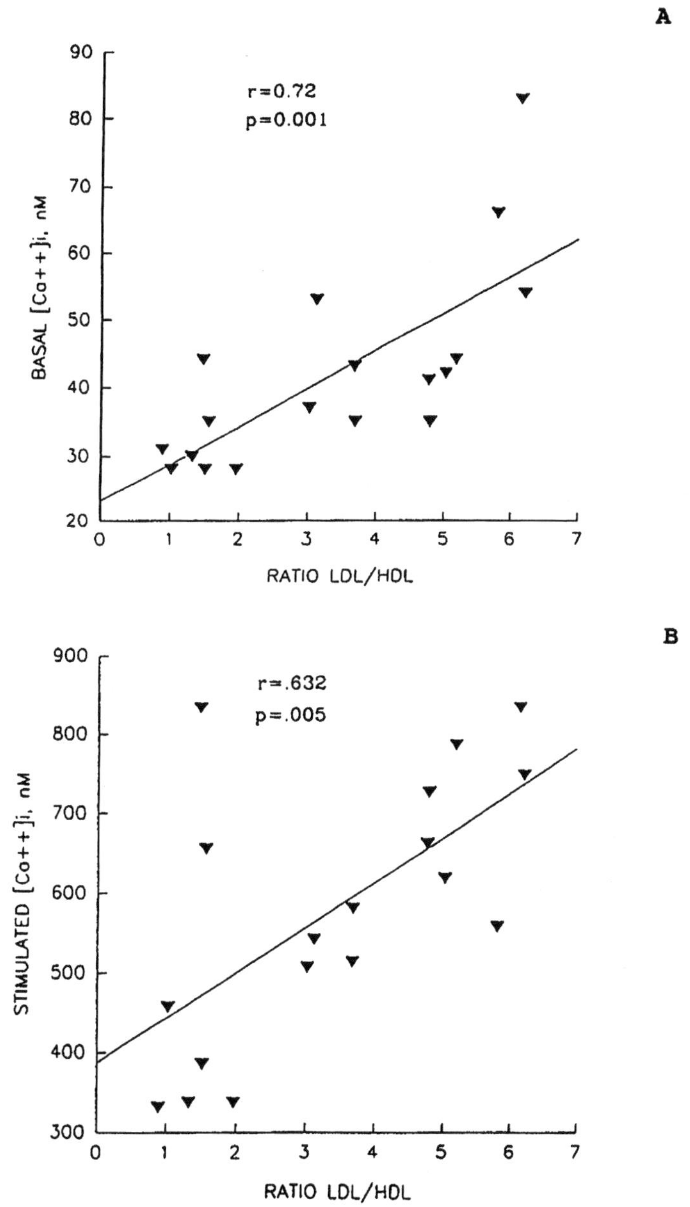

Figure 2. Direct correlation between basal (panel A) and thrombin-stimulated (0.2 u/ml) (panel B) intracellular free calcium concentrations ($[Ca^{2+}]_i$) in platelets from untreated hyperlipidemic patients and normolipidemic healthy controls and their serum LDL/HDL cholesterol ratio.

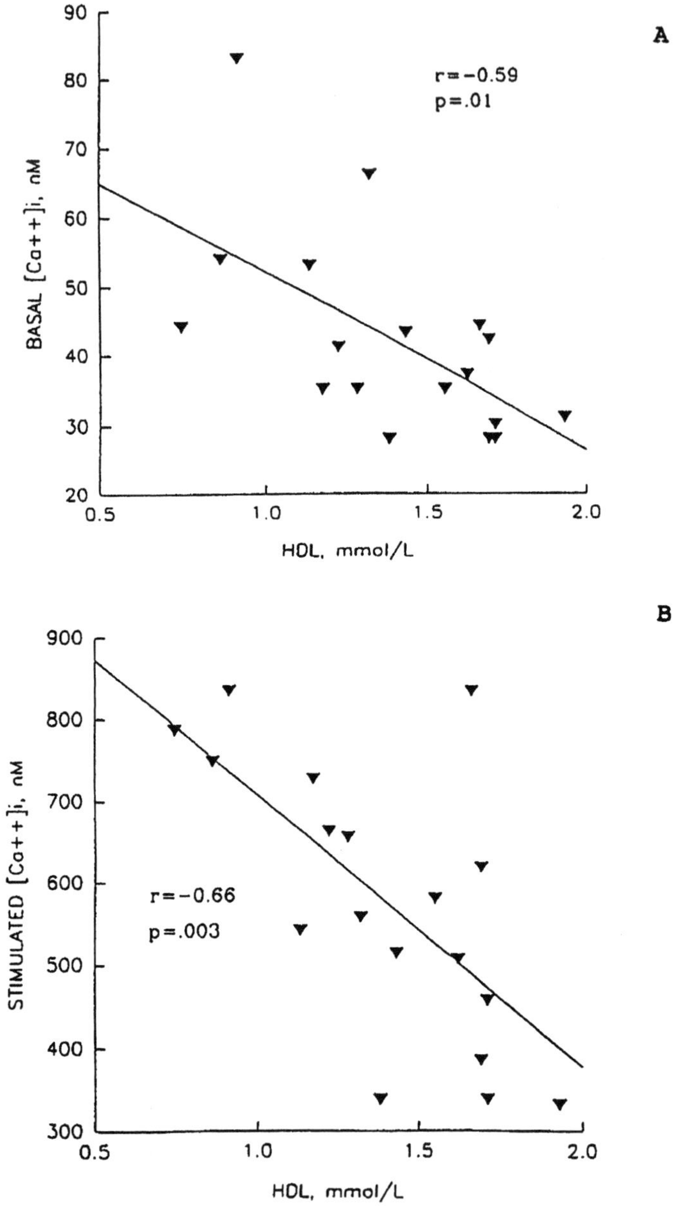

Figure 3. Inverse correlation between basal (panel A) and thrombin-stimulated (0.2 u/ml) (panel B) intracellular free calcium concentrations ($[Ca^{2+}]_i$) in platelets from untreated hyperlipidemic patients and normolipidemic controls and their serum HDL concentrations.

platelets were activated as a result of the elevated serum total and LDL concentrations. This reduction in platelet reactivity could reflect an improvement of endothelial function [6–10] or a lesser agonistic effect of LDL on its' platelet LDL receptor [16,17,21,22] or could be due to a normalization of platelet membrane fluidity as shown following treatment with lovastatin [34] and pravastatin [35]. The inverse correlation of serum HDL cholesterol concentration with platelet $[Ca^{2+}]_i$ could also be consistent with HDL cholesterol inhibiting LDL cholesterol binding to the platelet receptor [16].

Our results therefore, are in agreement with those of Hochgraf et al. [34] who found an increased platelet aggregability to collagen in type II hypercholesterolemic patients as compared to normolipidemic control subjects. Following treatment with lovastatin, the authors found that platelet aggregability was significantly lower in patients than in untreated normal controls although—as in our study—serum cholesterol concentrations remained significantly higher in treated patients than in controls. Our results are also supported by the findings of Lacoste et al. [36] where a lesser thrombus formation was observed when blood from patients following treatment with pravastatin was superfused over a pig aortic media preparation.

This would indicate that these drugs have a marked beneficial effect on platelets in addition to their effect on endothelial cells that occurs independent and beyond that of the degree of the lipid lowering effect [37]. This would help to explain in part the striking magnitude of cardiovascular risk reduction that has been observed in a number of secondary [38,39] and primary [40,41] prevention studies using HMG CoA reductase inhibitors even though there have been only small changes in the extent of plaque reduction in the coronary arteries [42]. It would also explain the observation that statins were able to reduce cardiovascular risk significantly even in patients with minor elevation of serum total and LDL concentrations [43] or when given to patients during unstable angina pectoris or non Q wave myocardial infarctions [44]. This notion is also supported by an improvement in endothelial function of the forearm arterial bed with pravastatin in patients with normal serum total cholesterol concentrations, an effect that appears to have been mediated by nitric oxide [45].

Although our studies were performed with platelets removed from their natural environment, they seem to have maintained their functional characteristics as has also been shown in relation to other clinical conditions such as hypertension [29]. On the other hand, heightened platelet responsiveness during the testing procedure could be a result of "pre-activation" due to platelet isolation procedures that could involve multiple centrifugation steps. However, our low basal intracellular free calcium concentration argues against significant platelet pre-activation using our isolation and storage methods. Although we demonstrated an exaggerated platelet activation response to thrombin and which correlated directly with the serum LDL cholesterol concentration, it is likely that other agonists such as catecholamines, could produce a similar effect.

In summary, we have shown that platelet hyper-reactivity as judged by a higher basal and thrombin stimulated $[Ca^{2+}]_i$ is present in untreated patients with hyperlipidemia compared to controls. Treatment with simvastatin reduced platelet reactivity significantly below that of normolipidemic controls even though the serum total and LDL cholesterol concentrations were not lowered to the level of normolipidemic controls. This indicates a beneficial effect of simvastatin treatment on platelet function that occurs independent of its' lipid lowering effect and could contribute to the reduction in risk for cardiovascular events beyond that of lowering of cholesterol. That platelets are activated in the presence of hyperlipidemia is also demonstrated by the direct correlation between serum LDL (LDL/HDL ratio) and the platelet $[Ca^{2+}]_i$. On the other hand the beneficial effect of a high serum HDL cholesterol is represented by an inverse relationship between serum HDL concentrations and platelet $[Ca^{2+}]_i$.

ACKNOWLEDGEMENTS

This work was supported by grants from the Manitoba Health Research Council, the P. Thorlakson Foundation and the Swedish Medical Research Council, the Nord-Västra Skånes Läkarförenings Research Foundation, and the Thelma Zoega Foundation (per L. Katzman). The authors express their thanks to Fran Geikie for typing the manuscript.

REFERENCES

1. Kannel WB, Castelli WP, Gordon T, McNamara PM. 1971. Serum cholesterol, lipoproteins, and the risk of coronary heart disease. Ann Int Med 74:1–12.
2. Ross R. 1993. The pathogenesis of atherosclerosis. A perspective for the 1990s. Nature 362:80–809.
3. Creager MA, Cooke JP, Mendelsohn ME, Gallagher SJ, Coleman SM, Loscalzo J, Dzau VJ. 1990. Impaired vasodilation of forearm resistance vessels in hypercholesterolemic humans. J Clin Invest 86:228–234.
4. Celemajer DS, Sorensen KE, Gooch VM, et al. 1992. Non-invasive detection of endothelial dysfunction in children and adults at risk of atherosclerosis. Lancet 340:1111–1115.
5. Seiler C, Hess OM, Buechi M, Suter TM, Krayenbuehl HP. 1993. Influence of serum cholesterol and other coronary risk factors on vasomotion of angiographically normal coronary arteries. Circulation 88(part 1):2139–2148.
6. Treasure CB, Klein JL, Weintraub WS, et al. 1995. Beneficial effects of cholesterol-lowering therapy on the coronary endothelium in patients with coronary artery disease. N Engl J Med 332:481–487.
7. Anderson TJ, Meredith IT, Yeung AC, Frei B, Selwyn AP, Ganz P. 1995. The effect of cholesterol lowering and antioxidant therapy on endothelium-dependent coronary vasomotion. N Engl J Med 332:488–493.
8. Laufs U, Wassmann S, Hilgers S, Ribaudo N, Bohm M, Nickenig G. 2001. Rapid effects on vascular function after initiation and withdrawal of atorvastatin in healthy, normo-cholesterolemic men. Am J Cardiol 88:1306–1307.
9. Egashira K, Hirooka Y, Kai H, Sugimachi M, Suzuki S, Inou T, Takeshita A. 1994. Reduction in serum cholesterol with pravastatin improves endothelium-dependent coronary vasomotion in patients with hypercholesterolemia. Circulation 89:2519–2524.
10. Nievelstein PFEM, de Groot PG. 1988. Interaction of blood platelets with the vessel wall. Haemostasis 18:342–359.
11. Ross R, Glomset J, Kariya B, Harker L. 1974. A platelet dependent serum factor that stimulates the proliferation of arterial smooth muscle cells in vitro. Proc Natl Acad Sci USA 71:1207–1210.
12. Vanhoutte PM. 1989. Endothelium, platelets, and vasospasm. In: P. Meyer and P. March, Blood cells and arteries in hypertension and atherosclerosis, page 1–14. Raven Press, New York.
13. Carvalho AC, Colman RW, Lees RS. 1974. Platelet function in hperlipoproteinemia. N Engl J Med 290:434–438.

14. Brook G, Winterstein G, Aviram M. 1983. Platelet function and lipoprotein levels after plasma exchange in patients with familial hypercholesterolemia. Cli Sci 64:637–642.
15. Hassall DG, Forrest LA, Bruckdorfer R, Marenah CB, Turner P, Cortese C, Miller E, Lewis B. 1983. Influence of plasma lipoproteins in a normal male population. Arteriosclerosis 3:332–338.
16. Knorr M, Locher R, Vogt E, Vetter W, Block LH, Ferracin F, Levkovits H, Pletscher A. 1988. Rapid activation of human platelets by low concentrations of low-density lipoprotein via phosphatidyl inositol cycle. Eur J Biochem 172:753–759.
17. Bochkov VN, Rozhkova TA, Matchin YuG, Lyakishev AA, Bochkova NA, Borisova YuL, Kukharchuk VV, Tchachuk VA. 1991. LDL and agonist-induced Ca^{2+} mobilization in platelets of healthy subjects and in patients with familial hyperlipoproteinemia type II. Thromb Res 61:403–409.
18. Aviram M, Brook JG. 1987. Platelet activation by plasma proteins. Progr Cardiovasc Dis 30: 61–72.
19. Curtiss LK, Plow EF. 1984. Interaction of plasma lipoprotein with human platelets. Blood 64: 365–374.
20. Kuo PT. 1981. Lipoproteins, platelets, and prostaglandins in atherosclerosis. Amer Heart J 102: 949–953.
21. Katzman PL, Bose R, Henry S, McLean DL, Walker S, Fyfe C, Perry Y, Mymin D, Bolli P. 1994. Serum lipid profile determines platelet reactivity to native and modified LDL—cholesterol in humans. Thrombosis Haemostasis 71:627–632.
22. Ardlie NG, Selley ML, Simons LA. 1989. Platelet activation by oxidatively modified low density lipoproteins. Atherosclerosis 76:117–124.
23. Meraji S, Moore CE, Skinner VO, Bruckdorfer KR. 1992. The importance of oxidation or glycosylation of low-density lipoproteins in relation to platelet activation. Platelets 3:155–162.
24. Koller E, Koller F, Doleschel W. 1982. Specific binding sites on human blood platelets for plasma lipo-proteins. Hoppe-Seyler Z Physiol Chem 363:395–405.
25. Katzman PL, Bose R, Walker S, Perry Y, Bolli P. 1991. Temperature-dependence of LDL binding and activation of human platelets. Thromb Res 64:503–508.
26. Lapetina EG. 1989. The biochemical messengers of activated platelets. In: P. Meyer and P. Marche, Blood cells and arteries in hypertension and atherosclerosis, pages 47–57. Raven Press, New York.
27. Friedewald WT, Levy RI, Frederickson DS. 1972. Estimation of the concentration of low-density lipoprotein cholesterol in plasma, without use of preparative ultracentrifuge. Clin Chem 18:499–502.
28. Standley PR, Gangasani S, Prakash R, Zemel MB, Sowers JR. 1991. Human platelet calcium measurements: Methodological considerations and comparisons with calcium mobilization in vascular smooth muscle cells. Am J Hypertension 4:546–549.
29. Erne P, Bolli P, Burgisser E, Buhler FR. 1984. Correlation of platelet calcium with blood pressure; effect of antihypertensive therapy. N Engl J Med 310:1084–1088.
30. Grynkiewicz G, Poenie M, Tsien RY. 1985. A new generation of Ca^{2+} indicators with greatly improved fluorescence properties. J Biol Chem 260:3440–3450.
31. Oshima T, Young EW, Bukosi RD, McCarron DA. 1990. Abnormal calcium handling by platelets of spontaneously hypertensive rats. Hypertension 5:606–611.
32. Livshits G, Weibort J, Meshulam N, Brunner D. 1989. Multivariate analysis of the twenty-year follow-up of the Donolo-Tel Aviv prospective coronary artery disease study and the usefulness of high density lipoprotein cholesterol percentage. Am J Cardiol 63:676–681.
33. Hamiwka L. 1994. Platelet derived growth factor release by human platelets in vitro: effects of thrombin, lipids and cyclosporine. B Med Sci Thesis.
34. Hochgraf E, Levy Y, Aviram M, Brook JG, Cogan V. 1994. Lovastatin decreases plasma and platelet cholesterol levels and normalizes elevated platelet fluidity and aggregation in hypercholesterolemic patients. Metabolism 43:11–17.
35. Le Quan Sang KH, Levenson J, Megnicu JL, Simon A, Devyuck MA. 1995. Platelet cytosolic Ca^{2+} and membrane dynamics in patients with primary hypercholesterolemia; Effects of pravastatin. Arterioscler Thromb Vasc Biol 15:759–764.
36. Lacoste L, Lam JYT. 1995. Hyperlipidemia and coronary artery disease: correction of the increased thrombogenic potential with cholesterol reduction. Circulation 92:3172–3177.
37. Rosenson RS, Tangney CC. 1998. Antiatherothrombic properties of statins. Implications of cardiovascular event reduction. JAMA 279:1643–1650.
38. Scandinavian Simvastatin Survival Study Group. 1994. Randomized trial of cholesterol lowering in 4444 patients with coronary heart disease: The Scandinavian Simvastatin Survival Study (4S). Lancet 344:1383–1389.

39. The Pravastatin Multinational Study Group for Cardiac Risk Patients. 1993. Effects of pravastatin in patients with serum total cholesterol levels from 5.2 to 7.8 mmol/liter plus two additional atherosclerotic risk factors. Am J Cardiol 72:1031–1037.
40. Salonen R, Nyyssonen K, Porkkala E, et al. 1995. Kuopio Atherosclerosis Prevention Study (KAPS): A population based primary primary prevention trial of the effect of LDL lowering on atherosclerotic progression in carotid and femoral arteries. Circulation 92:1758–1764.
41. Shepherd J, Cobb SM, Ford I, et al. 1995. Prevention of coronary heart disease with pravastatin in men with hypercholesterolemia. N Engl J Med 333:1301–1307.
42. Lansky AJ, Desai K, Leon MB. 2002. Quantative coronary angiography in regression trials: A review of methodologic considerations, endpoint selection, and limitations. Am J Cardiol 89(Suppl):4B–9B.
43. The Heart Protection Study. 2001. Presented at the 74th Scientific Sessions of the American Heart Association, Anaheim, Ca, November 13.
44. Schwartz GG, Olsson AG, Ezekowitz MD, Ganz P, Oliver MF, Waters D, Zeiher A, Chaitman BR, Leslie S, Stern T. 2001. Effects of atorvastatin on early recurrent ischemic events in acute coronary syndromes. The MIRACL Study: A randomized controlled trial. JAMA 285:1711–1717.
45. Masumoto A, Hirooka Y, Hironaga K, Eshima K, Setoguchi S, Egashira K, Takeshita A. 2001. Effect of pravastatin on endothelial function in patients with coronary artery disease (cholesterol-independent effect of pravastatin). Am J Cardiol 88:1291–1294.

G.N. Pierce, M. Nagano, P. Zahradka, and N.S. Dhalla (eds.).
ATHEROSCLEROSIS, HYPERTENSION AND DIABETES.

RAPAMYCIN-SENSITIVE SIGNAL TRANSDUCTION PATHWAYS AND THE CONTROL OF ADIPOGENESIS

ALEXANDER SORISKY, ANNEMARIE GAGNON, ANDREA BELL, and DARINE EL-CHAAR

Departments of Medicine and of Biochemistry, Microbiology, and Immunology, Ottawa Health Research Institute and the University of Ottawa, Ottawa, Canada K1Y 4E9

Summary. Adipose tissue development occurs in early life, followed by ongoing adipose tissue remodelling in the adult. Formation of new adipocytes (adipogenesis) occurs via the differentiation of committed progenitor cells, known as preadipocytes. In positive energy balance, existing adipocytes enlarge to a finite degree to store excess calories; adipogenesis then ensues to enlarge the reservoir capacity.

In vivo stimulators of adipogenesis have not been clearly identified, but may include insulin, IGF-1 (insulin-like growth factor 1), as well as certain fatty acids and/or their metabolites. Insulin/IGF-1 act on cell surface receptors, activating key intracellular signalling proteins. One of these, mTOR (mammalian target of rapamycin) is the focus of this review. mTOR binds to, and is inhibited by, rapamycin, an immunosuppressant that blocks T cell proliferation. Rapamycin also inhibits adipogenesis, and initial work suggested that it did so by interfering with the early proliferative clonal expansion stage of adipogenesis. Subsequent studies have revealed that rapamycin also inhibits adipogenesis by other routes that are independent of its anti-proliferative action. Rapamycin is proving to be a valuable tool to help dissect out the mTOR dependent signalling events that regulate adipogenesis.

Key words: Rapamycin, Adipogenesis, Insulin, Obesity

Corresponding Author: Alexander Sorisky MDCM, FRCPC, Ottawa Health Research Institute, Ottawa Hospital, 725 Parkdale Avenue, Ottawa ON K1Y 4E9 Canada. Tel: 613-798-5555 #17572; Fax: 613-761-5036; e-mail: asorisky@ohri.ca

INTRODUCTION

The critical time periods for adipose tissue development occur in fetal and neonatal life [1]. Healthy development of adipose tissue is crucial for energy storage, and the coordinated responses of lipogenesis and lipolysis are established vital functions of the adipocyte [2]. Recent discoveries in the field of adipocyte biology have revealed that adipocytes produce, and secrete, an array of bioactive molecules [3]. These "adipocytokines" include, but are not limited to, leptin, TNFα (tumour necrosis factor α), adiponectin, interleukin 6, PAI-1 (plasminogen activator inhibitor-1), and ASP (acylation stimulating protein). On this basis, it has been proposed that adipocytes might play a role in energy balance, insulin sensitivity, inflammation, fibrinolysis, and atherosclersosis. Adipose tissue remodelling continues throughout adult life, involving the formation of new adipocytes (adipogenesis) via the differentiation of committed progenitor fibroblast-like cells, known as preadipocytes [4]. In positive energy balance, existing adipocytes enlarge to a finite degree to house the excess calories. Adipogenesis follows to augment the reserve storage capacity of adipose tissue. Cellular turnover within the fat depot also appears to depend on apoptosis of adipose cells, either at the preadipocyte or adipocyte stage [5]. This review will focus on the preadipocyte signal transduction pathways that result in adipogenesis.

STAGES OF ADIPOGENESIS

Human preadipocytes are studied in primary culture, after isolation of stromal cells from adipose tissue by collagenase and filtration [6]. In addition, mammalian preadipocyte cell lines have been established that are fairly reliable models of adipogenesis [7]. They grow rapidly, and their differentiation response is robust and uniform. Their ultrastructural appearance resembles primary adipocytes, and when injected into athymic mice, they can form fat pads [8,9]. Of these, the embryonal murine 3T3-L1 cells have been extensively studied. Once grown to confluence, 3T3-L1 preadipocytes exit the cell cycle, and thereby become competent to differentiate. Treatment with insulin or IGF-1 results in a limited re-entry into the cell cycle, termed the clonal expansion phase, that lasts 3–4 days, after which the cells again exit the cell cycle. This is believed to facilitate the interaction of trans-acting factors with regulatory regions of adipogenic genes [10]. Members of three families of transcription factors appear to be important for differentiation, and these are SREBP1 (sterol regulatory element binding protein 1), C/EBP (CCAAT/enhancer binding protein) α, β, and δ, and PPARγ (peroxisome proliferator-activated receptor γ) [4]. SREBP1, whose induction is insulin-responsive, either directly stimulates the expression of PPARγ, and/or produces an endogenous ligand that activates PPARγ. C/EBPβ and C/EBPδ are transiently expressed, and are implicated in the upregulation of C/EBPα and PPARγ. Both C/EBPα and PPARγ are sufficient and necessary for adipogenesis, and act in a synergistic manner to promote adipose maturation [11]. Together with SREBP1, C/EBPα and PPARγ regulate a variety of genes that are important for the synthesis and storage of triacylglycerol and

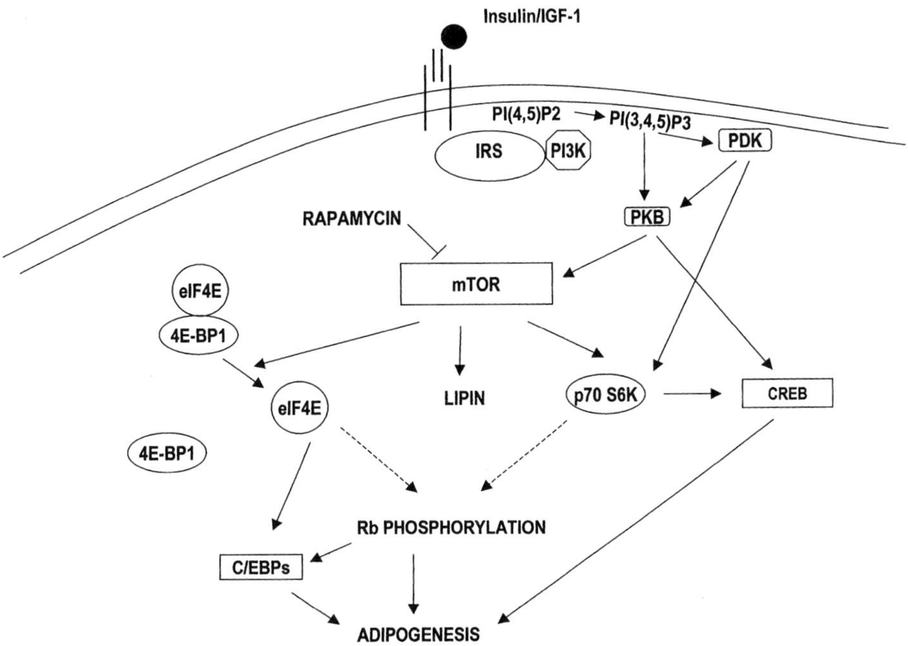

Figure 1. Model of mTOR-dependent adipogenic signalling. Insulin/IGF-1 engages the cell-surface receptor tyrosine kinase, resulting in the association of PI3K with IRS, the activation of PKB and mTOR. Downstream signals of mTOR include p70 S6 kinase (p70 S6K) and 4E-BP1, which indirectly regulate Rb phosphorylation and the clonal expansion phase of adipogenesis. These events are inhibited by rapamycin, which selectively interferes with mTOR action. Lipin is a recently identified insulin-responsive and rapamycin-sensitive phosphoprotein linked to adipogenesis. Dotted arrows indicate indirect effects. See text for details.

glucose transport, including glycerol phosphate dehydrogenase (GPDH), adipocyte lipid binding protein (aP2), fatty acid synthase (FAS), and glucose transporter 4 (GLUT4).

INSULIN/IGF-1 AND ADIPOGENIC SIGNAL TRANSDUCTION (see Fig. 1)

Both insulin and IGF-1 induce adipogenesis in these model systems, each binding to and activating their cognate receptor tyrosine kinase [12–15]. Autophosphorylation of the receptor β subunits further stimulates the tyrosine kinase catalytic function, leading to the tyrosine phosphorylation of multiple tyrosine residues on insulin receptor substrate (IRS) proteins, of which there are several members [16]. IRS serves as a pivotal docking protein, with certain of its C-terminal phosphotyrosine residues acting as high-affinity sites for signalling proteins that possess SH2 (Src homology 2) domains. SH2 domains are protein modules that specifically recognize phosphotyrosine residues in a sequence-specific context. IRS is required for adipogenesis [17].

PI3K (phosphoinositide 3-kinase) is an insulin-responsive lipid kinase [18]. The best understood form is a heterodimer consisting of a p85 adaptor subunit bound to a catalytic p110 subunit. p85 possesses two SH2 domains, allowing the p85-p110 dimer to bind to IRS. As a result, p110 is both directly activated through allosteric changes, as well as relocated closer to its substrate, PI(4,5)P2. Inhibition of PI3K by pharmacological or genetic strategies blocks adipogenesis [19–21]. The phosphorylation of PI(4,5)P2 generates PI(3,4,5)P3, which accumulates in the cell membrane, and attracts the serine/threonine protein kinase B (PKB; also known as Akt) by virtue of its pleckstrin homology (PH) domain [22]. When PKB binds PI(3,4,5)P3, its kinase activity is modestly activated. Full activation is achieved when it is phosphorylated by an upstream kinase known as 3-phosphoinositide-dependent kinase 1 (PDK) [23]. PDK1 also has a PH domain which directs it to the membrane where PI(3,4,5)P3 is produced. A PDK2 activity is also implicated in PKB activation, but the identity of this kinase is controversial. Expression of activated forms of PKB are sufficient to induce adipogenesis of confluent 3T3-L1 preadipocytes [24,25].

Several PKB substrates have now been identified, and include glycogen synthase kinase-3, phosphofructokinase, Bad, Forkhead family transcription factors, endothelial nitric oxide synthase, and CREB (cAMP response element binding protein) [26]. Phosphorylation of CREB by PKB activates it [27], and activated CREB has been shown to be sufficient and necessary for adipogenesis [28]. For the purposes of this review, we will concentrate on yet another PKB target, the serine/threonine kinase mTOR (target of rapamycin).

mTOR SIGNALLING

Two TOR genes were orginally cloned in yeast; when the proteins they encode are inhibited by rapamycin (see below), cell cycle arrest occurs [29]. The corresponding mammalian gene was named mTOR and it encodes for a large 289 kD protein. There is evidence that PKB appears to phosphorylate and activate mTOR, although other kinases may be involved [30–32]. Currently, it is conjectured that such regulatory kinases can only activate mTOR in the presence of sufficient nutrients (amino acids). The manner in which mTOR "senses" nutrient levels is not understood [33]. More recently, it has been reported that mTOR also senses ATP concentrations independently of amino acid abundance [34].

mTOR has a catalytic domain with homology to that of PI3K [35]. Although lipid kinase activity is not detectable, there are data that indicate mTOR directly phosphorylates and regulates two insulin-responsive proteins, p70 S6 kinase and 4E-BP1 (elongation initiation factor 4E binding protein) [32,36]. Others suggest that mTOR increases p70 S6 kinase phosphorylation indirectly by inhibiting the serine/threonine phosphatase, PP2A [37].

p70 S6 KINASE

This insulin-responsive serine/threonine kinase phosphorylates the S6 ribosomal protein. p70 S6 kinase has a counterpart, p85 S6 kinase, due to alternative mRNA splicing and alternative translation sites on one of the transcripts [38]. In addition to the central catalytic domain, there are important regulatory elements that include a N-terminal acidic region, a linker region distal to the catalytic region, and a C-terminal autoinhibitory domain. Serine/threonine residues that regulate the kinase appear in the catalytic and autoinhibitory domain. A three stage model of p70 S6 kinase activation includes [38]: 1) initial phosphorylations in the autoinhibitory domain which induce a conformational change, allowing, 2) phosphorylation of Thr389 (regulated by mTOR), and finally, 3) phosphorylation of Thr229 by PDK1. Protein kinase Cζ, another target of PI3K lipid products, can also phosphorylate p70 S6 kinase [39].

p70 S6 kinase stimulates the translation of mRNAs that contain 5′ terminal oligopyrimidine (5′TOP) tracts, encoding ribosomal proteins and elongation factors required for protein synthesis and for cell cycle progression [40]. It also regulates transcription by phosphorylating the CREB (cAMP response element binding protein) transcription factor on Ser 133 [28,41]. The importance of CREB for adipogenesis was noted above. The N-terminal region of p85 S6 kinase has a nuclear localization sequence, and this isoform resides in the nucleus [42]. Ample amounts of p70 S6 kinase are also present in the nucleus [41,43]. Both isoforms phosphorylate the protein S6 [38]. In the cytoplasm, S6 is part of the ribosomal complex regulating mRNA translation, and is acted upon by p70 S6 kinase. In the nucleus, S6 may influence mRNA processing, in coordination with subsequent translation in the cytoplasm by the ribosomal apparatus.

4E-BP1

4E-BP1 binds to and represses the activity of eIF4E (eukaryotic translation initiation factor 4E) by preventing its association with eIF4G [32]. eIF4E plays an essential role in translating a specific subset of mRNAs that have highly structured 5′ UTRs (untranslated regions), including cyclins and growth factors [35]. Phosphorylation of 4E-BP1 by mTOR in vitro occurs on Thr37 and Thr46, permitting further phosphorylation by unidentified kinases. The motif responsible for binding eIF4E is in the mid-region of 4E-BP1 (residues 35–85), and these phosphorylations disrupt its function. This results in the release of eIF4E and permits translation to proceed [32–33]. Constitutive overexpression of eIF4E in 3T3-L1 preadipocytes alters translational regulation of C/EBPα and β isoforms, and inhibits preadipocyte differentiation, apparently by inducing a transformed phenotype with reduced contact inhibition [44]. Recently, 4E-BP1-null mice were noted to have reduced amounts of adipose tissue, consistent with a possible role in fat metabolism [45].

RAPAMYCIN, mTOR, AND THE INHIBITION OF ADIPOGENESIS

The selective inhibition of mTOR by rapamycin has provided insights about its role in adipogenesis. Rapamycin is a macrolide that diffuses into cells and binds to FKBP12, its intracellular receptor. This complex binds to mTOR and inhibits the ability of mTOR to act on its downstream targets, perhaps in ways that go beyond direct inhibiton of mTOR kinase activity [33]. Its immunosuppressant action is due to interference with interleukin 2-dependent T cell proliferation [29]. Recently, it has received much attention as a key component of the immunosuppressive regimen used for human islet cell transplants in patients with type 1 diabetes [46]. Yeh et al. discovered that rapamycin could block 3T3-L1 adipogenesis, and concluded this was because it prevented the early clonal expansion phase [47].

DOWNSTREAM OF mTOR—A LINK TO ADIPOGENIC CLONAL EXPANSION

It appears that Retinoblastoma protein (Rb) is indirectly regulated by mTOR, and influences the clonal expansion phase of 3T3-L1 preadipocytes. Rb has been shown to be required for adipogenesis through required interactions with C/EBP transcription factors, based on gene deletion studies [48]. Another relevant Rb function is to maintain cell cycle arrest, and it is inhibited from doing so if it is phosphorylated by a cyclin D-cyclin-dependent kinase 4/6 complex. This permits clonal expansion of 3T3-L1 preadipocytes to proceed [49,50,51]. Rapamycin may interfere with the required Rb phosphorylation in two ways. By interfering with p70 S6 kinase activity, it can prevent the induction of cyclin D2 and D3, and via its interference with 4E-BP1 function, it can also block the translation of cyclin D1 [52]. These mechanisms, which perturb the cyclin D-cdk complex, might explain the ability of rapamycin to block clonal expansion in 3T3-L1 adipogenesis.

RAPAMYCIN-SENSITIVE PATHWAYS DISTINCT FROM CLONAL EXPANSION

Subsequent work has found that rapamycin is capable of attenuating 3T3-L1 preadipocyte differentiation even when it is added after the completion of clonal expansion [53]. In this study, it was established that clonal expansion was completed by day 4 of the 8 day differentiation protocol. Cells were treated with rapamycin for the first time on day 4, and the extent of adipogenesis was assessed on day 8. GPDH activity and triacylglycerol accumulation were significantly impaired, as was the induction of PPARγ and C/EBPα. The addition of rapamycin on day 4 essentially arrested any further differentiation. Therefore, rapamycin-sensitive signals that are required for continued adipogenesis operate after clonal expansion in 3T3-L1 preadipocytes. Rb is not expected to be involved at this phase, since its normal phosphorylation and dephosphorylation modifications are completed by day 4 [49,51].

Human preadipocytes in primary culture undergo adipogenesis without clonal expansion, unlike 3T3-L1 preadipocytes. As mentioned above, 3T3-L1 cells are embryonic and murine in origin. Possibly, human preadipocytes from adult humans are isolated at a later stage of development, perhaps already having passed through clonal expansion in vivo. We therefore explored whether rapamycin would be capable of abrogating differentiation of human preadipocytes. The absence of clonal expansion was confirmed under our experimental conditions. Rapamycin treatment severely inhibited human adipogenesis in cultures derived from men or women, and from abdominal sc fat or intra-abd omental fat. Adipogenesis was assessed by morphological appearance, and GPDH activity. This is further evidence that other mTOR-dependent pathways independent of clonal expansion must be operative [54].

Very recently, it was reported that mTOR regulated the phosphorylation of lipin [55]. A mutation in the lipin gene results in lipodystrophic mice that exhibit insulin resistance and dyslipidemia [56]. Based on its pattern of induction during adipogenesis, lipin might be a candidate for rapamycin action distinct from targets acting during clonal expansion.

CLOSING REMARKS

The use of rapamycin has provided new insights about mTOR and its downstream signals with respect to the regulation of adipogenesis. mTOR appears to be important for the clonal expansion phase, as well as other differentiation-inducing pathways in murine preadipocyte cell lines. Human preadipocyte differentiation (no clonal expansion phase) in culture is also rapamycin-sensitive. The potential connections between the nutrient-sensing functions of mTOR and its role in regulating the principal energy-storing tissue of the body are intriguing, and deserve further attention.

ACKNOWLEDGMENTS

This work was supported by a grants from the Heart and Stroke Foundation of Ontario (HSFO) and the Canadian Institutes of Health Research (CIHR). AS is a Career Investigator of the HSFO. AG is supported by a Premier's Research Excellence Award held by AS. AB is supported by a Doctoral Research Award co-funded by the HSFO and CIHR. DE-C was supported by a John D. Schultz Science Student Scholarship of the HSFO.

REFERENCES

1. Ailhaud G, Grimaldi P, Negrel R. 1992. Cellular and molecular aspects of adipose tissue development. Annu Rev Nutr 12:207–233.
2. Spiegelman BM, Flier JS. 1996. Adipogenesis and obesity: rounding out the big picture. Cell 87:377–389.
3. Wajchenberg BL. 2000. Subcutaneous and visceral adipose tissue: their relation to the metabolic syndrome. Endocrine Rev 21:697–738.
4. Rosen ED, Walkey CJ, Puigserver P, Spiegelman BM. 2000. Transcriptional regulation of adipogenesis. Genes Dev 14:1293–1307.
5. Sorisky A, Magun R, Gagnon AM. 2000. Adipose tissue apoptosis: death in the energy depot. Int J Obes 24 (Suppl 4):S3–S7.
6. Hauner H, Entenmann G, Wabitsch M, Gaillard D, Ailhaud G, Negrel R, Pfeiffer EF. 1989. Promoting effect of glucocorticoids on the differentiation of human adipocyte precursor cells cultured in a chemically defined medium. J Clin Invest 84:1663–1670.
7. Cornelius P, MacDougald OA, Lane MD. 1994. Regulation of adipocyte development. Ann Rev Nutr 14:99–129.
8. Novikoff AB, Novikoff PM, Rosen OM, Rubin CS. 1980. Organelle relationships in cultured 3T3-L1 preadipocytes. J Cell Biol 87:180–196.
9. Ross SE, Hemati N, Longo KA, Bennett CN, Lucas PC, Erickson RL, MacDougald OA. 2000. Inhibition of adipogenesis by Wnt signaling. Science 289:950–953.

10. Tang Q-Q, Lane MD. 1999. Activation and centromeric localization of CCAAT/enhancer-binding proteins during the mitotic clonal expansion of adipocyte differentiation. Genes Dev 13:2231–2241.
11. Rosen ED, Hsu C-H, Wang X, Sakai S, Freeman MW, Gonzalez FJ, Spiegelman BM. 2002. C/EBPα induces adipogenesis through PPARγ: a unified pathway. Genes Dev 16:22–26.
12. Smith PJ, Wise LS, Berkowitz R, Wan C, Rubin CS. 1988. Insulin-like growth factor-1 is an essential regulator of the differentiation of 3T3-L1 adipocytes. J Biol Chem 263:9402–9408.
13. Accili D, Taylor SI. 1991. Targeted inactivation of the insulin receptor gene in mouse 3T3-L1 fibroblasts via homologous recombination. Proc Natl Acad Sci USA 88:4708–4712.
14. Chaika OV, Chaika N, Volle DJ, Wilden PA, Pirrucello SJ, Lewis RE. 1997. CSF-1 receptor/insulin receptor chimera permits CSF-1-dependent differentiation of 3T3-L1 preadipocytes. J Biol Chem 272:11968–11974.
15. Gagnon AM, Sorisky A. 1998. The effect of glucose concentration on insulin-induced 3T3-L1 adipose cell differentiation. Obes Res 6:157–163.
16. Withers DJ, White M. 2000. The insulin signaling system—a common link in the pathogenesis of type 2 diabetes. Endocrinology 141:1917–1921.
17. Miki H, Yamauchi T, Suzuki R, Komeda K, Tsuchida A, Kubota N, Terauchi Y, Kamon J, Kaburagi Y, Matsui J, Akanuma Y, Nagai R, Kimura S, Tobe K, Kadowaki T. 2001. Essential role of insulin receptor substrate 1 (IRS-1) and IRS-2 in adipocyte differentiation. Mol Cell Biol 21:2521–2532.
18. Vanhaesebroeck B, Leevers SJ, Ahmadi K, Timms J, Katso R, Driscoll PC, Woscholski R, Parker PJ, Waterfield MD. 2001. Synthesis and function of 3-phosphorylated inositol lipids. Annu Rev Biochem 70:535–602.
19. Tomiyama K, Nakata H, Sasa H, Arimura S, Eisuke N, Watanabe Y. 1995. Wortmannin, a specific phosphatidylinositol 3-kinase inhibitor, inhibits adipocytic differentiation of 3T3-L1 cells. Biochem Biophys Res Comm 212:263–269.
20. Sorisky A, Pardasani D, Lin Y. 1996. The 3-phosphorylated phosphoinositide response of 3T3-L1 preadipose cells exposed to insulin, insulin-like growth factor-1, or platelet-derived growth factor. Obes Res 4:9–19.
21. Sakaue H, Ogawa W, Matsumoto M, Kuroda S, Takata M, Sugimoto T, Spiegelman BM, Kasuga M. 1998. Posttranscriptional control of adipocyte differentiation through activation of phosphoinositide 3-kinase. J Biol Chem 273:28945–28952.
22. Chan TO, Rittenhouse SE, Tsichlis PN. 1999. Akt/PKB and other phosphoinositide-regulated kinases: kinase activation by phosphoinositide-dependent phosphorylation. Annu Rev Biochem 68:965–1014.
23. Toker A, Newton AC. 2000. Cellular signaling: pivoting around PDK-1. Cell 103:185–188.
24. Magun R, Burgering BMT, Coffer PJ, Pardasni D, Lin Y, Chabot J, Sorisky A. 1996. Expression of a constitutively activated form of protein kinase B (c-Akt) in 3T3-L1 preadipose cells causes spontaneous differentiation. Endocrinology 137:3590–3593.
25. Kohn AD, Summers SA, Birnbaum MJ, Roth RA. 1996. Expression of a constitutively active Akt ser/thr kinase in 3T3-L1 adipocytes stimulates glucose uptake and glucose transporter 4 translocation. J Biol Chem 271:31372–31378.
26. Scheid MP, Woodgett JR. 2001. PKB/Akt: functional insights from genetic models. Nature Rev Molec Biol 2:760–768.
27. Du K, Montminy M. 1998. CREB is a regulatory target for the protein kinase Akt/PKB. J Biol Chem 273:32377–32379.
28. Reusch JEB, Colton LA, Klemm DJ. 2000. CREB activation induces adipogenesis in 3T3-L1 cells. Mol Cell Biol 20:1008–1020.
29. Cardenas ME, Zhu D, Heitman J. 1995. Molecular mechanisms of immunosuppression by cyclosporin, FK506, and rapamycin. Curr Opin Nephrol Hyper 4:472–477.
30. Scott PH, Brunn GJ, Kohn AD, Roth RA, Lawrence JC, Jr. 1998. Evidence of insulin-stimulated phosphorylation and activation of the mammalian target of rapamycin mediated by a protein kinase B signaling pathway. Proc Natl Acad Sci USA 95:7772–7777.
31. Nave BT, Ouwens DM, Withers DJ, Alessi DR, Shepherd PR. 1999. Mammalian target of rapamycin is a direct target for protein kinase B. Biochem J 344:427–431.
32. Gingras A-C, Raught B, Sonenberg N. 1999. eIF4 initiation factors. Annu Rev Biochem 68:913–963.
33. Raught B, Gingras A-C, Sonenberg N. 2001. The target of rapamycin (TOR) proteins. Proc Natl Acad Sci USA 98:7037–7044.
34. Dennis PB, Jaeschke A, Saitoh M, Fowler B, Kozma SC, Thomas G. 2001. Mammalian TOR: a homeostatic ATP sensor. Science 294:1102–1105.

35. Thomas G, Hall MN. 1997. TOR signalling and control of cell growth. Curr Opin Cell Biol 9: 782–787.
36. Isotani S, Hara K, Tokunaga C, Inoue H, Avruch J, Yonezawa K. 1999. Immunopurified mammalian target of rapamycin phosphorylates and activates p70 S6 kinase alpha in vitro. J Biol Chem 274:34493–34498.
37. Peterson RT, Desai BN, Hardwick JS, Schreiber SL. 1999. Protein phosphatase 2A interacts with the 70-kDa S6 kinase and is activated by the inhibition of FKBP12-rapamycin-associated protein. Proc Natl Acad Sci USA 96:4438–4442.
38. Dennis PB, Pullen N, Pearson RB, Kozma SC, Thomas G. 1998. Phosphorylation sites in the autoinhibitory domain participate in p70S6K activation loop phosphorylation. J Biol Chem 273: 14845–14852.
39. Romanelli A, Martin KA, Toker A, Blenis J. 1999. p70 S6 kinase is regulated by protein kinase Cζ and participates in a phosphoinositide 3-kinase-regulated signalling complex. Mol Cell Biol 19:2921–2928.
40. Jefferies HBJ, Fumagalli S, Dennis PB, Reinhard C, Pearson RB, Thomas G. 1997. Rapamycin suppresses 5′TOP mRNA translation through inhibition of p70S6K. EMBO J 16:3693–3704.
41. de Groot RP, Ballou LM, Sassone-Corsi P. 1994. Positive regulation of the cAMP-responsive activator CREM by the p70 S6 kinase. Cell 79:81–91.
42. Reinhard C, Fernandez A, Lamb NJC, Thomas G. 1994. Nuclear localization of p85S6K. EMBO J 13:1557–1565.
43. Kim S-J, Kahn CR. 1997. Insulin stimulates p70 S6 kinase in the nucleus of cells. Biochem Biophys Res Commun 234:681–685.
44. Calkhoven CF, Muller C, Leutz A. 2000. Translational control of C/EBPα and C/EBPβ isoform expression. Genes Dev 14:1920–1932.
45. Tsukiyama-Kohara K, Poulin F, Kohara M, DeMaria CT, Cheng A, Wu Z, Gingras AC, Katsume A, Elchebly M, Spiegelman BM, Harper ME, Tremblay ML, Sonenberg N. 2001. Adipose tissue reduction in mice lacking the translational inhibitor 4E-BP1. Nature Med 7:1128–1132.
46. Shapiro AM, Lakey JRT, Ryan EA, Korbutt GS, Toth E, Warnock GL, Kneteman NM, Rajotte RV. 2000. Islet transplantation in seven patients with type 1 diabetes mellitus using a glucocorticoid-free immunosuppressive regimen. New Engl J Med 343:230–238.
47. Yeh W-C, Bierer BE, McKnight SL. 1995. Rapamycin inhibits clonal expansion and adipogenic differentiation of 3T3-L1 cells. Proc Natl Acad Sci USA 92:11086–11090.
48. Chen PL, Riley DJ, Chen Y, Lee WH. 1996. Retinoblastoma protein positively regulates terminal adipocyte differentiation through direct interactions with C/EBPs. Genes Dev 10:2794–2804.
49. Shao D, Lazar MA. 1997. Peroxisome proliferator activated receptor g, CCAT/Enhancer-binding protein a, and cell cycle status regulate the commitment to adipocyte differentiation. J Biol Chem 272:21473–21478.
50. Classon M, Kennedy BK, Mulloy R, Harlow E. 2000. Opposing roles of pRB and p107 in adipocyte differentiation. Proc Natl Acad Sci USA 97:10826–10831.
51. Usui I, Haruta T, Iwata M, Takano A, Uno T, Kawahara J, Ueno E, Sasaoka T, Kobayashi M. 2000. Retinoblastoma protein phosphorylation via PI 3-kinase and mTOR pathway regulates adipocyte differentiation. Biochem Biophys Res Commun 275:115–120.
52. Schmelzle T, Hall MN. 2000. TOR, a central controller of cell growth. Cell 103:253–262.
53. Gagnon A, Lau S, Sorisky A. 2001. Rapamycin-sensitive phase of 3T3-L1 preadipocyte differentiation after clonal expansion. J Cell Physiol 189:14–22.
54. Bell A, Grunder L, Sorisky A. 2000. Rapamycin inhibits human adipocyte differentiation in primary culture. Obes Res 8:249–254.
55. Huffman TA, Mothe-Satney I, Lawrence JC, Jr. 2002. Insulin-stimulated phosphorylation of lipin mediated by the mammalian target of rapamycin. Proc Natl Acad Sci USA 99:1047–1052.
56. Peterfy M, Phan J, Xu P, Reue K. 2001. Lipodystrophy in the fld mouse results from mutation of a new gene encoding a nuclear protein, lipin. Nat Gen 27:121–124.

II. HYPERTENSION

G.N. Pierce, M. Nagano, P. Zahradka, and N.S. Dhalla (eds.).
ATHEROSCLEROSIS, HYPERTENSION AND DIABETES.

GENETIC PREDISPOSITION TO HYPERTENSION AND CARDIOVASCULAR DISEASE

TOSHIO OGIHARA, TOMOHIRO KATSUYA, and JITSUO HIGAKI

Departement of Geriatric Medicine, Osaka University Graduate School of Medicine

Summary. Essential hypertension occurs in individuals with a genetic predisposition who respond abnormally to environmental changes. A complex interplay of a number of genetic alterations and environmental factors is involved in the pathogenesis of hypertension. Therefore, hypertension does not follow a clear pattern of inheritance but exhibits familial aggregation of cases. A reverse genetic approach, which examines genetic factors underlying the root of pathogenesis first, is a powerful tool to clarify the complex interplay. To clarify the role of gene polymorphisms in hypertension, we have carried out case-control studies using a candidate gene approach. We mainly focused on gene components of the renin-angiotensin system as candidates, and obtained some suggestive positive results in the association with hypertension, but the estimated relative risk for hypertension was less than 2.0. These results led us to recognize the importance of investigation using a general population with a sufficient number of subjects. We collaborated in two large epidemiological cohort studies and examined the association between genetic factors and the participants' health status in each of them. To deal with a large number of samples, we established the TaqMan PCR method to save time and cost of genotyping. Our investigations revealed a small but significant effect of gene polymorphisms in increasing the risk for hypertension, and suggested interactions with environmental factors such as aging, sex, and salt intake. In this review, we discuss the consensus and controversy of genetic investigations for identification of hypertensive genes and consider the future of tailor-made medicine.

Correspondence: Toshio Ogihara, MD, PhD, Professor of Medicine, Department of Geriatric Medicine, Osaka University Graduate, School of Medicine, 2-2 #B6, Yamada-oka, Suita, Osaka 565-0871, Japan. Tel: +81-6-6879-3882; Fax: +81-6-6879-3859; e-mail: ogihara@geriat.med.Osaka-u.ac.jp

Key words: Genetics, Polymorphism, Renin-angiotensin system, Tailor-made medicine, TaqMan PCR

GENETIC APPROACHES FOR IDENTIFICATION OF HYPERTENSIVE GENES

Both environmental and genetic factors are involved in the pathogenesis of hypertension [1–3]. Some of the factors affect the cause of hypertension, while others affect the hypertensive complications in an organ-specific manner. There are three well known strategies to identify hypertensive genes; linkage analysis, sib-pair analysis and association study. Linkage analysis is a powerful shortcut approach to identify the exact causal gene of monogenic hypertension [4]. Lifton's group has succeeded several times to clone the causal gene of monogenic hypertension, in such conditions as Liddle syndrome [5] and glucocorticoid remediable aldosteronism [6] (Table 1). The next approach is the affected or discordant sib-pair method [7]. This is a sophisticated way to carry out genome screening, but its statistical power is not strong enough to identify the genetic risk for essential hypertension [8]. To detect genes in which the power of the genetic relative risk for hypertension is 2.0, the number of required sib-pairs is more than 4,000, suggesting that it is impossible to detect a common genetic risk for essential hypertension using the sib-pair method. In contrast, a case-control study has strong statistical power, and as a result, 1,000 cases and 1,000 controls should be enough for detection of a relative risk of 1.5 [9]. In addition to high blood pressure, essential hypertensive individuals have several interesting phenotypes, such as left ventricular hypertrophy and cerebral ischemia. In a future study, pharmacogenetic investigation or the correla-

Table 1. Monogenic hypertension and hypotension

Diseases	Causative gene	Chromosomal locus	Blood pressure
Hypertension exacerbated by pregnancy	Mineralocorticoid receptor	4q31.1	↑
GRA	Chimaeric 11β-hydroxylase/ aldosterone synthase	8q	↑
11β-hydroxylase deficiency	11β-hydroxylase (CYP11B1)	8q21	↑
17α-hydroxylase deficiency	17α-hydroxylase (CYP17)	10q24.3	↑
Liddle syndrome	ENaC, β, γ subunits	16p13–p12	↑
Gordon syndrome (PHA IIC)	WNK 1	12p13	↑
Gordon syndrome (PHA IIB)	WNK 4	17p11–q21	↑
AME (New syndrome)	11β-hydroxysteroid dehydrogenase	16q22	↑
PHA I (autosomal dominant)	Mineralocorticoid receptor	4q31.1	→, ↓
PHA I (autosomal recessive)	ENaC, α, β subunits	12p13	→, ↓
Gordon syndrome (PHA IIA)	?	1q31–q32	↑
Hypertension with brachidactyly	?	12p12.2–p11.2	↑

GRA: glucocorticoid remediable aldosteronism.
PHA: pseudo-hypoaldosteronism.
ENaC: amiloride sensitive epithelial sodium channel.
WNK: serine-threonine protein kinase, lysine deficient.
AME: apparent mineralocorticoid excess.

tion between a gene and cardiovascular complications can be examined using these cases. However, a case-control study also has several disadvantages. Cases with severe and early onset hypertension seem to have a high genetic risk for hypertension, but it is risky to define controls matched for sex and age as normotensives. Furthermore, the obtained results concerning the association with hypertension using case-control studies are frequently inconsistent. We think this disagreement has been due to the unreliable phenotypes of cases and differences in the background of controls [10]. Certainly, the criterion for hypertension is clear, and most of the cases were recruited from a medical institute. However, the phenotypes of the cases were often obtained while the subjects were receiving medication or subject to the white coat effect. In controls, subjects were obtained from various types of population, and their definition was based on exclusion criteria, suggesting that "controls" do not mean "healthy subjects". As a solution to these problems, we decided to use large general populations.

LARGE GENETIC EPIDEMIOLOGICAL STUDIES AND ACE GENE POLYMORPHISM

As the first large cohort epidemiological study, we collaborated with the National Cardiovascular Center, which has carried out a cohort study (the Suita study) using a population of urban residents since 1989 [11]. The greatest advantage of this study is that the participants were obtained from the residents' registration records at random. After obtaining informed consent for genetic analysis, the single nucleotide polymorphisms (SNPs) of participants were examined.

First of all, we focused on the renin-angiotensin system because this system determines fifteen to twenty percent of blood pressure variation. Several gene polymorphisms in the renin angiotensin system are already known and have been examined as candidate risk factors for cardiovascular disease. Among them, the homozygous deletion allele of the angiotensin converting enzyme gene (ACE/DD) has been shown to be a genetic risk for ischemic heart disease [12]. However, there has been some evidence showing an association between ACE gene polymorphisms and hypertension. In a rat cross model, the most famous BP-SP1 locus is mapped near the ACE locus on the chromosome 10 [13]. Furthermore, a report from the Framingham Study showed a unique male-specific association between the ACE I/D polymorphism and hypertension [14]. We evaluated the ACE I/D polymorphism in more than five thousand participants of the Suita Study. The insertion/deletion polymorphism in intron 16 of the ACE gene was determined by Rigat's protocol with minor modification [15]. Insertion allele specific amplification was performed to exclude misidentification of the ACE genotype. In comparison with the Framingham Study, the data of the Suita Study showed half the frequency of homozygous deletion of the ACE gene, and the same male-specific association with hypertension [16] (Fig. 1). Large genetic epidemiological studies are useful to compare results between different races. Now, we recognize the importance of large population-based studies, but the problem of genotyping a large number of samples has to be solved.

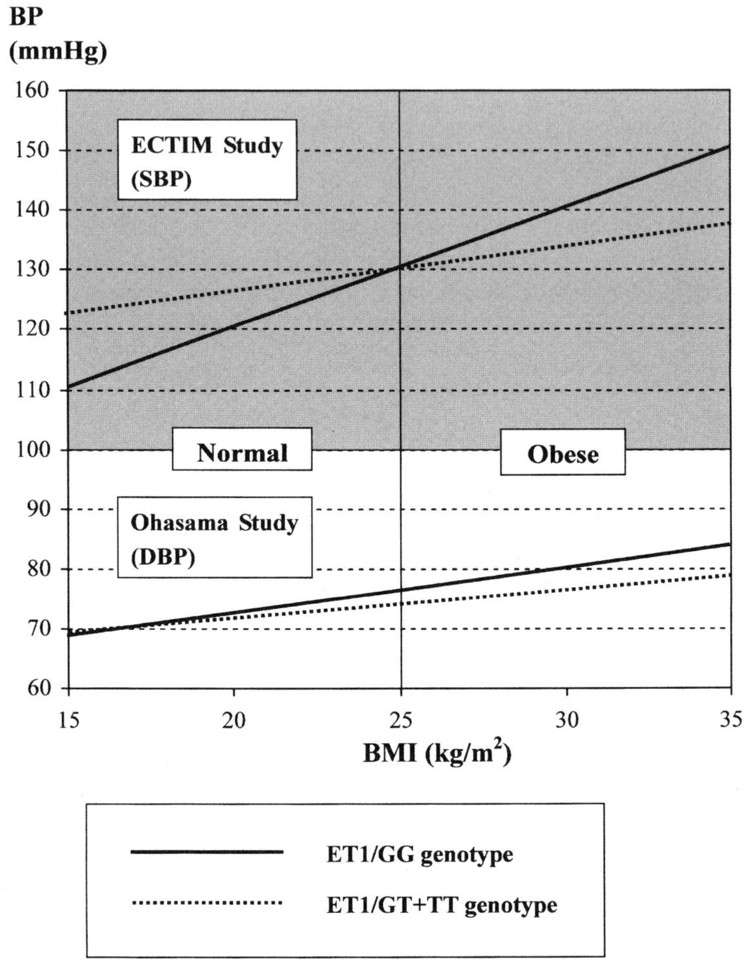

Figure 1. Genotype-specific regression slope of systolic blood pressure level on BMI

TAQMAN PCR METHOD AND ANGIOTENSINOGEN GENE VARIANTS

The TaqMan PCR method is a combination of PCR and allele-specific oligonucleotide hybridization [17]. After initial denaturation, an allele-specific probe with a fluorescent dye is hybridized with a specific sequence. The complementary fragment is extended from the primer by DNA polymerase, then the hydrolyzed probe produces fluorescence. Using a sequence detector, the genotype is easily detected by the difference in fluorescence. We applied this new technique for determination of angiotensinogen gene polymorphism. Because of difficulty in the design of primers and probes specific for the M235T (methionine to threonine substitution at codon

235) polymorphism of the angiotensinogen gene (AGT), we determined the T + 31C polymorphism which is located in intron 1 and is in complete linkage disequilibrium with M235T. The CC, CT and TT genotypes of this polymorphism and controls without DNA samples are clearly divided into four groups without digestion of PCR products using a restriction enzyme and gel electrophoresis. This approach markedly saved both time and cost of genotype determination. Using samples from the Suita Study, we examined the association between AGT/T + 31C and hypertension. AGT/T + 31C was associated with a family history of hypertension but not with the prevalence of hypertension [18]. The estimated odds ratio for a positive family history of hypertension in individuals with the C allele was 1.20 (95% CI: 1.06–1.35). Multiple logistic regression analysis revealed that the effect of the T + 31C polymorphism on increased risk for a family history of hypertension was significant (Wald $\chi^2 = 8.22$, $p = 0.016$). The estimated odds ratio for a family history of hypertension was 1.48 (1.12–1.97) in CC vs. TT and 1.08 (0.81–1.47) in CT vs. TT. Our results were compatible with the meta-analysis of Kunz and co-workers [19]. If cases were defined as those with a family history of hypertension, positive results were frequently obtained. Consequently, our current conclusion is that angiotensinogen polymorphism not directly but indirectly increases the risk for hypertension.

VARIOUS PHENOTYPES OF BLOOD PRESSURE AND GENE POLYMORPHISMS

Another large epidemiological study, the Ohasama Study which started with a cohort base in 1987, has focused on the importance of blood pressure measurements [20]. The Ohasama Study obtained 24 hour ambulatory blood pressure monitoring (ABPM) data from 802 subjects, and home blood pressure data were obtained from 1,245 subjects with informed consent for genetic analysis also. The various well-documented data concerning blood pressure allowed us to examine the interaction between genotype and blood pressure. In this study, we were able to examine three different types of blood pressure data, casual, ABPM and home blood pressure. Using the TaqMan PCR method, we evaluated about 802 participants of the Ohasama Study, and as a result, found no association between any parameter of blood pressure and the AGT/T + 31C polymorphism. However, focusing on the blood pressure difference between daytime and nighttime blood pressure, a significant difference between genotypes was observed. Blood pressure of subjects with the TT genotype significantly decreased at nighttime, suggesting that the AGT/C + 31 allele is a risk for non-dipping, which is considered a risk for cardiovascular complications [21]. This result seems to emphasize the importance of precise blood pressure measurements as the phenotype in the consideration of genetic predisposing factors for hypertension.

GENE-ENVIRONMENTAL INTERACTION AND OVERVIEW OF TAILOR-MADE MEDICINE

Another important issue is that the blood pressure is modulated by the interactions between environmental and genetic factors. It should always be kept in mind that the genetic effect is also modified by environmental factors, such as ageing, salt intake, and obesity. In the Suita Study, we examined the genetic involvement of the epsilon 4 allele in the apolipoprotein E gene (APOE/ε4), which has been shown to be a risk for hyperlipidemia and late onset type Alzheimer's disease, on the risk for hyperlipidemia and hypertension. Certainly, APOE/ε4 also significantly contributed to a 2.9% increase of total cholesterol, 11.8% increase of triglyceride and 3.2% decrease of HDL-cholesterol in the Suita Study. On the other hand, against our initial expectation, subjects with APOE/ε4 were significantly ($p < 0.03$) more frequent (19.7%) in normotensives than in hypertensives (16.9%), the estimated odds ratio for hypertension (with APOE/ε4 vs. without APOE/ε4) being 0.83 (95% CI: 0.70–0.98). Interestingly, the significance of the association (OR = 0.64, 95% CI: 0.48–0.86) was higher in young subjects (<60 years old) but disappeared in old subjects. A similar result in which the significance was enhanced in young subjects was observed in the association study between ACE/DD and hypertension. These results lead us to conclude that large scale of genetic epidemiological studies play a key role in examining these gene-environmental interactions.

In the Ohasama Study also, a unique association between the endothelin 1 gene (ET1) and hypertension was detected recently. The baseline characteristics (age, body mass index, systolic and diastolic blood pressure, antihypertensive treatment) of all subjects in the Ohasama Study were not significantly different according to the genotype of the G/T (Lys198Asn) polymorphism of ET1. In obese subjects ($\geq 25\,kg/m^2$), however, diastolic blood pressure was significantly associated with the G/T polymorphism of ET-1. After adjustment for confounding factors, a significant association remained; diastolic blood pressure in subjects carrying the T allele (GT + TT) was 1.8 mmHg higher ($p = 0.04$) than that in those with the GG genotype in overweight people [22]. Similar results were also obtained in ECTIM and the Glasgow Heart Scan Study [23] (Fig. 1). In addition, we showed in the Suita Study that the correlation between blood pressure and body mass index differed significantly according to the genotypes of a beta 2 adrenoceptor gene polymorphism.

As stated above, our recent investigations revealed an indirect effect of gene polymorphisms in the pathogenesis of hypertension and related disease. The aim of investigations concerning gene polymorphism seems to be distilled in the identification of certain environmental states that the polymorphism affects as risk factors. If a genotype is strongly effective in association with a high salt intake, restriction of salt intake should be the first recommendation by the physician. If a subject is considered to have a genetic predisposition to obesity, the physician should recommend dietary therapy and exercise. In the implementation of future tailored medication, information on single nucleotide polymorphisms must be useful in the prevention, care and treatment of common diseases in daily clinical practice.

ACKNOWLEDGEMENTS

We would like to express enormous gratitude to the following people for their continuous support of genetic epidemiological investigations: Drs. Jun Ogata, Toshifumi

Mannami, Nozomu Inamoto and Shunroku Baba (the Suita Study), Drs. Yutaka Imai, Takayoshi Ohkubo, Atsushi Hozawa, Mitsunobu Matsubara, Kenichi Nagai, Hirofumi Kitaoka, Ichiro Tsuji, Tsutomu Araki, Hiroshi Satoh, and Shigeru Hisamichi (the Ohasama Study). We are also grateful to Drs. Kazuhiko Ishikawa, Takashi Asai, Masayuki Fukuda, Noriyuki Sato, Seiju Takami, Yuxiao Fu, Yoshio Iwashima, Ken Sugimoto, Masaharu Motone, Shiori Takase, Yoshimi Kiuchi, Naoharu Iwai, Mitsuru Ohishi and Hiromi Rakugi, for their valuable support of the current studies.

The present study was supported by a Grant-in-Aid from the Japanese Ministry of Health, Labor, and Welfare, Grants-in-Aid for Scientific Research (12557063, 13770349, 13204050, 13670709) from the Ministry of Education, Science, Sports and Culture of Japan, and by research grants from the Uehara Memorial Foundation, the Takeda Medical Foundation, the Salt Science Research Foundation, the Osaka Medical Research Foundation for Incurable Diseases, the Yokoyama Foundation for Clinical Pharmacology and Therapeutics, the Kanae Foundation for Life and Socio-Medical Science and the Kurozumi Medical Foundation.

REFERENCES

1. Lalouel JM, Rohrwasser A. 2001. Development of genetic hypotheses in essential hypertension. J Hum Genet 46:299–306.
2. Timberlake DS, O'Connor DT, Parmer RJ. 2001. Molecular genetics of essential hypertension: recent results and emerging strategies. Curr Opin Nephrol Hypertens 10:71–79.
3. Higaki J, Katsuya T, Morishita R, Ogihara T. 2001. Symposium on the etiology of hypertension–summarizing studies in 20th century. 1. Hypertension and genes. Intern Med 40:144–147.
4. Lifton RP, Gharavi AG, Geller DS. 2001. Molecular mechanisms of human hypertension. Cell 104:545–556.
5. Lifton RP. 1995. Genetic determinants of human hypertension. Proc Natl Acad Sci USA 92: 8545–8551.
6. Lifton RP, Dluhy RG, Powers M, Rich GM, Cook S, Ulick S, Lalouel JM. 1992. A chimaeric 11 beta-hydroxylase/aldosterone synthase gene causes glucocorticoid-remediable aldosteronism and human hypertension. Nature 355:262–265.
7. Wilson AF, Elston RC, Tran LD, Siervogel RM. 1991. Use of the robust sib-pair method to screen for single-locus, multiple-locus, and pleiotropic effects: application to traits related to hypertension. Am J Hum Genet 48:862–872.
8. Xu X, Rogus JJ, Terwedow HA, Yang J, Wang Z, Chen C, Niu T, Wang B, Xu H, Weiss S, Schork NJ, Fang Z. 1999. An extreme-sib-pair genome scan for genes regulating blood pressure. Am J Hum Genet 64:1694–1701.
9. Risch NJ. 2000. Searching for genetic determinants in the new millennium. Nature 405:847–856.
10. Ogihara T, Katsuya T, Higaki J. 2000. Genetic analysis of essential hypertension in Japanese populations. Ann N Y Acad Sci 902:8–16.
11. Mannami T, Konishi M, Baba S, Nishi N, Terao A. 1997. Prevalence of asymptomatic carotid atherosclerotic lesions detected by high-resolution ultrasonography and its relation to cardiovascular risk factors in the general population of a Japanese city: the Suita study. Stroke 28:518–525.
12. Ohishi M, Rakugi H, Ogihara T. 1994. Association between a deletion polymorphism of the angiotensin-converting-enzyme gene and left ventricular hypertrophy [letter]. N Engl J Med 331: 1097–1098.
13. Jacob HJ, Lindpaintner K, Lincoln SE, Kusumi K, Bunker RK, Mao YP, Ganten D, Dzau VJ, Lander ES. 1991. Genetic mapping of a gene causing hypertension in the stroke-prone spontaneously hypertensive rat. Cell 67:213–224.
14. O'Donnell CJ, Lindpaintner K, Larson MG, Rao VS, Ordovas JM, Schaefer EJ, Myers RH, Levy D. 1998. Evidence for association and genetic linkage of the angiotensin-converting enzyme locus with

hypertension and blood pressure in men but not women in the Framingham Heart Study. Circulation 97:1766–1772.

15. Rigat B, Hubert C, Corvol P, Soubrier F. 1992. PCR detection of the insertion/deletion polymorphism of the human angiotensin converting enzyme gene (DCP1) (dipeptidyl carboxypeptidase 1). Nucleic Acids Res 20:1433.
16. Higaki J, Baba S, Katsuya T, Sato N, Ishikawa K, Mannami T, Ogata J, Ogihara T. 2000. Deletion allele of angiotensin-converting enzyme gene increases risk of essential hypertension in Japanese men: the Suita Study. Circulation 101:2060–2065.
17. Ibrahim MS, Lofts RS, Jahrling PB, Henchal EA, Weedn VW, Northrup MA, Belgrader P. 1998. Real-time microchip PCR for detecting single-base differences in viral and human DNA. Anal Chem 70:2013–2017.
18. Ishikawa K, Baba S, Katsuya T, Iwai N, Asai T, Fukuda M, Takiuchi S, Fu Y, Mannami T, Ogata J, Higaki J, Ogihara T. 2001. T + 31C polymorphism of angiotensinogen gene and essential hypertension. Hypertension 37:281–285.
19. Kunz R, Kreutz R, Beige J, Distler A, Sharma AM. 1997. Association between the angiotensinogen 235T-variant and essential hypertension in whites: a systematic review and methodological appraisal. Hypertension 30:1331–1337.
20. Imai Y, Satoh H, Nagai K, Sakuma M, Sakuma H, Minami N, Munakata M, Hashimoto J, Yamagishi T, Watanabe N, et al. 1993. Characteristics of a community-based distribution of home blood pressure in Ohasama in northern Japan. J Hypertens 11:1441–1449.
21. Fujiwara T, Katsuya T, Matsubara M, Mikami T, Ishikawa K, Kikuya M, Ohkubo T, Hozawa A, Michimata M, Suzuki M, Metoki H, Araki T, Tsuji I, Higaki J, Satoh H, Hisamichi S, Ogihara T, Imai Y. 2002. T + 31C polymorphism of angiotensinogen gene and nocturnal blood pressure decline: The Ohasama Study. J Hypertens 20:1779–1784.
22. Asai T, Ohkubo T, Katsuya T, Higaki J, Fu Y, Fukuda M, Hozawa A, Matsubara M, Kitaoka H, Tsuji I, Araki T, Satoh H, Hisamichi S, Imai Y, Ogihara T. 2001. Endothelin-1 gene variant associates with blood pressure in obese Japanese subjects: the Ohasama study. Hypertension 38:1321–1324.
23. Tiret L, Poirier O, Hallet V, McDonagh TA, Morrison C, McMurray JJ, Dargie HJ, Arveiler D, Ruidavets JB, Luc G, Evans A, Cambien F. 1999. The Lys198Asn polymorphism in the endothelin-1 gene is associated with blood pressure in overweight people. Hypertension 33:1169–1174.

G.N. Pierce, M. Nagano, P. Zahradka, and N.S. Dhalla (eds.).
ATHEROSCLEROSIS, HYPERTENSION AND DIABETES.
Kluwer Academic Publishers. Boston.

ROLE OF SYMPATHETIC NERVOUS SYSTEM IN HYPERTENSION

C.L. KAUL and P. RAMARAO

Department of Pharmacology and Toxicology, National Institute of Pharmaceutical Education and Research (NIPER), S.A. S. Nagar 160 062, Punjab, India

Summary. There is considerable evidence that sympathetic nervous system plays an important role in the pathogenesis of several cardiovascular diseases including hypertension. Most of the important evidence is based on the microneurographic method of intraneural recordings of sympathetic nerve activity and radiotracer techniques for the study of the norepinephrine kinetics. Three possible mechanisms for the long term regulation of arterial pressure proposed are antinatriuretic and renin stimulating effect of renal sympathetic nerves, sympathetic effects on the influence on the development of vascular membrane properties and lastly the trophic effects of the sympathetic nerves on the vascular smooth muscle. There is also some evidence regarding the role of SNS in different forms of experimental hypertension. Although the relationship between insulin resistance, hyperinsulinemia and hypertension is not very clear the possibility that the insulin resistance and compensatory hyperinsulinemia have major roles in susceptible subjects predisposed to hypertension by hereditary and environmental factors. Finally there is evidence that adrenergic activation may be involved in the progression of the structural alterations, which are prominent in hypertension including atherosclerosis. These findings lead further support to use of antihypertensive drugs which all interfere with the sympathetic functions.

Key words: Sympathetic nervous system, Hypertension, diabetes, Obesity, Renin angiotensin sytem

Address Correspondence to: C.L. Kaul, Department of Pharmacology and Toxicology, National Institute of Pharmaceutical Education and Research (NIPER), S.A. S. Nagar 160 062, Punjab, India. Fax: 91-172-214692; e-mail: kaulniper@yahoo.com

INTRODUCTION

The sympathetic nervous system (SNS) is of major importance in the regulation of numerous physiological functions including blood pressure. Its role in the genesis of hypertension has completed a full circle, an early enthusiasm, a period of neglect and strong evidence, which is being accumulated now. Although it is well established that SNS plays an important role in the acute regulation of blood pressure, it is not very clear whether alterations in the sympathetic activity contributes to long term arterial homeostasis [1]. This is partially related to the fact that assessing sympathetic functions in chronic state is not very easy. There is however, enough experimental and theoretical evidence to point out the involvement of renal sympathetic nerve as an important link between SNS and long-term arterial pressure control [2]. Recent studies of Mark [3] indicate increased sympathetic nerve activity in hypertension suggesting that SNS plays a primary role in the pathogenesis of hypertension and long term regulation of arterial pressure. Three possible mechanisms have been proposed to sustain the long-term sympathetic nerve influences in hypertension. These are antinatriuretic and renin stimulating effects of the renal sympathetic, nerve, sympathetic influence on the development of vascular membrane properties and tropic effects of the sympathetic nerves on vascular and cardiac muscle [3].

Hypertension being a multi-factorial disease, there is an imbalance between vasodilatory and vasoconstrictor mechanisms. Increased sympathetic nerve activity is one of the primary pathophysiological mechanisms in the development and maintenance of hypertension. This hyperactivity of SNS also contributes to progression of coronary artery diseases and may precipitate acute coronary events. The evidence supporting this concept comes largely from the studies performed in different animal models of hypertension where increased sympathetic drive to the heart and circulation was shown to either trigger persistent increased blood pressure or to the maintenance of blood pressure elevation originally produced by noradrenergic mechanisms [2,4–6].

Besides this the importance of SNS in the maintenance of hypertension is evident from the fact that all the drugs, which interfere with SNS on blood vessel can effectively lower the blood pressure to normotensive level [7]. The present review will summarize both experimental and clinical evidence to show involvement of SNS in hypertension.

Evidence for sympathetic activation

During the past two decades the situation has changed dramatically because a number of new techniques have been developed where direct and indirect quantification of adrenergic cardio-vascular influence has shown enhanced sympathetic nerve activity even in the humans. Increased cardiac sympathetic drive has also been reported in hypertensive subjects [8]. This evidence is based on the results where resting heart rate of borderline hypertensive patients was reduced by propranolol to marked degree than the lower heart rate of normotensive patients.

Previous studies reported have provided conflicting results regarding the changes in the catecholamines levels in hypertension. This was primarily related to the absence of accurate and sensitive methods for their estimation. However, with the advent of sensitive radio enzymatic method, it has been possible to measure accurately the circulating catecholamines levels as an index of sympathetic activity. Before the advent of this sensitive method, urinary excretion of catecholamines was used extensively to measure the adrenergic activity. However, the disadvantage in using this method was excretion of urinary catecholamines represents some of the events occurring in the body over a long period of time and minute and transitory changes in the sympathetic activity could not be correlated with urinary excretion. Some convincing evidence regarding the role of SNS in essential hypertension have come from the studies using radiotracer techniques for study of norepinephrine kinetics and microneurographic method for intraneural recording of sympathetic nerve activity. Using a sensitive method of estimation, it has been reported that norepinephrine levels are low during sleep, which increase progressively from supine to upright position and increase from mild to moderate and severe exercise. These changes seem to correlate with the behavioural changes in neural sympathetic drive in the cardiovascular system [9]. Although earlier studies reported comparing norepinephrine levels in normotensive and hypertensive individuals led to conflicting results, a meta-analysis published by Goldstein [10] showed that norepinephrine levels were higher in essential hypertensive patients when compared to normotensive control. These observations have also been further confirmed by other workers [11].

Using combined measurements of plasma catecholamines with responses to adrenergic agonists and antagonists on forearm vascular resistance in mild hypertensive subjects to dissect sympathetic nervous influences, Egan and coworkers [12] showed increased plasma catecholamine levels and greater reduction in the forearm vascular resistance in response to α-adrenoceptor blocker with no effect on the α-adrenoceptor sensitivity as determined by the norepinephrine response. These results seem to indicate that there is enhanced sympathetic vasoconstriction tone in young hypertensive subjects and this increased vasoconstrictor tone results from the increased sympathetic neural release of norepinephrine and not from increased α-adrenoceptor sensitivity to norepinephrine.

Although some studies have shown no evidence for increased muscle sympathetic nervous activity [13], there are number of reports where elevated muscle sympathetic nervous activity has been reported in mild hypertensive subjects which is consistent with the evidence for increased sympathetic neural influence on the forearm vascular resistance in mild hypertensive patients [14–18] . Even in accelerated essential and renovascular hypertension increase in the muscle sympathetic nervous activity has been reported [15,19].

Some of these discrepancies in the above results have been ascribed to diet, sodium and carbohydrate intake and body mass, since some of these parameters were not carefully controlled and these features are an important determinant to muscle sympathetic nervous activity [20–22].

Involvement of SNS in the long-term regulation of arterial pressure

It is well accepted that SNS via baroreceptor reflex plays an important role in the short-term regulation of blood pressure [23,24]. There are, however, several arguments against its role in the long-term regulation. One of the major arguments is that the baroreceptors reset or adapt to the chronic changes in the arterial pressure. Although resetting of arterial baroreceptors is well established, it is not very clear whether cardio pulmonary receptors also play role. Further studies of Miki et al. [25,26] have shown that increase in the arterial pressure for 30–60 minutes produce sustained decrease in the renal afferent nerve activity and concluded that arterial stretch receptors do not reset. Another argument against the role of baroreflex in the long-term regulation of sympathetic activity is that the chronic impairment of afferent baroreflex pathways does not result in significant changes in the arterial pressure. It has been argued that the chronic changes in the sympathetic efferent pathways do not consistently affect the arterial pressure. These observations are further supported by experiments in which chronic intravenous infusion of norepinephrine in conscious dogs do not produce hypertension [27] and long term sympathetic blockade produced by 6-hydroxydopamine (6-OHD) [28] or α-adrenoceptor antagonist do not produce a sustained fall in arterial pressure [29]. It has also been argued that sympathetic over activity may not alone be significant to increase arterial pressure since certain pathological states like heart failure and cirrhosis where increased sympathetic activity is seen are not characterized with hypertension. The same analogy cannot however, apply to rennin angiotensin system (RAS) where the importance of the system in chronic hypertension can be questioned.

One of the mechanisms proposed to explain the long-term regulation of arterial pressure is the pressure-natriuresis mechanism [30–32]. This theory basically predicts, the maintenance of arterial pressure is attained by changes in the renal excretion of sodium and water. Although there is some controversy regarding this mechanism, there is enough evidence to support it [30–32].

Although most of these arguments do not favour the role of SNS in the long-term regulation of hypertension, these negative results do not rule out its possibility [33–36]. The argument against the role of baroreflex in the long tem control of blood pressure is recognized and it is quite likely that baroreceptor independent pathways can even regulate the sympathetic activity. Secondly failure to produce chronic hypertension after intravenous infusion of norepinephrine in conscious dogs may be related to the fact that continuous infusion do not mimic bursting pattern of sympathetic nerve discharge. It is also well recognized that other neurotransmitters are present (neuropeptide Y) with norepinephrine in the sympathetic nerve terminals, which can modulate arterial pressure independently or with norepinephrine. Although neuropeptide Y (NPY) released from sympathetic nerve terminals has very little effect on the sympathetic target tissues, it enhances the response of peripheral targets to noradrenergic stimulation [37,38]. Further NPY may produce hypertension by increasing the response of norepinephrine on the target tissue. Increasing levels of NPY are reported to parallel increased plasma norepinephrine in DOCA-Salt and pulmonary hypertensive models [38]. The vasoconstrictor effect of ATP, which is released in response to sympathetic stimulation and coexists in the synapse with norepinephrine potentiates the vascular responses of norepinephrine [39]. Under normal conditions, the role of epinephrine as a modulator in hypertension is not very significant, but in hypertensive individuals, release of epinephrine seems to be higher from target organs and thereby increasing sympathetic transmission and thus contributing to increased arterial pressure [40].

It is, therefore likely that the intravenous infusion of norepinephrine may not exactly mimic sympathetic nerve stimulation and increase arterial pressure but intrarenal administration does. Intrarenal administration of norepinephrine does increase the arterial pressure by increasing peripheral resistance and such doses of norepinephrine are ineffective when given intravenously [41,42]. Even low doses of norepinephrine, which do not affect renal blood flow, also produce hypertension [43,44], which supports the concept that increased sympathetic activity of the kidney specifically produce hypertension. Further support to the role of SNS in the long-term regulation of blood pressure comes from the findings that renal sympathetic neural activation can effect long term arterial pressure regulation. Activation of renal sympathetic nerve promotes antinatriuresis and stimulates the release of renin [45,46] resulting in increased renal vascular resistance and circulating concentration of angiotensin-II, a powerful vasoconstrictor. Antinatriuresis effect is seen at low frequency renal nerve stimulation, which do not influence renal blood flow or glomerular filtration rate. It seems that the renal sympathetic nerves have a multiple actions on renal functions and have a pathophysiological role in the long-term regulation of arterial pressure. The role of central neural α_2-adrenoceptors which control the sympathetic neural outflow seems to be involved in altering regulation of renal sympathetic nerve activity in spontaneous hypertensive rats [47–50].

Some evidence also exists that SNS can influence the vascular membrane properties. Increase in the passive permeability of vascular muscle to sodium has been reported in spontaneous hypertensive rats, which results in augmented response to norepinephrine [51]. Further evidence supporting the role of SNS in the long term maintenance of hypertension comes from the studies where SNS like RAS is reported to promote the growth of vascular [52,53] and cardiac muscle [54,55]. Tropic effects of SNS, cardiac myocytes are independent of contractile and haemodynamic effects, which are mediated by α-adrenoceptors [54], whereas the tropic effect on the vascular smooth muscle increase vascular resistance and response to vasoconstriction stimuli resulting in hypertension. These tropic effects of SNS on blood pressure are greater during growth and development [52], which seems to suggest that the increased sympathetic nerve activity is greater during the early stages of hypertension at a time when it is most likely to effect the structure and membrane properties of blood vessels resulting in the long-term regulation of blood pressure.

From the above discussion it seems pertinent to conclude that SNS does have a role in the long-term regulation of blood pressure. A few studies have also been reported where chronic changes in sympathetic activity have an impact on pressure regulation, eg renal dennervation shifts the acute renal function curve to a lower pressure level [56] and if these changes can be extrapolated to long term changes in renal functions and arterial pressure seem to suggest that renal sympathetic neural activation has an impact on the long term regulation of arterial pressure. Activation of renal sympathetic nerve stimulates the renin release and increase the circulation of angiotensin II, a powerful vasoconstrictor [45]. Chronic stimulation of sympathetic ganglia is also reported to produce hypertension [57–59]. All these studies seem to suggest the haemostatic control of arterial pressure needs a chronically responsive nervous system.

Considerable evidence also exists that rats rendered hypertensive by DOCA saline showed hyperactivity of SNS which is reflected by increased turnover of norepinephrine, increased levels of circulating norepinephrine [60,61]. Further, there is decreased retention and storage of endogenous norepinephrine in the sympathetic nerve terminal in these animals [62], which suggest that there is an enhanced release of norepinephrine from sympathetic nerve terminals [63]. These alterations are characterized by decreased endogenous norepinephrine contained in a number of sympathetically innervated tissues [60]. These results seem to indicate that there is a defect in the storage and retention of norepinephrine in the sympathetic nerves in this type of hypertension and thereby increase the availability of the neurotransmitter at the receptor site. Changes in the turnover of norepinephrine have also been reported in other forms of experimental hypertension e.g. neurogenic type [64] and perinephritic type [65] in hypertension associated with kidney infarction [66] and hypertension produced by unilateral renal artery stenosis with contralatral nephrectomy [60].

Central regulation of the SNS also plays an important role in the maintenance of blood pressure but its contribution to chronic arterial pressure is less clear. The major pathway of the nervous system contributing to hypertension is SNS. Many clinical studies have shown that peripheral SNS are intimately involved in hypertension and recent studies have characterized the abnormality in the brain that seems to predispose animal models to overacting of SNS and hypertension. The data suggests that the brain via the SNS directly contributes to some forms of hypertension and indirectly contribute to all of them [67]. Over action of the SNS may result either by an appropriate elevated sympathetic drive from brain centers and increase in the release of neurotransmitter in the periphery or amplification of neurotransmitter signal at the target tissue.

SNS, hypertension and diabetes

Insulin resistance and hyperinsulinemia with obesity have been postulated to mediate human associated hypertension [68]. Association of diabetic mellitus and hypertension predispose an individual to atheroslerotic cardiovascular diseases. It has been postulated that hyperinsulinemia may be an important factor to cause hypertension in patients with diabetic mellitus and this is based on the facts that hyperinsulinemia can cause (a) sodium and water retention (b) increased sympathetic nerve activity and reduced catecholamine clearance, (c) increased intracellular calcium concentration and reduced magnesium concentration, (d) increased vascular responsiveness for the vasoactive substances. Evidence supporting this hypothesis has come mainly from epidemiological studies showing correlation between insulin resistance, hyperinsulinemia and blood pressure. Further, it has also been suggested from short-term studies that insulin has renal and sympathetic effects that could raise blood pressure if these effects are sustained. Although this evidence has been accumulative over a period of time, there are no studies, which demonstrate direct correlation between chronic hypertension and insulin resistance or hyperinsulinemia in humans. Some long-term studies reported in dogs and humans do not support the hypothesis. In fact many studies in dogs and humans suggest the vasodialatory effect of insulin, which leads to reduction in blood pressure. Although resistance to metabolic effects of insulin has been suggested for hyperinsulinemia to cause hypertension, chronic increase in plasma concentration of insulin does not cause hypertension in dogs and humans. Studies with antihyperglycemic therapy intended to lower blood pressure by decreasing insulin resistance, may be unrelated to the effects on insulin sensitivity. Obesity seems to be the key factor to account for the correlation between hypertension, insulin resistance and hyperinsulinemia but increased blood pressure in obesity is not mediated through insulin resistance and hyperinsulinemia.

Although there is no direct correlation between hyperinsulinemia, insulin resistance and hypertension, there is enough evidence that indicate metabolic abnormalities associated with diabetic mellitus may increase the risk of cardiovascular complications, which may be associated with hypertension and diabetes [68].

Experimental evidence for humans and animals support the concept that adrenergic neural factors may be involved in development of hypertensive related cardiovascular complications. The role of neural sympathetic factors in the pathophysiology of hypertension and its complications suggest that the modulation of sympathetic activity should be an important target for anti-hypertensive therapy to reduce blood pressure and cardiovasucular complications [69].

Despite the clinical importance of this association the nature of the relationship between blood pressure and insulin resistance remains obscure. It is likely that some other factors like environmental or genetic are involved in their relationship since hypertension does not develop any of the insulin resistance subjects and hyperinsulinemia does not always cause rise in blood pressure [70].

SNS, obesity and hypertension

Obesity has been reported to account for 75% of human essential hypertension. Renal sodium reabsorption and a hypertensive shift of renal pressure, natriuresis plays a key role in modulating this type of hypertension. Activation of SNS contributes to obesity-induced hypertension by excessive sodium retention because adrenergic blockade or renal denncrvation markedly attenuates this effect [71]. Some of the recent observations also suggest that leptin with its multiple interaction with other neurochemical pathways in the hypothalamus may be a link between excess weight gain and increased sympathetic nerve activities. These observations are based on experiments where short-term administration of leptin into cerebral ventricle increases sympathetic activity whereas long-term infusion in nonobese rodents can cause increased heart rate and arterial pressure through adrenergic activation. A number of studies reported show a correlation between plasma leptin concentration and high blood pressure [72,73]. However, not all studies have confirmed this correlation [74]. There is also some evidence that hyperlipidemia increases sympathetic activity in obesity [68]. It may therefore be concluded that activation of SNS may not be the only factor by which obesity measures blood pressure. The role of RAS and the physical compression of the kidney may be an important factor in measuring blood pressure in obesity [75,76]. Since obesity accounts for about 75% of human essential, hypertension it is important that unraveling mechanism by which weight gain increases the sympathetic activity, alters renal functions and raises arterial pressure may provide the better understanding in essential hypertension.

ROLE OF RENIN ANGIOTENSIN SYSTEM (RAS)

In any discussion on the mechanisms involved in hypertension the two important factors, which need to be differentiated, are (a) initiating and (b) sustaining of hypertension. The etiological role of plasma rennin in initiation and maintenance of renovascular hypertension has been subject of controversy in animal studies. Experimental hypertension induced by clamping one or both renal arteries, the pressor substance released [77] from the kidney appears only for about a week in rats [78] and 3 to 4 days in dogs [79] although chronic hypertension develops. These results indicate that RAS is important only for initiation of experimentally induced hypertension and may not be necessary for its chronic maintenance. Although RAS does not seems to have precise role in essential hypertension, the heterogenicity of plasma renin value in this type of hypertension may be of pathophysiologial and prognostic importance. Although the role of RAS in the long-term regulation of arterial pressure is reasonably established [1], it is not very clear whether SNS also plays a similar role in body fluid volume and arterial pressure homeostasis.

The renal nerves are thought to play an important role in cardiovascular regulation under normotensive and hypertensive conditions. Although renal dennervation does not alter basal plasma renin activity (PRA) in normotensive animals, it prevents increased renin release in neurogenic hypertension suggesting that increased PRA may be one of the several factors that contribute to increased blood pressure after baroreceptor deafferentation [80]. There is also some direct and indirect evidence that increase in blood pressure or blood volume produces sustained changes in renin release. Decrease in renal perfusion pressure (4 days) increase in the plasma renin activity suggesting that renal baroreceptors do not reset to this chronic stimulus [81]. Further chronic sodium and water depletion sustained increase in plasma rennin activity and angiotensin II concentration. Conversely increase in sodium intake produces suppression of rennin and angiotensin II [45].

Since the renal nerve activity stimulates renin release, Reinhart et al. [81] have studied the role of RAS in mediating the long-term hypertensive effects of renal adrenergic stimulation. The results reported by these authors seem to suggest that the tubular effects of Angiotensin II increases sodium reabsorption which plays an important role in mediating hypertension by low levels of adrenergic stimulation. These results will have relevance to the human essential hypertension, which is characterized by high rate of renal norepinephrine spillover and increased PRA [82]. There is growing evidence implicating the role of SNS in the pathogenesis and renovascular hypertension in humans. Increase in plasma norepinephrine and urinary excretion of catecholamines and their metabolites have been reported in patients with renovascular hypertension [83–85]. Similar observations have been reported for one kidney and one clip hypertension [65,86–92]. Intracisternal administration of 6-OHD or creation of leision in the posterior hypothalamus prevents hypertension in one-kidney, one-clip model [86,87]. In one-kidney, one-clip hypertensive rats, renal dennervation is reported to significantly lower blood pressure without any significant change in sodium and water intake, sodium excretion, PRA and a decrease in plasma catecholamines levels [93]. These requests indicate that in this type of hypertension the fall in blood pressure following renal dennervation is in part secondary to a decrease in peripheral sympathetic activity.

Even in the genetic models (SHR of the Okamoto strain) there is evidence that SNS via the efferent renal nerve activity plays an important role in the pathogenesis and hypertension by causing sodium retention [94]. Renal dennervation delays the development and blunts the severity of hypertension [94–96], which is an accompanied by increased urinary sodium excretion suggesting a renal efferent mechanism. However, the effect of renal dennervation on the development and maintenance of hypertension in SHR in dependent upon the age of the animals when the kidneys are dennervated [94]. Similar to SHR increased renal efferent nerve activity contributes to the development of hypertension. In the DOCA saline hypertensive rats, hypertension is caused by renal sodium retention. Renal dennervation carried out prior to starting DOCA- saline treatment delays the development and blunts the severity of hypertension [97,98].

The role of vascular RAS and its interaction with sympathetic neurotransmission has been investigated in hypertensive patients [99]. In the animal studies vascular angiotension II increases the vasoconstriction produced by stimulation of noradrenaline release at the presynaptic level and this effect is mediated by β-adrenoeptor activation. All these results seem to indicate that SNS via the renal nerves play an important role in the pathogenic of renovascular hypertension in laboratory animals and even the humans.

Role of SNS in experimental hypertension

Role of SNS in experimental hypertension has been investigated using immunosympathectomized rats, DOCA-saline rats and rats sympathectomized with 6-OHD and guanethidine. The results reported in the literature are conflicting 6-OHD when given to weanling rats failed to develop hypertension in bilaterally clamped renal hypertensive rats. In these weanling rats there was a marked destruction of sympathetic nervous system as judged by the cardiac catacholamine concentration [7,100]. Adult rats given 6-OHD with bilateral clamping or DOCA treatment did not prevent development of hypertension [101]. Although these authors reported that there is a considerable lag time in the development of hypertension, which has not been confirmed by other authors [100]. In the adult rats given 6-OHD cardiac catecholamine levels where 40% of control when measured after 8 weeks although when measured after one week in the same group the catecholamines levels were undetected. These results seems to indicate that in the adult rats there is certain amount of re-generation of SNS following 6-OHD treatment which is not seen in the weanling rats. This has some similarity to immunosympathectomy where neurons are most vulnerable during first two weeks after birth [102]. Immunosympathectomy has also been reported to prevent the development of hypertension in the rat [103,104]. The failure of 6-OHD to prevent the development of hypertension in the adult rats may be related to the re-generation of adrenergic nerve terminals [105,106]. Intracerebroventricular or intracisternal injection of 6-OHD is also reported to prevent the rise in blood pressure that follows renal artery clamping in the rats [107] and cellophane perinephritis in rabbits [108]. After 4 weeks treatment with DOCA and saline centrally administered 6-OHD does not influence the blood pressure [109] indicating the importance of central neurogenic component in the early stages of development but may be not essential when the hypertension is developed. The development and maintenance of DOCA Saline hypertension could be due to various factors like early increase in peripheral sympathetic neuronal activity, circulating catecholamine levels in the presence of sodium retention and increased vascular reactivity. Increased renal sympathetic tone in the DOCA Saline hypertension has also been reported, which facilitate sodium retention and is necessary for the development of hypertension [110].

Neonatal administration of guanethedine to LH rats is reported not to alter blood pressure levels at the adult age indicating thereby their peripheral sympathetic fibers are not essential for the development of hypertension in LH Rats [28,111]. These authors further showed marked supersensitivity to α- & β- adrenoceptor stimulation and reducing catecholamines are derived mostly from the adrenal medulla, which play only a minor role in the control of blood pressure Lo et al. [111]. In sympathectomized animals using guanethedine Lo et al. [111] have shown stimulation of α adrenoceptors by circulating catecholamines play a significant role in the maintenance of blood pressure. Longe et al. [112] using DOCA-saline treated model of hypertension have demonstrated that adrenal medulla contribute more to the maintenance of blood pressure in male than female rats. The literature reports on the effect of neonatal sympathectomy on the development of genetic hypertension in rats are rather confusing because of the difference in the method of sympathectomy and the techniques used for measurement of blood pressure. In some of the earlier studies where guanethadine treatment is reported to completely prevent the development of hypertension, the method of measuring blood pressure was tail cuff technique [113]. Recent studies have however shown that restraining sympathectomized animals results in hypotension whereas control animals demonstrate hypertension under identical conditions [114].

Intracerebroventricular or intracisternal administration of 6-OHD has been reported to prevent rise in blood pressure that follows clamping of renal arteries [107,115]. Since central administration of 6-OHD is known to influence the fluid consumption and adequate saline intake is essential for the development of DOCA saline hypertension, the interference with the development at the time of hypertension resulting from destruction of catecholamine neurons cannot be accounted completely by diminished fluid intake [115]. Immunosympathetic with anti-body to nerve growth factor has also been reported to prevent both renal and DOCA Saline hypertension [104].

Sympathetic activation and organ damage

Considerable evidence exists in both animal models of hypertension and essential hypertension that sympathetic factors are involved in the progression of the cardiovascular structural alterations accompanying hypertension [3–6]. It has been reported that adrenergic agonists stimulate the growth of myocytes and replication of vascular smooth muscle cell in vitro, which is blocked by adrenoceptor antagonist [116,117]. Further beside the blood pressure, the cardiac sympathetic drive is also reported to be involved in the progression and regulation of left ventricular hypertrophy [118,119]. The arteriolar remodeling, which is seen in hypertension results in the increase in the total peripheral resistance i.e. increase in wall to lumen ratio and this reported to be much less marked in blood vessels which are subjected to sympathetic dennervation [117,120]. It thus seems that by promoting the vascular smooth muscle cell replication, activation of SNS can promote atherogenic process leading to established atherosclerotic plague [121]. Further in sympathectomised rats distensibility of carotid and femoral artery is increased [122]. Even in humans the distensibilities of femoral and radial arteries is markedly increased after removal of adrenergic tone by various procedures [123]. The contraction of the vascular smooth muscle is sympathetically mediated since the contracted muscle tissue is much less prone to distension for the intravascular pressure than the muscle, which is in relaxed state [117].

REFERENCES

1. Lohmeier TE. 2001. The sympathetic nervous system and long-term blood pressure regulation. Am J Hyperts 14:147S–154S.
2. DiBona GF. 2000. Nervous kidney. Interaction between renal sympathetic nerves and the renin angiotensin system in the control of renal function. Hypertension 36:1083–1088.
3. Mark AL. 1996. The sympathetic nervous system in hypertension: a potential long term regulator of arterial pressure. J Hypertens 14(Suppl. 5):S159-S165.
4. Folkow B. 1982. Physiological aspects of primary hypertension. Physiol Rev 62:347–504.
5. Oparil S. 1986. The sympathetic nervous system in clinical and experimental hypertension. Kidney Int 30:437–452.
6. Mancia G. 1997. Bjorn Folkow Award lecture: the sympathetic nervous system in hypertension. J Hypertens 15:1553–1565.

7. Kaul CL. 1999. Role of sympathetic nervous system in experimental hypertension and diabetes mellitus. Clin Exp Hypertens 21:95–112.
8. Julius S, Pascual AV, London R. 1971. Role of parasympathetic inhibition in the hyperkinetic type of borderline hypertension. Circulation 44:413–418.
9. Watson RD, Hamilton CA, Reid JL, Littler, WA. 1979. Changes in plasma norepinephrine blood pressure and heart rate during physical activity in hypertensive men. Hypertension 1:341–346.
10. Goldstein DS. 1983. Plasma catecholamines and essential hypertension. An analytical review. Hypertension 5:86–99.
11. Grassi G, Cattaneo BM, Seravalle G, Lanfranchi A, Mancia G. 1998. Baroreflex control of sympathetic nerve activity in essential and secondary hypertension. Hypertension 31:68–72.
12. Egan B, Panis R, Hinderliter A, Schork N, Julius S. 1987. Mechanism of Increased alpha adrenergic vasoconstriction in human essential hypertension. J Clin Invest 80:812–817.
13. Wallin BG, Sundlof G. 1979. A quantitative study of muscle nerve sympathetic activity in resting normotensive and hypertensive subjects. Hypertension 1:67–77.
14. Anderson EA, Sinkey CA, Lawton WJ, Mark AL. 1989. Elevated sympathetic nerve activity in borderline hypertensive humans. Evidence from direct intraneural recordings. Hypertension 14: 177–183.
15. Miyajima E, Yamada Y, Yoshida Y, Matsukawa T, Shionoiri H, Tochikubo O, Ishii M. 1991. Muscle sympathetic nerve activity in reno-vascular hypertension and primary aldosteronism. Hypertension 17:1057–1062.
16. Matsukawa T, Gotoh E, Hasegawa O, Miyajima E, Shionoiri H, Tochikubo O, Ishii M. 1991. Reduced arterial baroreflex control of muscle sympathetic nerve activity in young borderline hypertensives. Funct Neurol 6:113–120.
17. Yamada Y, Miyajima E, Tochikubo O, Matsukawa T, Ishii M. 1989. Age-related changes in muscle sympathetic nerve activity in essential hypertension. Hypertension 13:870–877.
18. Floras JS, Hara K. 1993. Sympathoneural and haemodynamic characteristics of young subjects with mild essential hypertension. J Hypertens 11:647–655.
19. Matsukawa T, Mano T, Gotoh E, Ishii M. 1993. Elevated sympathetic nerve activity in patients with accelerated essential hypertension. J Clin Invest 92:25–28.
20. Somers VK, Mark AL, Abboud FM. 1988. Potentiation of sympathetic nerve responses to hypoxia in borderline hypertension subjects. Hypertension 11:608–612.
21. Rea RF, Hamdan M. 1990. Baroreflex control of muscle sympathetic nerve activity in borderline hypertension. Circulation 82:856–862.
22. Scherrer U, Randin D, Tappy, Vollenweider P, Jequier E, Nicod P. 1994. Body fat and sympathetic nerve activity in healthy subjects. Circulation 89:2634–2640.
23. Spyer KM. 1990. The central nervous organization of reflex circulatory control. In central regulation of Autonomic functions. Ed AD Loewy and KM Spyer 168–188.
24. Stekiel WJ, Contney SJ, Lombard JH. 1991. Sympathetic neural control of vascular muscle in reduced renal mass hypertension. Hypertension 17:1185–1191.
25. Miki K, Hayashida Y, Shiraki K. 1991. Quantitative and sustained suppression of renal sympathetic nerve activity by left atrial distension in conscious dogs. Pflugers Arch 419:610–615.
26. Miki K, Hayashida Y, Shiraki K. 1993. Cardiac-renal-neural reflex plays a major role in natriuresis induced by left atrial distension. Am J Physiol 264:R369–R375.
27. King BD, Sack D, Kichuk MR, Hintze TH. 1987. Absence of hypertension despite chronic marked elevations in plasma norepinephrine in conscious dogs. Hypertension 9:582–590.
28. Julien C, Kandza P, Barres C, Lo M, Cerutti C, Sassard J. 1990. Effects of sympathectomy on blood pressure and its variability in conscious rats. Am J Physiol 259:H1337–H1342.
29. Osborn JW, Provo BJ, Montana III JS, Trostel KA. 1993. Salt-sensitive hypertension caused by long-term α-adrenergic blockade in the rat. Hypertension 21:995–999.
30. Cowley AW Jr, 1992. Long-term control of arterial blood pressure. Physiol Rev 72:231–300.
31. Guyton AC, Coleman TG, Cowley AW Jr., Scheel KW, Manning RD Jr, Norman RA Jr. 1972. Arterial pressure regulation: overriding dominance of the kidneys in long-term regulation and in hypertension. Am J Med 52:584–594.
32. Hall JE, Guyton AC, Coleman TG, Mizelle HL, Woods LL. 1986. Regulation of arterial pressure: role of pressure natriuresis and diuresis. Fed Proc 45:2897–2903.
33. Alexander N, Velasquez MT, Decuir M, Maronde RF. 1980. Indices of sympathetic activity in the sinoaortic-denervated hypertensive rat. Am J Physiol 238:H521–H526.

34. Alper RH, Jacob HJ, Brody MJ. 1987. Regulation of arterial pressure liability in rats with chronic sinoaortic deafferentation. Am J Physiol 253:H466–H474.
35. Barres C, Lewis SJ, Jacob HJ, Brody, MJ. 1992. Arterial pressure liability and renal sympathetic nerve activity are dissociated in SAD rats. Am J Physiol 263:R639–R646.
36. Osborn JW, England SK, Provo BJ. 1990. Normalization of arterial pressure after baroreceptor denervation (BD): role of body fluid balance and autonomic tone. FASEB J 4:A555.
37. Edvinsson L, Hakanson R, Wahlestedt C, Uddman, R. 1987. Effect of neuropeptide Y on the cardiovascular system. Trends Pharmacol Sci 8:231–235.
38. Westfall TC, McCullough LA, Vickery L, Naos L, Yang CL, Han SP, Egan T, Chen X, MacArthur H. 1998. Effects of neuropeptide Y at sympathetic neuroeffector junctions. Adv Pharmacol 42:106–110.
39. Oberhauser V, Vonend O, Rump LC. 1999. Neuropeptide Y and ATP interact to control renovascular resistance in the rat. J Am Soc Nephrol 10:1179–1185.
40. Rumantir MS, Jennings GL, Lambert GW, Kaye DM, Seals DR, Esler MD. 2000. The adrenaline hypothesis of hypertension revisited: evidence for adrenaline release from the heart of patients with essential hypertension. J Hypertens 18:717–723.
41. Cowley AW Jr, Skeleton M, Merrill DC. 1986. Are hypertensive effects of aldosterene, angiotension vasopressin and norepinephrine chemically additive. Hypertension 8:332–343.
42. Katholi RE, Carey RM, Ayers CR, Vaughan ED Jr, Yancey MR, Morton CL. 1977. Production of sustained hypertension by chronic intrarenal norepinephrine infusion in conscious dogs. Circ Res 40(Suppl. 1):I-118–I-126.
43. Osborn JL, Gordin E. 1991. Sodium intake and renal neuroadrenergic hypertension. (Abstact) Hypertension 18:384.
44. Osborn JL, Gordon E, Drysdale P. 1991. Low level intrarenal norepinephrine causes hypertension in dogs. (Abstract) Amer J Hyperten 4:74A.
45. Keeton TK, Campbell WB. 1980. The pharmacologic alteration of renin release. Pharmcol Rev 32:81–227.
46. DiBona GF. 1989. Sympathetic nervous system influences on the kidney. Role in hypertension. Am J Hypertens 2:119S–124S.
47. Koepke JP, Jones S, DiBona GF. 1987. Alpha2-adrenoceptors in amygdala control renal sympathetic nerve activity and renal activity in conscious spontaneously hypertensive rats. Brain Res 404: 80–88.
48. Koepke JP, Jones S, DiBona GF. 1988. Sodium responsiveness of central α-2 adrenoceptors in spontaneously hypertensive rats. Hypertension 11:326–333.
49. Kapusta DR, Knardahl S, Koepke JP, Johnson AK, DiBona GF. 1989. Selective central α-2 adrenoceptor control of regional haemodynamic responses to air jet stress in conscious spontaneously hypertensive rats. J Hypertens 7:189–194.
50. DiBona GF, Jones SY, Sawin LL. 1996. Renal sympathetic neural mechanisms as intermediate phenotype in spontaneously hypertensive rats. Hypertension 27:626–630.
51. Hermsmeyer K. 1976. Cellular basis for increased sensitivity of vascular smooth muscle in spontaneously hypertensive rats. Circ Res 38(Suppl. II):II53–II57.
52. Bevan RD. 1984. Trophic effects of peripheral adrenergic nerves on vascular structure. Hypertension 6(Suppl. III): III19–III26.
53. Hart MN, Heistad DD, Brody MJ. 1980. Effect of chronic hypertension and sympathetic denervation on wall/lumen ratio of cerebral vessels. Hypertension 2:419–423.
54. Simpson P. 1983. Norepinephrine-stimulated hypertrophy of cultured rat myocardial cells is an alpha 1 adrenergic response. J Clin Invest 72:732–738.
55. Simpson PC, Kariya K, Karns LR, Long CS, Karliner JS. 1991. Adrenergic hormones and control of cardiac myocyte growth. Mol Cell Biochem 104:35–43.
56. Roman RJ, Cowley AW Jr. 1985. Characterization of a new model for the study of the pressure-natriuresis in the rat. Am J Physiol 248:F190–F198.
57. Kottke FJ. 1945. The production of arterial hypertension by chronic renal artery nerve stimulation. Am J Physiol 145:38–47.
58. Kubicek WG, Kottke FJ. 1953. Renal function during arterial hypertension produced by chronic splanhnic nerve stimulation in the dog. Am J Physiol 174:397–400.
59. Liard JF, Tarazi RC, Ferrario, CM, Manger WM. 1975. Hemodynamic and humoral characterstics of hypertension induced by prolonged stellate ganglion stimulation in conscious dogs. Circ Res 36:455–464.

60. De Champlain J, Mueller RA, Axelrod J. 1969. Turnover and synthesis of norepinephrine in experimental hypertension in rats. Circ Res 25:285–291.
61. De Champlain J, Farley L, Cousineau D, Van Ameringen MR. 1976. Circulating catecholamine levels in human and experimental hypertension. Circ Res 38:109–114.
62. De Champlain J, Krakoff LR, Axelrod J. 1968. Interrelationship of sodium intake, hypertension norepinephrine storage in the rat. Circ Res 23:479–490.
63. Crabb GA, Head RJ, Hempstead, J, Berkowitz BA. 1980. Altered disposition of vascular catecholamines in hypertensive (DOCA-salt) rats. Clinical Exp Hypertension 2:129–138.
64. Dequattro V, Nagatsu T, Maronde R, Alexander N. 1969. Catecholamine synthesis in rabbits with neurogenic hypertension. Circ Res 24:545–555.
65. Volicer L, Sheer E, Hilse H, Visweswaram D. 1968. The turnover of norepinephrine in the heart during experimental hypertension in rats. Life Sci 7:525–532.
66. Henning M. 1969. Noradrenaline turnover in renal hypertensive rats. J Pharm Pharmacol 21:61–63.
67. Wyss JM, Carlson SH. 1999. The role of central nervous system in hypertension. Curr Hypertens Rep 3:246–253.
68. Hall JE, Brands MW, Zappe DH, Alonso Galcia M. 1995. Insulin resistance, hyperinsulinemia and hypertension: causes, consequences or merely correlations. J Cardiovascular Pharmacol 24(suppl. 2):S39–S49.
69. Reaven GM, Lithell H, Landsberg L. 1996. Hypertension and associated metabolic abnormalities: the role of insulin resistance and the sympatho-adrenal system. N Engl J Med 334:374–381.
70. Greco D, Sinagra D. 1995. Hyperinsulinism/insulin resistance: cause, effect or marker of essential arterial hypertension. J Hypertens 2:163–173.
71. Hall JE, Hildebrandt DA, Kuo J. 2001. Obesity hypertension: Role of leptin and sympathetic nervous system. Am J Hypertens 14:103S–115S.
72. Hirose H, Saito I, Tsujioka M, Mori M, Kawabe H, Saruta T. 1998. The obese gene product, leptin: possible role in obesity-related hypertension in adolescents. J Hypertens 16:2007–2012.
73. Suter PM, Locher R, Hasler, E, Vetter W. 1998. Is there a role for the ob gene product leptin in essential hypertension? Am J Hypertens 11:1305–1311.
74. Rutkowski MP, Klanke CA, Su YR, Reif M, Menon AG. 1998. Genetic markers at the leptin (ob) locus are not significantly linked to hypertension in African Americans. Hypertension 31:1230–1234.
75. Hall JE. 2000. Pathophysiology of obesity hypertension. Curr Hypertens Rep 2:139–147.
76. Hall JE, Brands MW, Henegar JR. 1999. Mechanism of hypertension and kidney disease in obesity. Ann NY Acad Sci 892:91–107.
77. Goldblatt H, Lynch J, Hauzal RF. 1934. Studies on experimental hypertension. J Expt Med 59:347–349.
78. Blaquier P, Bohn DF, Houbler SW. 1960. Evidence against an increase in circulating pressure material in renal hyperensive rats. Am J Physiol 198:1148–1152.
79. Brown TC, Davis JO, Olichney MT, Johnson CI. 1966. Relation of plasma renin to sodium balance and arterial pressure in experimental renal hypertension. Circ Res 18:475–483.
80. Ciricello J, Siman JK, Mercer, PF. 1991. Effect of renal dennervation on plasma renin activity after aortic baroreceptor deafferentiation. Can J Physiol Pharmacol 18:475–483.
81. Reinhart GA, Lohmeier TE, Hord CE Jr. 1995. Hypertension induced by chronic renal adrenergic stimulation is angiotensin dependent. Hypertension 25:940–949.
82. Esler M. 1995. Sympathetic nervous system: Contribution to human hypertension and related cardiovascular diseases. J Cardiovasc Pharmacol 26:524–528.
83. Gordon RD, Bachmann AW, Jackson RV, Saar N. 1992. Increased sympathetic activity in renovascular hypertension in man. Clin Exp Pharmacol Physiol 9:277–281.
84. Izumi Y, Honda M, Shiratsuchi T, Hatano M. 1980. A case of renovascular hypertension with high urinary noradrenaline excretion. Jpn Circ J 44:893–898.
85. Januszewicz W, Wocial B. 1978. Urinary excretion of catecholamines and their metabolites in patients with renovascular hypertension. Jpn Heart J 19:468–478.
86. Bunag R, Eferakeya A. 1976. Immediate hypotensive after effects of posterior hypothalamic lesion in awake rats with spontaneous, renal or DOCA hypertension. Cardiovasc Res 10:663–671.
87. Dargie HJ, Franklin SS, Reid JL. 1976. The sympathetic nervous system in renovascular hypertension in the rat. Br J Pharmcol 56:365.

88. Douglas JR Jr, Johnson EM Jr, Heist JF, Marshall GR, Needleman P. 1976. Is the peripheral sympatho-adrenal nervous system necessary for renal hypertension? J Pharmacol Exp Ther 196: 35–43.
89. Dargie HJ, Franklin SS, Reid JL. 1977. Plasma noradrenaline concentration in experimental renovascular hypertension in the rat. Clin Sci Mol Med 52:477–483.
90. Estrugamou M, De La Riva IJ. 1977. Cardiovascular reactivity and neurogenic tone in hypertension derived from renal artery stenosis and contralateral nephrectomy in the rat. Acta Physiol Lat Am 27:231–238.
91. Petty MA, Reid JL. 1977. Changes in noradrenaline concentration in brain stem and hypothalamus nuclei during the development of renovascular hypertension. Brain Res 136:376–380.
92. Eide I, Myers MR, DeQuattro V, Kolloch R, Eide K, Whigham H. 1980. Increased hypothalamus noradrenaline activity in one-kidney one-clip renovascular hypertensive rats. J Cardiovasc Pharmcol 2:833–841.
93. Katholi RE, Winhernitz SR, Oparil S. 1982. Decrease in peripheral sympathetic nervous activity following renal denervation or unclipping in the one-kidney, one-clip Goldblatt hypertensive rats. J Clin Invest 69:55–62.
94. Winternitz SR, Katholi RE, Oparil S. 1980. Role of renal sympathetic nerves in the development and maintenance of hypertension in the spontaneously hypetensive rats. J Clin Invest 66:971–978.
95. Kline RL, Kelton PM, Mercer PF. 1978. Effect of renal denervation on the development of hypertension in spontaneously hypertensive rats. Can J Physiol Pharmacol 56:818–822.
96. Liard JF. 1977. Renal denervation delays blood pressure increase in the spontaneously hypertensive rats. Experientia 33:339–340.
97. Winternitz SR, Katholi RE, Oparil S. 1982. Importance of the renal nerves in the pathogenesis of experimental hypertension. Hypertension 4(Suppl. III): 108–114.
98. Katholi RE, Naftilan AJ, Oparil S. 1980. Importance of renal sympathetic tone in the development of DOCA-slt hypertension in the rat. Hypertension 2:266–273.
99. Taddei S, Virdis A, Mattei P, Sudano I, Ghiadoni L, Salvetti A. 1994. Vascular renin angiotensin system and sympathetic nervous system activity in human hypertension. J Cardiovascular Pharmacol 23(Suppl. 1): S1–S8.
100. Grewal RS, Kaul CL. 1970. Mechanism of the antagonism of the hypotensive effect of guanethidine by propranolol. Br J Pharmacol 38:771–775.
101. Finch L, Leach GD. 1970. The contribution of sympathetic nervous system to the development and maintenance of experimental hypertension in the rat. Br J Pharmacol 39:317–324.
102. Hamberger B, Levi MR, Norberg KA. 1965. Monoamines in immunosympathectomized rats. Int J Neuropharmacol 4:91–95.
103. Ayiety-Smith E, Varma DR. 1970. An assessment of the role of the sympathetic nervous sytem in experimental hypertension using normal and immunosympathectomised rats. Br J Pharmacol 40:175–185.
104. Beilin LJ, Wade DN, Honour AJ, Cole TJ. 1970. Vascular hyper-reactivity with sodium loading and with desoxycorticosterone induced hypertension in the rat. Clin Sci 39:793–810.
105. Finch L, Haeusler G, Thoenen H. 1973a. A comparison of the effects of chemical sympathectomy by 6-hydroxydopamine. Br J Pharmacol 47:249–260.
106. Finch L, Haeusler G, Kuhn H, Thoenen H. 1973b. Rapid recovery of vascular adrenergic nerves in the rat after chemical sympathectomy with 6-hydroxydopamine. Br J Pharmacol 48:59–72.
107. Haeusler G, Finch L, Thoenen, H. 1972. Central adrenergic neurons and the intiation and development of experimental hypertension. Experentia 28:1200–1203.
108. Chalmers JP, Dollery CT, Lewis PJ, Reid, JL. 1974. The importance of central adrenergic neurons in renal hypertension in rabbits. J Physiol 238:403–411.
109. Mayers MG, Lewis PJ, Reid, JL, Reid JL. 1974. Central noradrenergic and serotonergic neurons in DOCA-saline hypertension in the rat (abstract). Eur J Clin Invest 4:322.
110. Katholi RE, Naftilan AJ, Oparil S. 1980. Importance of renal sympathetic tone in the development of DOCA-salt hypertension in the rat. Hypertension 2:266–273.
111. Lo M, Julein C, Barres C, Boomsma F, Cerutti C, Vincent M, Sassard J. 1991. Blood pressure maintenance in hypertensive sympathectomized rats. I. Adrenal medullary catecholamines. Am J Physiol 261:R1045–R1051.
112. Longe DL, Hayward JR, Hinojosa-Laborde C. 1998. Role of he adrenal medullae in male and female DoCA-salt hypertensive rats. Hypertension 31:403–408.

113. Lee RM, Triggle CR, Cheung DW, Coughlin MD. 1987. Structural and functional consequence of neonatal sympathectomy on the blood vessels of spontaneously hypertensive rats. Hypertension 10:328–338.
114. Barron BA, Van Loon GR. 1989. Role of sympathoadreno medullary system in cardiovascular response to stress in rats. J Auton Nerv Syst 28:179–188.
115. Reid L, Zivin JA, Kopin IJ. 1975. Central and peripheral adrenergic mechanisms in the development of deoxycorticosterone-saline hypertension rats. Circ Res 37:569–579.
116. Sen S, Tarazi RC, Khairaillah P, Bumpus FM. 1974. Cardiac hypertrophy in spontaneously hypertensive rats. Circ Res 35:775–781.
117. Heagerty AM. 1997. Structural changes in resistance arteries. In: Hand book of Hypertension, vol. 17: Pathophysiology of Hypertension. Eds. Zanchetti A, Mancia G. 426–437, Amsterdam, Elsevier Science.
118. Frohlich ED, Tarazi RC. 1979. Is arteria pressure the sole factor responsible for hypertensive cardiac hypertrophy? Am J Cardiol 44:959–963.
119. Morgan HE, Baker KM. 1991. Cardiac hypertrophy, mechanical, neural and endocrine dependence. Circulation 83:13–25.
120. Folkow B. 1978. The fourth Volhard Lecture: Cardiovascular structural adaptation: Its role in the initiation and maintenance of primary hypertension. Clin Sci Mol Med 4:3S–22S.
121. Clarkson TB, Kaplan IR, Adams MR. 1987. Psychological influences on the pathogenesis of arteriosclerosis among nonhuman primates. Circulation 76 (Suppl. I): I-29–I-40.
122. Mangoni AA, Mircoli L, Giannattasio, C, Mancia G, Ferrari AU. 1997. Effects of sympathectomy on mechanical properties of common carotid and femoral arteries. Hypertension 30:1085–1088.
123. Fallia M, Grappiolo A, Emanuelli G, Vitale G, Fraschini N, Giannattasio C, Mancia G. 1999. J. Sympathetic tone restrains arterial distensibility of healthy and atherosclerotic subjects. J Hypertens 17:I117–I123.

G.N. Pierce, M. Nagano, P. Zahradka, and N.S. Dhalla (eds.).
ATHEROSCLEROSIS, HYPERTENSION AND DIABETES. Copyright © 2003.
Kluwer Academic Publishers. Boston.

ROLE OF HYPOTHALAMIC PEPTIDES IN THE DEVELOPMENT OF HYPERTENSION

PALLAB K. GANGULY and MANOJ CHAKRAVARTY

Department of Anatomy, College of Medicine and Medical Sciences, Arabian Gulf University, P.O. Box 22979, Manama, Bahrain

Summary. Hypertensive animals show remarkable changes in neurotransmitter activities in hypothalamus. The changes appear to have direct effects on the sympathetic nervous system and may have a causal relationship with most forms of hypertension. Although it is generally agreed that catecholamine-containing neurons are concentrated in specific nuclei in hypothalamus and project to preganglionic neurons of spinal sympathetic system, the precise mechanisms by which these neurons are modulated are less settled. Over the past two decades various reports suggest that peptides play major role in the development of hypertension by modulating catecholamine-containing neurons in specific areas of hypothalamus. Since an increased sympathetic activity is the hallmark of both animal and human forms of hypertension, a thorough knowledge of peptidergic control of hypothalamic catecholaminergic neurons is crucial. This article will briefly review some of the peptides (particularly neuropeptide Y) which take part in the activation of the sympathetic system through a common central circuitry resulting in the chronic elevation of blood pressure. Attempts will be made to implicate sodium as possible initiating mechanisms for such hypothalamic changes and hypertension.

***Key words*:** Sympathetic system, Hypothalamic nuclei, Hypertension, Sodium ion

SYMPATHETIC SYSTEM AND HYPERTENSION

It is now generally agreed that alterations of sympathetic activity is an integral problem in a variety of cardiovascular diseases and their complications [1]. This

Corresponding Author: Dr. P. K. Ganguly, MBBS, MD, FACA, Professor, Arabian Gulf University, P. O. Box 22979, Manama, Bahrain. Telephone: (00973) 239711; Fax: (00973) 271090; e-mail: paul_ganguly@hotmail.com

understanding has been reached as various anti-sympathetic drugs work therapeutically in cardiovascular disorders. Althought some controversy exists, plasma concentrations of norepinephrine (NE) has been suggested to reflect this alteration of the sympathetic activity in cardiovascular diseases. In this respect, there is unequivocal agreement implicating sympathetic activity in hypertension, the focus of the present article. In fact, several factors are known to increase sympathetic outflow and increased total peripheral resistance in clinical essential hypertension. These factors such as genetic constitution, baroreflex resetting, stress and renin-angiotensin-aldosterone systems have been studied in great detail in the recent past to provide some insight into the progress of hypertension [2]. All of them are known to interact with the sympathetic nervous system to produce abnormal sodium handling, the root cause of increased and prolonged blood pressure [3].

Given the multiplicity of factors regulating blood pressure, the contribution of increased autonomic activity to essential hypertension must be, therefore, addressed in order to resolve the key issue about the etiology of hypertension. The data on plasma norepinephrine and epinephrine levels, norepinephrine kinetics, direct nerve traffic recordings (in certain individuals) augment the accuracy of identifying patients with an increased sympathoneural contribution to blood pressure [4]. The question still remains as to what initiates the increased sympathetic tone in hypertension? The following sections will partly address this issue.

CENTRAL CONTROL OF BLOOD PRESSURE: ROLE OF HYPOTHALAMUS

The central nervous system plays a major role in the short-and long-term regulation of arterial pressure [5]. It is now well known that such regulation is exerted by modulation of the activity of sympathetic neurons. Whereas the medulla oblongata is the central integrative area of the brain which generates the tonic excitatory background projected to spinal preganglionic sympathetic neurons that maintain normal resting levels of arterial pressure, suprasegmental control involving higher centres have gained much attention in the recent past. It is believed that the rich interconnection may play a pivotal role supporting the often-sustained activity of centrally generated sympathetic drive.

The hypothalamus is known to control the autonomic nervous system and integrates the autonomic and neuroendocrine systems, thus preserving body homeostasis. Researchers have shown that stimulation of the posterior and lateral nuclei causes sympathetic responses, which include elevation of blood pressure, hyperglycemia, acceleration of the heart rate and inhibition of peristalsis in the gastrointestinal tract. Accordingly, the hypothalamus is regarded as a higher nervous center for the control of lower sympathetic centers in the brainstem and spinal cord.

HYPOTHALAMIC NUCLEI CONTAINING CATECHOLAMINERGIC NEURONS

The hypothalamus is generally divided by the fornix into medical and lateral zones. For better clarity the areas are also divided into anterior (ventral) and posterior (dorsal) zone (Fig. 1). The axons of neurons in the paraventricular nucleus, the lateral

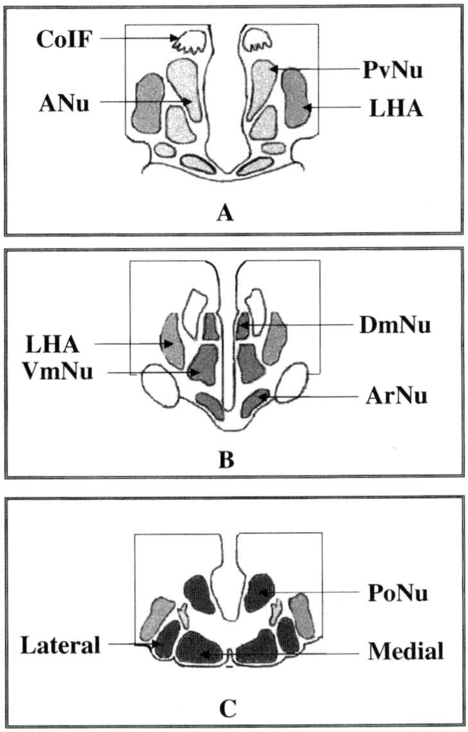

Figure 1. Coronal sections of the hypothalamus showing the anatomical distribution of the various nuclei. A Anterior (ventral) B. Middle C. Posterior (dorsal) views. ColF-Column of fornix. PVNu-Paraventricular nucleus. LHA-Lateral hypothalamic area. VmNu-Ventromedial nucleus. ArNu-Arcuate nucleus. PoNu-Posterior nucleus. ANu-Anterior nucleus.

hypothalamic area and the posterior hypothalamus project into autonomic spinal cord nuclei (sympathetic) of the intermediolateral cell column (Fig. 2). Neurons from hypothalamus also project into cranial nerve nuclei in the brain stem (vagus) and the sacral cell column (parasympathetic). Via these connections, the hypothalamus exerts control over autonomic system related to blood pressure and other functions [6]. Since there is a direct evidence for an increase in sympathetic nervous activity in nearly all forms of hypertension in animals including renovascular hypertension, Dahl salt-sensitive rats and spontaneously hypertensive rats, the hypothalamic nuclei containing catecholamine neurons have been studied in great detail.

More recently it has been shown that hypothalamus contains a variety of neuropeptides, which have direct effect on autonomic activities. In fact, neuropeptides are integral to the sympathetic system and modulate the transmission of norepinephrine [7]. This observation is substantiated by the fact that many of the neuropeptides are co-localized with the catecholaminergic neurons. Functional changes

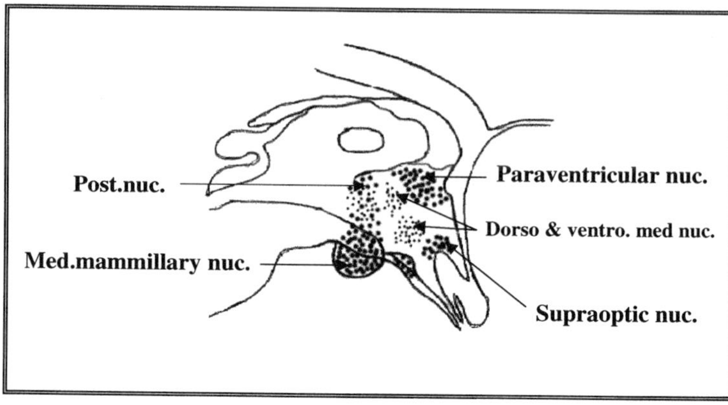

Figure 2. Sagittal section of the hypothalamus showing various nuclei involved in the autonomic activities.

in natriuretic peptides, neuropeptide Y, angiotensin, vasopressin, vasoactive intestinal polypeptide, opioids and many other substances including nitric oxide, gamma amino butyric acid, bradykinin, ouabain-like substance are seen throughout the hypothalamus but are particularly evident rostrally. It is believed that these changes lead to an increase in sympathetic nervous activity, which is responsible for increased blood pressure (for a detail description of the various changes of each of these substances, the readers are referred to the review article by De Wardener, H.E [8]). Although the exact cause of these peptidergic changes in the hypothalamus is unknown at the present time, it is apparent that the hypothalamic changes begin as the pressor rises. Interestingly, sympathetic activation appears to mediate obesity-induced hypertension and leptin and its multiple interactions with neuropeptides in the hypothalamus may link excess weight gain with increased sympathetic activity [9]. Therefore, hypothalamus remains one of the most important areas for further investigation in hypertension.

CHANGES IN HYPOTHALAMIC PEPTIDE CONCENTRATIONS IN HYPERTENSION

Experiments have revealed that hypothalamic changes have a specific direction and are reflected on the specific alteration in arterial pressure. Therefore, in a hypertensive situation, an increase in activity of a peptide or a substance at one site may stimulate blood pressure while the same increase occurring simultaneously at another site may depress blood pressure [8]. In spontaneously hypertensive rats there is an increase in norepinephrine content in the paraventricular nuclei, which may rise blood pressure but the same increase in norepinephrine in the anterior hypothalamus may depress blood pressure. These results are interpreted to mean that there is both pressor and compensatory depressor changes which are mediated by hypo-

Table 1. Effect of NPY (10^{-9}M) on the release of norepinephrine in the paraventricular nucleus

	Norepinephrine Levels (percent changes from pre-drug level)
Control	−51 ± 3
Hypertensive rats	−8 ± 1*

The values are means ± SE of 5 experiments. Norepinephrine release is expressed as the percent change from the pre-drug baseline levels. Spontaneously hypertensive rats were used in the experiments. The hypertensive rats had higher levels of norepinephrine but the response of NPY effect in these animals was significantly low. *$p < 0.05$.

Table 2. NPY receptors in the paraventricular nucleus

	NPY receptors (optical density units)
Control	0.39 ± 0.05
Hypertensive rats	0.12 ± 0.01*

Specific binding was determined as the difference in binding observed in the absence and presence of 1.0 μm NPY. Aortic-banded rats were used for the experiments. *$p < 0.05$.

thalamus but the ultimate effect is the increase in sympathetic nervous activity that probably initiates the rise in blood pressure [8].

The question, therefore, arises as to what stimulates the rise in catecholamine level in selected areas such as paraventricular nuclei. Catecholamines are frequently co-localized with other active peptides, which have biological importance. In order to focus on one such peptide, neuropeptide Y (NPY) the release of norepinephrine from the paraventricular nucleus of spontaneously hypertensive rats was monitored using in vivo microdialysis technique [10 & 11]. It may be pointed that the hypothalamus is rich in NPY-containing fibers, and therefore it is possible that a functional interaction between NPY and norepinephrine may exist. Within the hypothalamus norepinephrine levels in hypertensive rats were markedly elevated when compared with control animals. Interestingly, these hypertensive animals demonstrated no changes in norepinephrine after exposure to NPY, whereas decreases of more than 50% of norepinephrine level were seen in control animals (Table 1). The density of NPY receptors was decreased in hypothalamus of hypertensive rats (Table 2). The cause of this decreased responsiveness of PVN to the inhibitory effect of NPY in hypertension is still speculative. It is reasonable to believe that heightened sympathetic activity may be precipitated due to a defect in the NPY receptor acting centrally (Y2 receptor). This could be due to an intrinsic problem or a down-regulation of Y2 receptors in the presence of heightened NPY level. Many other peptides controlling norepinephrine secretion are also increased in hypothalamus [8]. In fact, functional changes in these substances occur in the

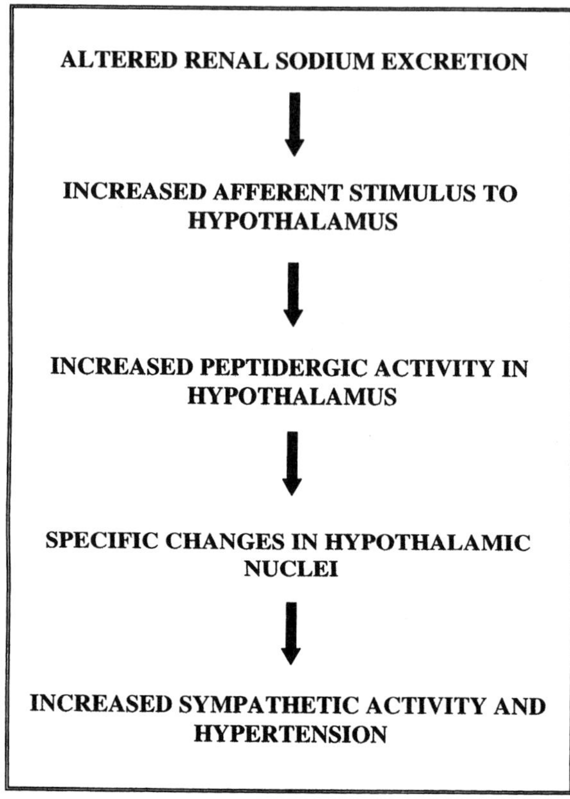

Figure 3. The possible mechanism in the initiation of the development of hypertension.

hypothalamus but are particularly prominent rostrally; most lead to an increase in sympathetic activity believed to be responsible for increased blood pressure.

POSSIBLE INITIATING MECHANISMS FOR THE HYPOTHALAMIC CHANGES: ROLE OF SODIUM

The origin of the peptidergic changes on hypothalamus during the development of hypertension is unknown. Many reports now suggest that the pressor hypothalamic changes in hypertension are part of the kidney's impaired ability to excrete sodium [12]. Since blood pressure and hypothalamic function are sensitive to local changes in sodium concentration in various areas of hypothalamus, it is tempting to suggest that sodium plays a major role in initiating hypertension [8]. It may be pointed out that changes in vascular volume including central venous pressure and stretch of the auricles initiate changes in hypothalamic function. Therefore, the cardiopulmonary afferents to hypothalamic nuclei should provide additional insight into the hypertension-associated trigger mechanisms. If most forms of hypertension are associated with an impaired ability to excrete sodium, it is essential therefore that the future research must establish the missing link between kidney and hypothalamus in hypertension (Fig. 3). Since a high sodium intake causes significant increase in NPY level, research on sodium effect should establish this missing link and has great potential in understanding the etiology of hypertension.

REFERENCES

1. Goldstein DS. 1991. Levels of catechols and clinical assessment of sympathoadrenal activity. In: Catecholamine and Heart Disease, Ed. P.K. Ganguly, 45–71. Boca Raton, Florida: CRC Press.
2. Goldstein DS. 1993. Autonomic nervous dysfunction in essential hypertension. In: Hypertension Primer, Eds. J. L. Izzo Jr, H.R. Black, 61–63. Dallas: American Heart Association.
3. Nakamura K, Cowley AW. 1989. Sequential changes of cerebrospinal fluid sodium during the development of hypertension in Dahl rats. Hypertension 13:243–249.
4. Goldstein DS, McCarty R, Polinsky RJ, Kopin IJ. 1983. Relationship between plasma norepinephrine and sympathetic neural activity. Hypertension 5:552–565.
5. Chalmers JP, Kapoor V, Llewellyn-Smith IJ, Minson JB, Pilowsky PM. 1992. Central control of blood pressure. Eur Heart J 13 (suppl. A):2–9.
6. Loewy AD. 1990. Central autonomic pathways. In: Central regulation of alutonomic function. Eds. AD Loewy, KM Spyer, 88–103, New York: Oxford University Press.
7. Benarroch EE. 1994. Neuropeptides in the sympathetic system: presence, plasticity, modulation and implications. Ann Neurol 36:6–13.
8. De Wardener HE. 2001. The hypothalamus and hypertension. Physiol Rev 81:1599–1658.
9. Hall JE, Brands MW, Hildebrandt DA, Kuo J, Fitzgerald S. 2000. Role of sympathetic nervous system and neuropeptides in obesity hypertension. Braz J Med Biol Res 33:605–618.
10. Woo ND, Mukherjee K. Ganguly PK. 1993. Norepinephrine levels in paraventricular nucleus of spontaneously hypertensive rats: role of neuropeptide Y. Am J Physiol 265:H893–H898.
11. Woo ND, Ganguly PK. 1994. Altered neuropeptide Y effects on noradrenaline levels in the paraventricular nucleus of rats following aortic constriction. Can J Cardiol 10:471–476.
12. Cowley AW. 1992. Long-term control of arterial blood pressure. Physiol Rev 72:231–300.

G.N. Pierce, M. Nagano, P. Zahradka, and N.S. Dhalla (eds.).
ATHEROSCLEROSIS, HYPERTENSION AND DIABETES. Copyright © 2003.
Kluwer Academic Publishers. Boston.

MYOSIN LIGHT CHAIN KINASE IN ENDOTHELIAL CELL CALCIUM SIGNALING AND ENDOTHELIAL FUNCTIONS

QUANG-KIM TRAN, MD, PHD and HIROSHI WATANABE, MD, PHD

Department of Clinical Pharmacology and Therapeutics, Hamamatsu University School of Medicine, Hamamatsu, Japan

Summary. Many important functions of vascular endothelial cells are closely coupled to changes in intracellular calcium concentration. In this context, myosin light chain kinase (MLCK) has been receiving increasing attention in recent years. Evidence is accumulating to show involvement of MLCK endothelial cell calcium signaling and important functions of endothelial cells including barrier function and regulation of vascular tone.

Key words: Myosin light chain kinase, Endothelial cell, Calcium, Endothelium-derived relaxing factors

INTRODUCTION

Tremendous research over the past two decades has expanded the importance of the endothelium well beyond its anatomically termed name. Much more than being a simple semi-permeable barrier that interfaces the blood and the vascular smooth muscle, the endothelium is now recognized as a multifunctional organ involved in various physiological and pathological processes. Endothelial cells regulate systemic and regional vascular tone with the production of vasorelaxing autacoids including nitric oxide and PGI_2 and vasoconstricting substances such as endothelin; they modulate blood coagulation states with the expression of antithrombotic molecules on their surface such as thrombomodulin and heparin sulfate; and they control cell-cell

Corresponding Author: Hiroshi Watanabe, MD, PhD, Department of Clinical Pharmacology and Therapeutics, Hamamatsu University School of Medicine, 1-20-1 Handayama, Hamamatsu 431-3192, Japan. Tel: +81 53 435 2385; Fax: +81 53 435 2384; e-mail: hwat@hama-med.ac.jp

adhesion with the expression of adhesion molecules such as ICAM and VCAM. The endothelium is also involved in wound healing, cellular proliferation and angiogenesis. Endothelial cell dysfunction has been implicated in many cardiovascular diseases, which renders modulation of endothelial functions a promising therapeutic approach. Many important functions of endothelial cells depend on changes in intracellular Ca^{2+} concentration ($[Ca^{2+}]i$). Activation of endothelial nitric oxide synthase and production of nitric oxide, for example, is largely dependent on store-operated Ca^{2+} entry (SOCE) [1]. Production of other autacoids, biosynthesis of von Willebrand factor and tissue plasminogen activator, and control of intercellular permeability, cell proliferation and angiogenesis also require Ca^{2+} entry [2–4]. Autocrine functions of endothelial cells such as stimulation of von Willebrand factor release by prostacyclin also depend on Ca^{2+} entry [5].

In this context of the endothelium as a regulator of many vascular functions via fluctuations in intracellular Ca^{2+} concentration, myosin light chain kinase (MLCK) has been receiving increasing attention in recent years. Activation of MLCK and the resultant phosphorylation of myosin light-chain (MLC) are key events in the initiation of smooth muscle cell contraction [6,7]. Endothelial cells possess a modest amount of MLC and thus endothelial MLCK had received little attention. However, the past few years have seen demonstrations of significant roles of MLCK in endothelial cell biology from calcium signaling, endothelial barrier function, regulation of endothelium-derived relaxing factors, and cell-cell interaction. The present writing is intended to give a brief overview of MLCK's roles in the regulation of Ca^{2+} signaling and other functions of endothelial cells.

THE ENDOTHELIAL MLCK GENE AND ACTIVATION OF MLCK

The MLCK gene is a member of the inmmunogloblin gene superfamily. The human MLCK gene (7.7 kb) is more than 95% homologous to the rabbit and bovine smooth muscle MLCK and 65–70% homologous to the avian nonmuscle MLCK. The endothelial MLCK gene was first cloned and expressed in 1997 [8]. More than 95% homology exists between the C termini of the endothelial and the smooth muscle isoforms. The C termini of both smooth muscle and endothelial MLCK isoforms contain a domain known as kinase-related protein (KRP) or telokin. This region facilitates binding of the enzyme to the unphosphorylated MLC or myosin and consequently promotes MLCK contractile activities [9,10]. The N terminus of the endothelial MLCK isoform, however, contains a 922-amino acid stretch which is not found in the smooth muscle isoform. This suggests that smooth muscle and endothelial MLCK isoforms may have different regulatory mechanisms and cellular functions [11], and that endothelial MLCK could interact with unique contractile proteins as compared to the smooth muscle MLCK. The MLCK gene is located on chromosome 3 in the q26–q27 region [12], containing two promoters that initiate transcription of mRNAs for KRP (2.6 kb), smooth muscle MLCK (5.8 kb), and nonmuscle MLCK (8.1 kb) [13–15]. Interestingly, the human endothelial MLCK contains consensus sequences for a variety of protein kinases including highly conserved potential phosphorylation sites for cAMP-dependent protein kinase A (PKA) in the CaM-binding region. Increases in intracellular cAMP levels have been shown to enhance MLCK phosphorylation 2.5-fold and reduce kinase activity in MLCK immunoprecipitates 4-fold.

Recently four more variants of the nonmuscle MLCK gene were identified with different deletion regions compared with the original MLCK gene, adding up the nonmuscle MLCK isoforms identified to five in total: MLCK1, MLCK2, MLCK 3a, MLCK 3b and MLCK4. The main differences known among the isoforms are the deletion regions in comparison with the first isoform identified, MLCK1. Whether these isoforms encode proteins with different functions is presently not known.

MLCK possesses a protein kinase catalytic core followed by a regulatory segment consisting of autoinhibitory and calmodulin-binding sequences [16]. The catalytic domain contains residues on its surface that bind a regulatory segment resulting in autoinhibition through an intrasteric mechanism, prevents MLC binding and catalysis [17]. Upon a rise in cytosolic Ca^{2+}, Ca^{2+}/calmodulin binding induces a significant movement of the regulatory segment away from the surface of the catalytic core necessary for binding and phosphorylating myosin regulatory light chain. Recent evidence suggests that activation of muscle MLCK requires translocation of bound calmodulin to a position at the end of the C-terminal lobe of the enzyme, allowing substrate binding to the exposed catalytic cleft [18]. Unlike the muscle form of MLCK, which is activated by a rise in intracellular Ca^{2+} concentration, the endothelial isoform of MLCK may require more than a rise in Ca^{2+} to get activated [19].

MLCK IN ENDOTHELIAL CELL CA^{2+} SIGNALING

Endothelial cells express a vast array of Ca^{2+} channels [20]. Ca^{2+} signaling mechanisms in endothelial cells have been reviewed recently [21]. The first suggestion of MLCK's involvement in the regulation of Ca^{2+} entry in endothelial cells was demonstrated in primary cultured porcine aortic endothelial cells, where ML-9 and wortmannin, strong inhibitors of MLCK, completely inhibited the entry portion of the Ca^{2+} response provoked by both IP_3-dependent and -independent mechanisms [22] (Fig. 1). These findings are supported by a recent study, in which ML-9 inhibited both Ca^{2+} release and entry in rat pulmonary endothelial cells examined by fluorescent microscopy and patch-clamp electrophysiology [23]. ML-9 is a selective inhibitor of MLCK that acts by competing with ATP for binding to the enzyme [24]. The observations that application of ML-9 during Ca^{2+} entry abolishes the ion influx almost immediately [24] and removal of ML-9 from the medium instantly restores Ca^{2+} entry [22] suggest that MLCK inhibition with ML-9 may block activity of a transmembrane Ca^{2+} entry channel or alter endothelial cell membrane potential. Whether inhibition of MLCK affects release from intracellular stores is controversial, based on different data from different laboratories using different sources for endothelial cells. Ion channels and gene expression in endothelial cells, even in the same cell type, are highly variable depending on cell isolation, culture and growth conditions [8], and thus controversial data observed from different

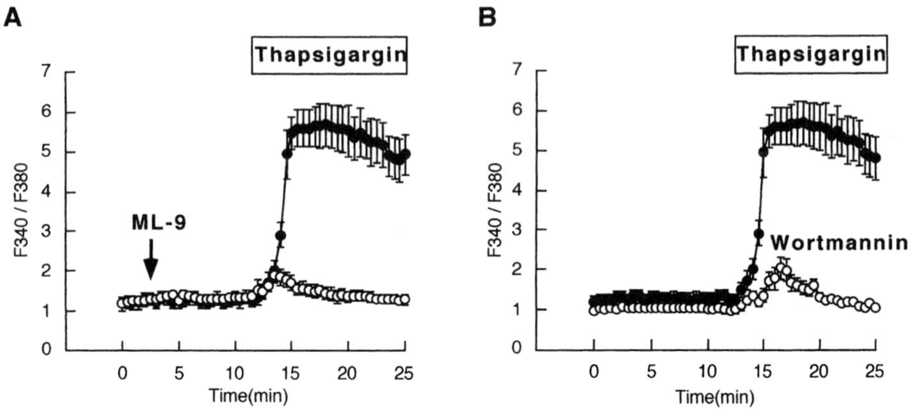

Figure 1. Effects of MLCK inhibitors, ML-9 (A) and wortmannin (B), on thapsigargin-stimulated Ca^{2+} response in the presence of extracellular Ca^{2+} in endothelial cells. Closed circles represent treatment with thapsigargin (1 µM) only and open circles represent treatment with thapsigargin (1 µM) and the inhibitor. (A) Fura-2 loaded cells were pretreated for 10 min with ML-9 (100 µM) prior to the administration of thapsigargin. (B) Cells were pretreated for 30 min with wortmannin (100 µM) prior to the administration of thapsigargin. Values are means ± SD; n = 14 cells from 3 separate experiments. [Reproduced from Biochem Biophs Res Commun 1996; 225: 777–784]

endothelia with different methods of isolation and culture seems unavoidable. In human platelets, wortmannin inhibited significantly thrombin-induced Ca^{2+} entry and MLC phosphorylation without affecting intracellular store release [25], and in human monocytes, MLCK inhibitors also inhibit Ca^{2+} entry but not Ca^{2+} release from intracellular stores [26]. Based on the use of inhibitors, MLCK was shown to control endothelial cell Ca^{2+} entry more strongly than tyrosine kinase, such that inhibitors of MLCK, at maximal inhibitory concentrations, inhibit bradykinin- and thapsigargin-induced Ca^{2+} entry in porcine aortic endothelial cells to a greater extent than do tyrosine kinase inhibitors [27]. MLCK was also demonstrated to play a role in the chloride influx that partly influences Ca^{2+} influx in porcine aortic endothelial cells [28]. Further pharmacological evidence supporting involvement of MLCK in the regulation of store-operated Ca^{2+} entry in endothelial cells was provided with the use of a series of different MLCK inhibitors including HA 1077, wortmannin, ML-5, ML-7, and ML-9. ML-5 and ML-7 are synthetic analogs of ML-9, but with different specificities for MLCK. These three inhibitors inhibit agonist-induced Ca^{2+} entry according to their potencies to inhibit the enzyme [29]. ML-9 was also shown to inhibit MLC phosphorylation to the same extent as it did store-operated Ca^{2+} entry. Involvement of MLCK in store-operated Ca^{2+} entry in endothelial cells was further consolidated with experiments in which transfection of MLCK antisense attenuated bradykinin- and thapsigargin-stimulated Ca^{2+} entry whereas MLCK sense transfection did not [30].

Ca^{2+} entry stimulated by shear stress is also completely prevented by MLCK inhibition (Fig. 2). Here again, application of ML-9 immediately inhibits the plateau

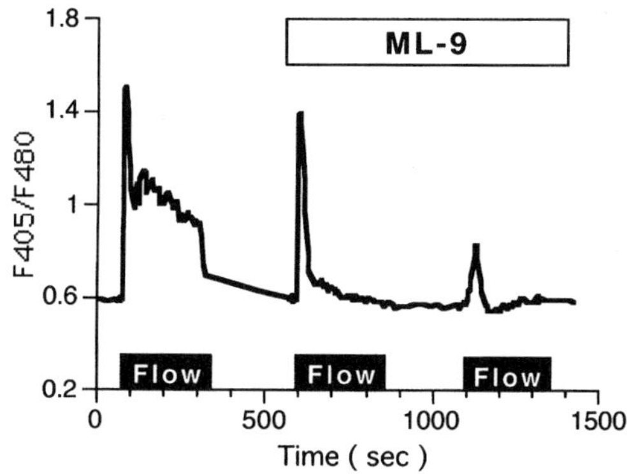

Figure 2. Representative traces showing the effect of ML-9 (100 μM) on fluid- flow-stimulated Ca^{2+} response in endothelial cells in the presence of 1 mM extracellular Ca^{2+} and 500 nM ATP. Indo-1 loaded cells were exposed to fluid flow (shear stress = 5 dynes/cm^2) with and without ML-9. Fluid flow stimulation caused peak & plateau Ca^{2+} increase. Treatment with ML-9 blocked plateau phases of the Ca^{2+} response to fluid flow stimulation. [Reproduced from FASEB J 1998; 12: 341–348, with permission]

portion of the Ca^{2+} response to shear stress, leaving the initial peak little or not at all affected. Shear stress activation of Ca^{2+} entry in endothelial cells is a phenomenon of great physiological importance. Mechanistically, fluid flow transfers blood-borne agonists to the cell surface; flow can activate phospholipase C and increase inositol triphosphate. In addition, the permeability of the cell membrane to extracellular Ca^{2+} increases upon exposure to flow. Shear stress also activates heterotrimeric G-proteins and small G proteins, which participate in Ca^{2+} signaling. Recently, shear stress was shown to activate Ca^{2+} entry in endothelial cells via activation of P2X4 purinoceptors [31]. Now the observation that MLCK inhibition prevents this Ca^{2+} entry has important physiological significance, as shear stress is one of the most constant physiological stimuli that control the production of endothelium-derived relaxing factors and factors, expression of antithrombotic molecules on the endothelial cell surface and regulation of gene expression in endothelial cells.

Phosphorylation of MLC is an important function of MLCK. It is involved in the control of cell shape, cellular permeability and cell motility. Generally, the level of MLC phosphorylation may be considered as a marker for cellular MLCK activity. In studies of the role of MLCK in Ca^{2+} entry in endothelial cells, MLCK inhibitors were shown to inhibit MLC phosphorylation to the same extent as they did store-operated Ca^{2+} entry [29]. This served to correlate MLCK activity with activation of Ca^{2+} entry in endothelial cells. At the same time, it raised the question of whether MLCK activates Ca^{2+} entry in endothelial cells by phosphorylating MLC, in other words, whether phosphorylated MLC is the substrate for MLCK in its activation of Ca^{2+} entry. Subsequent studies showed that phosphorylation of MLC is strictly dependent on Ca^{2+} entry, such that bradykinin-stimulated phosphorylation

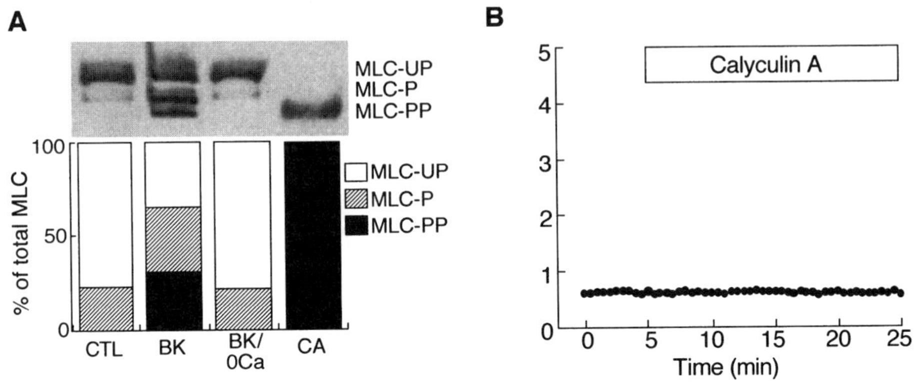

Figure 3. MLC phosphorylation-independent control of endothelial Ca^{2+} signaling by MLCK. (A) Immunostaining of MLC in cultured porcine aortic ECs revealed unphosphorylated (upper bands, MLC-UP or open areas), monophosphorylated (middle bands, MLC-P or shaded areas) and diphosphorylated MLC (lower bands, MLC-PP or closed areas), respectively. The degree of phosphorylation is expressed as percentage of the total extracted MLC. In the presence of 1 mM extracellular Ca^{2+}, BK (10 nM, 2 min) stimulated the formation of diphosphorylated MLC, which was abolished by the removal of extracellular Ca^{2+} (BK/ 0 Ca). Calyculin A (1 μM, 10 min) converted all MLC to diphosphorylated form (Caly A). Data were from 3 separate experiments. [Reproduced from FASEB J 2001; 15: 282–284, with permission] (B) Effect of calyculin A (1 μM) on endothelial cell Ca^{2+} signaling in the presence of 1 mM extracellular Ca^{2+}. Calyculin A did not affect cytosolic Ca^{2+} concentration in endothelial cells.

of MLC is completely prevented by removal of extracellular Ca^{2+}, whereas increasing phosphorylated MLC by inhibiting phosphatase activity with calyculin A does not affect $[Ca^{2+}]_i$ [30] (Fig. 3). These findings were supported by another study in which thapsigargin and thrombin activated MLC phosphorylation only in the presence of Ca^{2+} entry in bovine pulmonary artery endothelial cells [32]. Thus, rather than being a substrate for the activation of Ca^{2+} entry by MLCK in endothelial cells, phosphorylated MLC probably is involved solely in contractile events of these cells.

At this stage, pharmacological studies have provided plenty of evidence for a role of MLCK in the regulation of store-operated Ca^{2+} entry in endothelial cells. No data are presently available, however, to show that store-operated Ca^{2+} entry is increased in endothelial cells overexpressing MLCK or decreased in endothelial cells isolated from MLCK (-/-) transgenic animals. In addition, with the finding that MLC phosphorylation is secondary to Ca^{2+} entry, it is completely unknown at present how MLCK activates Ca^{2+} entry in endothelial cells. Much more is expected to be done in this exciting area of signal transduction.

REGULATION OF ENDOTHELIAL FUNCTIONS BY MLCK

MLCK and endothelial cell barrier function

As noted above, non-muscle endothelial cells contain a fairly small amount of MLC. This, however, enables endothelial cells to contract and remain contracted, hence the hypothesis that agonists stimulate actin-myosin interaction enough to pull cells apart at their sites of adhesion, increasing transendothelial permeability [33,34]. A key endothelial cell contractile event in models of agonist-induced barrier dysfunction is the phosphorylation of regulatory MLCs catalyzed by MLCK and/or through the activity of the Rho/Rho kinase pathway. MLCK phosphorylates MLC at Ser-19 and secondarily at Thr-18, increasing myosin activity [35,36]. It is a common observation that increases in $[Ca^{2+}]i$ induce inter-endothelial cell gap formation and increase macromolecule permeability [37]. With the classic role of MLCK in phosphorylating MLC and its newly described role in the regulation of Ca^{2+} entry in endothelial cells, it is likely that the enzyme could act to translate changes in $[Ca^{2+}]i$ into alterations in endothelial barrier function. In fact, several studies have shown that inhibition of MLCK prevent agonists from decreasing both intercellular adhesion and endothelial barrier integrity [38–40]. These studies, however, conflict with studies reporting that inhibition of MLCK did not prevent agents that directly increase $[Ca^{2+}]i$ from increasing endothelial permeability [35,41]. Whether these discrepancies reflect recently discovered differences in endothelial MLCK gene isoforms remains to be the work of the years to come. Avoiding the paradigm of agonist stimulation, a nice recent study has shown that transference of activated MLCK protein into coronary venule endothelial cells causes phosphorylation of MLC and contraction, resulting in gap formation and concomitant increases in permeability [42].

MLCK and endothelium-dependent vasodilatation

Production of endothelium-derived vasorelaxing factors (EDRFs) is an important physiological feature of the endothelial cells. Activation of endothelial nitric oxide synthase leading to the production of nitric oxide is dependent on SOCE [1,43,44]. NO released from endothelial cells induces relaxation of underlying smooth muscle cells by increasing cyclic GMP levels, whereas EDHF relaxes smooth muscle cells through hyperpolarization by opening K^+ channels. Although several molecules have been proposed as EDHF, there is indication that EDHF is mediated in part by increases in $[Ca^{2+}]i$. In fact, acetylcholine binds to muscarinic receptors and triggers Ca^{2+} release and Ca^{2+} entry the same way as does bradykinin [45]; the Ca^{2+} ionophore A23187 could induce endothelium-dependent hyperpolarization [46]; and endothelium-dependent hyperpolarization elicited by TG and cyclopiazonic acid was abolished by removal of extracellular Ca^{2+} [47,48]. The involvement of MLCK in the activation of SOCE in endothelial cells raised the likelihood that the enzyme also could be involved in the production of EDRFs and EDHF. We have thus shown that MLCK inhibitors ML-9 and wortmannin abolished bradykinin- and thapsigargin-stimulated NO production in porcine aortic endothelial cells (Fig. 4).

The role of MLCK in EDHF production was tested in experiments measuring smooth muscle cell membrane potential in rat mesenteric artery under acetylcholine stimulation. Endothelial denudation did not affect resting membrane potential, but deprived acetylcholine of its ability to hyperpolarize the membrane. ML-9 and wortmannin inhibit the hyperpolarization response in both dose- and time-dependent

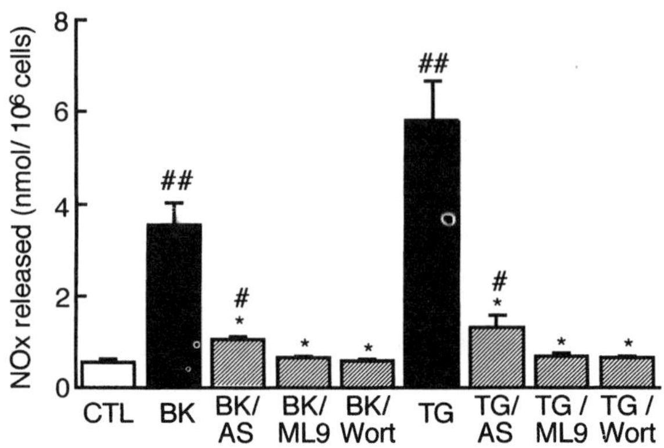

Figure 4. Regulation by MLCK of BK- and TG-stimulated NO production from ECs. Treatment for 10 min with BK (10 nM) and TG (1 μM) greatly increased NO production from basal level (CTL), which was strongly inhibited by either transfection with MLCK antisense (BK/AS or TG/AS), or pretreatment with ML-9 (100 μM, 10 min) (BK/ML9 or TG/ML9) or wortmannin (100 μM, 30 min) (BK/Wort or TG/Wort), respectively. Data were from 4 separate experiments. ⋆, $P < 0.01$ vs either BK in BK-treated group or TG in TG-treated group; #, $P < 0.05$; ##, $P < 0.01$ vs control. [Reproduced from FASEB J 2001; 15: 282–284, with permission]

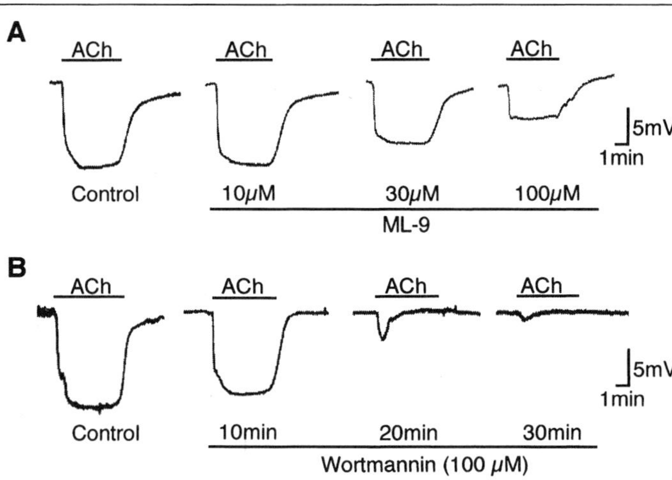

Figure 5. Regulation by MLCK of ACh-induced hyperpolarization of SMCs. (A) Dose-dependent inhibition by ML-9 of ACh-induced hyperpolarization of SMCs. Rat mesenteric arterires were pretreated for 10 min with the specified concentrations of ML-9 before application of ACh (1 μM). (B) Time-dependent inhibition by wortmannin of ACh-induced SMC hyperpolarization. Rat mesenteric arteries were pre-incubated with wortmannin (100 μM) for the specified periods before application of ACh (1 μM). [Reproduced from FASEB J 2001; 15: 282–284, with permission]

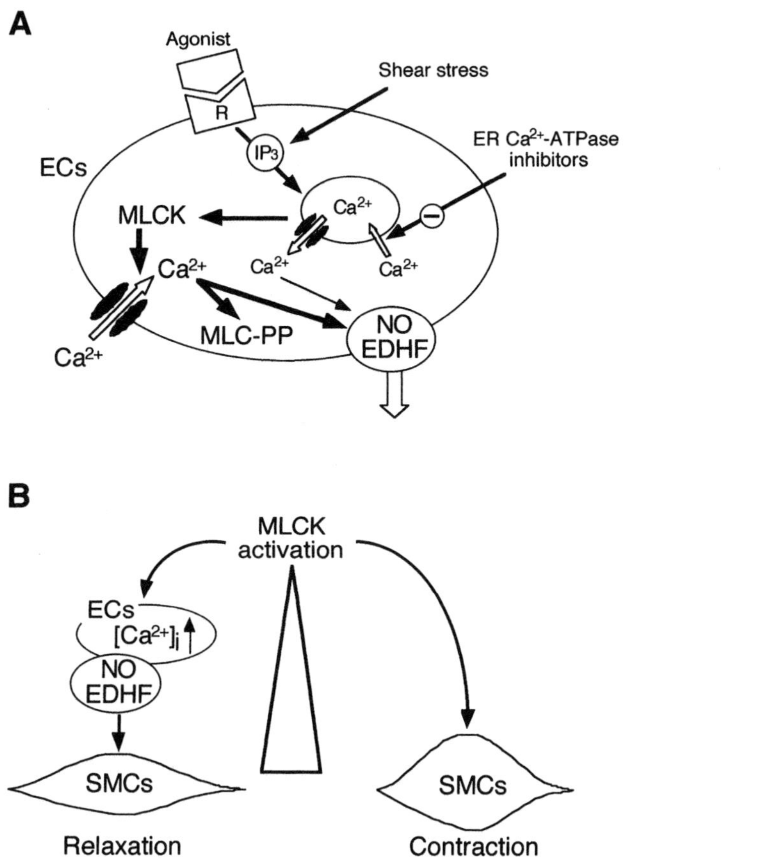

Figure 6. Schematic diagrams for the regulation by MLCK of endothelial Ca^{2+} entry (CE) and endothelium-dependent vasodilation. (A) MLCK, activated following internal Ca^{2+} store depletion in ECs by agonists, shear stress or endoplasmic reticulum Ca^{2+} ATPase inhibitors, triggers CE, which causes MLC diphosphorylation and stimulates production of NO and EDHF. (B) Activation of MLCK in ECs causes vascular relaxation via increased $[Ca^{2+}]_i$, NO and EDHF, thereby counter-balancing its well-known vasoconstrictor effects in smooth muscle cells. [Reproduced from FASEB J 2001; 15: 282–284, with permission]

manners (Fig. 5). These data are backed up by a study in which ML-9 and wortmannin were found to reduce active stress of swine carotid smooth muscle in a dose-dependent manner [49]. Endothelial NO production has been shown to be correlated more with transmembranous Ca^{2+} influx than intracellular store Ca^{2+} release [1,3]. Although further studies are necessary to determine if there is a direct effect of MLCK on endothelial nitric oxide synthase or its assembling structures, there likely exists a cause-effect relationship between the inhibitory effects exerted by blocking MLCK on endothelial cell Ca^{2+} entry and NO production. This hypothesis seems to fit well into an MLCK-activation-NO-deactivation mechanism, as the NO-induced relaxation has been attributed to cGMP-mediated decreases in $[Ca^{2+}]i$ and MLCK activity [50]. Endogenous NO is known to relax large arteries while EDHF mainly works on small resistance arteries [51]. Our data unveil a hitherto unknown physiological function of MLCK and establish a counter-balancing role for MLCK in the regulation of vascular tone: vasoconstriction via direct action on smooth muscle cells and vasodilation via action on endothelial cells (Fig. 6).

CONCLUDING REMARKS

The past few years have seen increased recognition of the role of MLCK in vascular biology. MLCK is now known to involve in endothelial cell Ca^{2+} signaling and important functions of endothelial cells including barrier function and regulation of vascular tone. It is also involved in the regulation of other processes including volume-regulated anion channel [52], Ca^{2+} signaling in monocytes [26], and adhesion and transendothelial migration of neutrophils [53,54], suggesting an important role for the enzyme in inflammation and atherosclerosis. MLCK and MLC phosphorylation are also implicated in endothelial apoptosis [55,56]. With the identification of endothelial MLCK gene and MLCK's involvement in endothelial Ca^{2+} signaling and endothelium-dependent vasodilatation, the ground is laid for further work on the role of MLCK in the physiology and pathophysiology of the endothelium.

REFERENCES

1. Lin S, Fagan KA, Li KX, Shaul PW, Cooper DM, Rodman DM. 2000. Sustained endothelial nitric-oxide synthase activation requires capacitative Ca^{2+} entry. J Biol Chem 275:17979–17985.
2. Kruse HJ, Grunberg B, Siess W, Weber PC. 1994. Formation of biologically active autacoids is regulated by calcium influx in endothelial cells. Arterioscler Thromb 14:1821–1828.
3. Lückhoff A, Pohl U, Mulsch A, Busse R. 1988. Differential role of extra- and intracellular calcium in the release of EDRF and prostacyclin from cultured endothelial cells. Br J Pharmacol 95:189–196
4. Hallam TJ, Pearson JD, Needham A. 1988. Thrombin-stimulated elevation of human endothelial-cell cytoplasmic free calcium concentration causes prostacyclin production. Biochem J 251:243–249.
5. Vischer UM, Lang U, Wollheim CB. 1998. Autocrine regulation of endothelial exocytosis: von Willebrand factor release is induced by prostacyclin in cultured endothelial cells. FEBS Lett 424:211–215.
6. Adelstein RS, Eisenberg E. 1980. Regulation and kinetics of the actin-myosin-ATP interaction. Annu Rev Biochem 49:921–956.
7. Kamm KE, Stull JT. 1985. The function of myosin and myosin light chain kinase phosphorylation smooth muscle. Annu Rev Pharmacol Toxicol 25:593–620.
8. Garcia JG, Lazar V, Gilbert-McClain LI, Gallagher PJ, Verin AD. 1997. Myosin light chain kinase in endothelium: molecular cloning and regulation. Am J Respir Cell Mol Biol 16(5):489–494.
9. Shirinsky VP, Vorotnikov AV, Birukov KG, Nanaev AK, Collinge M, Lukas TJ, Sellers JR, Watterson DM. 1993. A kinase-related protein stabilizes unphosphorylated smooth muscle myosin minifilaments in the presence of ATP. J Biol Chem 268:16578–16583.
10. Silver DL, Vorotnikov AV, Watterson DM, Shirinsky VP, Sellers JR. 1997. Sites of interaction between kinase-related protein and smooth muscle myosin. J Biol Chem 272:25353–25359.
11. Verin AD, Gilbert-McClain LI, Patterson CE, Garcia JG. 1998. Biochemical regulation of the non-muscle myosin light chain kinase isoform in bovine endothelium. Am J Respir Cell Mol Biol 19:767–776.

12. Potier MC, Chelot E, Pekarsky Y, Gardiner K, Rossier J, Turnell WG. 1995. The human myosin light chain kinase (MLCK) from hippocampus: cloning, sequencing, expression, and localization to 3qcen-q21. Genomics 29:562–570.
13. Gallagher PJ, Herring BP. 1991. The carboxyl terminus of the smooth muscle myosin light chain kinase is expressed as an independent protein, telokin. J Biol Chem 266:23945–23952.
14. Collinge M, Matrisian PE, Zimmer WE, Shattuck RL, Lukas TJ, Van Eldik LJ, Watterson DM. 1992. Structure and expression of a calcium-binding protein gene contained within a calmodulin-regulated protein kinase gene. Mol Cell Biol 12:2359–2371.
15. Gallagher PJ, Herring BP, Griffin SA, Stull JT. 1991. Molecular characterization of a mammalian smooth muscle myosin light chain kinase. J Biol Chem 266:23936–23944.
16. Hanks SK, Quinn AM. 1991. Methods Enzymol. 200:38–62.
17. Stull JT, Lin PJ, Krueger JK, Trewhella J, Zhi G. 1998. Myosin light chain kinase: functional domains and structural motifs. Acta Physiol Scand 164:471–482.
18. Krueger JK, Gallagher SC, Zhi G, Geguchadze R, Persechini A, Stull JT, Trewhella J. 2001. Activation of myosin light chain kinase requires translocation of bound calmodulin. J Biol Chem 276: 4535–4538.
19. Garcia JG, Schaphorst KL, Shi S, Verin AD, Hart CM, Callahan KS, Patterson CE. 1997. Mechanisms of ionomycin-induced endothelial cell barrier dysfunction. Am J Physiol 273:L172–L184.
20. Nilius B, Droogmans G. 2001. Ion channels and their functional role in vascular endothelium. Physiol Rev 81:1415–1459.
21. Tran QK, Ohashi K, Watanabe H. 2000. Calcium signalling in endothelial cells. Cardiovasc Res 48:13–22.
22. Watanabe H, Takahashi R, Zhang XX, Kakizawa H, Hayashi H, Ohno R. 1996. Inhibition of agonist-induced Ca^{2+} entry in endothelial cells by myosin light-chain kinase inhibitor. Biochem Biophys Res Commun 225:777–784.
23. Norwood N, Moore TM, Dean DA, Bhattacharjee R, Li M, Stevens T. 2000. Store-operated calcium entry and increased endothelial cell permeability. Am J Physiol Lung Cell Mol Physiol 279: L815–L824.
24. Saitoh M, Ishikawa T, Matsushima S, Naka M, Hidaka H. 1987. Selective inhibition of catalytic activity of smooth muscle myosin light chain kinase. J Biol Chem 262:7796–7801.
25. Hashimoto Y, Ogihara A, Nakanishi S et al. 1992. Two thrombin-activated Ca^{2+} entry channels in human platelets. J Biol Chem 267:17078–17081.
26. Tran QK, Watanabe H, Le HY, Pan L, Seto M, Takeuchi K, Ohashi K. 2001. Myosin light chain kinase regulates capacitative Ca^{2+} entry in human monocytes. Arterioscler Thromb Vasc Biol 21:509–515.
27. Takahashi R, Watanabe H, Zhang XX, Kakizawa H, Hayashi H, Ohno R. 1997. Roles of inhibitors of myosin light chain kinase and tyrosine kinase on cation influx in agonist-stimulated endothelial cells. Biochem Biophys Res Commun 235:657–662.
28. Tran QK, Watanabe H, Zhang XX, Takahashi R, Ohno R. 1999. Involvement of myosin light-chain kinase in chloride-sensitive Ca^{2+} influx in porcine aortic endothelial cells. Cardiovasc Res 44:623–631.
29. Watanabe H, Takahashi R, Zhang XX, Goto Y, Hayashi H, Ando J, Isshiki M, Seto M, Hidaka H, Niki I, Ohno R. 1998. An essential role of myosin light-chain kinase in the regulation of agonist-and fluid flow-stimulated Ca^{2+} influx in endothelial cells. FASEB J 12:341–348.
30. Watanabe H, Tran QK, Takeuchi K, Fukao M, Liu MY, Kanno M, Hayashi T, Iguchi A, Seto M, Ohashi K. 2001. Myosin light-chain kinase regulates endothelial calcium entry and endothelium-dependent vasodilation. FASEB J 15:282–284.
31. Yamamoto K, Korenaga R, Kammiya A, Ando J. 2000. Fluid shear stress activates Ca^{2+} influx into human endothelial cells via P2X4 purinoceptors. Cir Res 87:385–391.
32. Moore TM, Norwood NR, Creighton JR, Babal P, Brough GH, Shasby DM, Stevens T. 2000. Receptor-dependent activation of store-operated calcium entry increases endothelial cell permeability. Am J Physiol Lung Cell Mol Physiol 279:L691–L698.
33. Wysolmerski RB, Lagunoff D. 1990. Involvement of myosin light chain kinase in endothelial cell retraction. Proc Natl Acad Sci USA 87:16–20.
34. Lum H, Malik AB. 1994. Regulation of vascular endothelial barrier function. Am J Physiol Lung Cell Mol Physiol 267:L223–L241.
35. Ikebe M, Hartshorne DJ. 1985. Phosphorylation of smooth muscle myosin at two distinct sites by myosin light chain kinase. J Biol Chem 260:10027–10031.

36. Ikebe M, Hartshorne DJ, Elzinga M. 1986. Identification, phosphorylation and dephosphorylation of a second site for myosin light chain kinase on the 20,000-dalton light chain of smooth muscle myosin J Biol Chem 261:36–39.
37. Curry FE. 1992. Modulation of venular microvessel permeability by calcium influx into endothelial cells. FASEB J 6:2456–2466.
38. Garcia JG, Verin AD, Schaphorst KL. 1996. Regulation of thrombin-mediated endothelial cell contraction and permeability. Semin Thromb Hemost 22:309–315.
39. Moy AB, Shasby SS, Scott BD, Shasby DM. 1993. The effect of histamine and cyclic adenosine monophosphate on myosin light chain phosphorylation in human umbilical vein endothelial cells. J Clin Invest 92:1198–1206.
40. Sheldon R, Moy A, Lindsley K, Shasby S, Shasby DM. 1993. Role of myosin light-chain phosphorylation in endothelial cell retraction. Am J Physiol Lung Cell Mol Physiol 265:L606–L612.
41. Moore TM, Chetham PM, Kelly JJ, Stevens T. 1998. Signal transduction and regulation of lung endothelial cell permeability. Interaction between calcium and cAMP. Am J Physiol Lung Cell Mol Physiol 275:L203–L222.
42. Tinsley JH, de Lanerolle P, Wilson E, Ma W, Yuan SY. 2000. Myosin light chain kinase transference induces myosin light chain activation and endothelial hyperpermeability. Am J Physiol Cell Physiol 279:C1285–C1289.
43. Ignarro LJ. 1989. Endothelium-derived nitric oxide: actions and properties. FASEB J 3:31–36.
44. Furchgott RF, Vanhoutte PM. 1989. Endothelium-derived relaxing and contracting factors. FASEB J 3:2007–2018.
45. Nathanson NM. 1987. Molecular properties of the muscarinic acetylcholine receptor. Annu Rev Neurosci 10:195–236.
46. Chen GF, Suzuki H. 1990. Calcium dependency of the endothelium-dependent hyperpolarization in smooth muscle cells of the rabbit carotid artery. J Physiol (Lond) 421:521–534.
47. Fukao M, Hattori Y, Kanno M, Sakuma I, Kitabatake A. 1997. Sources of Ca^{2+} in relation to generation of acetylcholine-induced endothelium-dependent hyperpolarization in rat mesenteric artery. Br J Pharmacol 120:1328–1334.
48. Fukao M, Hattori Y, Kanno M, Sakuma I, Kitabatake A. 1995. Thapsigargin- and cyclopiazonic acid-induced endothelium-dependent hyperpolarization in rat mesenteric artery. Br J Pharmacol 115:987–992.
49. Wingard CJ, Murphy RA. 1999. Inhibition of Ca^{2+}-dependent contraction in swine carotid artery by myosin kinase inhibitors. Gen Pharmacol 32:483–494.
50. Lincoln TM, Komalavilas P, Cornwell TL. 1994. Pleiotropic regulation of vascular smooth muscle tone by cyclic GMP-dependent protein kinase. Hypertension 23:1141–1147.
51. Gerland CJ, Plane F, Kemp BK, Cocks TM. 1995. Endothelium-dependent hyperpolarization: a role in the control of the vascular tone. Trends Pharmacol Sci 16:23–30.
52. Nilius B, Prenen J, Walsh MP, Carton I, Bollen M, Droogmans G, Eggermont J. 2000. Myosin light chain phosphorylation-dependent modulation of volume-regulated anion channels in macrovascular endothelium. FEBS Lett 466:346–350.
53. Saito H, Minamiya Y, Kitamura M, Saito S, Enomoto K, Terada K, Ogawa J. 1998. Endothelial myosin light chain kinase regulates neutrophil migration across human umbilical vein endothelial cell monolayer. J Immunol 161(3):1533–1540.
54. Garcia JG, Verin AD, Herenyiova M, English D. 1998. Adherent neutrophils activate endothelial myosin light chain kinase: role in transendothelial migration. J Appl Physiol 84(5):1817–1821.
55. Mills JC, Stone NL, Erhardt J, Pittman RN. 1998. Apoptotic membrane blebbing is regulated by myosin light chain phosphorylation. J Cell Biol 140:627–636.
56. Petrache I, Verin AD, Crow MT, Birukova A, Liu F, Garcia JG. 2001. Differential effect of MLC kinase in TNF-alpha-induced endothelial cell apoptosis and barrier dysfunction. Am J Physiol Lung Cell Mol Physiol 280:L1168–L1178.

G.N. Pierce, M. Nagano, P. Zahradka, and N.S. Dhalla (eds.).
ATHEROSCLEROSIS, HYPERTENSION AND DIABETES. Copyright © 2003.
Kluwer Academic Publishers. Boston.

SARPOGRELATE INHIBITS GENES INVOLVED IN VASCULAR NEOINTIMAL HYPERPLASIA AND REMODELING

SUSHIL K. SHARMA,[1] NOBUAKIRA TAKEDA, AMARJIT S. ARNEJA, and NARANJAN S. DHALLA

[1] *University of North Dakota School of Medicine and Health Sciences, Department of Physiology, Pharmacology, and Therapeutics, Grand Forks, ND, U.S.A., Institute of Cardiovascular Sciences, St. Boniface Hospital Research Centre, University of Manitoba, Departments of Physiology and Medicure, Winnipeg, Manitoba, Canada, and Aoto Hospital, Jikei University, Tokyo, Japan*

Summary. Although basic molecular mechanisms of vascular neointimal hyperplasia leading to vascular remodeling remain unknown, it is generally held that various genes are upregulated or inhibited during this process. We have recently discovered that a specific serotonin receptor (5-HT2A) antagonist, sarpogrelate, inhibits vascular remodeling by suppressing the serotonin-induced c-fos and c-jun heterodimerization. By conducting RT-PCR and cell transfection studies, we have shown that over-expression of the 5-HT2A receptor enhanced while sarpogrelate inhibited vascular neoinitmal hyperplasia and remodeling by binding with the ligand binding domain (localized in the third intra-cytoplasmic loop) of the 5-HT2A receptor. These data are interpreted to suggest the therapeutic potential of sarpogrelate in cardiovascular diseases such as atherosclerosis, myocardial ischemia, and coronary artery restenosis.

Key words: Vascular neointimal hyperplasia, Vascular remodeling, Sarpogrelate 5-HT2A receptor, c-fos-c-jun heterodimerization, Serotonin, Cardiovascular diseases

INTRODUCTION

Basic molecular mechanism of vascular neointimal hyperplasia (NIH) leading to restenosis and vascular remodeling remains unknown. Serotonin (a vasoactive neurotransmitter) causes cell proliferation, cell survival, as well as hypertrophy of many

Address for Correspondence: Dr. Sushil K. Sharma, PhD, Department of Physiology, Pharmacology, and Therapeutics, University of North Dakota, 501 North Columbia Road, Grand Forks, ND 58203, USA. Tel.: (701) 777-3280; Fax: (701) 777-4490; e-mail: Sharmas64@Hotmail.Com

cells in culture, including vascular smooth muscle cells. Thus, it is considered a potential candidate in the pathogenesis of atherosclerosis and hypertension [1]. Whether the mitogenic effect of serotonin is mediated through cell surface receptors, serotonin transporters or both depending on the cell type, remains unresolved. Serotonin-induced hyperplasia and hypertrophy in cultured bovine pulmonary artery smooth muscle cells [2] through signaling pathway that utilizes its transport system and O_2 formation [3]. Furthermore, serotonin plays an important role in pulmonary and cardiovascular remodeling through these signaling mechanisms [4]. Recently, Lee et al. [5] have reported that serotonin-induced hyperplasia and hypertrophy in bovine pulmonary artery smooth muscle cells but not in endothelial cells and occurred through high affinity uptake mechanism. The proliferative effect of serotonin was synergistic with other mitogens. Whereas, a specific 5-HT2A receptor antagonist, sarpogrelate (Anplag or MCI-9042) was found to abolish the serotonin-induced hyperplasia in cultured rat aortic smooth muscle cells (RASMC), suggesting that the chemotectic effect of serotonin may be mediated through the 5-HT2A receptor pathway [6]. These studies indicated that platelet-derived serotonin plays an important role in neointimal hyperplasia [6]. Pakala and Benedict [7] have also reported that regenerating endothelial cells at the site of vascular injury release growth factors including serotonin, leads to smooth muscle cell proliferation and neointimal hyperplasia. This review has been focussed to highlight the functional significance of serotonin in the progression of NIH following injury and its possible prevention by pre-treatment with a specific 5-HT2A receptor antagonist, sarpogrelate.

SEROTONIN AND VASCULAR NIH

Peripheral and central physiological effects of serotonin are routed through the binding to multiple receptor subtypes [8]. Among them, serotonin 5-HT2A receptors are known to activate the phospholipase C-β second messenger pathways [9]. The mitogenic effect of serotonin was abolished by phospholipase C inhibitor U73122, suggesting that 5-HT2A receptor-mediated signal of serotonin was transduced by PLC. The potent vasoactive substances, 5-HT, angiotensin-II, and bradykinin bind to G-protein coupled receptor and activated phospholipase C-β [10]; these agonists induce transient increase in intracellular calcium. Cellular cyclic nucleotides also play an important role in the intracellular signaling process for growth regulation by serotonin and recent studies point to protein phosphorylation pathways as being important in the mitogenic response. The tendency to release EDCF (superoxide anions, endoperoxidase, thromboxane A2 and endothelin) is preserved or even enhanced in damaged vessels, which favors vasospasm, thrombus and cell proliferation. As such, serotonin did not induce SMC migration, but rather a stimulatory chemotectic influence in the presence of other migration factors such as SMC-derived migration factor, platelet-derived migration factor, and fibronectin. It has been suggested that the combined use of 5-HT and TXA2 receptor antagonists might inhibit growth of endothelial cells at the site of vascular injury which may also inhibit neointimal hyperplasia. Sarpogrelate significantly reduced intimal hyperplasia in rabbit left carotid artery which was de-endothelialized following balloon injury. Receptor-activated increase in $[Ca^{+2}]_i$ in smooth muscle cells might be coupled to receptor activated increase in protein tyrosine phosphorylation of ras GAP120. Ketanserin, a 5-HT receptor antagonist in drinking water (100 mg/kg/day), significantly reduced post-transplant arteriosclerotic thickening of the intima by a mechanism other than the inhibition of platelet function, decrease in blood pressure, or immunosuppression. Serotonin has been shown to enhance tyrosine phosphorylation of GTPase activating protein P120, which occurs in smooth muscle cells but not in endothelial cells, and to enhance cell proliferation. Tyrosine kinase and 5-HT uptake inhibitor, 8 bromoadenosine 3′5′ cyclic monophosphate, blocked both serotonin-induced DNA synthesis and tyrosine phosphorylation.

5-HT2A receptor was detected on plasma membrane in myoblasts at the level of T-tubules in contracting myotubes. Binding of serotonin to this receptor increased the expression of genes involved in myogenic differentiation. Furthermore, 5-HT2A receptor was able to activate another signaling pathway. It triggered a rapid and transient tyrosine phosphorylation of JAK2 kinase in response to serotonin. JAK2 autophosphorylation was followed by the tyrosine phosphorylation of JAK2 kinase in response to serotonin. JAK2 autophosphorylation was followed by the tyrosine phosphorylation of STAT3 (signal transducers and activators of transcription) and its transcription into the nucleus. Previous studies have shown that 5-HT2A receptor and STAT3 cooperate with JAK2, indicating that they are physically associated. Serotonin receptor (5-HT2A) in skeletal muscle myoblasts was able to activate the intracellular phosphorylation pathways used by cytokines. The survival effect was mimicked by the 5-HT2A/2C-receptor agonist, α-methyl 5-HT, and blocked by the 5-HT2A receptor antagonist, cinanserin. Similarly, ketanserine reduced post-transcriptional atherosclerotic thickening of the intima. Because of its antiatherosclerotic effect, ketanserin therapy may prove beneficial for the long-term survival of vascular allografts.

5-HT2A RECEPTOR ANTAGONISM AND NIH

Recently, we have established that serotonin-induced cellular hyperplasia was inhibited by a novel and specific 5-HT2A receptor antagonist, sarpogrelate, in a time and concentration-dependent manner [11,12]. Heparin also inhibited serotonin-induced cellular hyperplasia and hypertrophy in SMC, through its inhibition of a phosphorylated intermediate protein (GTPase activating protein) [5]. In vein grafts 5-HT produced significantly larger contractions than control veins, which were inhibited by methiothepin but not by sarpogrelate [13]. Recently, Kuga et al. [14] have reported that coronary hyperconstriction response to serotonin, one week after injury, resulted primarily from hyperactivity of vascular smooth muscle cells. It was suggested that functional impairments of vasoreactivity in the vessel wall as a result of mechanical stretching of the smooth muscle cell layer plays an important role in the immediate dilation produced in vasospastic arteries [15]. Pre-incubation with protein tyrosine kinase inhibitors, genistein or tyrphostin, significantly inhibited serotonin or phenylephrine-induced transient rise in $[Ca^{2+}]_i$ in smooth muscle cells [16]. Insulin also attenuated serotonin-induced Ca^{2+} influx, the intracellular calcium transients and contraction in cultured VSMC from dog femoral artery while phloridzin blocked this effect [17]. It has also been demonstrated that serotonin receptor antagonist ketanserin diminished arteriosclerotic development by its effect on platelet function and on vascular smooth muscle cells proliferation. Serotonin-induced increase in growth response was associated with an early increase in the c-myc and α-actin gene expression and was blocked by agents that elevate cellular adenosine 3′5′ cyclic monophosphate or inhibit 5-HT transport or tyrosine phosphorylation [2]. Serotonin caused a concentration-dependent accumulation of intracellular cAMP in the circular muscles [18].

Tamura et al. [6] have studied the chemotectic role of serotonin in cultured rat aortic smooth muscle cells. Their studies indicate that serotonin as such may not be involved in cell migration but that it exerts its effect at physiological concentrations in the presence of other migration factors such as smooth muscle-derived migration factor, platelet-derived migration factor, and fibronectin. The mitogenic effect of serotonin was completely abolished by a selective 5-HT2A receptor antagonist sarpogrelate. We have now established that protein tyrosine kinase inhibitor, genestein inhibited serotonin-induced increase in $[Ca^{2+}]_i$ and cell proliferation. Furthermore, we have observed that serotonin-induced increase in light chain myosine kinase expression was inhibited by sarpogrelate. Serotonin-induced cell proliferation was totally inhibited by tyrosine kinase inhibitors, genestein and tyrphostin. Semenchuk and Salvo [16] demonstrated that receptor activated increase in $[Ca^{2+}]_i$ is evoked by serotonin or phenylpherine in cultured smooth muscle cells. It was suggested that tyrosine phosphorylation may act as an intermediate signal in 5-HT-induced mitogenesis of smooth muscle cells, which requires cellular internalization of serotonin rather than its action on membrane receptors [5]. The vasoactive effects of various mitogens involving intravascular neointimal hyperplasia, plaque formation, platelet aggregation and thrombogenesis in the cardiovascular system is triggered by an increase in the intracellular free ionized calcium $[Ca^{2+}]_I$; whereby others have reported that this transient increase in $[Ca^{2+}]_i$ was insufficient to induce human vascular cell proliferation [10]. These investigators suggested that transient increase in $[Ca^{2+}]_i$ and subsequent PKC activity by a vasoconstrictive agent might be insufficient to induce vascular smooth muscle cell proliferation [10]. Recent studies have shown that vascular 5-HT2A receptor signaling and contractions are associated with activation of L-type calcium channels, phospholipase C, and tyrosine kinase C activation [19]. It was suggested that 5-HT2A-receptor activates all the three pathways independently to elicit contraction and that one of the tyrosine kinases activated by 5-HT is mitogen-activated protein kinase. The presence of serotonin receptor in T-tubules suggested a role for serotonin in excitation-contraction coupling and/or effect in skeletal muscle fiber repair [20]. It has also been reported that serotonin receptor antagonist ketanserin (5-HT2A receptor) diminished the atherosclerotic development by its effect on the platelet function and on vascular smooth muscle cells. These data suggested that stimulation of a vascular 5-HT2A receptor activates

Ca^{2+} channels and PLC as well as MEK to cause rat aortic contractions and that MEK activation was at least partially independent of two signaling pathways associated with 5-HT2A receptor [19].

Recent studies have discovered two active ingredients in methanolic extracts of the plant Garcinia Mangostana i.e α-mangostin and γ-mangostin which were histamine H1 and serotonin 5-HT2A receptor antagonists, respectively. γ-mangostin significantly inhibited 5-HT-induced vascular smooth muscle cell contractions, platelet aggregation, and inhibited 5-HT2A receptor binding. These responses were similar to those observed with sarpogrelate as earlier reported by Hara et al. [21], Hara et al. [22], and Kanamori et al. [23]. Serotonin caused a concentrations-dependent accumulation of intracellular cAMP in the circular muscle [18] and reduced cell death was noticed in cultures exposed to serotonin. These observations indicated that serotonin did not exert its effect on dividing neuroepithilial cells in the developing cortex, but rather it affected the postmitotic neurons. It has been reported that through the tyrosine kinase signaling pathways, serotonin plays an important role in remodeling of both the pulmonary and systemic circulation [4]. Recently, Pakala and Benedict [7] have suggested that regenerating endothelial cells at the site of vascular injury might release growth factors for vascular smooth muscle cells leading to neointimal hyperplasia and combined use of serotonin and TXA2 receptor antagonists may inhibit the growth of endothelial cells at the site of vascular injury and attenuate neointimal hyperplasia.

$[Ca^{2+}]_i$ AND NIH

Measurement of intracellular free ionized calcium $[Ca^{2+}]_i$ can be used as a hallmark of 5-HT2A receptor activation/inactivation and cell proliferation in RASMC. We have established that pre-incubation with sarpogrelate inhibited specifically 5-HT-mediated increase in $[Ca^{2+}]_i$, suggesting its specificity at the 5-HT2A receptor. Sarpogrelate could inhibit exclusively 5-HT-induced increase in $[Ca^{2+}]_i$ in coronary artery smooth muscle cells [12]. Various other vasoactive agents such as angiotensin-II, PDGF, phorbol 12, myristate 13, acetate (PMA), and endothelin induced an increase in $[Ca^{2+}]_i$, however sarpogrelate could not influence this increase in $[Ca^{2+}]_i$. Our studies suggest that sarpogrelate is a novel 5-HT2A receptor antagonist, which exclusively influence 5-HT-induced increase in $[Ca^{2+}]_i$ in RASMC. Recently, we have discovered that sarpogrelate inhibited serotonin-induced increase in DNA, RNA and protein synthesis, that may occur due to the inhibition of 5-HT2A receptor and hence the levels of $[Ca^{2+}]_i$ may modulate the protooncogenes involved in cell proliferation [11]. Serotonin, angiotensin-II and bradykinin were unable to induce cell proliferation or act as co-mitogens with platelet-derived growth factor (PDGF) in human vascular smooth muscle cells. In RASMC, 5-HT increase $[Ca^{2+}]_i$ via 5-HT2A receptor subtype by inducing influx of extracellular Ca^{2+} partially through L-type voltage-operated Ca^{2+} channels as well as by mobilizing Ca^{2+} from its intracellular stores. Previous studies have reported no proliferation in response to serotonin, angiotensin-II and bradykinin in human vascular smooth muscle cells; however it could act as a co-mitogen with platelet-derived growth factor.

Serotonin, α-methyl 5-HT and 2,5, dimethoxy 4-indol amphetamine all contracted the rat aorta, whereas 5-HT2A receptor antagonist, ketanesrin, inhibited contractions due to 5-HT. The tyrosine kinase inhibitor, genestein, shifted the 5-HT-induced contraction curve to the right, while daidzein, an inactive isomer of genestein, was ineffective. PD098058, an inhibitor of MEK, shifted contraction due to 5-HT to the right. Serotonin-induced increase in $[Ca^{2+}]_i$ was completely inhibited by ketanserine, while diltiazem partially suppressed 5-HT-induced increase in $[Ca^{2+}]_i$. Serotonin stimulation induced an increase in $[Ca^{2+}]_i$ and increased the production of inositol trisphosphate which was significantly inhibited by staurosporine and H-7. Phorbol 12, myristate 13, acetate induced increase in $[Ca^{2+}]_i$ was abolished by removal of extracellular Ca^{2+} but was not affected by pre-treatment with PTX; this change was not accompanied by changes in cAMP content [24]. In RASMC, 5-HT increased $[Ca^{2+}]_i$ via 5-HT2A receptor subtype by inducing influx of extracellular Ca^{2+} as well as by moblilizing Ca^{2+} from its intracellular stores. It was suggested that activation of PKC might be involved in this process whereas PTX sensitive G-protein and cAMP were not involved [24].

PROTEIN TYROSINE PHOSPHORYLATION AND NIH

Recent studies have indicated that protein phosphorylation plays an important role in the mitogenic response. Related to this is the observation that sarpogrelate significantly reduced NIH in the left carotid artery, denuded endothelial cells by inflated balloon in the hypercholestrolemic rabbits by inhibiting proliferation of smooth muscle cells and cholesterol uptake by macrophages. Similarly, Heparin inhibited both hyperplastic and hypertrophic effect of serotonin on smooth muscle cells through the inhibition of a phosphorylated intermediate protein [25] named as GTPase activating protein. In vein grafts, serotonin produced significantly larger contractions than control veins; these effects were inhibited by methiothepin but not by 5-HT2A receptor antagonist, sarpogrelate [13]. According to Kuga et al. [14], coronary hyperconstriction response to serotonin one week after the injury resulted primarily from hyperactivation of smooth muscle cells. Previous studies by Chan et al. [15] have suggested that functional impairment of vasoreactivity in the vessel wall as a result of mechanical stretching of the smooth muscle cell layer exerts a greater influence than structural alterations in the immediate dilation produced in vasoactive agents. A rapid enhancement of tyrosine phosphorylation of a 120 kD protein P120 was associated with the serotonin-induced mitogenesis [2]. Nitric oxide (NO)-generating agent sodium nitropruside dose-dependently inhibited serotonin-induced ^{3}H-thymidine incorporation by smooth muscle cells. These data suggested that serotonin acts as a mitogen for smooth muscle cells through a signal transduction cascade involving tyrosine phosphorylation. Sodium nitropruside prevented the serotonin-induced mitogenesis of SMC through elevation of intracellular cyclic GMP and inhibition of tyrosine phosphorylation of P120 [2]. Recent studies by Di Salvo et al. [26] have demonstrated that tyrosine phosphorylation of PLC gamma-1 is not required for tyrosine kinase-dependent increase in $[Ca^{2+}]_i$ which resulted from stimulation of diverse G-protein coupled receptors in vascular smooth muscle cells. Furthermore, enhancement of tyrosine phosphorylation of P120 by 5-HT was prevented by pre-incubation with sodium nitropruside or exogenously added cyclic GMP.

Vascular smooth muscle cell reactivity to serotonin (neointimal hyperplasia) is significantly increased in hypertension and atherosclerosis [27]. Tyrosine kinase activation was found to mediate partial changes in contractility, due to 5-HT in arterial smooth muscle cells, while tyrphostin-23 was somewhat nonselective. It was suggested that these observations have significant implications, not only in understanding a novel pathway of 5-HT signal transduction but also in vascular diseases in which growth and/or contractility to 5-HT is increased [27]. It has been reported previously that the synthetic platelet-activating factor (PAF) potentiated anoxic contraction in rat aortic rings through the release of serotonin. Serotonin induced both hyperplasia and hypertrophy of pulmonary artery smooth muscle cells through its high affinity uptake [28] and enhanced tyrosine phosphorylation of proteins including GTPase activating protein (P120) within minutes; this effect occurred in smooth muscle cells but not in endothelial cells thus it preceded the other crucial events associated with 5-HT-induced mitogenesis. Tyrosine kinase inhibitors and 5-HT uptake inhibitors blocked both the 5-HT-induced DNA synthesis and tyrosine phosphorylation, while vandate increased DNA synthesis and tyrosine phosphorylation in both control and serotonin-treated cells. Stimulation of cellular proliferation and hypertrophy produced by 5-HT were totally abolished by tyrosine kinase inhibitors which did not affect 5-HT uptake [25]. These studies suggested that tyrosine phosphorylation of protein P120 may act as an intermediate signal in 5-HT-induced mitogenesis of smooth muscle cells which require cellular internalization of 5-HT rather than its action on a membrane receptor [25]. Tyrosine kinase, enzyme is an important candidate for serotonin-induced mitogenesis and could play an important role in serotonin-induced vascular smooth muscle cell contractility. Tyrosine kinase inhibitors, genistein as well as tyrphostin decreased the potency of serotonin approximately 4 fold and reduced maximal contraction to 5-HT in carotid arteries [1]. Serotonin induced time and concentration-dependent increase in the phosphotyrosine immunoreactivity of the 42kD protein (MAP kinase) in RASMC. Recent studies have indicated that serotonin-activated increase in $[Ca^{2+}]_i$ in vascular smooth muscle cells was associated with enhanced protein tyrosine phosphorylation. These responses were blocked by protein tyrosine kinase inhibitors genistein and tyrphostin, suggesting that the increase in $[Ca^{2+}]_i$ and tyrosine phosphorylation are functionally coupled. The potent vasoconstrictor substances, 5-HT, angiotensin II and bradykinin bind to G protein coupled receptors and activated phospholipase C beta [10]. Florian and Watts [19] have illustrated that vascular 5-HT2A receptor signaling, contraction and cell proliferation are associated with the activation of L-type of calcium channels, phospholipase C and protein tyrosine kinase activation (One of the tyrosine kinase that is activated by serotonin is mitogen-activated protein kinase, MEK). It was demonstrated that serotonin, α-methyl serotonin and 2, 5 dimethoxy 4 indol amphetamine, all contracted rat aorta, whereas 5-HT2A receptor antagonist, ketanserin, blocked contraction to 5-HT. The tyrosine kinase inhibitor, genistein, shifted contraction to 5-HT, α-methyl serotonin and DOI approximately 10 fold to the right whereas deidzein, an inactive isomer of genistein, was unable to shift 5-HT-induced contraction. PD 098059, an inhibitor of MEK, shifted contraction to 5-HT approximately 7 fold right. In cultured smooth muscle cells, 5-HT stimulated tyrosine phosphorylation of 42 kD and 44 kD proteins, identified as ERK and MAPKs. This phosphorylation was reduced by PD 098059. Neither nifedipine nor NCDC reduced serotonin-induced ERK, MAPK tyrosine phosphorylation, but the combination of nifedipine, NDCD and PD 098059 abolished serotonin-induced ERK and MAPK tyrosine phosphorylation [19]. It has also been demonstrated that tyrosine phosphorylation of PLC gamma-1 is not required for tyrosine kinase-dependent increase in $[Ca^{2+}]_i$ resulting from stimulation of diverse G-protein coupled receptors in VSMC [26].

FREE RADICALS AND NIH

Previous studies by Lee et al. [29] reported that serotonin stimulated tyrosine phosphorylation of bovine pulmonary artery smooth muscle cells through its active transport via serotonin transporter. Recently they have established that serotonin elevates O_2^- formation within 10 min. The O_2^- free radical scavenger Tiron and N-acetyl cysteine, a substrate for glutathione, blocked the 5-HT-induced O_2^- formation and cell proliferation. Serotonin transporter inhibitor, imipramine or diphenyliodonium, a NADPH oxidase inhibitor, blocked both 5-HT-induced elevation of O_2^- and cellular proliferation. It was emphasized that endothelial cells did not exhibit either 5-HT-induced proliferation or O_2^- formation [3]. They concluded that the 5-HT-induced cellular proliferation of SMC through signaling pathways utilizes 5-HT transporter and O_2^- formation [3]. Hydrogen peroxide also induced contractions of rat aortic segments at pathophysiological concentrations, which were Ca^{2+}-dependent. These investigations confirmed that hydroxyl radicals (OH), cycloxygenase products, protein kinases and products of protein tyrosine phosphorylation appear to play some role in H_2O_2-induced SMC contractions. Furthermore, metabolites catalysed by cytochrome P-450 dependent enzyme upon treatment with H_2O_2 exerted a vasodilatory effect on rat aortic segments. It was suggested that some unidentified product, produced by cytochrome P-450 inhibitor (Prodifen) during H_2O_2 treatment, appears to play some role in vascular smooth muscles of rat aortic rings, whereas nitric oxide (NO) donating agent sodium nitroprusside inhibited serotonin-induced ^{3}H-thymidine incorporation by smooth muscle cells. Bromo-cyclic GMP mimicked the antimitogenic action of sodium nitropruside that was inhibited by hemoglobin and potentiated by SOD suggesting the involvement of NO in serotonin-induced NIH. Recent studies have also suggested that a reactive oxygen species might be involved in the regulation of vascular tone. However the underlying mechanism remains unknown. Hydrogen peroxide (H_2O_2)-induced contraction of the denuded rat aortic ring was more pronounced than those of intact rat aorta. The contractile effect of H_2O_2 was completely inhibited by 1,200 U/ml of catalase whereas the presence of 1 μM Fe^{2+} or 10 μM prodifen, a cytochrome P-450 monooxygenase inhibitor, potentiated the contractile effect of H_2O_2 on isolated rat aortic segments. 1 mM of defroxamine (a Fe^{2+} chelator) attenuated the vessel contraction, induced by H_2O_2 and/or Fe^{2+}. Removal of extracellular calcium, addition of verapamil, administration of protein kinase inhibitor (staurosporine), treatment with an inhibitor of protein tyrosine phosphorylation (genistein) or employment of indomethacin resulted in a significant attenuation of contractile response of the vessel to H_2O_2. H_2O_2 can induce contraction of rat aortic segments at physiological concentrations which are Ca^{2+}-dependent. Some unidentified mediator, produced by cytochrome P-450 inhibitor (Prodifen) during H_2O_2 treatment, appears to play some role in contraction of vascular smooth muscle of rat aortic segment in vitro. NG-Nitro L arginine abolished the relaxing effect of bradykinin and 5-HT in the presence of ketanserine. It was concluded that both the contractile function of the smooth muscle cells and the endothelial production or action of NO is preserved or slightly enhanced in coronary arteries from pigs with chronic myocardial remodeling.

PROTO-ONCOGENES AND NIH

The exact molecular mechanism and crucial steps involved in the transcriptional regulation of cell proliferation and NIH remain unknown. Two important protooncogenes involved in cell proliferation are c-*fos* and c-*jun* which heterodimerize at the CCAAT region to initiate intracellular signal transduction cascade involved in DNA replication and hence cell proliferation [30–37]. In our study we hypothesized that sarpogrelate could inhibit heterodimerization in order to exert its antiproliferative effect. We have established that serotonin-induced NIH was associated with the induction of immediate early genes (c-fos and c-jun) and 5-HT2A receptor mRNA expression which was confirmed using radioimmunoprecipitation, immunoblotting and RT-PCR analysis. Inhibition of serotonin-induced increase in 5-HT2A receptor and *fos/jun* mRNA expression by sarpogrelate confirmed that it is a potent 5-HT2A receptor antagonist and its antiproliferative action is routed through 5-HT2A receptor blockade followed by inhibition of *fos-jun* heterodimerization. The most striking feature of this study was the finding that sarpogrelate induced a partial yet significant inhibition of *fos/jun* mRNA expression, as compared to 5-HT2A receptor that was completely inhibited by sarpogrelate. It is suggestive of the fact that the protooncogenes, *c-fos/c-jun* may receive peripheral inputs from diverse variety of signaling pathways, whereas serotonin 5HT2A receptor gene was modulated exclusively by either 5-HT and/or sarpogrelate. Previous studies by Lee et al. [38] have reported that serotonin-induced hyperplasia and hypertrophy via activation of c-*myc* and α-actin gene expression in bovine pulmonary artery smooth muscle cells was blocked by agents elevating cyclic AMP and inhibiting 5-HT transport or tyrosine phosphorylation.

Serotonin, angiotensin-II, platelet-derived growth factor (PDGF) and endothelin are four major mitogens involved in intravascular NIH [39–45]. Sarpogrelate, a novel specific 5-HT2A receptor antagonist, inhibited specifically the mitogenic response in RASMC which was triggered by the agonist, 5-HT. Mitogenic response induced by the other receptor agonists such as angiotensin-II, PDGF and endothelin was not influenced by sarpogrelate. These data confirmed our recent study in which we established that sarpogrelate did not influence DNA, RNA, and protein synthesis induced by these vasoactive agents, suggesting its specificity exclusively at the 5HT2A receptor. Sarpogrelate inhibited DNA synthesis at G2-M phase of the DNA cell cycle which was confirmed by Flow Cytometry [11]. Radioimmunoprecipitation, immunoblotting and RT-PCR data suggest that sarpogrelate inhibited 5-HT2A receptor expression, c-*fos* and c-*jun* mRNA expressions at the transcriptional level. RT-PCR data suggests that sarpogrelate binds specifically at the catalytic domain, localized in the third intracytoplasmic loop of the 5-HT2A receptor. These events inhibit 5-HT-induced increase in $[Ca^{2+}]_i$ channel activity, hence *fos-jun* heterodimerization which is involved in the intracellular signal transduction events such as DNA replication, cell proliferation and apoptosis. DNA, RNA, and protein synthesis was inhibited at any given dose of sarpogrelate. In general, lower doses of sarpogrelate (10^{-12}–10^{-6} M) induced inhibition in DNA, RNA, and protein synthesis while higher doses of (>40 μM) induced selective apoptosis of hyperproliferative vascular smooth muscle cells. Still higher doses (100 μM or above) induced a cytotoxic effect. These observations suggest that sarpogrelate (a highly specific 5-HT2A receptor antagonist) could have a great therapeutic potential in the prevention and treatment of NIH, observed in angina pectoris or in other coronary and cerebrovascular insufficiencies such as stroke and epilepsy [46]. In general, it is suggested that serotonin triggered, while sarpogrelate inhibited *fos-jun* heterodimerization and hence cell proliferation through 5-HT2A receptor modulation in RASMC.

ACKNOWLEDGEMENTS

The work reported in this article was supported by a grant from the Canadian Institutes of Health Research (CIHR) Group in Experimental Cardiology. NSD hold a Canadian Institutes of Health Research/Pharmaceutical Research Development Chair in Cardiovascular Research supported by Merck Frosst Canada. Sarpogrelate was kindly supplied by Mr. Tsutomu Iwasa, Mitsubishi Pharma Corp, Tokyo, Japan.

REFERENCES

1. Watts SW, Yeum CH, Campbell G, Webb RC. 1996. Serotonin stimulates protein tyrosyl phosphorylation and vascular contraction via tyrosine kinase. J Vasc Res 33:288–298.
2. Lee SL, Wang WW, Fanburg BL. 1996. Nitroprusside inhibits serotonin-induced mitogenesis and tyrosine phosphorylation of smooth muscle cells. Am J Physiol 270:L362–L367.
3. Lee SL, Wang WW, Fanburg BL. 1998. Superoxide as an intermediate signal for serotonin-induced mitogenesis. Free Rad Biol Med 24:855–858.
4. Fanburg BL, Lee SL. 1997. A new role for an old molecule: serotonin as a mitogen. Am J Physiol 272:L795–806.
5. Lee SL, Wang WW, Joseph PM, Hales CA, Fanburg BL. 1997. Inhibitory effect of heparin on serotonin-induced hyperplasia and hypertrophy of smooth muscle cells. Am J Respir Cell Mol Biol 17:78–83.
6. Tamura K, Kanzaki T, Saito Y, Otabe M, Morisaki N. 1997. Serotonin (5-hydroxytryptamine, 5-HT) enhances migration of rat aortic smooth muscle cells through 5-HT2 receptors. Atherosclerosis 132:139–143.
7. Pakala R, Benedict CR. 1998. Effect of serotonin and thromboxane A2 on endothelial cell proliferation: effect of specific receptor antagonists. J Lab Clin Med 131:527–537.

8. Hoyer D, Hannon JP, Martin GR. 2002. Molecular, pharmacological and functional diversity of 5-HT receptors. Pharmacol Biochem Behav 71:533–554.
9. Ramage AG. 2001. Central cardiovascular regulation and 5-hydroxytryptamine receptors. Res Bull 56:425–439.
10. Assender JW, Irenius E, Fredholm BB. 1997. 5-Hydroxytryptamine, angiotensin and bradykinin transiently increase intracellular calcium concentrations and PKC-alpha activity, but do not induce mitogenesis in human vascular smooth muscle cells. Acta Physiol Scand 160:207–217.
11. Sharma SK, Zahradka P, Chapman D, Kumamoto H, Takeda N, Dhalla NS. 1999. Inhibition of serotonin-induced vascular smooth muscle cell proliferation by sarpogrelate. J Pharmacol Exp Therapeut 290:1475–1481.
12. Sharma SK, Del Rizzo DF, Zahradka P, Bhangu SK, Werner JP, Kumamoto H, Takeda N, Dhalla NS. 2001. Sarpogrelate inhibits serotonin-induced proliferation of porcine coronary artery smooth muscle cells: Implications for long term graft potency. Ann Thorac Surg 71:1856–1865.
13. Mawatari K, Komori K, Kuma S, Yamamura S, Ishii T, Sugimachi K. 1997. Effects of serotonin and endothelin on the smooth muscle cells of autogenous vein grafts. Br J Surg 84:1419–1424.
14. Kuga T, Kadokami T, Kuwata K, Hata H, Ohara Y, Egashira K, Shimokawa H, Takeshita A. 1997. Central role of vascular smooth muscle hyperreactivity in coronary hyperconstriction after balloon injury in miniature pigs. Coron Artery Dis 8:69–75.
15. Chan PD, Findlay JM, Vollrath B, Cook DA, Grace M, Chen MH, Ashforth RA. 1995. Pharmacological and morphological effects of in-vitro transluminal balloon angioplasty on normal and vasospastic canine basilar arteries. J Neurosurg 83:522–530.
16. Semenchuk LA, Di Salvo J. 1995. Receptor-activated increases in intracellular calcium and protein tyrosine phosphorylation in vascular smooth muscle cells. FEBS Lett 370:127–130.
17. Kahn AM, Allen JC, Seidel CL, Song T. 1994. Insulin inhibits serotonin-induced Ca2+ influx in vascular smooth muscle. Circulation 90:384–390.
18. Kitagawa S, Yamaguchi Y, Kunitomo M, Imaizumi N, Fujiwara M. 1993. Altered vasoconstrictor responsiveness in vitamin D-induced arteriosclerotic rat aortas. Jpn J Pharmacol 61:283–289.
19. Florian JA, Watts SW. 1998. Integration of mitogen-activated protein kinase kinase activation in vascular 5-hydroxytryptamine2A receptor signal transduction. J Pharmacol Exp Ther 284:346–355.
20. Guillet-Deniau I, Burnol AF, Girard J. 1997. Identification and localization of a skeletal muscle secrotonin 5-HT2A receptor coupled to the Jak/STAT pathway. J Biol Chem 272:14825–14829.
21. Hara H, Oskabe M, Kitajima A, Tamao Y, Kikumoto R. 1991. MCI-9042, a new antiplatelet agent is a selective S2-serotonergic receptor antagonist. Thromb Haemost 65:415–420.
22. Hara H, Kitajima A, Shimada H, Tamao Y. 1994. Antithrombotic effect of MCI-9042, a new antiplatelet agent on experimental thrombosis models. Thromb Haemost 66:484–488.
23. Kanamori A, Matoba K, Yajima Y. 1994. Effects of sarpogrelate on serotonin-induced increase in cytosolic Ca^{2+} in cultured rat mesangial cells. Life Sci 55:PL 365–370.
24. Hirafuji M, Nezu A, Kanai Y, Ebihara T, Kawahara F, Tanimura A, Minami M. 1998. Effect of 5-hydroxytryptamine on intracellular calcium dynamics in cultured rat vascular smooth muscle cells. Res Commun Mol Pathol Pharmacol 99:305–319.
25. Lee SL, Wang WW, Fanburg BL. 1997. Association of Tyr phosphorylation of GTPase-activating protein with mitogenic action of serotonin. Am J Physiol 272:C223–C230.
26. Di Salvo J, Raatz Nelson S. 1998. Stimulation of G-protein coupled receptors in vascular smooth muscle cells induces tyrosine kinase dependent increases in calcium without tyrosine phosphorylation of phospholipase C gamma-. FEBS Lett 422:85–88.
27. Watts SW, Baez M, Webb RC. 1996. The 5-hydroxytryptamine2B receptor and 5-HT receptor signal transduction in mesenteric arteries from deoxycorticosterone acetate-salt hypertensive rats. J Pharmacol Exp Ther 277:1103–1113.
28. Lee SL, Wang WW, Lanzillo JJ, Fanburg BL. 1994. Serotonin produces both hyperplasia and hypertrophy of bovine pulmonary artery smooth muscle cells in culture. Am J Physiol 266:L46–L52.
29. Lee SL, Wang WW, Moore BJ, Fanburg BL. 1991. Dual effect of serotonin on growth of bovine pulmonary artery smooth muscle cells in culture. Circ Res 68:1362–1368.
30. Verma IM, Ransone LJ, Visvader J, Sassone-Corsi P, Lamph WW. 1990. fos-jun conspiracy: implications for the cell. Ciba Found Symp 150:128–137.
31. McKnight SL. 1991. Molecular Zippers in Gene Regulation. Sci American 264:54–64.
32. Ng KW, Ridgway P, Cohen DR, Tremethick DJ. 1997. The binding of a Fos/Jun heterodimer can completely disrupt the structure of a nucleosome. EMBO J 16:2072–2085.

33. Kerppola TK, Curran T. 1997. The transcription activation domains of Fos and Jun induce DNA bending through electrostatic interactions. EMBO J 16:2907–2916.
34. Leonard DA, Rajaram N, Kerppola TK. 1997. Structural basis of DNA bending and oriented heterodimer binding by the basic leucine zipper domains of Fos and Jun. Proc Natl Acad Sci (USA) 94:4913–4918.
35. McGill G, Fisher DE. 1998. DNA bending and the curious case of Fos/Jun. Chem Biol 5:R29–R38.
36. Sitlani A, Crothers DM. 1998. DNA-binding domains of Fos and Jun do not induce DNA curvature: an investigation with solution and gel methods. Proc Natl Acad Sci (USA) 95:1404–1409.
37. Chen L, Glover JN, Hogan PG, Rao A, Harrison SC. 1996. Structure of the DNA-binding domains from NFAT, Fos and jun bound specifically to DNA. Nature 392:42–48.
38. Lee SL, Wang WW, Lanzillo JJ, Fanburg BL. 1994. Regulation of serotonin-induced DNA synthesis of bovine pulmonary artery smooth muscle cells. Am J Physiol 266:L53–L60.
39. Yang H, Lu D, Yu K, Raizada MK. 1996. Regulation of neuromodulatory actions of angiotensin II in the brain neurons by the Ras-dependent mitogen-activated protein kinase pathway. J Neurosci 16:4047–4058.
40. Yang H, Lu D, Raizada MK. 1997. Angiotensin II-induced phosphorylation of the AT1 receptor from rat brain neurons. Hypertension 30:351–357.
41. Yang H, Lu D, Vinson GP, Raizada MK. 1997. Involvement of MAP kinase in angiotensin II-induced phosphorylation and intracellular targeting of neuronal AT1 receptors. J Neurosci 17:1660–1669.
42. Watts SW, Cohen ML, Mooney PQ, Johnson BG, Schoepp DD, Baez M. 1994. Disruption of potential alpha-helix in the G loop of the guinea pig 5-hydroxytryptamine2 receptor does not prevent receptor coupling to phosphoinositide hydrolysis. J Neurochem 62:934–943.
43. Watts SW. 1996. Serotonin activates the mitogen-activated protein kinase pathway in vascular smooth muscle: use of the mitogen-activated protein kinase kinase inhibitor PD098059. J Pharmacol Exp Ther 279:1541–1550.
44. Assender JW, Southgate KM, Hallett MB, Newby AC. 1992. Inhibition of proliferation, but not of Ca^{2+} mobilization, by cyclic AMP and GMP in rabbit aortic smooth-muscle cells. Biochem J 288:527–532.
45. Assender JW, Irenius E, Fredholm BB. 1996. Endothelin-1 causes a prolonged protein kinase C activation and acts as a co-mitogen in vascular smooth muscle cells. Acta Physiol Scand 157:451–460.
46. Lafont A, Libby P. 1998. The smooth muscle cell: Sinner or saint in restenosis and the acute coronary syndrome? J Am Coll Cardiol 32:283–285.

G.N. Pierce, M. Nagano, P. Zahradka, and N.S. Dhalla (eds.).
ATHEROSCLEROSIS, HYPERTENSION AND DIABETES. Copyright © 2003.
Kluwer Academic Publishers. Boston.

A NUTRITIONAL APPROACH TO PREVENT HIGH BLOOD PRESSURE

SUDESH VASDEV,[1] CAROL ANN FORD,[1] LINDA LONGERICH,[2] and SUSHIL PARAI[3]

Department of Medicine[1], Laboratory Medicine[3] and Division of Community Health[2] The Health Sciences Centre, Memorial University of Newfoundland St. John's, Newfoundland, Canada A1B 3V6

Summary. In essential hypertension, excess endogenous aldehydes bind sulfhydryl groups of membrane proteins, altering membrane Ca^{2+} channels and increasing cytosolic free calcium and blood pressure. Abnormalities in carbohydrate metabolism may underlie the etiology of the clinical course of hypertension. Insulin resistance and glucose intolerance is a common feature of hypertension in humans and in animal models. Elevated endogenous aldehydes in spontaneously hypertensive rats may be due to increased production of reactive aldehydes such as methylglyoxal, when the glycolytic pathway of glucose metabolism is impaired. The thiol compound, N-acetyl cysteine, normalizes elevated blood pressure by binding excess endogenous aldehydes and normalizing Ca^{2+} channels and cytosolic free calcium. Dietary supplementation with nutrients which can increase endogenous cysteine and glutathone may improve carbohydrate metabolism, lower blood pressure and normalize associated biochemical and histopathological changes. This nutritional approach to lower blood pressure has been demonstrated in spontaneously hypertensive rats, a model of human essential hypertension using supplementation with either vitamin B6, vitamin C, N-acetyl cysteine or lipoic acid.

Key words: Hypertension, Dietary supplements

INTRODUCTION

At present, available antihypertensive drugs normalize blood pressure by various means without removing the cause which is not known [1]. Over the past several

Correspondence to: Dr. Sudesh Vasdev, DVM, PhD, FACB, Professor of Medicine, Room H4310, Department of Medicine, Health Sciences Centre, Memorial University of Newfoundland, St. John's, Newfoundland, Canada A1B 3V6. Telephone No.: (709) 777-7260; Fax No.: (709) 777-7010; e-mail: svasdev@mun.ca

years, we have been investigating the underlying mechanism of essential hypertension and exploring the possibility of its prevention by nutritional supplementation. We have suggested that some of these nutritional supplements act to prevent one of the underlying causes of essential hypertension, elevated tissue aldehydes [2–6].

Role of aldehydes in hypertension

Aldehydes are formed as intermediate metabolites in humans and animals [1–3]. One major source of aldehydes in the body comes from the metabolism of fructose and glucose. If glucose metabolism via the glycolytic pathway is impaired, as in insulin resistance, there will be a build up of glyceraldehyde, glyceraldehyde-3-phosphate and dihydroxyacetone phosphate with further metabolism to methylglyoxal, a highly reactive ketoaldehyde [7–12]. Methylglyoxal itself also inhibits the glycolytic pathway [13] which can lead to increased insulin resistance. Aldehydes react nonenzymatically with sulfhydryl and amino groups of proteins and inhibit their function. Protein disulphide bonds and sulfhydryl groups have been shown to be involved in the functioning of L-type Ca^{2+} channels [14,15]. Excess metabolic aldehydes can lead to the formation of aldehyde protein conjugates [16,17], altering sulfhydryl (SH) groups of calcium channels and vascular membrane calcium handling. Disruption of vascular calcium channels can raise cytosolic free calcium $[Ca^{2+}]i$ levels and lead to increased peripheral vascular resistance and hypertension (Fig. 1). We have shown that elevated tissue aldehydes are one of the causes of hypertension in spontaneously hypertensive rats (SHRs), a model of insulin resistance and essential hypertension [2].

Antihypertensive mechanisms of cysteine

Under normal physiological conditions, tissue levels of aldehydes are maintained at a low level. This is accomplished through further catabolism or by binding to soluble sulfhydryl compounds like cysteine. Cysteine reacts with aldehydes forming a hemimercaptal which is further converted to a thiazolidine-carboxylic acid, which is excreted in bile and urine [16]. In addition to reacting directly with aldehydes, cysteine is also a precursor of glutathione. Glutathione (γ-glutamyl-cysteinyl glycine), a tripeptide, represents 90% of the total non-protein low molecular weight thiols in the body and is present in all cells [18]. It is a storage form of cysteine and is a cofactor in the enzymatic catabolism of methylglyoxal, an aldehyde produced when glucose metabolism is altered as a result of insulin resistance [10,11].

Hypertensive SHRs have elevated tissue aldehydes and cytosolic free Ca^{2+} and display hyperplasia of the smooth muscle cell, thickening of the wall and narrowing of the lumina of the small arteries and arterioles in the kidney. We have shown that N-acetyl-cysteine, an analogue of cysteine, when given in the diet to SHRs, normalizes tissue aldehydes, cytosolic free Ca^{2+} and adverse renal vascular changes and lowers blood pressure to levels similar to those of normotensive Wistar-Kyoto (WKY) rats used as controls [2]. Because the dietary amino acid cysteine proved to be an effective antihypertensive agent, we have investigated other dietary agents

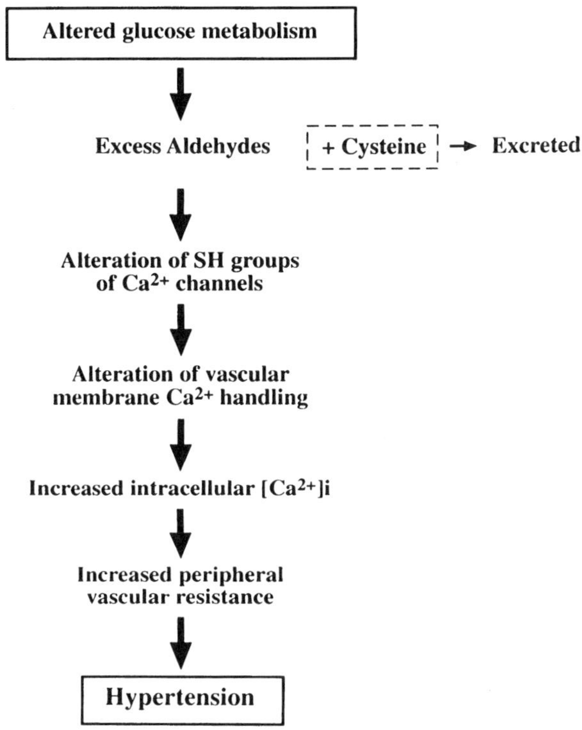

Figure 1. Role of aldehydes in the development of hypertension.

which could produce similar effects by increasing endogenous cysteine levels [4–6]. We report here the results of studies investigating dietary supplementation with vitamin B6, vitamin C and lipoic acid.

The role of vitamin B6 in the conversion of methionine to cysteine

In addition to a dietary source, cysteine is also synthesized metabolically from dietary methionine [19–20]. For the endogenous synthesis of cysteine, the first step in this process involves the demethylation of methionine to homocysteine. Homocysteine then combines with serine to yield cystathionine in a reaction catalyzed by cystathionine β-synthase. Finally, cystathionine is converted to cysteine and α-ketoglutarate by the enzyme cystathionase. Both cystathionine β-synthase and cystathionase are vitamin B6 requiring enzymes. A diet deficient in vitamin B6, when given chronically to rats, leads to decreased activity of these two enzymes in the liver [21,22]. Rats on a vitamin B6 deficient diet also had lower plasma cysteine levels and higher plasma homocysteine levels [20]. Dietary supplementation of vitamin B6 should stimulate the activity of these enzymes and increase the endogenous synthesis of cysteine from methionine. In hypertensive animals and humans,

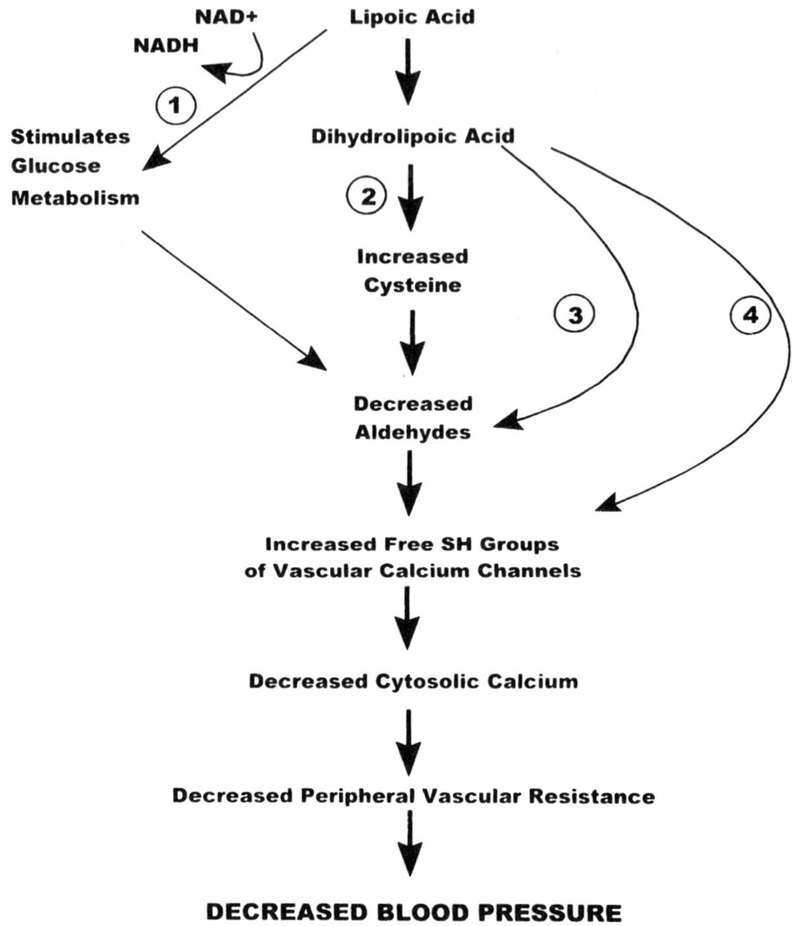

Figure 2. Antihypertensive effect of lipoic acid: four sites of action.

increased production of cysteine would lead to more efficient excretion of excess metabolic aldehydes, normalizing vascular calcium channels and lowering blood pressure [6,23].

The role of vitamin C in maintaining adequate cysteine levels

Ascorbic acid (vitamin C) is needed as a cofactor in various enzymatic reactions including the conversion of cystine to cysteine [24]. Dietary supplementation of ascorbic acid in mice, rats, guinea pigs and humans leads to increased tissue levels of glutathione, the stable storage form of cysteine [24–27]. Glutathione is depleted in the tissues of SHRs and human hypertensives [28,29]. Plasma levels of ascorbic

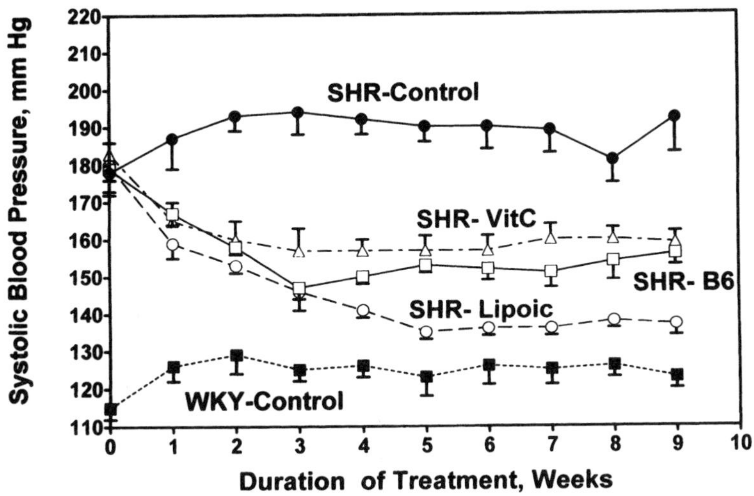

Figure 3. The line graph shows the effect of vitamin B6, vitamin C and lipoic acid supplemented diet on systolic blood pressure in SHR rats. Starting at 12 weeks of age, animals were divided into five groups of six animals each. Animals in WKY-control group [■– – –■] and SHR-control group [●—●] were given a normal diet and SHR-vitamin B6 group [□—□], a diet supplemented with 20 mg of vitamin B6; SHR-vitamin C group [△– – –△], a diet supplemented with 100 mg of vitamin C; and SHR-lipoic acid group [○– – –○], a diet supplemented with 50 mg of lipoic acid per 100 gm of diet, for the next nine weeks. All animals were given normal drinking water. Values are mean ± SD of six animals in each group for each week. Each mean value of systolic blood pressure from weeks 1–9 in the SHR-vitamin B6 group, SHR-vitamin C group or SHR-lipoic acid group is significantly different from the mean values of SHR-controls and from the mean values of WKY-controls.

acid are low in human hypertensives [27,28,30,31]. Dietary supplementation of ascorbic acid may act to lower blood pressure by increasing the tissue levels of glutathione and the aldehyde binding compound cysteine.

The role of lipoic acid in lowering aldehydes and normalizing vascular Ca^{2+} channels

Alpha-lipoic acid is a unique short chain fatty acid with two sulphur atoms which are converted to sulfhydryl (SH) groups in dihydrolipoic acid (DHL), its reduced form. It is metabolically active in both the oxidized and reduced form [32–34]. Lipoic acid may act at four sites (Fig. 2) to lower tissue aldehydes and normalize vascular Ca^{2+} channels. First, lipoic acid as a component of coenzyme A stimulates glucose metabolism leading to decreased formation of reactive aldehydes. Second, the redox partner dihydrolipoic acid converts cystine to cysteine. Third, as DHL has two SH groups, it will act similar to cysteine and bind excess aldehydes leading to their excretion. Fourth, lipoic acid may act directly on vascular Ca^{2+} channels to increase free sulfhydryl groups and normalize Ca^{2+} transport.

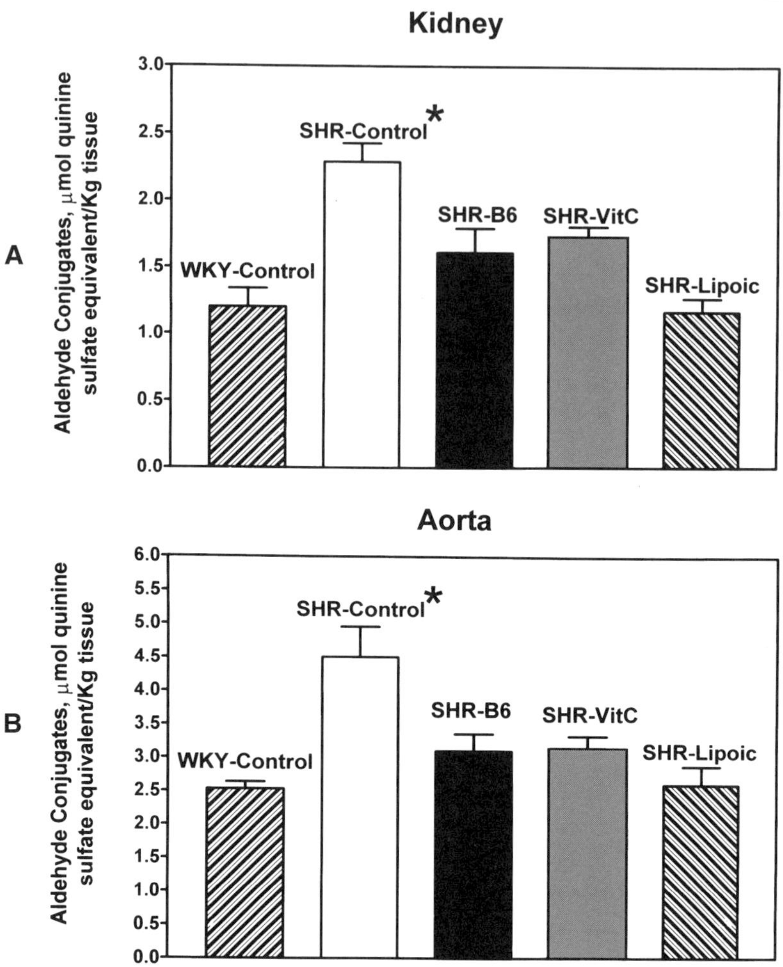

Figure 4. Bar graph shows the effect of vitamin B6, vitamin C and lipoic acid supplemented diet on kidney (A) and aorta (B) aldehyde conjugates in SHR rats. Starting at 12 weeks of age, animals were divided into five groups of six animals each. Animals in the WKY-control group and SHR-control group were given a normal diet and SHR-vitamin B6 group, a diet supplemented with 20 mg of vitamin B6, SHR-vitamin C group, a diet supplemented with 100 mg of vitamin C; and SHR-lipoic acid group, a diet supplemented with 50 mg of lipoic acid per 100 gm of diet, for the next nine weeks. All animals were given normal drinking water. All tissue values are mean ± SD of six animals in each group at completion of the study age 21 weeks. The symbol (*) indicates that values are significantly different from other groups.

Antihypertensive effect of dietary vitamin B6, vitamin C and lipoic acid in SHRs

In our laboratory, we investigated the antihypertensive effects of these three supplements in the diet of SHRs, an animal model of human hypertension. Before

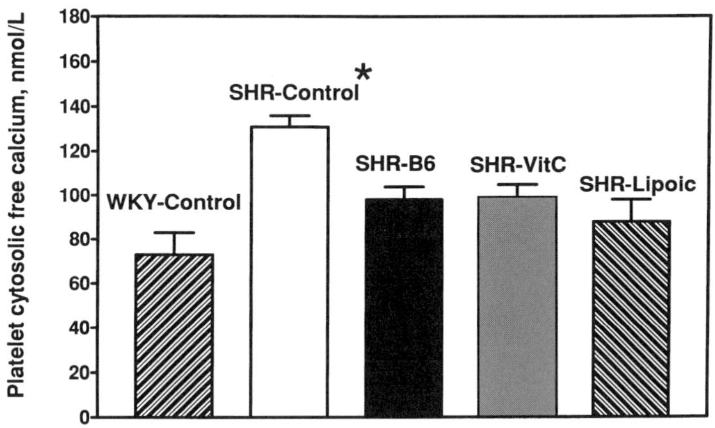

Figure 5. Bar graph shows the effect of vitamin B6, vitamin C and lipoic acid supplemented diet on platelet cytosolic free calcium in SHR rats. Starting at 12 weeks of age, animals were divided into five groups of six animals each. Animals in the WKY-control group and SHR-control group were given a normal diet and SHR-vitamin B6 group, a diet supplemented with 20 mg of vitamin B6; SHR-vitamin C group, a diet supplemented with 100 mg of vitamin C; and SHR-lipoic acid group, a diet supplemented with 50 mg of lipoic acid per 100 gm of diet, for the next 9 weeks. All animals were given normal drinking water. All values are mean ± SD of six animals in each group at completion of the study age 21 weeks. The symbol (*) indicates that values are significantly different from other groups.

treatment, systolic blood pressure (SBP) at 12 weeks of age was significantly higher in SHRs compared with WKY rats of similar age. When SHRs were given a diet supplemented with vitamin C, vitamin B6 or lipoic acid, their SBP decreased significantly at one through nine weeks of treatment compared with SHR-controls of the same age but was still significantly higher than the WKY-controls of the same age (Fig. 3). Aldehyde conjugate levels were significantly higher in the kidney and aorta of untreated hypertensive SHRs as compared with WKY control rats at age 21 weeks. Vitamin B6, vitamin C and lipoic acid treatment for nine weeks significantly decreased both kidney and aortic aldehyde conjugates as compared with SHR-control rats (Fig. 4). We also found significantly higher platelet $[Ca^{2+}]i$ in untreated hypertensive rats than normotensive WKY rats. Vitamin B6, vitamin C and lipoic acid treatment for nine weeks significantly decreased these levels (Fig. 5). It has been suggested that cytosolic free calcium concentration in platelets reflects tone and structural changes of resistance vessels [32]. Platelets were chosen because, besides being an easily accessible tissue, they represent abnormalities in calcium handling similar to those described in vascular tissue [33].

In hypertensive SHRs, we found smooth muscle cell hyperplasia, thickening of the wall and narrowing of the lumen in the small arteries and arterioles of the kidney. Vitamin B6, vitamin C and lipoic acid treatment attenuated these changes [4–6].

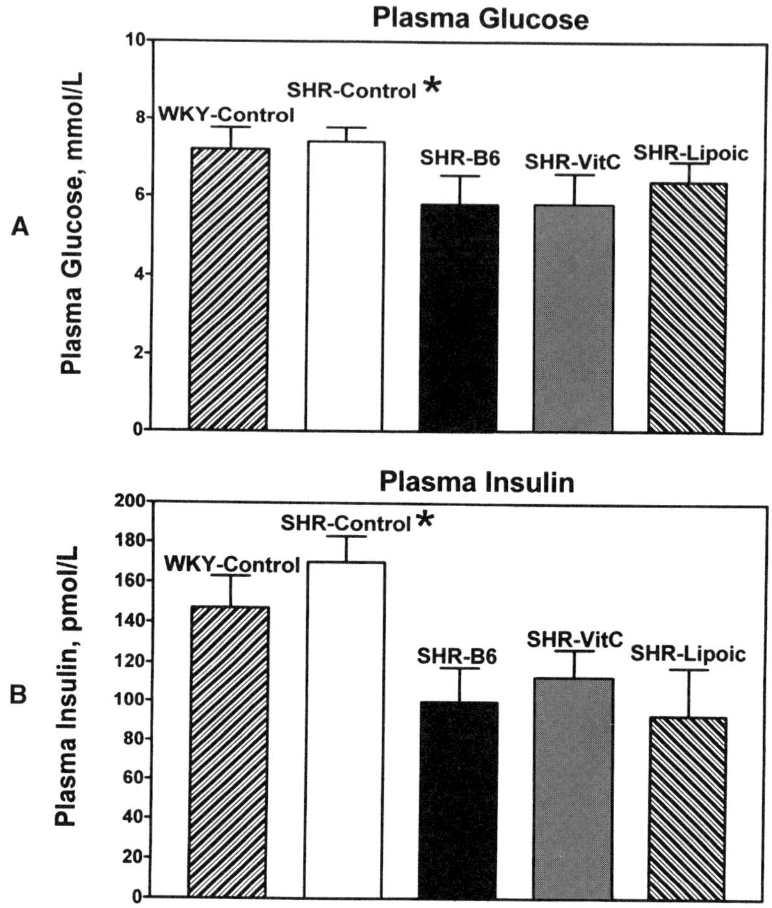

Figure 6. Bar graph shows the effect of vitamin B6, vitamin C and lipoic acid supplemented diet on plasma glucose (A) and insulin levels (B) in SHR rats. Starting at 12 weeks of age, animals were divided into five groups of six animals each. Animals in WKY-control group and SHR-control group were given a normal diet and SHR-vitamin B6 group, a diet supplemented with 20 mg of vitamin B6; SHR-vitamin C group, a diet supplemented with 100 mg of vitamin C; and SHR-lipoic acid group, a diet supplemented with 50 mg of lipoic acid per 100 gm of diet, for the next 9 weeks. All animals were on normal drinking water. All values are mean ± SD of six animals in each group at completion of the study age 21 weeks. The symbol (*) indicates that values are significantly different from other SHR groups.

SHRs, with insulin resistance, have increased secretion of insulin and elevated plasma levels in order to maintain normal plasma glucose concentration. Supplementation with vitamin B6, vitamin C and lipoic acid stimulated glucose metabolism and lowered both plasma glucose and insulin in SHRs (Fig. 6). The stimulation of carbohydrate metabolism through the glycolytic pathway leads to decreased formation of the metabolic aldehydes which adversely affect calcium channels. This would aid in the normalization of membrane Ca^{2+} channels, leading to decreased cytosolic free calcium and lower blood pressure.

CONCLUSION

In conclusion, treatment with either vitamin B6, vitamin C or lipoic acid lowers blood pressure in SHRs by lowering tissue aldehydes and correcting altered glucose metabolism. We suggest that nutritional supplementation could be a simple and effective treatment for essential hypertension in humans.

ACKNOWLEDGEMENTS

We gratefully acknowledge the staff of the Division of Anatomic Pathology and Division of Biochemical Pathology and Renal Laboratory of the Department of Laboratory Medicine, Health Sciences Centre for technical assistance and Ms. Janice Petten for typing the manuscript. We also thank the Medical Research Council of Canada for financial support to carry out this study.

REFERENCES

1. Julius S. 2000. Five decades of antihypertensive treatment: the unresolved issues. J Hypertens 18 (suppl 3):S3–S7.
2. Vasdev S, Mian T, Ford CA, Longerich L, Parai S. 1996. Role of endogenous aldehydes in spontaneously hypertensive and disulfiram-induced hypertensive rats. Nutr Metab Cardiovasc Dis 6:130–140.
3. Vasdev S, Ford CA, Longerich L, Parai S, Gadag V. 1999. Antihypertensive effect of low ethanol intake in spontaneously hypertensive rats. Mol Cell Biochem 200:85–92.
4. Vasdev S, Ford CA, Parai S, Longerich L, Gadag V. 1999. Dietary vitamin B6 supplementation attenuates hypertension in spontaneously hypertensive rats. Mol & Cell Biochem 200:155–162.
5. Vasdev S, Ford CA, Parai S, Longerich L, Gadag V. 2000. Dietary α-lipoic acid supplementation lowers blood pressure in spontaneously hypertensive rats. J Hypertens 18:567–573.
6. Vasdev S, Ford CA, Parai S, Longerich L, Gadag V. 2001. Dietary vitamin C supplementation lowers blood pressure in spontaneously hypertensive rats. Mol Cell Biochem 218:97–103.
7. Brandt RB, Siegel SA. 1979. Methylglyoxal production in human blood. Submolecular biology and cancer. Excerpta Medica, CIBA Foundation Symposium 67:211–223.
8. Kashiwagi A, Obata T, Suzaka M, Takagi Y, Kida Y, Igawa T, Tanaka Y, Asahina T, Ikebuchi M, Saeki Y, Kikkawa R, Shigeta Y. 1992. Increase in cardiac muscle fructose content in streptozotocin-induced diabetic rats. Metabolism 41:1041–1046.
9. Kondoh Y, Kawase M, Ohmori S. 1992. D-lactate concentrations in blood, urine and sweat before and after exercise. Eur J Appl Physiol 65:88–93.
10. Thornalley PJ. 1993. Modification of the glyoxalase system in disease processes and prospects for therapeutic strategies. Biochem Soc Trans 21:531–534.
11. Phillips SA, Mirrlees D, Thornalley PJ. 1993. Modification of the glyoxalase system in streptozotocin-induced diabetic rats. Effect of the aldose reductase inhibitor statil. Biochem Pharmacol 46:805–811.
12. Vander Jagt DL, Hunsaker LA. 1993. Substrate specificity of reduced and oxidized forms of human aldose reductase. In: H Weiner (ed) Enzymology and Molecular Biology of Carbonyl Metabolism 4. Plenum Press, New York, pp 279–288.
13. Leoncini G, Maresca M, Buzzi E. 1989. Inhibition of the glycolytic pathway of methylglyoxal in human platelets. Cell Biochem Function 7:65–70.
14. Murphy BJ, Washkurak AW, Tuana BS. 1990. Dihydropyridine binding to the L-type Ca^{2+} channel in rabbit heart sarcolemma and skeletal muscle transverse-tubules: role of disulfide, sulfhydryl and phosphate groups. Biochim Biophys Acta 1052:333–339.

15. Zaidi NF, Lagenaur CF, Abramson JJ, Pessah I, Salama G. 1989. Reactive disulfides trigger Ca^{2+} release from sarcoplasmic reticulum via an oxidation reaction. J Biol Chem 264:21725–21736.
16. Schauenstein E, Esterbauer H, Zollner S. 1977. In: Aldehydes in biological systems, their natural occurrence and biological activities. Pion Limited, 207 Brondes Bury Park, London, pp 1–7.
17. Vasdev S, Barrett B, Longerich L, Ford CA. 1996. Ethanol-induced hypertension: the role of acetaldehyde. In: NS Dhalla (ed) Pathophysiology of Heart Failure. Kluwer Academic Publishers, Norwell, MA, USA, pp 77–93.
18. Meister A, Anderson ME, Hwang O. 1986. Intracellular cysteine and glutathione delivery systems. J Am Col Nutr 5:137–151.
19. Lehninger AL. 1978. Biochemistry: the molecular basis of cell structure and function. 2nd ed. Worth Publishers, Inc, New York, pp 698.
20. Smolin LA, Benevenga NJ. 1982. Accumulation of homocyst(e)ine in vitamin B-6 deficiency: A model for the study of cystathionine β-synthase deficiency. J Nutr 112:1264–1272.
21. Finkelstein JD, Chalmers FT. 1970. Pryidoxine effects on cystathionine synthase in rat liver. J Nutr 100:467–469.
22. Takeuchi F, Izuta S, Tsubouchi R, Shibata Y. 1991. Glutathione levels and related enzyme activities in vitamin B-6 deficient rats fed a high methioinine and low cystine diet. J Nutr 121:1366–1373.
23. Aybak M, Sermet A, Ayyildiz MO, Karakilcik S. 1995. Effect of oral pyridoxine hydrochloride supplementation on arterial blood pressure in patients with essential hypertension. Arzeimittel-forschung 45:1271–1273.
24. Meister A. 1992. Commentary on the antioxidant effects of ascorbic acid and glutathione. Biochem Pharmacol 44:1905–1915.
25. Paolisso G, Balbi V, Volpe C, Varricchio G, Gambardella A, Saccomanno F, Ammendola S, Varricchio M, D'Onofrio F. 1995. Metabolic benefits deriving from chronic vitamin C supplementation in aged non-insulin dependent diabetics. J Am Coll Nutr 14:387–392.
26. Meister A. 1994. Glutathione-ascorbic acid antioxidant system in animals. J Biol Chem 269: 9397–9400.
27. Johnston CS, Meyer CG, Srilakshmi JC. 1993. Vitamin C elevates red blood cell glutathione in healthy adults. Am J Clin Nutr 58:103–105.
28. Janero DR, Burghadt B. 1989. Cardiac membrane vitamin E and malon-dialdehyde levels in heart muscle of normotensive and spontaneously-hypertensive rats. Lipids 24:33–38.
29. Uysal M, Bulur H, Sener D, óz H. 1986. Lipid peroxidation in patients with essential hypertension. Int J Clin Pharmacol Ther Toxicol 24:474–476.
30. Wen Y, Killalea S, McGettigan P, Feely J. 1996. Lipid peroxidation and antioxidant vitamins C and E in hypertensive patients. Irish J Med Sci 165:210–212.
31. Pierdomenico SD, Costantini F, Bucci A, De Cesare D, Cuccurullo F, Mezzetti A. 1998. Low-density lipoprotein oxidation and vitamins E and C in sustained and white-coat hypertension. 31:621–626.
32. α-lipoic acid. 1998. Alternative Medicine Review 3(4):308–310.
33. Packer L, Witt EH, Tritschler HJ. 1995. Alpha-lipoic acid as a biological antioxidant. Free Radical Biology & Medicine 19(2):227–250.
34. Han D, Handelman G, Marcocci L, Sen CK, Roy S, Kobuchi H, Tritschler HJ, Flohé L, Packer L. 1997. Lipoic acid increases *de novo* synthesis of cellular glutathione by improving cystine utilization. BioFactors 6:321–338.
35. Bolli P, Erne P, Hulthen UL, Ritz R, Kiowski W, Ji BH, Buhler FR. 1984. Parallel reduction of calcium-influx-dependent vasoconstriction and platelet-free calcium concentration with calcium entry and β-adrenoceptor blockade. J Cardiovasc Pharmac 6:S996–S1001.
36. Pollard TD. 1975. Electron microscopy of synthetic myosin filaments. J Cell Biol 67:93–104.

G.N. Pierce, M. Nagano, P. Zahradka, and N.S. Dhalla (eds.).
ATHEROSCLEROSIS, HYPERTENSION AND DIABETES. Copyright © 2003.
Kluwer Academic Publishers. Boston.

CARDIOVASCULAR AND RENAL ACTIONS OF LEPTIN

PRABAL K. GUHA, MD,[1] DANIEL VILLARREAL, MD,[1] GARRY P. REAMS, MD,[2] and RONALD H. FREEMAN, PHD[2]

[1] *SUNY—Upstate Medical University, Syracuse, New York, USA;* [2] *University of Missouri School of Medicine, Columbia, Missouri USA*

Summary. Leptin is a recently isolated circulating peptide hormone that is primarily synthesized and secreted by the adipocytes. A major function of this hormone is the control of energy balance by binding to receptors in the hypothalamus, leading to reduction in food intake, as well as elevation in temperature and energy expenditure. In addition, increasing pharmacological evidence suggests that leptin, through its direct and indirect actions, may play an important role in cardiovascular and renal functions. While the relevance of endogenous leptin needs further clarification, it appears to be a potential pressure and volume regulating factor, and may function pathophysiologically as a common link to obesity and hypertension.

***Key words*:** Natriuresis, Systemic and renal hemodynamics, Hypertension

INTRODUCTION

Leptin, the product of the Ob gene is a recently isolated circulating peptide hormone whose structure is highly conserved amongst vertebrates [1]. It is primarily synthesized and secreted into the circulation by adipocytes [1,2], although the brain [3] placenta [4], gastrointestinal tract [5,6], and the skeletal muscle [7] appear to be additional sources. As a regulatory hormone, the first described major action of leptin was on the hypothalamus, acting as adipostat, to control body weight

Correspondence: Daniel Villarreal, MD, FACC, FAHA, Division of Cardiology, Department of Medicine, SUNY Upstate Medical University, Rm 6142, 750 East Adams Street, Syracuse, NY, 13210, USA. Tel: (315) 464-9578; Fax: (315) 464-9571; e-mail: villarrd@upstate.edu

and fat deposition through its effects on appetite inhibition, as well as stimulation of the metabolic rate and thermogenesis [1,2].

In the last several years, however, it has become apparent that the functions of leptin are more extensive than that of an anti-obesity hormone. Leptin also affects several neuroendocrine mechanisms and regulates multiple hypothalamic—pituitary axes [8,9]. In addition, there is increasing evidence suggesting that the biology of leptin extends to other organs including the kidney, the sympathetic nervous system and the systemic vasculature, where it may have prominent effects [10–12].

This review is primarily directed to the consideration of the potential role of leptin as a regulatory mechanism to produce adjustments of body fluid balance and pressures in physiological and pathophysiological conditions, including hypertension. A number of excellent reviews are available for other various endocrine functions of leptin and the interested reader is referred to these for detailed knowledge [11,13,14].

BIOLOGY OF LEPTIN RECEPTORS

The leptin receptor is a member of the extended class I cytokine receptor family having at least six splice variants Ob-R (a–f) [1,2,15]. The ob-Ra variant has been postulated to transport leptin across the blood-brain barrier [16–18]. Ob-Rc and Ob-Rd have been implicated in the clearance of leptin from the circulation, and the Ob-Re variant is a putative soluble receptor [15–17]. The Ob-Rb variant encodes a receptor with a long intracellular domain, which is essential for intracellular signal transduction; and finally, the recently recognized Ob-Rf variant has as yet no identified function [16–18].

High tissue levels of leptin receptor gene expression occur in the lung, moderate levels in the kidney, and low levels in the heart, brain, spleen, liver, and muscle [18–20], as demonstrated by reverse transcription-polymerase chain reaction analysis and Southern blot analysis. Expression of the extracellular domain of the leptin receptor Ob-R and the short splice variant Ob-Ra has been shown in many peripheral tissues; however, the long splice variant Ob-Rb has been detected in fewer organ systems including the adrenal gland, kidney and heart [20,21]. This long splice variant with long intracellular domain possess two peptide motifs which interact with an intracellular glycoprotein gp 130, which in turn activates Janus Kinases (family of tyrosine kinases) to promote transcription thru phosphorylation of the STAT (signal transducer and activator of transcription) pathway. Within the kidney, in situ hybridization using the Ob-R probe localized the mRNA to the inner zone of the medulla and the pyramid, appearing to be associated with collecting tubules and ducts [20]. Moreover, recent immunohistochemical studies by Martinez et al. [22] utilizing a monoclonal antibody 3H10, IgG2b against rat leptin demonstrated intense labeling of the hormone in the apical membrane and the cytoplasm of the inner medullary collecting duct cells in the normal rat. Similar renal localization has been shown with autoradioagraphy studies in the same species [23]. Thus, these evidence are suggestive of role of leptin on renal physiology as well as the involvement of the kidney in the degradation and clearance of the hormone [14,22,24].

EFFECT OF LEPTIN ON SYMPATHETIC NERVOUS SYSTEM AND SYSTEMIC HEMODYNAMICS

It is now well demonstrated that circulating leptin crosses the blood brain barrier and act on the lateral and medial region of the hypothalamus to regulate energy balance via the stimulation of the sympathetic nervous system [10,11]. Relevant to these information is that the well known fact that the circulating levels of leptin vary in direct proportion to the adipose tissue mass [25], and consistent elevations in plasma leptin have been found in humans and animal models of obesity. This disease of ever increasing proportions, in turn is frequently characterized by elevations in arterial blood pressure. Though the association between hypertension and obesity has been previously described, the pathophysiological basis of obesity-induced hypertension remains unclear [20,26]. Mechanisms suggested to be involved include increased plasma volume and cardiac output, hyperinsulinemia and insulin resistance, enhanced sympathetic nervous system activity, and sodium retention with dysfunction of salt-regulating hormones [20,26]. Although the renal mechanisms that lead to obesity related sodium retention have not been fully evaluated, these do not appear to be related to either renal vasoconstriction or decreased filtered sodium load. Obesity, however, is associated with an enhanced absolute and fractional sodium reabsorption that may occur at distal nephron sites [27].

As an additional potential pathophysiological mechanism, recent studies have focused on the potential effects of leptin on sympathetic nervous system-induced elevations of arterial blood pressure. It is now well established that leptin infusion can activate the sympathetic nervous system both by local peripheral actions as well as centrally mediated effects on the hypothalamus. Leptin alters the secretion of various neuromodulators including Neuropetide Y, alpha MSH, Melanin concentrating hormone and the Agouti related peptide, which in turn, have regulatory actions on sympathetic activation and tone [28]. Leptin administration reduces the level of Neuropeptide Y expression in the hypothalamus and may therefore lead to blood pressure elevation [11]. Studies with direct intracerebral perfusion of leptin have demonstrated a rise in lumbar and adipose sympathetic nerve activity. In addition, sympathetic nerve activity in various organs in response to intravenous leptin has been studied in normal Sprague Dawley rats and the lean and obese variant of Zucker rats [10]. In this investigation, incremental doses of murine leptin produced a slow, dose-dependent increase in the sympathetic discharge from the renal nerves and the brown adipose tissue in the Sprague Dawley rat. Sympathoactivation was maintained even on transecting nerve distal to the recording site, although it was significantly inhibited by ganglionic blockade, indicating an efferent rather than afferent nerve activation [10,11]. Similar responses were seen in the lean Zucker rats; however the sympathetic nerve activation was markedly blunted in the obese Zucker rats [10]. This attenuated response was interpreted to be related to a leptin receptor defect characteristic of the obese Zucker strain. It is important to point out that although the higher doses used in this set of experiments raised the leptin concentration to supraphysiologic levels, an effect was evident at lower doses [10]. In this regard it is of interest that the leptin induced early activation of the sympathetic nervous tone did not appear to be accompanied by parallel elevation in arterial blood pressure when the hormone was acutely infused intravenously in normotensive and hypertensive rats [12,29,30].

In contrast to the lack of acute systemic leptin effect on arterial blood pressure are the studies with direct local infusion of the hormone in the cerebral ventricles of normal rats [11]. Dunbar et al. reported that with this infusion mode of leptin leads to a slow increase of mean arterial pressure (MAP) by approximately 10% at the end of 90 min recording period. However significant blood pressure elevations were seen as early as 10 minutes. Consistent with this effect, the lumbar sympathetic nerve activity also increased progressively to a maximum of 10% over baseline. On the other hand, the response in the renal nerve activity was slower in onset and reached statistical significance only after 45 minutes of infusion [11]. Interestingly, the observed lack of change in renal flow in spite of the rise in the renal sympathetic nerve activity could have been related to concurrent renal vasodilation. Thus, in the context of available information, it is evident that central administration of leptin acutely increases the sympathetic outflow similar to the peripheral leptin administration. The absence of arterial blood pressure elevation in the latter case raises the possibility of the simultaneous local activation of counterregulatory vasodilatory mechanisms to help maintain systemic hemodynamics. In support of this concept, in vitro studies performed by Lembo et al. [31] in the aortic rings of Wistar Kyoto rats have demonstrated a dose dependent leptin-induced vasorelaxation. In this investigation, leptin's effect in the aortic ring was abolished by N^{ω}-nitro-L-arginine methyl ester (L-NAME) administration or endothelial denudation, suggesting that at least in part, nitric oxide (NO) mediated the vasodilatory response. In addition endothelium-derived hyperpolarizing factor (EDHF) also appears to contribute to this phenomenon. Pertinent to these findings, it is relevant to point out that the expression of the Ob-Rb receptor has been demonstrated in vascular endothelium [32,33], indicating that the endothelium is the target of leptin's activity. More recently, a seminal study by Fruhbeck [34] demonstrated a dose dependent elevation in plasma NO produced by intravenous administration of synthetic leptin in normal rats. The effect required an intact leptin receptor, as it could not be elicited in the fa/fa rat model, which lacks a functional leptin receptor [12]. Of major interest in this study, blockade of NO production with L-NAME produced leptin-induced enhancement of arterial blood pressure. Conversely, blockade of the sympathetic nervous system with chlorisondamine lead to leptin mediated reduction in blood pressure [34]. Thus, it is possible to suggest that during acute systemic administration of leptin, the hormone's lack of effect on arterial blood pressure may represent a balanced action on the peripheral vascular resistance. In this context, it is also possible to suggest that in pathophysiological conditions such as obesity or hypertension, independent alteration of vasodilatory mechanisms involving NO production and metabolism could result in the disruption of this balanced effect of the hormone.

CHRONIC HYPERLEPTINEMIA AND HYPERTENSION

In chronic hyperleptinemic conditions, the potential balanced effects of acute leptin infusion on peripheral vascular resistance may not remain. In a recent investigation, the effects of chronic infusion of leptin were evaluated in groups of normal conscious Sprague Dawley rats by Shek et al. [35]. Following control observations, leptin was continuously infused either intravenously or into the carotid artery, at a dose 0.1 μg/kg/min for 5 days followed by 1 μg/kg/min for 7 days. With the low dose infusion there was minimal rise in blood pressure, but with the higher dose there was a significant 6–10 mm Hg elevation detected at 5 days of infusion by either route. The hypertensive effect rapidly reversed on cessation of the hormone infusion. The heart rate response followed a similar pattern with a significant rise during the higher infusion dose. In support of the concept of hypertensinogenic effects of chronic hyperleptinemia are the studies by Aizawa et al. [36] in transgenic mice overexpressing leptin. In these animals, endogenous leptin was elevated twenty fold and this was associated with significant increases in the systolic blood pressure of approximately 15–20 mm Hg compared to the control mice. Importantly the hypertension was abolished with the intraperitoneal injection of an alpha-blocker, indicating the major involvement of the sympathetic system in the leptin-induced elevations in blood pressure.

LEPTIN AND RENAL REGULATION OF SODIUM-VOLUME BALANCE

As outlined previously, in vitro studies have strongly indicated that the renal medulla and in particular the inner medullary collecting duct [20,22] contain the long tail Ob-Rb leptin receptor which in turn, suggests a functional role of this hormone in renal biology. To this end it is important to point out that at least in the rat, 3–6 fold elevations of plasma leptin occurs postprandially [5,6], a condition characterized by intravascular sodium and volume surfeit. Accordingly, the renal effects of leptin may not only be viewed as the result of plasma hormone level elevation, but also highly dependent on the underlying systemic and renal vascular hemodynamic conditions. Initial studies performed by independent laboratories, have demonstrated that acute administration of synthetic leptin in the rat produced a significant elevation in urinary sodium and water excretion. Serrdeil-Le Gal et al. [23] reported that intraperitoneal injections of synthetic murine leptin in normal hydrated conscious rats at a dose of 0.5 mg/kg was associated with a significant two to three fold increase in urinary volume when compared to vehicle infused rats. This effect was most apparent within two hours of leptin administration. More recently, Jackson and Li [29] reported that acute ipsilateral intrarenal infusions of synthetic human leptin in increasing doses of 0.3 to 30 μg/min into anesthetized rats produced a significant two to three fold elevation in urinary sodium and volume excretion without significant effects on renal or systemic hemodynamics. Since the natriuresis and diuresis were confined to the infused kidney, these results suggested a direct local effect. Importantly, the renal excretory actions of leptin required approximately 1.5 hrs to be fully expressed [29]. This delayed time course is consistent with alterations at the level of gene transcription with the de novo synthesis of proteins and turnover of existing proteins to achieve the biological response. This in turn, is consonant with the JAK-STAT signal transduction pathway characteristic of the Ob-Rb isoform of the leptin receptor that predominates in the kidney. For reasons that are unclear, Jackson and Li did not observe diuretic or natriuretic responses with the acute infusion of murine leptin in these rats [29], which is in contrast the result of several other studies [12,23,30]. In this regard, it is important to note that the amino-acid sequence homology between murine and rat leptin is 96% [37], whereas the homology of human and rat leptin is only 84% [37]. It is also pertinent to mention that synthetic murine leptin exerts other predictable biological functions in the central nervous system of the rat [10]. Of specific relevance, studies by Haynes et al. [10] recently demonstrated that synthetic murine leptin produced a dose related significant elevation in efferent sympathetic nerve activity to kidney, adrenal gland, brain, adipose tissue, and hindlimb of the normal rat.

More recently, Villarreal et al. [12] examined the hemodynamic and renal actions of acute infusions of synthetic murine leptin in rat models of normotension (Sprague Dawley rat), hypertension (Spontaneously Hypertensive rats) and obesity (lean and obese Zucker rats). As depicted in Fig. 1, in the normotensive animals, an intravenous bolus of 400 μg/kg of leptin produced a robust six to seven fold elevation in urinary sodium excretion (UNaV) and the fractional excretion of sodium (FENa). In contrast, the hypertensive rats were refractory to the renal effects of leptin when infused either with 400 or 1,600 μg/kg (Fig. 1). Interestingly, while the lean Zucker rats responded very similarly to the Sprague Dawley rats (SDR), the natriuretic effect was attenuated in the obese Zucker animals (Fig. 2). Indeed, at 400 μg/kg no natriuresis was elicited, but at 1,600 μg/kg a modest but significant two to three fold increment in UNaV was observed. Mean arterial pressure, creatinine clearance, urinary potassium excretion, plasma renin activity and plasma aldosterone concentration remained unchanged in all of the rat strains with the acute infusion of the hormone. Collectively, these findings were interpreted to suggest that leptin might be a natriuretic hormone primarily acting at the tubular level for promotion of sodium excretion in normal rats, and that it may function pathophysiologically in obesity and hypertension. However, the mechanism(s) underlying the natriuresis and the nature of blunted responses to leptin in obesity and hypertension were not determined.

Nevertheless, based on these initial information, it was hypothesized that the lack of a natriuretic response to leptin could have been related, at least in part, to the activation of a counterregulatory antinatriuretic mechanism involving the efferent renal sympathetic nerve activity (ERSNA) [10,38]. Thus, in a subsequent study, Villarreal et al. [12,39] examined the hemodynamic and renal excretory effects of synthetic murine leptin in anesthetized and uninephrectornized Spontaneously

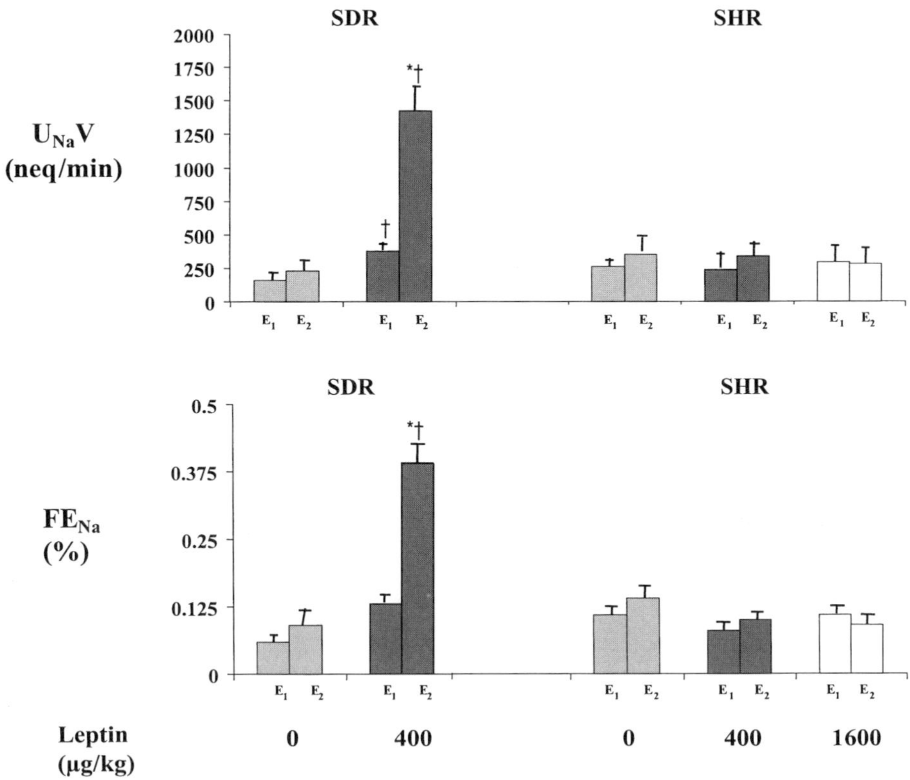

Figure 1. Renal effects of leptin in Sprague Dawley rats (SDR) and Spontaneously Hypertensive rats (SHR). *Top*: Urinary sodium excretion ($U_{Na}V$). *Bottom*: Fractional excretion of sodium (FE_{Na}). Control (0 dose, $n = 8$); leptin 400 µ/kg ($n = 8$); leptin 1,600 µg/kg (n = 8). Values are means ± SE. E_1 and E_2, experimental periods (45 min each). $^{\star}P < 0.05$ vs E_1. $^{\dagger}P < 0.05$ vs control of corresponding experimental period. (From Villarreal D, Reams G, Freeman RH, Taraben A. Am J Physiol 1998;275:R2056–R2060. Reproduced by permission of the American Physiological Society).

Hypertensive rats (SHR) with either acute, chronic (7 days) or sham renal denervation. As shown in Fig. 3, in the Spontaneously Hypertensive rats with acute renal denervation, an intravenous bolus of 1600 µg/kg of leptin produced a significant two to four fold elevation in UNaV compared to vehicle control group, but did not elicit a natriuresis in the sham denervated animals. Importantly, chronic renal denervation was associated with qualitatively and quantitatively similar increases in sodium excretion in response to leptin (Fig. 3). In a different part of the study, urinary norepinephrine excretion as an index of ERSNA, was examined in groups of intact normal Sprague Dawley rats and Spontaneously Hypertensive rats. As demonstrated in Fig. 4, in both strains of rats the administration of leptin was associated with significant elevations in urinary norepinephrine excretion, corroborat-

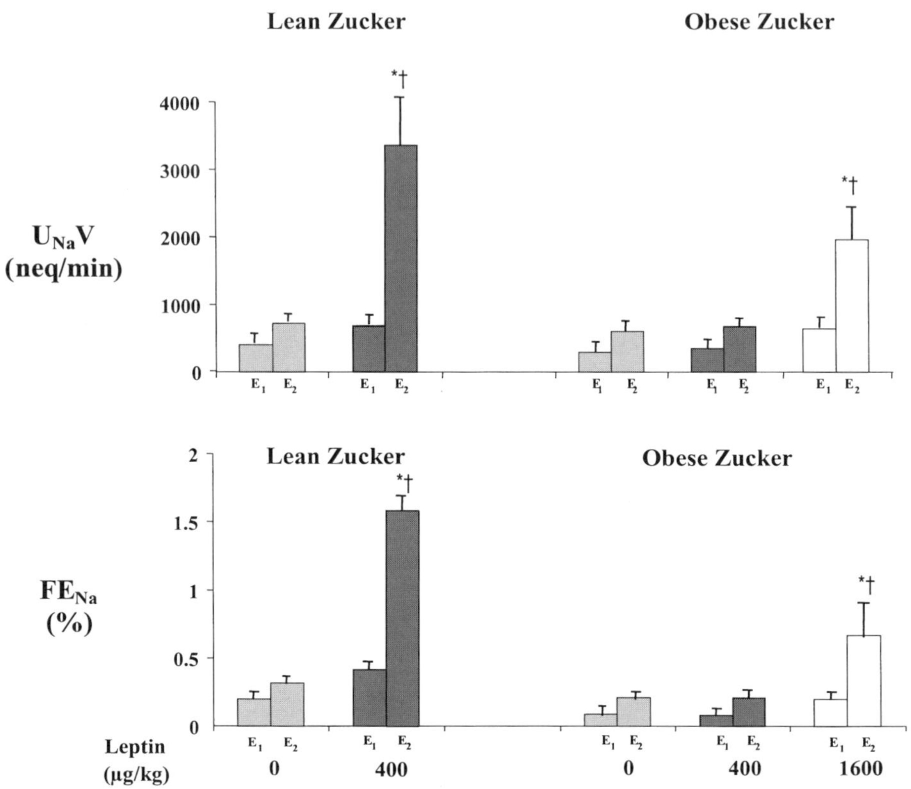

Figure 2. Renal effects of leptin in lean and obese Zucker rats. *Top*: $U_{Na}V$. *Bottom*: FE_{Na}. Control (0 dose, $n = 8$); leptin, 400 µg/kg ($n = 8$); leptin, 1,600 µg/kg ($n = 8$). Values are means ± SE. E_1 and E_2 , experimental periods (45 min each). $^{*}P < 0.05$ vs E_1. $†P < 0.05$ vs control of corresponding experimental period. (From Villarreal D, Reams G, Freeman RH, Taraben A. Am J Physiol 1998;275:R2056–R2060. Reproduced by permission of the American Physiological Society).

ing the concept of a leptin-induced activation of sympathetic nervous system. In the aggregate then, the studies by Villarreal et al. [12] suggest that leptin's net effect on sodium excretion may reflect both direct natriuretic and indirect antinatriuretic actions. Moreover, modulation of responsivity to leptin may differ under various physiological and pathophysiological states to determine the overall magnitude of leptin induced urinary sodium excretion. For this latter effect, however, specific renal tubular mechanisms of action of the hormone remain incompletely defined.

In contrast to the aforementioned studies indicating natriuretic/diuretic actions of leptin is the report from Shek et al. [35] with chronic administration of murine leptin in normal conscious Sprague Dawley rats. In this investigation with continuous leptin infusion at a dose of 1 µg/kg/min either directly into the carotid artery

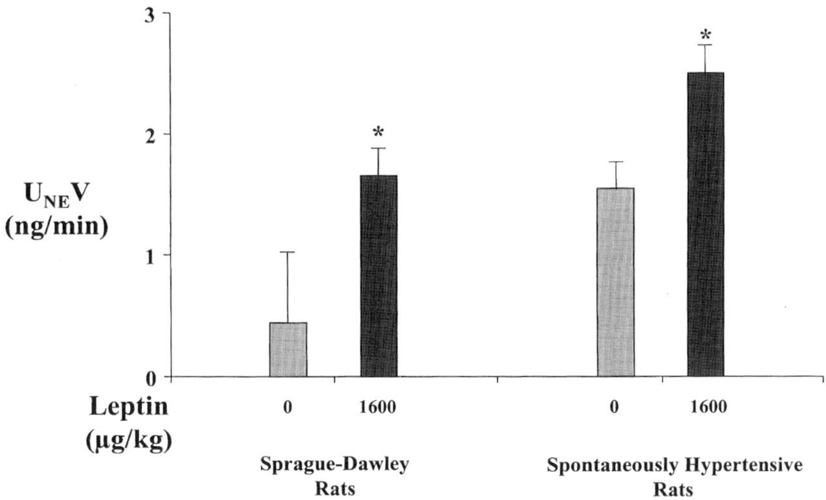

Figure 3. Effects of leptin on urinary norepinephrine excretion ($U_{Ne}V$) in groups of anesthetized rats. Control (0 dose, $n = 5$ for each group); leptin 1,600 µg/kg ($n = 5$ for each group). Urine was collected for 90 min each. Values are means ± SE. $*P < 0.05$ vs control (0 dose).

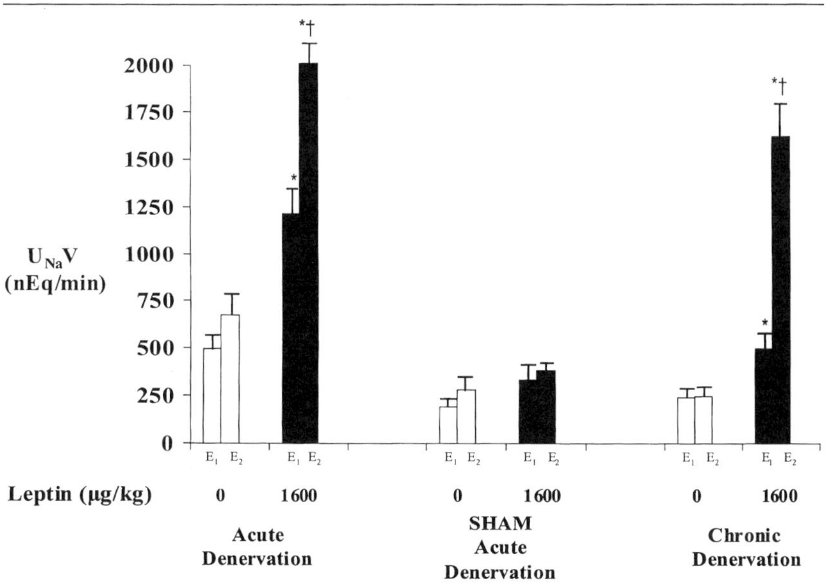

Figure 4. Natriuretic ($U_{Na}V$) effects of leptin in SHR's with acute denervation ($n = 8$ for each group), sham acute denervation ($n = 6$ for each group), and chronic denervation ($n = 8$ for each group). Symbols are (□) vehicle (0 dose); (■) leptin (1,600 µg/kg). Values are means ± SE. E_{1-2} are the experimental periods of 45 minutes each. $*P < 0.05$ vs the corresponding period at 0 dose within each experimental series; $†P < 0.05$ vs E_1. (From Villarreal D, Reams G, Freeman RH. Kidney Int 2000;58:989–994. Reproduced by permission of Blackwell Science Ltd.)

or intravenously for 7 days, there was appetite suppression and marked reduction in food intake of approximately 65–70%. The animals were maintained in sodium balance with the continuous administration of sodium chloride in approximate dose of 3 mEq/day, although potassium was not supplemented. In both groups of rats, mean arterial pressure significantly increased 6–10 mmHg during leptin infusion. Although there was a tendency for elevation in urine flow, sodium excretion remained unchanged, in spite of the increases in arterial pressure. The reasons for the absence of a natriuretic effect are unclear but, as noted earlier, may imply an antinatriuretic effect of leptin-induced sympathetic nervous system activation, which was also considered to be responsible for the elevation in arterial pressure [10,35]. Also, it is pertinent to note that these animals were in marked negative potassium balance [35] and this effect could have influenced the absence of leptin-induced natriuresis [40]. Indeed, previous studies in animals and humans have demonstrated that chronic dietary potassium restriction is associated with significant sodium and chloride retention [40]. Although the mechanisms responsible for this phenomenon are not clear, Gallen et al. [40] have suggested that an adaptive response to potassium restriction is an increase in Na^+, K^+: $2Cl^-$ reabsorptive co-transport in the thick ascending limb. More recently, studies in rats have suggested that low potassium diet produces intrarenal hypoxia with reductions in NO and prostaglandin E2, which favor salt retention and blood pressure elevation [41]. Also relevant and interesting to the lack of leptin-induced natriuresis in the study of Shek et al. was the approximate 50% reduction in plasma aldosterone but not plasma renin [35]. Although it is possible that the fall in aldosterone was related to hypokalemia, it is also possible that at least in part, this effect could be leptin-induced, as has been demonstrated to occur with corticosterone [42]. Important to this concept is the previous demonstration of abundant long isoform leptin receptors (Ob-Rb) in the cortex and medulla of the adrenal gland [20,42].

LEPTIN, NITRIC OXIDE AND RENAL EXCRETORY FUNCTION

Based on the data of Lembo et al. [31] and Fruhbeck et al. [34], who demonstrated that leptin had vasorelaxant properties mediated at least in part by vascular endothelial NO release, and the well known role of NO in tubular sodium excretion [43,44], Villarreal et al. [45] have conducted initial studies to examine whether natriuretic responses to leptin in normotensive rats could be mediated by NO. In this study, the hemodynamic and renal excretory effects of synthetic murine leptin were examined in anesthetized rats treated chronically with L-NAME (185 μmol/kg IP every 12 h for 4 days) to inhibit NO production. As depicted in Table 1, an intravenous bolus of 400 μg/kg of leptin to L-NAME treated rats failed to produce a significant natriuresis compared to vehicle control group. These results are in contrast to the robust natriuresis induced by leptin at the same dose in other experiments (See Fig. 1). In additional studies in rats treated chronically with L-NAME, sodium nitroprusside (SNP) was infused continuously (average dose 5 μg/kg/min) to restore NO and arterial pressure. The dose of SNP was titrated to maintain MAP between 110

Table 1. Hemodynamic and renal effects of leptin in sprague dawley rats with chronic nitric oxide inhibition

	Control		Leptin	
	E_1	E_2	E_1	E_2
MAP (mmHg)	160 ± 4	156 ± 6	158 ± 6	164 ± 9
$U_{Na}V$ (nEq/min)	224 ± 65	248 ± 153	252 ± 34	204 ± 35

Values are means ± SE; $n = 5$ rats in control group (0 dose of leptin) and $n = 5$ rats in leptin (400 μg/kg) group.
E_{1-2} experimental periods (45 min each). MAP, mean artrial pressure. Other abbreviations as in Fig. 1.

Table 2. Hemodynamic and renal effects of leptin in sprague dawley rats with chronic nitric oxide inhibition before and after sodium nitroprusside

	Control	Leptin
MAP (mmHg) (before SNP)	160 ± 6	164 ± 9
MAP (mmHg) (after SNP)	122 ± 4	126 ± 5
$U_{Na}V$ (nEq/min)	160 ± 32	468 ± 38*

Values are means ± SE; $n = 6$ rats in control group (0 dose of leptin) and $n = 6$ rats in leptin (400 μg/kg) group. The experimental period in each group lasted 45 min. *$P < 0.05$ vs control. SNP, sodium nitroprusside. Other abbreviations as in Table 1.

and 130 mmHg. As shown in table 2 the data indicated three to fourfold elevation in UNaV induced by leptin with restoration of NO by SNP [45]. Importantly this natriuretic effect occurred in spite of 40 mm Hg reduction in MAP and consequently reduced renal perfusion pressure (Table 2). Thus, similar to the vasculature, these observations suggest that NO may play an important mechanistic role in the natriuretic effects of leptin.

It is pertinent to point out that the in vivo studies which have addressed the renal actions of leptin have consisted of pharmacological infusions of the hormone and the relevance of endogenous leptin as a sodium-volume regulatory hormone remains undetermined. Recently, with the development of a polyclonal antibody against leptin, Villarreal et al. have addressed this question. Studies were conducted experiments in normal Sprague Dawley rats that chronically received water ad libitum containing 0.9% saline for 7 consecutive days to produce sodium/volume expansion. On the day of the acute experiment and following anesthesia with inactin, the rats received polyclonal leptin antibody (0.5 μl/gm) or antibody vehicle (0.5 μl/gm sheep serum). Over a ninety minutes observation period, urinary volume excretion was significantly reduced by approximately 20–25% in rats receiving the antibody (unpublished data). Thus, these initial results indicate that, under conditions of water surfeit, blockade of endogenous leptin significantly reduced diuresis, suggesting a role for this hormone in the renal control of volume excretion, at least under these experimental conditions. Clearly however, additional studies are necessary to establish the importance of leptin as a renal regulatory hormone.

EFFECTS OF LEPTIN ON RENAL STRUCTURE AND CARDIAC FUNCTION

In addition to its actions on renal excretion, leptin may also function pathophysiologically as a growth and profibrogenic factor in the kidney. Studies conducted by Wolf et al. [46] in normal rats have suggested that recombinant murine leptin promoted mRNA expression and activated secretion of TGFβ as well as proliferation of glomerular endothelial cells. Based on these observations, the authors have suggested that the chronic hyperleptinemia of morbid conditions such as obesity and diabetes mellitus type 2 could contribute at least in part, to the development of glomerulosclerosis and progressive renal damage characteristic of these diseases.

More recently, investigations by Nickola et al. [47] have examined the role of leptin as potential link between obesity and cardiac dysfunction. Contractile responses which were evaluated in isolated ventricular myocytes of normal rats indicated that leptin induced a dose dependent inhibition in myocyte shortening with maximal contractility reduction of approximately 22% [47]. Interestingly, and similar to the information on the renal excretory function outlined earlier, the effect of leptin on contractile shortening appeared to be mediated, at least in part through the increased production of NO [47]. Whether these observations are relevant to obesity-induced cardiomyopathy or cardiac dysfunction in other hyperleptinemic conditions requires further study and clarification. However, it is pertinent to point out that in a follow up study by the same group of investigators [48], similarly isolated ventricular myocytes of spontaneous hypertensive rats failed to demonstrate a leptin induced reduction in myofiber shortening, which in part could have been related to the significantly attenuated generation of NO promoted by leptin in this hypertensive animal strain [48].

SUMMARY AND CONCLUSIONS

It is now well established that cardiovascular and renal functions require the activation of multiple neuro-hormonal mechanisms designed to maintain stability. The recently discovered hormone leptin has multiple actions that may be important not only in the control of body fat and energy metabolism, but also in physiological and pathophysiological cardio-renal regulation. Potentially prominent are its effects on renal sodium excretion, sympathetic nervous system activation, vascular tone, NO stimulation and potentially myocardial contractility. Further research awaits the characterization of mechanisms of action and the relevance of the direct and indirect effects of leptin, including its interaction with other prominent hormonal systems, in both health and disease, particularly obesity and hypertension.

ACKNOWLEDGEMENT

The authors wish to acknowledge the expert technical assistance of Bonnie Backus.

REFERENCES

1. Misra A, Garg A. 1996. Leptin: Its receptor and obesity. J Invest Med 44:540–548.
2. Lonnqvist F. 1996. The obese (ob) gene and its product leptin: A new route towards obesity treatment in man? Q J Med 89:327–332.
3. Esler M, Vaz M, Collier G, Nestel P, Jennings G, Kaye D, Seals D, Laubert G. 1998. Leptin in human plasma is derived in part from the brain and cleared by the kidneys. Lancet 351:879.
4. Masuzaki H, Ogawa Y, Sagawa N. 1997. Non-adipose production of leptin; leptin as a novel placenta-derived hormone in humans. Nat Med 3:1029–33.
5. Saladin R, De Vos P, Guerre-Millo M, Leturgue A, Girard J, Staels B, Aumerx J. 1995. Transient increase in obese gene expression after food intake or insulin administration. Nature 377:527–529.
6. Bado A, Levasseur S, Attoub S, Kermoglant S, Laigneau J-P, Bartoluzzi M-N, Molzo L, Lehy T, Guerre-Millo M, LeMarchang-Brustel Y, Lewin MJM. 1998. The stomach is a source of leptin. Nature 394:790–793.
7. Wang J, Liu R, Hawkins M, Barzalai N, Rossetti L. 1998. A nutrient sensing pathway regulates leptin gene expression in muscle and fat. Nature 393:684–688.
8. Banks WA, Kastin AJ, Huang W, Jaspan JB, Maness LM. 1996. Leptin enters brain by saturable system independent of insulin. Peptide 17:305–311.
9. Barash IA, Cheung CC, Weigle DS, Ren H, Kabigting EB, Kuijper EB, Clifton DK, Steiner RA. 1996. Leptin is a metabolic system to the reproductive system. Endocrinology 137:3144–3147.
10. Haynes WG, Morgan DA, Walsh SA, Mark AL, Sivitz WI. 1997. Receptor-mediated regional sympathetic nerve activation by leptin. J Clin Invest 100:270–278.
11. Dunbar JC, Hu Y, Lu H. 1997. Intracerebroventricular leptin increases lumbar and renal sympathetic nerve activity and blood pressure in normal rats. Diabetes 46:2040–2043.
12. Villarreal D, Reams G, Freeman RH, Taraben A. 1998. Renal effects of leptin in normotensive and hypertensive and obese rats. Am J Physiol 275:R2056–R2060.
13. Ahima RS, Flier JS. 2000. Leptin. Annu Rev Physiol 62:413–437.
14. Sharma K, Considine RV. 1998. The Ob protein (leptin) and the kidney. Kidney Int 53:1483–1487.
15. Caro JF, Sinha MK, Kolazynki JW, Zhang PL, Considine RV. 1996. Leptin: the tale of an obesity gene. Diabetes 45:1455–1462.
16. Chen H, Charlat O, Tartaglia LA, Woolf EA, Weng X, Ellis SJ, Lakes ND, Culpepper J, Moore KJ, Breitbart RE, Duyk GM, Culpepper RI, Morgenstern JP. 1996. Evidence that diabetes gene encodes leptin receptor: Identification of leptin receptor gene in db/db mice. Cell 84:491–495.
17. Lee GH, Proenca R, Montez JM, Carroll KM, Darvishzadeh JG, Lee JL, Friedman JM. 1996. Abnormal splicing of the leptin receptor in diabetic mice. Nature 379:632–635.
18. Tartaglia LA, Dembski M, Weng X, Deng N, Culpepper J, Devos R, Richards GJ, Campfield LA, Clark FT, Deeds J, Muir C, Sanker D, Moriarty A, Woolf EA, Monroe CA. 1995. Identification and expression cloning of leptin receptor Ob-R. Cell 83:1263–1271.
19. Cioffi JA, Shafer AW, Zypanci TJ, Smithgom J, Mikhail A, Platika D, Snodgrass HR. 1996. Novel B219-/OB receptor isoforms: possible role of leptin in hematopoiesis and reproduction. Nat Med 2:586–589.
20. Hoggard N, Mercer JG, Rayner DV, Moar K, Trayhurn P, Williams LM. 1997. Localization of leptin receptor mRNA splice variants in murine peripheral tissues by RT-PCR and in situ hybridization. Biochem Biophys Res Commun 232:383–387.
21. Emilsson V, Liu YL, Cawthorne MA, Morton NM, Davenport M. 1997. Expression of leptin receptor mRNA in pancreatic islets and direct inhibitory action of leptin on insulin secretion. Diabetes 46:313–316.
22. Martinez Anso E, Lostao MP, Martinez JA. 1995. Immunohistochemical localization of leptin in rat kidney. Kidney Int 55:1129–30.
23. Serrardeil-Le Gal C, Raufaste D, Brossard G, Pouzet B, Marty E, Maffrand J-P, LeFur G. 1997. Characterization and localization of leptin receptors in the rat kidney. FEBS Lett 404:185–191.
24. Fogteloo AJ, Meinders AE, Pijl H, Kroon AA, Frolich M, De Leeuw PW. 2001. Renal clearance of endogenous leptin in hypertensive humans with or without renal artery stenosis. Am J Physiol Endocrinol Metab 281:E400–E404.
25. Considine RV, Sinha MK, Heiman ML, Kriauciunas A, Stephens TW, Nyce MR, Ohannesian JP, Marco CC, McKee LJ, Bauer TL, Caro JF. 1996. Serum immunoreactive leptin levels in normal weight and obese humans. N E J M 334:292–295.

26. Hall JE. 1994. Renal and cardiovascular mechanisms of hypertension and obesity. Hypertension 23:381–394,
27. Hall JE, Brands MW, Dixon WN, Smith Jar JR 1993. Obesity-induced hypertension. Renal function and systemic hemodynamics. Hypertension 22:292–299.
28. Hall JE, Brand MW, Hildebrandt DA, Kuo J, Fitzgerald S. 2000. Role of sympathetic nervous system and neuropeptides in obesity hypertension. Brazilian J Med and Biol Res 33:605–618.
29. Jackson EK, Li P. 1997. Human leptin has natriuretic activity in the rat. Am J Physiol 272:F333–F338.
30. Shimizu K, Izumiya Y, Keaton T, Takakowa H, Yokoyoma H, Kobayashi K. 2000. Renal effects of leptin: Interrelationship between natriuresis sympathoactivation. J Hypertens 18:515. (Abstract)
31. Lembo L, Vecchione C, Fratta L, Marino G, Trimarco V, d'Amati G, Trimarco B. 2000. Leptin induces direct vasodilation through distinct endothelial mechanisms. Diabetes 49:293–297.
32. Parhami F, Tintut Y, Ballard A, Fogelman AM, Demer LL. 2001. Leptin enhances the calcification of vascular cells: Artery wall as a target of leptin. Circ Res 88:954–960.
33. Bouloumie A, Drexler CAH, Lafontan M, Busse R. 1998. Leptin, the product of ob gene promotes angiogenesis. Circ Res 83:1059–1066.
34. Fruhbeck G. 1999. Pivotal role of nitric oxide in the control of blood pressure after leptin administration. Diabetes 48:903–908.
35. Shek EW, Brands MW, Hall JE. 1998. Chronic leptin infusion increases arterial pressure. Hypertension 31:409–414.
36. Aizawa-Abe M, Ogawa Y, Masuzaki H, Ebihara K, Satoh N, Matsouka N, Hayashi T, Hosoda K, Inoue G, Yoshimasa Y, Nakao K. 2000. Pathophysiological role of leptin in obesity-related hypertension. J Clin Invest 105:1243–1252.
37. Murakami T, Shima K. 1995. Cloning of rat obese cDNA and its expression in obese rats. Bioche Biophys Res Commun 209:994–952.
38. DiBona GF. 1985. The kidney in pathogenesis of hypertension: the role of renal nerves. Am J Kidney Dis 5:A27–A31.
39. Villarreal D, Reams G, Freeman RH. 2000. Effects of renal denervaton on the sodium excretory action of leptin in hypertensive rats. Kidney Int 58:989–994.
40. Gallen IW, Rosa RM, Esparaz DY, Young JB, Robertson JL, Battle D, Epstein FH, Landsberg L. 1998. On mechanism of the effects of potassium restriction on blood pressure and renal sodium retention. Am J Kidney Dis 31:19–27.
41. Suga S, Phillips MI, Kim Y-G, Gordon KL, Johnson RI. 1999. Potassium deficiency induces renal hypoxia, tubulointerstitial injury and salt-sensitivity. J Am Soc Nephrol 10:356A.
42. Pralong FP, Roduit R, Waeber G, Castillo E, Mosimann F, Thorens B, Gaillard RC. 1998. Leptin inhibits directly glucocorticoid secretion by normal human and rat adrenal gland. Endocrinology 139:4264–4268.
43. Kone BE, Baylis C. 1997. Biosynthesis and homeostatic roles of nitric oxide in the normal kidney. Am J Physiol 272:F561–F578.
44. Zou A-P, Cowley Jr AW. 1999. Role of nitric oxide in the control of renal function and salt sensitivity. Current Hypertension Reports 1:178–186.
45. Freeman RH, Villarreal D, Reams G. 2001. Effects of nitric oxide on the renal excretory action of leptin. FASEB J 15:A135.
46. Wolf G, Hamann A, Han DC, Helmchen U, Thaiss F, Ziyadeh FN, Stahl RAK. 1999. Leptin stimulates proliferation and TGF-β expression in renal glomerular endothelial cells: Potential role in glomerulosclerosis. Kidney Int 56:860–872.
47. Nickola MW, Wold LE, Colligan PB, Wang G-J, Samson WK, Ren J. 2000. Leptin attenuates cardiac contraction I rat ventricular myocytes: Role of NO. Hypertension 36:501–505.
48. Wold LE, Relling DP, Duan J, Norby FL, Ren J. 2002. Abrogated leptin-induced cardiac contractile response in ventricular myocyte under spontaneous hypertension. Role of JAK/STAT pathway. Hypertension 39:69–74.

G.N. Pierce, M. Nagano, P. Zahradka, and N.S. Dhalla (eds.).
ATHEROSCLEROSIS, HYPERTENSION AND DIABETES.
Kluwer Academic Publishers. Boston.

BRAIN Na,K-ATPase ENZYMATIC ACTIVITY AND CARDIOVASCULAR REGULATION[1]

MARY-ANNE H. KENT, JAMES W. VAN HUYSSE,[2] and FRANS H.H. LEENEN[3]

Hypertension Unit, University of Ottawa Heart Institute, Ottawa, Ontario, Canada K1Y 4W7

[1] This research was supported by operating grant MOP-11897 from the Canadian Institutes of Health Research (to FHH Leenen) and operating grant T-4170 from the Heart and Stroke Foundation of Ontario (to JW Van Huysse); [2] Supported by a scholarship from the Canadian Institutes of Health Research/Pharmaceutical Manufacturer's Association (PMAC) of Canada (Pfizer Canada); [3] Supported by a career investigator award of the Heart and Stroke Foundation of Ontario

Summary. Na,K-ATPase enzymatic activity, by maintaining intracellular cation homeostasis regulates many cellular functions. This review focuses on the role of brain Na,K-ATPase activity in cardiovascular regulation. Na,K-ATPase activity in cardiovascular/osmo-regulatory nuclei may regulate cardiovascular function by modulating neurotransmitter release and/or cell responsiveness. Inhibition of Na,K-ATPase activity in cardiovascular/osmo-regulatory nuclei increases blood pressure and causes hypertension. Inversely, an increase in Na,K-ATPase activity in nuclei involved in cardiovascular/osmo-regulation decreases blood pressure in normotensive and hypertensive rats. A decrease in brain Na,K-ATPase activity is associated with several cardiovascular diseases such as salt-sensitive hypertension, heart failure post myocardial infarction (MI) and hypertension induced by suprarenal aortic constriction (SRC). In hypertension induced by SRC, brain Na,K-ATPase isozyme expression and activity decrease in the early phase but increase in the established phase of the hypertension. The decrease in brain Na,K-ATPase activity in salt-sensitive hypertension appears to be mediated by a direct inhibitory action of brain ouabain-like-compounds (OLCs) and reflects mainly a decrease in α_2/α_3 isozyme activity. In rats post MI, brain OLCs decrease both α_1 and α_2/α_3 Na,K-ATPase isozyme activity by direct and indirect mechanisms that may not involve a change in expression. Brain OLCs may indirectly modulate Na,K-ATPase activity by increasing the release of neurotransmitters such as NE and ACh that regulate Na,K-ATPase activity. The neurotrans-

Address for Correspondence: Frans H.H. Leenen, MD, PhD, FRCPC, Hypertension Unit, University of Ottawa Heart Institute, H360, 40 Ruskin Street, Ottawa, Ontario, Canada K1Y 4W7. Telephone and Fax: (613) 761 4521; e-mail: fleenen@ottawaheart.ca

mitters involved in mediating the changes in Na,K-ATPase activity in rats post MI or in hypertension are not yet known. However, these studies suggest that brain α_2/α_3 as well as α_1 Na,K-ATPase isozymes may play a role in the central control of the circulation.

Key words: Brain, Na,K-ATPase enzymatic activity, α subunit isoform expression, Cardiovascular regulation, Endogenous ouabain-like-compounds

INTRODUCTION

The Na, K-ATPase is a highly conserved plasma membrane protein that, by generating Na^+ and K^+ transmembrane electrochemical gradients, maintains resting membrane potential and regulates cell volume, pH, and excitability and Na^+-dependent transport of sugars and amino acids. Using the energy released from the hydrolysis of intracellular ATP, the Na,K-ATPase transports three Na^+ ions out of and two K^+ ions into the cell against their respective electrochemical gradients.

The Na,K-ATPase, by maintaining intracellular cation homeostasis, regulates many cellular functions. This review focuses on the role of brain Na,K-ATPase enzymatic activity in cardiovascular regulation. We first discuss the enzyme structural properties and distribution in the brain and then summarize the evidence for the role of brain Na,K-ATPase activity in the regulation of sympathetic nerve activity and blood pressure. This is then followed by a review of the studies on changes in brain Na,K-ATPase enzymatic activity and/or expression in cardiovascular diseases such as hypertension and a discussion of central mechanisms which may be involved in regulating brain Na,K-ATPase enzymatic activity.

ENZYME STRUCTURE AND DISTRIBUTION

The Na,K-ATPase is a heterodimer composed of an α catalytic subunit and β subunit. The α subunit (100 kDa) contains the binding sites for Na^+, K^+, ATP, P_i, and is responsible for the ion transport and catalytic properties of the enzyme [1,2]. The β subunit (45–55 kDa) is a highly glycosylated protein that regulates the level of enzyme transported to the plasma membrane, modulates Na^+ and K^+ affinity and is essential for a stable and functional enzyme [1]. There are four α (α_1, α_2, α_3 and α_4) and three β (β_1, β_2 and β_3) subunit isoforms known to be expressed in mammals [1,2]. Each isoform is a product of a different gene and exhibits a tissue/cell-specific and developmental pattern of expression [1,2]. In the brain, the α_1 and all three β isoforms are present in neurons and glia [2]. The α_2 isoform is expressed mainly in glia and is expressed only in some neurons, whereas the α_3 isoform is expressed exclusively in neurons [2,3]. Neuronal axons/ nerve terminals express predominantly the α_3 isozyme, whereas dendrites express mainly the α_1 isozyme [3,4,5]. Neuronal cell bodies appear to express α_1 and/or α_3, depending on neuronal cell type. Immuno-fluorescence studies demonstrate that neuronal cell bodies of pyramidal cells of the neocortex and hippocampus and cerebellar purkinje cells express predominantly the α_3 isozyme, whereas cell bodies of cerebellar granule cells express mainly the α_1 isozyme [3,6]. In contrast, neuronal cell bodies in telencephalic and dorsal root ganglia cultures express both the α_1 and α_3 isozyme [5,7]. The expression of α_1 versus α_3 in cell bodies of hypothalamic neurons has not yet been studied. It is likely that in hypothalamic neuronal cell bodies, the expression of the α_1 and α_3 isozyme and the α_1/α_3 ratio is nucleus specific.

FUNCTIONAL CONSEQUENCES OF INHIBITION OR ACTIVATION OF BRAIN Na,K-ATPase ACTIVITY

Inhibition of Na,K-ATPase activity

Na,K-ATPase enzymatic activity can be inhibited directly by cardiac glycosides such as ouabain or by a decrease in substrate availability including $[Na^+]_i$ or $[K^+]_o$ [8,9]. Ouabain binds directly to the α subunit when the enzyme is in its phosphorylated state bound to Mg^{++} and Na^+ and inhibits enzymatic activity by preventing both the release of Na^+ into the extracellular space and subsequent binding of and transport of K^+ into the cell [10]. The inhibitory effect of ouabain on Na,K-ATPase activity can be mimicked by a decrease in extracellular $[K^+]$. An increase in $[K^+]_o$ decreases the binding of cardiac glycosides to the α subunit most likely by facilitating the enzyme conformational change required for the binding and subsequent transport of K^+ into the cell [10]. Thus, the binding of cardiac glycosides to the Na^+/K^+ pump is promoted by cytosolic Na^+, Mg^{++} and ATP, but inhibited by high $[K^+]_o$ [10].

In rodents, the Na,K-ATPase α subunit isoforms possess different affinities for ouabain. The α_3 and α_2 isoforms have high affinities (IC_{50} = 10–500 nM) and the α_1 isoform has a low affinity ($IC_{50} = 10^{-5}$ M) for ouabain [11,12,13]. Thus, at low concentrations, ouabain will selectively inhibit the activity of the α_2 and α_3 isozymes, whereas at high concentrations, ouabain will inhibit the activity of the α_2 and α_3 as well as the α_1 isozyme. The functional significance of the ouabain resistance of the α_1 isoform in rodents has not yet been determined. In this review, the cardiovascular responses to inhibition of brain Na,K-ATPase enzymatic activity will be outlined using ouabain as a prototype inhibitor.

Acute intracerebroventricular (icv) injections of ouabain increase sympathetic nerve activity (SNA), mean arterial pressure (MAP) and heart rate (HR) in normotensive rats [14]. In rats, ouabain injected directly into hypothalamic nuclei including the paraventricular nucleus (PVN), the anterior and posterior hypothalamic nucleus, the nucleus medianus [15] or median preoptic nucleus (MnPO) [16], or brainstem rostral ventral medulla (RVLM) [17] increases MAP. This suggests that the action of ouabain in cardiovascular regulatory nuclei in the hypothalamus or brainstem most likely contributes to the sympatho-excitatory and pressor responses to icv ouabain.

Chronic icv infusion of ouabain causes hypertension in normotensive rats [18], and is associated with decreases in both α_1 and combined α_2/α_3 Na,K-ATPase isozyme activity in hypothalamic and pons/medulla homogenates, but not with changes in Na,K-ATPase isozyme expression [19]. Surprisingly, the decrease in Na,K-ATPase enzymatic activity is mediated, only to a minor extent, by a direct inhibitory action of ouabain. These findings suggest that ouabain may decrease α_1

and α_2/α_3 Na,K-ATPase isozyme activity by direct and indirect mechanisms that may not involve a change in enzyme expression. Ouabain may indirectly decrease brain Na,K-ATPase activity by increasing the release of neurotransmitters that regulate Na,K-ATPase enzymatic activity (see section: Regulators of brain Na,K-ATPase enzymatic activity and/or expression).

Ouabain may increase SNA and MAP by directly increasing the release of neurotransmitters in sympatho-excitatory nuclei. Na,K-ATPase enzymatic activity is inversely related to neurotransmitter release [20]. At the presynaptic terminal, a decrease in Na,K-ATPase activity is associated with an increase in neurotransmitter release [20]. Conditions (such as decreased $[K^+]_o$) or drugs (such as cardiac glycosides) known to inhibit Na,K-ATPase activity increase the release of various neurotransmitters including GABA, NE, 5HT and ACh [20–29]. In presynaptic nerve terminals (synaptosomes) isolated from the cerebral cortex, ouabain, at a high concentration (10^{-4} M), increases the release of ACh [20,28,29]. In rat cortical synaptosomes, ouabain (10^{-8} M to 10^{-4} M) induces a concentration-dependent increase in ACh release, reflecting a 2-fold increase in ACh release at 10^{-4} M ouabain [28]. Ouabain, at high concentrations (10^{-4} M) also increases the release of ACh from depolarized nerve terminals, but to a lesser extent than in non-depolarized nerve terminals [29]. In nerve terminals depolarized with 25 mM K^+, the increase in ACh release induced by ouabain (10^{-4} M) is generally about 50% less than that observed under resting conditions in the presence of external Ca^{++} [29]. However, the enhanced release of ACh in response to ouabain may also depend on how the nerve terminal is depolarized, as ouabain (10^{-4} M) has no effect on the release of ACh in nerve terminals depolarized by veratrine (100 μM) in the presence of $[Ca^{++}]_o$ [29]. These studies suggest that ouabain, by acting at the presynaptic terminal, may be capable of inducing the release of neurotransmitters in vivo, even at low concentrations. Furthermore, the extent of neurotransmitter release induced by ouabain in vivo may depend on the concentration of ouabain, as well as whether the nerve terminal is in a resting or stimulated state.

Another possible mechanism through which ouabain may increase SNA and MAP may be by increasing neuron/glia cell responsiveness to neurotransmitters/modulators [8]. The ouabain-sensitive α_2 and α_3 Na,K-ATPase isozymes may regulate cell responsiveness by modulating Ca^{++} stores indirectly via the Na^+/Ca^{++} exchanger [30,31]. In cultured astrocytes and in cultured hippocampal neurons, the Na,K-ATPase α_3 or α_2 isoform and the Na^+/Ca^{++} exchanger are confined to the region of the plasma membrane overlying the endoplasmic reticulum [30]. This region is termed the plasmerosome [30]. The α_2 and α_3 Na,K-ATPase isozymes may regulate $[Na^+]$ in the restricted cytosolic space between the plasma membrane and endoplasmic reticulum and thereby modulate Ca^{++} stores indirectly via the Na^+/Ca^{++} exchanger. In contrast, the Na,K-ATPase α_1 isoform is uniformly distributed in the plasma membrane and is not colocalized with the Na^+/Ca^{++} exchanger, suggesting that the α_1 Na,K-ATPase isozyme may regulate bulk cytosolic $[Na^+]$ [30]. Inhibition of the α_3 Na,K-ATPase isozyme with low concentrations of ouabain (3–100 nM) enhances the hormone-evoked mobilization of stored Ca^{++} in rat mesenteric arterial myocytes [31]. Similar to neurons, the α_3 Na,K-ATPase isozyme in these arterial myocytes is expressed at the plasmerosome colocalized with the Na^+/Ca^{++} exchanger [30]. The ouabain mediated increase in hormone-evoked Ca^{++} mobilization depends on external Na^+, but not external Ca^{++} indicating that the increase in $[Ca^{++}]_i$ does not arise from an increase in Ca^{++} influx via Ca^{++} channels, but arises from the mobilization of Ca^{++} from internal stores [31]. Thus, in arterial myocytes, nanomolar concentrations of ouabain increase hormone-evoked Ca^{++} mobilization, most likely by disrupting the Na^+ gradient necessary to drive the efflux of Ca^{++} via the Na^+/Ca^{++} exchanger, leading to an increase in Ca^{++} levels in the plasmerosome and consequently an increase in Ca^{++} stores. It is likely that ouabain, at low concentrations, may also increase neuron and glia excitability by a similar mechanism.

In vivo, ouabain located in the synaptic cleft can therefore increase neurotransmitter release by acting at the presynaptic terminal or increase cell responsiveness by acting at the neuronal cell body membrane. What determines whether ouabain acts at the presynaptic terminal or neuronal cell body is not known. In vitro, ouabain appears to increase cell responsiveness at a slightly lower concentration than is required to enhance neurotransmitter release [28,31]. Furthermore, it is not known whether the release of neurotransmitters in response to low concentrations of ouabain, under resting conditions, would stimulate the post-synaptic neuron/glia cell and cause physiological effects. Thus, it is possible that low concentrations of ouabain ($<10^{-7}$ M) in vivo may increase cell responsiveness, and higher concentrations of ouabain may increase both cell responsiveness and neurotransmitter release, especially when the nerve terminal is in a resting state. However, the effects of ouabain on cell responsiveness may depend on the isozymes expressed at the neuronal cell body membrane. Thus, low concentrations of ouabain may not regulate the responsiveness of neurons that express predominantly the α_1 Na,K-ATPase isozyme.

From these studies, it can be concluded that a decrease in Na,K-ATPase enzymatic activity in nerve terminals and/or neuronal/glia cell bodies in cardiovascular regulatory nuclei increases SNA, MAP and HR. Thus, central mechanisms leading to a decrease in Na,K-ATPase enzymatic activity in cardiovascular regulatory nuclei may contribute to sympathetic hyperactivity in cardiovascular diseases such as salt-sensitive hypertension and heart failure post myocardial infarction (MI).

Activation of Na,K-ATPase activity

An increase in Na,K-ATPase activity decreases neurotransmitter release and cell responsiveness in vitro [22,32]. Thus, an increase in Na,K-ATPase enzymatic activity in sympatho-excitatory nuclei may decrease MAP and HR, while an increase in enzyme activity in sympatho-inhibitory nuclei would likely increase MAP and HR. Na,K-ATPase enzymatic activity can be increased directly by increasing $[Na^+]_i$ or $[K^+]_o$ and indirectly by hormones such as insulin [9,33,34]. Central administration of KCl or insulin has been shown to decrease BP and HR in normotensive rats presumably by increasing brain Na,K-ATPase enzymatic activity [35–37]. These studies will therefore be reviewed to outline the cardiovascular responses to a putative increase in brain Na,K-ATPase enzymatic activity.

Acute icv injections of KCl cause a concentration dependent decrease in arterial pressure and HR, which can be significantly attenuated by a prior icv injection of a subpressor dose of ouabain [35,36]. This suggests that the depressor and bradycardic responses to icv KCl may be mediated, at least in part, by an increase in brain Na,K-ATPase enzymatic activity. It is not known whether icv KCl indeed increases brain Na,K-ATPase activity. Acute increases in $[K^+]_o$ increase Na,K-ATPase enzymatic activity in cultured mouse astrocytes [9]. The cardiovascular responses to icv KCl are unlikely mediated by cell depolarization as 1) the estimated increases in K^+ concentrations in the CSF are not sufficient to cause depolarization and 2) ouabain would enhance rather than block the effects of icv KCl if they were mediated by cell depolarization [38]. It is possible therefore that icv KCl may decrease MAP and HR by increasing Na,K-ATPase activity in brain nuclei involved in sympatho-excitation.

Insulin injected icv decreases BP and HR as well as renal SNA in a dose-dependent manner in normotensive anesthetized rats [37]. Chronic icv infusion of insulin for 5 days decreases BP and HR in spontaneously hypertensive rats (SHR) [37]. Insulin increases Na,K-ATPase enzymatic activity in cultured rat astrocytes and rat synaptosomes [33,34]. The cardiovascular responses to icv insulin may therefore be mediated by an increase in Na,K-ATPase activity. Insulin receptors are present in cardiovascular/osmo-regulatory nuclei including the OVLT, SFO, outer layer of the median eminence and ventromedial hypothalamic nucleus (VMH) [39]. Insulin injected directly into the VMH decreases BP, HR and renal SNA in normotensive rats, suggesting that the VMH may contribute to the cardiovascular responses to icv insulin [37]. Since insulin increases Na,K-ATPase activity in vitro and insulin receptors are present in cardiovascular/osmo-regulatory nuclei, it is tempting to conclude that insulin induces its cardiovascular effects by increasing Na,K-ATPase activity in sympatho-excitatory nuclei. However, the effects of icv insulin on Na,K-ATPase enzymatic activity in different brain regions remain to be determined.

In summary, the depressor and bradycardic responses to icv KCl and insulin are consistent with the concept that an increase in Na,K-ATPase enzymatic activity in sympatho-excitatory nuclei may decrease BP and HR.

BRAIN Na,K-ATPase ENZYMATIC ACTIVITY AND CARDIOVASCULAR DISEASE

A decrease in brain Na,K-ATPase enzymatic activity appears to contribute to cardiovascular diseases such as salt-sensitive hypertension and heart failure (HF) post myocardial infarction (MI) [19,40,41]. Hypertension induced by suprarenal aortic constriction and the genetic form of hypertension in spontaneously hypertensive rats (SHR) have also been associated with a change in brain Na,K-ATPase enzymatic activity [42,43]. However, the brain areas and/or central mechanisms mediating the changes in brain Na,K-ATPase activity appear to depend on the type of cardiovascular disease. For instance, salt-sensitive hypertension is associated with a decrease in Na,K-ATPase activity in the hypothalamus in Dahl salt-sensitive (Dahl

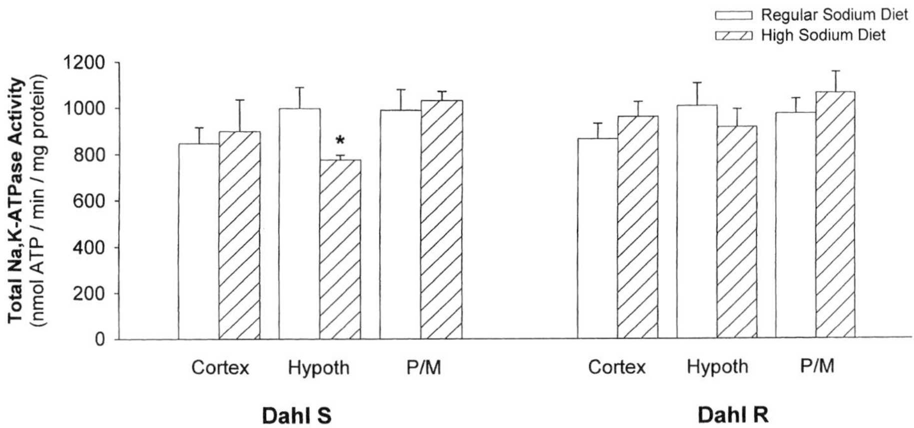

Figure 1. Effects of high sodium diet from 4 to 7 weeks of age on brain Na,K-ATPase enzymatic activity in Dahl S and Dahl R rats. Hypoth: hypothalamus; P/M: pons/medulla. Values are mean ± SEM $*P < 0.05$ vs regular sodium diet. (Adapted from Abdelrahman et al. [40].)

S) rats, but in the pons/medulla in SHR [40,41]. Furthermore, the decrease in brain Na,K-ATPase enzymatic activity in salt-sensitive hypertension appears to be caused by a direct inhibitory action of endogenous ouabain-like-compounds (OLCs), whereas in hypertension induced by suprarenal aortic constriction, the changes in brain Na,K-ATPase activity appear to be related to a change in isozyme expression [40,41,42]. This suggests that brain Na,K-ATPase enzymatic activity can be regulated by more than one mechanism. We will therefore review central mechanisms that may be contributing to the changes in brain Na,K-ATPase enzymatic activity in cardiovascular diseases such as salt-sensitive hypertension, hypertension induced by suprarenal aortic constriction and HF post MI.

Salt-sensitive hypertension

In Dahl S rats and SHR, a high sodium diet increases brain OLCs and causes sympatho-excitation and hypertension [44,45]. Intracerebroventricular (icv) infusions of antibody Fab fragments that bind ouabain and related steroids including OLCs with high affinity (Fab fragments) [46] prevent/reverse the salt-induced hypertension in Dahl S and SHR, demonstrating that brain OLCs mediate salt-sensitive hypertension in these models [47,48]. Brain OLCs may directly bind to and inhibit Na,K-ATPase isozyme activity in cardiovascular and osmo-regulatory nuclei leading to increased sympathetic outflow and thereby hypertension.

A high sodium diet from 4–7 weeks of age increases MAP and decreases total Na,K-ATPase activity in hypothalamic homogenates in Dahl S rats and in pons/medulla homogenates in SHR (Figs. 1 and 2A) [40,41]. In SHR, the decrease in total Na,K-ATPase activity in the pons/medulla in response to high salt intake

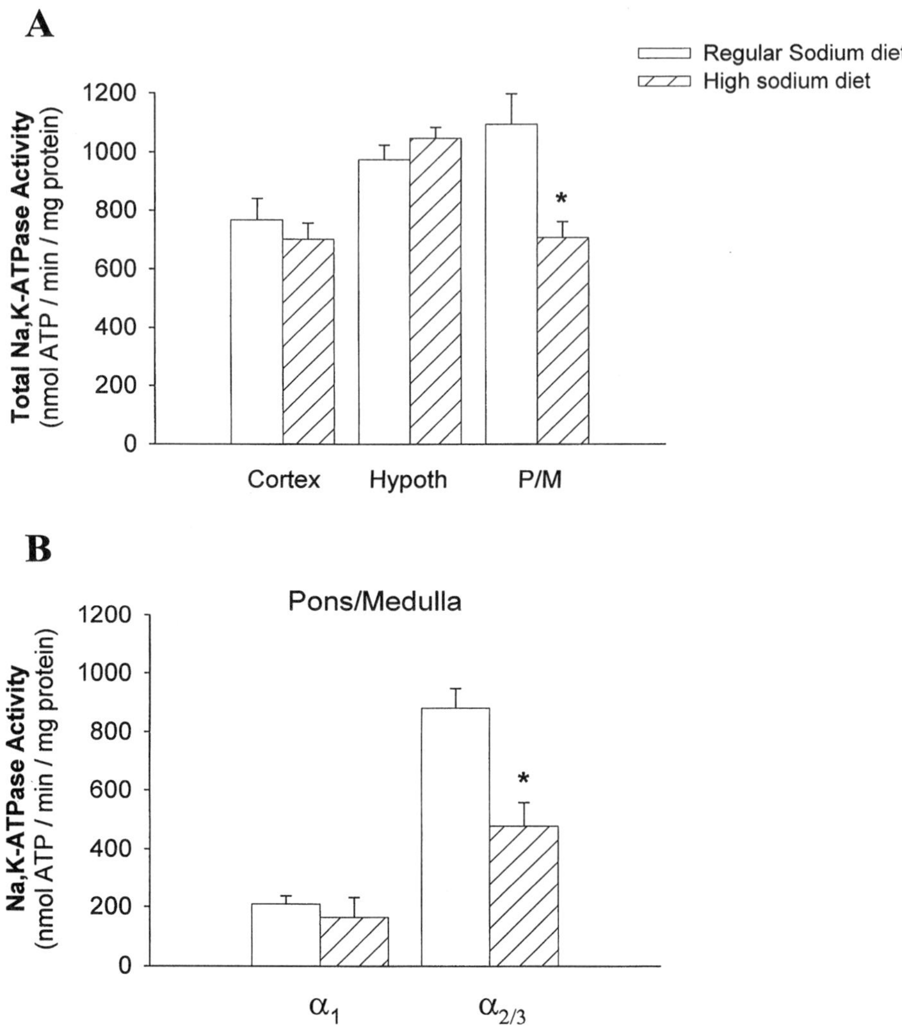

Figure 2. Effects of high sodium diet from 4 to 7 weeks of age on brain Na,K-ATPase enzymatic activity in SHR. **A:** Total Na,K-ATPase activity in the cortex, hypothalamus and pons/medulla. **B:** α_1 and α_2/α_3 Na,K-ATPase activity in the pons/medulla. Hypoth: hypothalamus; P/M: pons/medulla. Values are mean ± SEM *$P < 0.05$ vs regular sodium diet. (Adapted from Ou et al. [41].)

reflects a decrease in the activity of the ouabain-sensitive α_2/α_3 isozymes (Fig. 2B) [41]. Antibody Fab fragments in vitro markedly increase total Na,K-ATPase activity in the pons/medulla of SHR fed a high sodium diet and almost completely reverse the decrease in Na,K-ATPase activity observed in response to high sodium intake (Table 1 and Fig. 3) [41]. Antibody Fab fragments in vitro also markedly

Table 1. Effects of antibody Fab Fragments in vitro on total Na,K-ATPase enzymatic activity in SHR and Dahl S vs Dahl R rats on a regular and high sodium diet from 4–7 weeks of age

	Hypothalamus	Pons/Medulla	Cortex
SHR			
R-Na	4 ± 3	22 ± 4*	4 ± 2
H-Na	3 ± 4	46 ± 7*	13 ± 5
Dahl S			
R-Na	18 ± 7*	15 ± 3*	−2 ± 4
H-Na	32 ± 11*	5 ± 4	−1 ± 3
Dahl R			
R-Na	13 ± 8	−4 ± 3	8 ± 9
H-Na	15 ± 7*	−2 ± 2	−1 ± 2

Values are percent changes in total activity from that in the absence of antibody Fab fragments (Fab). R-Na: regular sodium diet; H-Na: high sodium diet. Values are expressed as mean ± SEM *$P < 0.05$ vs the absence of Fab (n = 5–6). [Fab] = 10^{-5} M. (Adapted from Abdelrahman et al. [40] and Ou et al. [41]).

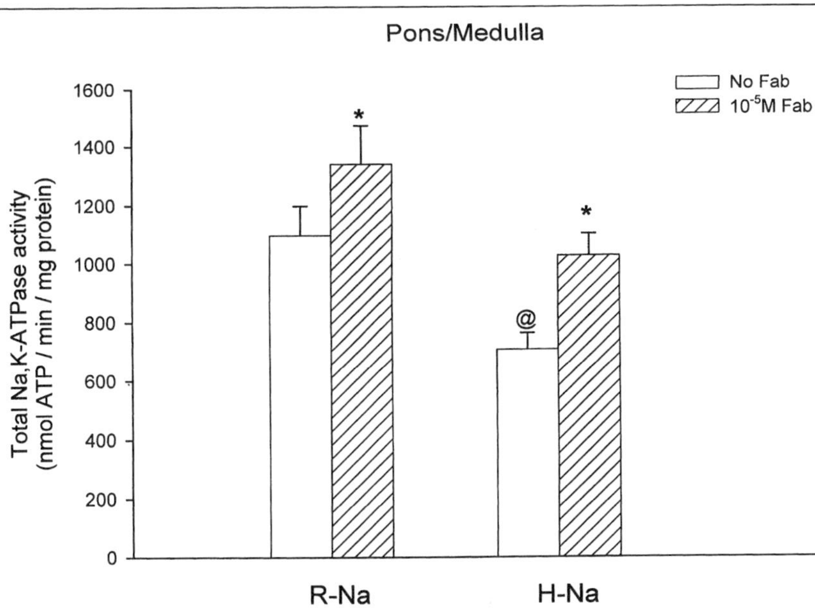

Figure 3. Effects of antibody Fab fragments on total Na,K-ATPase enzymatic activity in the pons/medulla in SHR fed a regular or high sodium diet. R-Na: regular sodium diet; H-Na: high sodium diet. Values are mean ± SEM (n = 5–6) ©$P < 0.05$ vs regular sodium diet (t-test) *$P < 0.05$ vs no Fab (paired t-test). (Adapted from Ou et al. [41].)

increase total Na,K-ATPase activity in hypothalamic homogenates of Dahl S rats fed a high sodium diet (Table1) [40]. This suggests that the decrease in Na,K-ATPase enzymatic activity in response to a high sodium diet in these genetic models of salt-sensitive hypertension is mediated mainly by the direct inhibitory action of brain OLCs and is not due to a decrease in Na,K-ATPase isozyme protein expression. Interestingly, a small increase in total Na,K-ATPase activity by Fab fragments in vitro is also observed in the hypothalamus in Dahl S rats and in the pons/medulla in SHR fed a regular sodium diet (Table 1) [40,41]. Even on a regular sodium diet, OLCs may therefore cause some inhibition of Na,K-ATPase enzymatic activity in both strains of rats. The functional significance of this is not clear since Fab fragments icv do not change sympathetic nerve activity and blood pressure in SHR or Dahl S rats fed a regular sodium diet [47,48].

In deoxycorticosterone (DOC)-salt hypertension, no changes in Na,K-ATPase enzymatic activity are observed in whole brain homogenates [49]. However, DOC-salt modulates Na,K-ATPase enzymatic activity in specific nuclei in the hypothalamus and brainstem [50]. In the hypothalamus of rats treated with DOC-salt for 8 days, total Na,K-ATPase activity is decreased in the lateral hypothalamic area, but unchanged in the PVN, SFO, arcuate nucleus or VMH [50]. In contrast, in the brainstem, total Na,K-ATPase activity is increased in the periventricular gray (PVG) [50]. Changes in total Na,K-ATPase activity are not associated with a change in Na,K-ATPase expression in all brain areas studied [50]. This suggests that DOC-salt hypertension may be associated with a change in Na,K-ATPase enzymatic activity in specific nuclei which is not detectable in homogenates of large brain regions such as the hypothalamus, pons/medulla, or whole brain.

Suprarenal aortic constriction induced hypertension and spontaneously hypertensive rats (SHR)

Hypertension induced by suprarenal aortic constriction and SHR are two models of hypertension where a change in brain Na,K-ATPase enzymatic activity is associated with a change in isozyme protein expression [42,43]. Total Na,K-ATPase enzymatic activity decreases in the cortex in mature SHR compared to age-matched WKY rats, as well as young SHR and is associated with a decrease in high affinity ouabain binding sites, as determined by ^{3}H-ouabain binding [43]. This suggests that the decrease in total Na,K-ATPase activity in the cortex in SHR is due to a decrease in the expression of the α_2/α_3 isozyme. Na,K-ATPase isozyme activity or expression, however, were not measured in brain areas containing cardiovascular regulatory nuclei such as the hypothalamus and pons/medulla. Suprarenal aortic constriction rapidly increases MAP and causes isoform-specific and time-dependent changes in brain Na,K-ATPase activity and expression (Figs. 4 and 5) [42]. At 1 week following aortic constriction, mRNA and protein levels of all three α Na,K-ATPase isoforms are decreased in whole brain homogenates, but only the enzymatic activity of the α_1 isozyme is decreased (Fig. 4) [42]. In contrast, at 4 weeks after aortic constriction, mRNA and protein levels of all three α Na,K-ATPase isoforms are increased in whole brain homogenates, but only the α_2/α_3 isozyme enzymatic

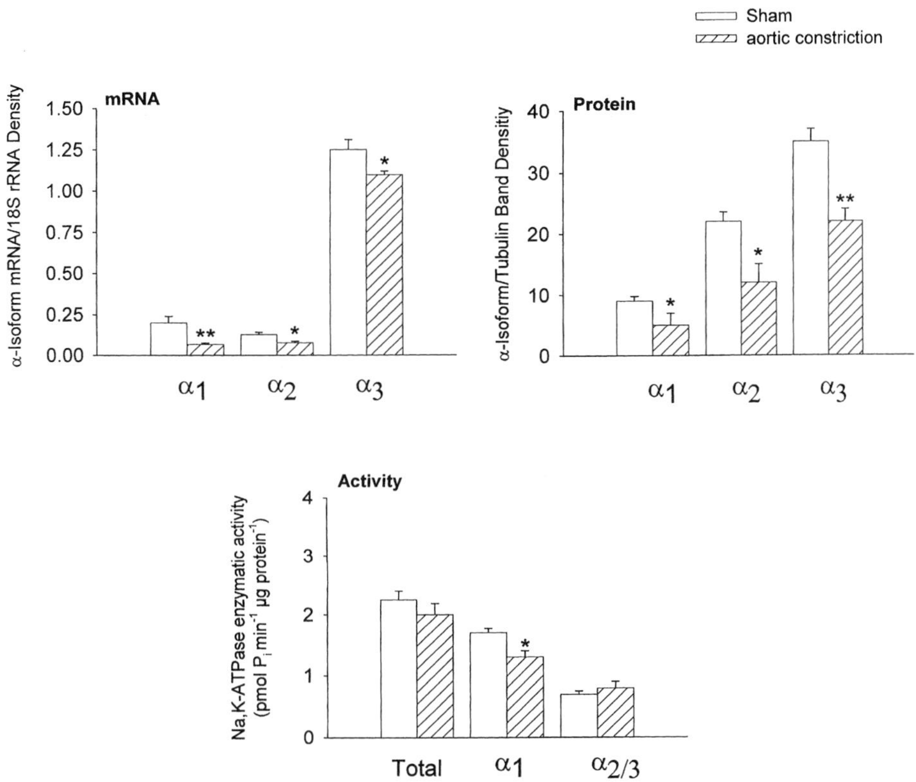

Figure 4. Effects of suprarenal aortic constriction on brain Na,K-ATPase isozyme mRNA and protein expression and enzymatic activity 1 week following aortic constriction. Values are mean ± SEM (n = 3–6) *P < 0.05 and **P < 0.01 vs Sham. (Adapted from Chow et al. [42].)

activity is increased (Fig. 5) [42]. Changes in the α_1, α_2 and α_3 Na,K-ATPase isoform protein expression in whole brain homogenates appear to be mediated by brain regions outside the hypothalamus, as no changes in α isoform protein expression were observed in the hypothalamus at 1 or 4 wks following aortic constriction [42]. The functional significance of these opposite changes in Na,K-ATPase expression and activity in the early versus established phase of this form of hypertension has not yet been assessed.

Heart failure post myocardial infarction (MI)

Sympathetic nerve activity increases in rats post MI and contributes to the progression of left ventricular dysfunction [51,52]. Brain OLC increases in rats post MI [51]. Furthermore, blockade of brain OLCs normalizes sympathetic activity and improves cardiac function [51,52]. Thus, brain OLCs, by mediating an increase in

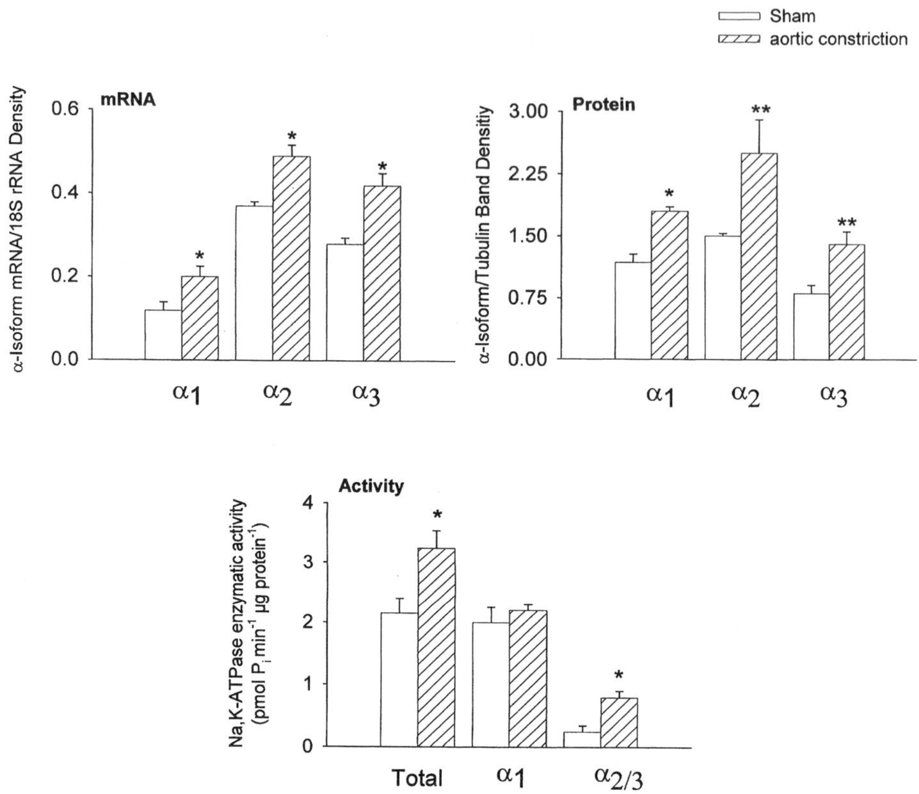

Figure 5. Effects of suprarenal aortic constriction on brain Na,K-ATPase isozyme mRNA and protein expression and enzymatic activity 4 weeks following aortic constriction. Values are mean ± SEM (n = 3–6) *P < 0.05 and **P < 0.01 vs Sham. (Adapted from Chow et al. [42].)

sympathetic nerve activity, contribute to the progression of left ventricular dysfunction in rats post MI. Recently, our lab has shown that both α_1 and the combined α_2/α_3 Na,K-ATPase isozyme activity are decreased in hypothalamic homogenates in rats at 3 months post MI [19]. However, in hypothalamic homogenates, total Na,K-ATPase enzymatic activity increases only slightly by in vitro Fab fragments [19]. Furthermore, the decrease in Na,K-ATPase isozyme activity in rats post MI is not associated with a change in isozyme protein expression [19]. This suggests that the decrease in Na,K-ATPase activity in the hypothalamus in rats post MI is mediated only, in part, by the direct inhibitory action of brain OLCs and does not reflect a decrease in isozyme protein expression. Exogenous ouabain administered chronically icv decreases α_1 and α_2/α_3 Na,K-ATPase activity by direct and indirect mechanisms (see section: Inhibition of Na,K-ATPase activity) This suggests that endogenous brain OLCs may also decrease Na,K-ATPase activity by indirect as well as direct mechanisms. Thus, in rats post MI, OLCs may directly decrease α_2/α_3 isozyme activity and indirectly decrease α_1 and possibly further decrease α_2/α_3 isozyme. Endogenous OLCs may indirectly modulate Na,K-ATPase activity by increasing the release of neurotransmitters that regulate Na,K-ATPase activity (see section: Regulators of Na,K-ATPase expression and/or activity). Thus, in rats post MI, the decrease in Na,K-ATPase enzymatic activity may reflect direct inhibition by brain OLCs as well as indirect inhibition by neurotransmitters/modulators released in response to OLCs.

Conclusion

The studies reviewed here demonstrate that the enzymatic activity attributable to individual Na,K-ATPase α isozymes is altered in cardiovascular diseases associated with sympathetic hyperactivity including salt-sensitive hypertension, heart failure post MI and hypertension secondary to suprarenal aortic constriction. The alterations in brain Na,K-ATPase activity either correlate with changes in α-subunit expression or relate to indirect and/or direct action of brain OLCs. Particularly intriguing are the alterations in α_1 Na,K-ATPase isozyme activity in rats post MI and in rats following aortic constriction, since the α_1 subunit has been previously considered to be a housekeeping protein and as such its expression and enzymatic activity ought to be relatively stable. These studies suggest that the brain α_1 Na,K-ATPase isozyme is actively regulated and may not only function as a housekeeping protein. The possible implications for the roles of the different Na,K-ATPase isozymes in cardiovascular regulation, however, requires further investigation.

REGULATORS OF BRAIN Na,K-ATPase ENZYMATIC EXPRESSION AND/OR ACTIVITY

Neurotransmitters such as norepinephrine and acetylcholine and second messengers such as PKA and PKC can modulate brain Na,K-ATPase activity and/or expression [53–59]. The effects of these neurotransmitters and second messengers on Na,K-ATPase enzymatic activity in the brain will be briefly reviewed.

Norepinephrine (NE) and both α and β-adrenoreceptor agonists/antagonists modulate brain Na,K-ATPase activity in vivo [53–56]. Stimulation of central α_1 and/or β adrenergic receptors by chronic icv infusions of NE, phenylephrine or the β-adrenoreceptor agonist isoproterenol or by peripheral (ip) injections of the α_2-adrenoreceptor antagonist yohimbine increase total Na,K-ATPase activity and α_2/α_3 expression in the rat cerebral cortex [53,54]. The increase in total Na,K-ATPase enzymatic activity in response to α_1 and/or β-adrenoreceptor stimulation most likely reflects an increase in α_2/α_3 isozyme activity [54]. Similarly, an ip injection of desipramine, an inhibitor of NE uptake increases total Na,K-ATPase activity in hypothalamic homogenates and α_2/α_3 expression in the ventromedial hypothalamic area, possibly by indirectly stimulating central α_1 and/or β adrenergic receptors [55,56]. Chronic activation of brain adenylate cyclase by icv infusions of forskolin also increases Na,K-ATPase α_2/α_3 expression and activity in the cortex.

[59] Activation of adenylate cyclase increases cAMP [58]. Since α or β-adrenoreceptor stimulation in the rat brain increases cAMP [60], it is likely that α_1 and/or β-adrenoreceptors stimulation increases α_2/α_3 Na,K-ATPase expression and enzymatic activity by increasing the production of cAMP. Stimulation of central α_2-adrenoreceptors by chronic icv infusions of the α_2-adrenoreceptor agonist clonidine decreases Na,K-ATPase α_2/α_3 expression in the cerebral cortex [54]. Consistent with a functional role for endogenous α_2-adrenoreceptor stimulation, α_2-adrenoreceptor antagonists increase α_2/α_3 Na,K-ATPase expression and activity in the cortex [53]. In the brain, stimulation of α_2-adrenoreceptors inhibits NE release, while α_2-adrenoreceptor antagonists increase NE release [61–64]. These studies suggest that activation of brain α_2-adrenoreceptors may decrease α_2/α_3 Na,K-ATPase expression and presumably enzymatic activity by decreasing the release of NE leading to a decrease in α_1 and/or β-adrenoreceptor stimulation and cAMP production. Thus, in the brain, NE regulates α_2/α_3 Na,K-ATPase enzymatic activity and expression via cAMP. The functional significance of changes in Na,K-ATPase activity and α_2/α_3 isozyme expression in response to adrenoreceptor stimulation, however, has not been assessed.

Acetylcholine (ACh) decreases total Na,K-ATPase enzymatic activity in vivo [57]. Physostigmine (ip), an inhibitor of the ACh metabolizing enzyme acetylcholine esterase, decreases total Na,K-ATPase enzymatic activity in the cerebral cortex, caudate, thalamus, hippocampus and medulla in rats [57]. The effects of physostigmine on the enzymatic activity of the individual Na,K-ATPase isozymes is not known. Stimulation of ACh receptors in the rat parietal cortex increases PKC [65]. In dissociated rat striatal neurons, the PKC activator phorbol 12,13-dibutyrate decreases α_2/α_3 activity by ~30%, and only slightly decreases α_1 activity by ~15% [66]. It is possible that the decrease in Na,K-ATPase activity in response to ACh may be mediated by PKC activation and therefore may reflect a decrease in the activity of all three Na,K-ATPase isozymes.

In summary, neurotransmitters via second messengers differentially regulate brain Na,K-ATPase isozyme expression and/or activity. Norepinephrine modulates α_2/α_3 Na,K-ATPase activity and expression via cAMP, whereas ACh may decrease the activity of all three Na,K-ATPase isozymes via PKC.

CONCLUSION

Brain Na,K-ATPase isozyme expression and/or enzymatic activity is clearly altered in heart failure post MI and in hypertension. Both brain OLCs and neurotransmitters regulate brain Na,K-ATPase isozyme expression and/or activity. It seems likely that besides OLCs neurotransmitters contribute to the changes in brain Na,K-ATPase enzymatic activity in cardiovascular diseases such as heart failure post MI and in hypertension. However, the neurotransmitters involved and their interaction with OLCs remain to be determined. It is possible that the search for the mechanisms underlying changes in Na,K-ATPase enzymatic activity associated with cardiovascular diseases may turn up heretofore unknown brain Na,K-ATPase sympathetic and cardiovascular regulatory systems.

REFERENCES

1. Blanco G, Mercer R. 1998. Isozymes of the Na,K-ATPase: Heterogeneity in structure, diversity in function. Am J Physiol 275:F633–F650.
2. Mobasheri A, Avila J, Cozar-Castellano I, Brownleader MD, Trevan M, Lamb JF, Martin-Vasallo P. 2000. Na^+,K^+-ATPase Isozyme diversity; Comparative biochemistry and physiological implications of novel functional interactions. Biosci Rep 20:51–91.
3. McGrail KM, Phillips JM, Sweadner KJ. 1991. Immunofluorescent localization of the three Na,K-ATPase isozymes in the rat central nervous system: Both neurons and glia can express more than one Na,K-ATPase. The J Neurosci 11:381–391.
4. Brines ML, Gulanski BI, Gilmore-Herbert M, Greene AL, Benz Jr EJ, Robbins RJ. 1991. Cytoarchitectural relationships between [^{3}H]ouabain binding and mRNA for isoforms of the sodium pump catalytic subunit in rat brain. Mol Brain Res 10:139–150.
5. Brines ML, Robbins RJ. 1993. Cell-type specific expression of the Na^+,K^+-ATPase catalytic subunits in cultured neurons and glia: evidence for polarized distribution in neurons. Brain Res 631:1–11.
6. Peng L, Martin-Vasallo P, Sweadner KJ. 1997. Isoform of the Na,K-ATPase α and β subunits in the rat cerebellum and in granule cell cultures. The J Neurosci 17:3488–3502.
7. Dobretsov M, Hastings SL, Stimers HR. 1999. Non-uniform expression of α subunit of the Na^+/K^+ pump in rat dorsal root ganglia neurons. Brain Res 821:212–217.
8. Blaustein MP. 1993. Physiological effects of endogenous ouabain: control of intracellular Ca^{2+} stores and cell responsiveness. Am J Physiol 264:C1367–C1387.
9. Hajek I, Subbarao KVS, Hertz L. 1996. Acute and chronic effects of potassium and noradrenaline on Na^+,K^+-ATPase activity in cultured mouse neurons and astrocytes. Neurochem Int 28:335–342.
10. Katz AM. 1985. Effects of digitalis on cell biochemistry: Sodium pump inhibition. J Am Coll Cardiol 5:16A–21A.
11. Sweadner KJ. 1989. Isozyme of the Na,K-ATPase. Biochim Biophys Acta 988:185–220.
12. Therien AG, Nestor NB, Ball WJ, Blostein R. 1996. Tissue-specific vs isoform specific differences in cation activation kinetics of the Na,K-ATPase. J Biol Chem 271:7104–7112.
13. Ewart HS, Klip A. 1995. Hormonal regulation of the Na,K-ATPase: mechanisms underlying rapid and sustained changes in pump activity. Am J Physiol 269:C295–C311.
14. Huang BS, Harmsen E, Yu H, Leenen FHH. 1992. Brain ouabain-like activity and the sympathoexcitatory and pressor effects on central sodium in rats. Circ Res 71:1059–1066.
15. Jones DL, Lo S. 1990. Ouabain injected into the hypothalamus elicits pressor responses in anaesthetized rats. A mapping study. Pharmac Biochem Behav 36:979–983.
16. Budzikowski AS, Leenen FHH. 1997. Brain ouabain in the median preoptic nucleus mediates salt-sensitive hypertension in spontaneously hypertensive rats. Hypertension 29:599–605.
17. Teruya H, Yamazato M, Muratani H, Sakima A, Takishita S, Terano Y, Fukiyama K. 1997. Role of ouabain-like-compound in the rostral ventral medulla in rats. J Clin Invest 99:2791–2798.
18. Huang BS, Huang X, Harmsen E, Leenen FHH. 1994. Chronic central versus peripheral ouabain, blood pressure and sympathetic nerve activity in rats. Hypertension 23:1087–1090.
19. Kent MA, Van Hyusse JW, Leenen FHH. 2002. The effects of ouabain and endogenous ouabain like compounds on Na,K-ATPase activity and expression. The FASEB J 16:A465.
20. Meyer EM, Cooper JR. 1981. Correlation between Na,K-ATPase activity and acetylcholine release in rat cortical synaptosomes. J Neurochem 36:467–475.
21. Vizi ES. 1978. Na,K-activated adenosinetriphosphatase as a trigger in neurotransmitter release. Neurosci 3:367–384.
22. Vizi ES, Oberfrank F. 1992. Na^+/K^+-ATPase, its endogenous ligands and neurotransmitter release. Neurochem Int 20:11–17.
23. Torok TL. 1989. Neurochemical transmission and the sodium pump. Progress Neurobiol 32:11–76.
24. Santos MS, Goncalves PP, Carvalho AP. 1991. Release of γ-[^{3}H]aminobutyric acid from synaptosomes: effect of external cations and ouabain. Brain Res 547:135–141.
25. Blasi JMV, Cena V, Gonzalez-Garcia C, Marsal J, Solsona C. 1988. Ouabain induces acetylcholine release from pure cholinergic synaptosomes independently of extracellular calcium concentrations. Neurochem Res 13:1035–1041.
26. Sweadner KJ. 1985. Ouabain-evoked norepinephrine release from intact rat sympathetic neurons: evidence for carrier mediated release. J Neurosci 5:2397–2406.
27. Schoffelmeer ANM, Mulder AH. 1983. [^{3}H]Noradrenaline release from brain slices induced by an increase in intracellular sodium concentration: role of intracellular calcium stores. J Neurochem 40:615–621.

28. Satoh E, Nakazato Y. 1989. [^{3}H]Acetylcholine release and the change in cytosolic free calcium level induced by high K^+ and ouabain in rat synaptosomes. Neurosci Lett 107:284–288.
29. Vyas S, Marchbanks RM. 1981. The effect of ouabain on the release of [^{14}C]acetylcholine and other substances from synaptosomes. J Neurochem 37:1467–1474.
30. Juhaszova M, Blaustein MP. 1997. Na^+ pump low and high ouabain affinity α subunit isoforms are differently distributed in cells. Prot Natl Acad Sci USA 94:1800–1805.
31. Arnon A, Hamlyn JM, Blaustein MP. 2000. Ouabain augments Ca^{2+} transients in arterial smooth muscle without raising cytosolic Na^+. Am J Physiol 279:H679–H691.
32. Phillis JW. 1992. Na^+/K^+-ATPase as an effector of synaptic transmission. Neurochem Int 20:19–22.
33. Matsuba T, Murata Y, Kawamura N, Hayashi M, Tamada K, Takuma K, Maeda S, Baba A. 1993. Selective induction of α_1 isoform of ($Na^+ + K^+$)-ATPase by insulin/insulin-like growth factor-1 in cultured rat astrocytes. Arch Biochem Biophys 307:175–182.
34. Brodsky JL. 1990. Insulin activation of brain Na^+,K^+-ATPase is mediated by α_2 isoform of the enzyme. Am J Physiol 258:C812–C817.
35. Shah Jui, Jandhyala S. 1991. Role of the Na^+,K^+-ATPase in the centrally mediated hypotensive effects of potassium in anaesthetized rats. J Hypertension 9:167–170.
36. Shah J, Jandhyala B. 1993. Physiological significance of the Na^+/K^+-ATPase activity in the central nervous system and endogenous sodium-pump inhibitors in the neural regulation of arterial blood pressure. J Cardiovasc Pharm 22(Supp 2):S13–S15.
37. Nishimura M, Takahashi H, Matsusawa M, Ikegaki I, Nakanishi T, Yoshimura M. 1991. The effects of insulin-like materials in the brain on central cardiovascular regulation: with special reference to the central effects of sodium chloride. J Hypertension 9:509–517.
38. Shah J, Jandhyala BS. 1995. Age-dependent alterations in Na^+,K^+-ATPase in the central nervous system of spontaneously hypertensive rats: Relationship to the development of high blood pressure. Clin Exper Hypertension 17:751–767.
39. Baski DG, Davidson DA, Corp ES, Lewellen T, Graham M. 1986. An inexpensive microcomputer digital imaging system for densitometry; quantitative autoradiography of insulin receptors with I^{125} and LKB Ultrofilm. J Neurosci Methods 16:119–129.
40. Abdelrahman AM, Harmsen E, Leenen FHH. 1992. Dietary sodium and Na,K-ATPase activity in Dahl salt-sensitive versus salt-resistant rats. J Hypertens 13:517–522.
41. Ou C, Harmsen E, Leenen FHH. 1993. Effects of high sodium on Na^+/K^+-ATPase activity in Wistar Kyoto (WKY) and spontaneously hypertensive rats (SHR). The FASEB J 7:A547
42. Chow MK, Shao Q, Ren B, Leenen FHH, Van Huysse JW. 2002. Changes in brain Na,K-ATPase isoform expression and enzymatic activity after aortic constriction. Brain Res 944:124–134.
43. Chen CC, Lin-Shiau SY. 1986. Decreased Na^+-K^+-ATPase activity and [^{3}H]ouabain binding sites in various tissues of spontaneously hypertensive rats. Eu J Pharmacol 122:311–319.
44. Leenen FHH, Harmsen E, Yu H, Ou C. 1993. Effects of dietary sodium on central and peripheral ouabain-like activity in the spontaneously hypertensive rats. Am J Physiol 264:H2051–H2055.
45. Leenen FHH, Harmsen E, Yu H. 1994. Dietary sodium and central vs peripheral ouabain-like activity in Dahl salt-sensitive vs salt-resistant rats. Am J Physiol 267:H1916–H1920.
46. Balzan, S, Montali U, Biver P, Ghione S. 1991. Digoxin-binding antibodies reverse the effect of endogenous digitalis-like compounds on Na,K-ATPase in erythrocytes. J Hypertension 9:S304–S305.
47. Huang BS, Leenen FHH. 1994. Brain "ouabain" mediates the sympathoexcitatory and hypertensive effects of high sodium intake in Dahl salt-sensitive rats. Circ Res 74:586–595.
48. Huang BS, Leenen FHH. 1996. Blockade of brain "ouabain" prevents sympathoexcitatory and pressor responses to high sodium in SHR. Am J Physiol 271(40):H103–H108.
49. Sahin-Erdemli I, Medford RM, Songu-Mize E. 1995. Regulation of Na^+,K^+-ATPase α subunit isoforms in rat tissues during hypertension. Eu J Pharmacol 292:163–171.
50. Grillo C, Coirini H, McEwen BS, De Nicola AF. 1989. Changes of salt intake and of (Na+K)-ATPase activity in brain after high dose treatment with deoxycorticosterone. Brain Res 499:225–233.
51. Leenen FHH, Huang BS, Yu H, Yuan B. 1995. Brain ouabain mediates sympathetic hyperactivity in congestive heart failure. Cir Res 77:993–1000.
52. Leenen FHH, Yuan B, Huang BS. 1999. Brain ouabain or angiotensin II contribute to cardiac dysfunction after myocardial infarction. Am J Physiol 277:H1786–H1792.
53. Swann AC. 1983. Stimulation of brain Na^+,K^+-ATPase by norepinephrine in vivo: prevention by receptor antagonists and enhancement by repeated stimulation. Brain Res 260:338–341.
54. Swann AC, Steketee JD. 1989. Subacute noradrenergic agonist infusions in vivo increase Na^+,K^+-ATPase and ouabain binding in rat cerebral cortex. J Neurochem 52:1598–1604.

55. Viola MS, Antonelli MC, Enero MA, Rodriguez de Lores Arnaiz G. 1997. Desipramine modulates ^{3}H-ouabain binding in rat hypothalamus. J Neurosci Res 47:77–89.
56. Viola MS, Bojorge G, Rodriguez de Lores Arnaiz G, Enero MA. 1989. Stimulation of Na^{+},K^{+}-ATPase activity in certain membranes of the rat central nervous system by acute administration of desipramine (DMI). Cell Mol NeuroBiol 9:263–271.
57. Stojanonic T, Djuricic BM, Mursulja BB. 1980. The effect of physostigmine on (Na^{+}+K^{+})-ATPase activity in different rat brain regions. Experientia 36:1348–1350.
58. Therien AG, Blostein R. 2000. Mechanisms of sodium pump regulation. Am J Physiol 279:C541–C566.
59. Swann AC, Steketee J. 1989. Forskolin infusions in vivo increase ouabain binding in brain. Brain Res 476:351–355.
60. Daly JW, Pagett W, Crevelin CR, Cantacuzene D, Kirk KL. 1981. Cyclic AMP-generating systems: regional differences in activation by adrenergic receptors in rat brain. J Neurosci 1(1):49–59.
61. Dubocovich ML. 1984. Presynaptic alpha-adrenoreceptors in the central nervous system. Ann NY Acad Sci 430:7–35.
62. Langer SZ. 1981. Presynaptic regulation of the release of catecholamines. Pharmacol Rev 32:337–362.
63. L'Heureux R, Dennis T, Curet O, Scatton B. 1986. Measurement of endogenous noradrenaline release in the rat cerebral cortex in vivo by transcortical dialysis: Effects of drugs affecting noradrenergic transmission. J Neurochem 46:1794–1801.
64. Taube HD, Starke K, Borowski E. 1977. Presynaptic receptor systems on the noradrenergic neurons in rat brain. Naunyn-Schmiedeberg's Arch Pharmacol 299:123–141.
65. Van der Zee EA, Strosberg AD, Bohus B, Luiten PG. 1993. Colocalization of muscarinic acetylcholine receptors and protein kinase C gamma in rat parietal cortex. Brain Res Mol Brain Res 18:152–162.
66. Nishi A, Fisone G, Snyder GL, Dulubova SI, Aperia A, Nairn AC, Greengard P. 1999. Regulation of Na,K-ATPase isoforms in rat neostriatum by dopamine and protein kinase C. J Neurochem 73:1492–1501.

G.N. Pierce, M. Nagano, P. Zahradka, and N.S. Dhalla (eds.).
ATHEROSCLEROSIS, HYPERTENSION AND DIABETES. Copyright © 2003.
Kluwer Academic Publishers. Boston.

DEVELOPMENT OF TRANSDERMAL AND TRANSBUCCAL DRUG DELIVERY SYSTEMS FOR CARDIOACTIVE DRUGS WITH SPECIAL REFERENCE TO ANTI-HYPERTENSIVE AGENTS

S.S. AGRAWAL

Dept. of Pharmacology, College of Pharmacy Pushp Vihar, Sector-3, New Delhi-110017, India

Summary. The effectiveness and better patient compliance is driving a steady increase in the use of transdermal patches and buccal films that deliver an array of drugs ranging from hormones to pain relievers and drugs acting on cardiovascular system.

Transdermal and transmucosal drug delivery systems are self contained dosage forms which permit absorption of drug from the tissue surface, through its layers into the general circulation, at controlled rates, resulting in sustained blood levels.

Through a patch placed on the skin, transdermal drug delivery can be customized to deliver medication up to seven days. These non-invasive, sustained release dosage forms can prevent the hepatic first pass metabolism of drugs and provide steady flow of medication with the benefit of reducing adverse drug reactions and leads to better patient compliance.

In particular, the simplicity and compliance aspects of patches especially with the paediatric and geriatric patients and also patients who cannot swallow the oral solid dosage forms and no longer want a daily commitment in the administration of their medication will make them popular in the near future.

The reason for the less popularity of these systems was due to the irritation caused because of sweating and decrease in the adhesion of the patches. However, these have been popular in elite countries because of the favourable temperature conditions there, with increasing facilities of controlling environmental conditions in most countries around the world, it is likely that these systems will gain further popularity in future.

Correspondence: Prof. S.S. Agrawal, Dept. of Pharmacology, College of Pharmacy Pushp Vihar, Sector-3, New Delhi-110017, India. Phone: 91-11-26519649, 26563771; Fax: 91-11-26868503; e-mail: agrawal_shyam@hotmail.com

***Key words*:** Transdermal drug delivery systems (TDS), Transmucosal delivery (TMD) Carvedilol, Verapamil HCl (VHCl), Diltiazem HCl (DTZHCl), Atenolol

I INTRODUCTION

Cardiovascular drugs have always been in the forefront of research because the cardiovascular disorders are on an increase globally, millions of people suffer from cardiac diseases and these drugs require chronic administration to get symptomatic relief.

Hypertension especially, has become more prevalent in most parts of the world. On an average 25% of the adult population suffers from hypertension and the most important pre-disposing factors of hypertension are anxiety, stress, tension etc. Amidst all such problems there is every possibility of forgetting the dose due to complicated dose regime (due to busy, mechanical life) and thus patient non-compliance has become quite common. Frequent dosing and unpredictable absorption of conventional delivery systems have led to the popular concept of transdermal and transmucosal drug delivery systems for drug therapy of hypertension—the silent killer.

The oral route of administration has certain disadvantages such as hepatic first pass metabolism and enzymatic degradation within the gastrointestinal tract. Continuous intravenous administration at a programmed rate has been recognized as a superior mode of drug delivery not only to bypass hepatic first pass effect, but also to maintain a constant, prolonged and therapeutically effective drug level in the body. A closely monitored i.v. infusion can provide the advantages of direct entry of drug into the systemic circulation and control of circulating drug levels. However, this mode of drug delivery entails certain risks and necessitates hospitalization and close medical supervision of the patient. These advantages, however, can be closely duplicated, without the potential hazards, by the transdermal drug delivery system.

The transdermal and buccal drug delivery systems are devoid of all these disadvantages, in addition, their potential benefits include easy termination of drug input in case of adverse effects, permits use of drugs with a short biological half life, avoidance of absorption variability and differential metabolism associated with oral therapy. Pre-programmed drug delivery diminishes chance of over and/or under dosage, minimizes inter- and intra-patient variation. These drug delivery systems will certainly permit lower daily dose (since hepatic first pass metabolism is avoided), provide simplified dosage regimen by reducing frequency of dosing, provide predictable and extended duration of action by effective maintenance of steady state drug concentration, enhanced therapeutic efficacy, improved patient compliance as self administration is advocated [1].

Transdermal and transmucosal drug delivery systems are self contained dosage forms which permit absorption of drug from the tissue surface, through its layers into the general circulation at controlled rates, resulting in sustained blood levels.

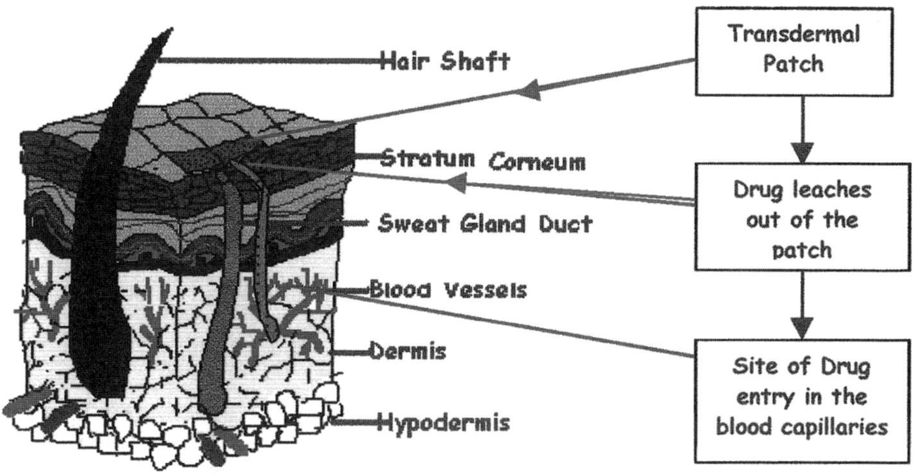

Figure 1. Drug Delivery through the skin.

Owing to the importance of cardiovascular diseases, the development of transdermal and transmucousal drug delivery system of various drugs especially anti-hypertensive agents is of paramount importance in the present era.

Skin as a site for drug administration

The drug through transdermal drug delivery system diffuses and enters into stratum corneum (the outermost layer of the epidermis) before partitioning into viable epidermis; from where it is absorbed via the dermal microcirculation into the systemic circulation & subsequent elimination [1].

Buccal mucosa as a site for drug delivery

It is estimated that the permeability of the buccal mucosa is **4 to 4000 times** greater than that of skin. Even though the sublingual mucosa is relatively more permeable than the buccal mucosa, it is not suitable for a sustained release oral transmucosal drug delivery [2].

The buccal mucosa possesses an expanse of smooth and immobile mucosa, making placement of device easier. Thus the buccal mucosa (Fig. 2) is a favourable site for retentive TMD, sustained and controlled drug delivery applications, delivery of less permeable molecules and peptide drugs [3,4].

The cells of the oral epithelia are surrounded by mucus, consisting of proteins and carbohydrate complexes, that play a role in cell-cell adhesion and bioadhesion of mucoadhesive drug delivery systems [5,6]. The saliva rich environment of the oral cavity favors the selection of hydrophilic polymers as vehicles [2]. The buccal

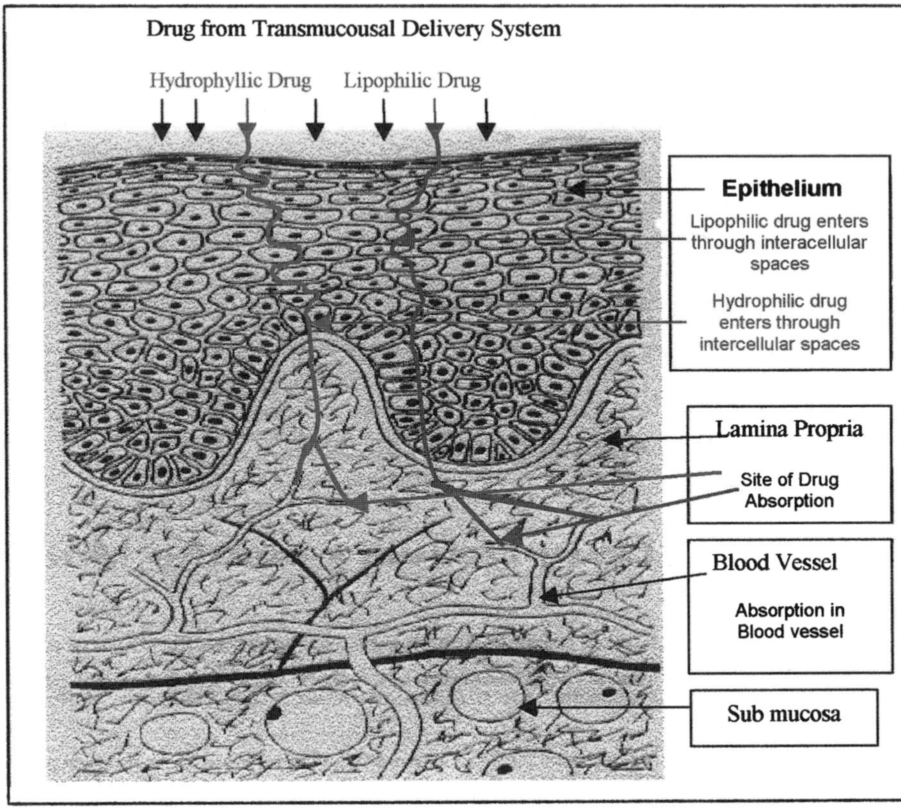

Figure 2. Drug Delivery through Buccal Mucosa [2].

epithelium is non keratinised and may limit the rate at which some drugs (e.g. beta-blockers) are absorbed [7]. The blood flowing through the vessels in the lamina propria acts as a sink for drugs delivered transmucosally [8].

II COMPONENTS OF TRANSDERMAL AND TRANSMUCOSAL PATCHES

The selection of drug candidates for transdermal delivery is of paramount importance. All drugs cannot be given transdermally. Feasibility of a drug for transdermal and transmucosal delivery is based on three relevant parameters [9–11]. (a) Biological properties of the drug i.e. drug should be potent, as concentration in ng/ml only can be achieved through transdermal route. Drugs, which undergo extensive hepatic first pass metabolism, can be given transdermally to avoid drug inactivation and the drug should have short half life as attainment of steady state plasma levels gets delayed for drugs with longer half life (percutaneous absorption being a slow process). (b) physico-chemical properties of the drug effects the drug release from the delivery system, the most common mechanism being diffusion and partition i.e. drug diffusion within the delivery system to the device–skin interface and diffusion of drug across stratum corneum. The transport characteristics of a drug are determined primarily by its size and level of interaction with delivery systems, stratum corneum and viable epidermis. Partitioning of the drug from delivery system into stratum corneum and drug partitioning from stratum corneum into the viable epidermis. For better penetration of drug, the molecule must favour the stratum corneum over the device. Moreover, partitioning of drug molecule from the stratum corneum to viable tissue must be reasonably balanced to ensure adequate penetration of the drug into systemic circulation. Extreme partitioning characteristics are not conducive to successful drug delivery via the skin. (c) Pharmacokinetic behavior of the drug also determines the release of the drugs.

The following kinetic parameters are associated with the release of drug from TDD systems F (K_1) describes the input kinetics from transdermal system, K_B shows competition between the device and the stratum corneum for the drug, smaller value indicates better design of transdermal system; K_1 and K_2 are the first order rate constants which describe drug transport across the stratum corneum and viable tissue respectively. They are found to be proportional to the corresponding diffusion coefficients through these layers; K_3 describes the affinity of the drug for stratum corneum in comparison to viable epidermis. The ratio of K_3/K_2 for a drug may be viewed as an effective partition coefficient between stratum corneum and viable epidermis and has been shown to be linearly correlated with n-octanol water partition (K) of the drug, K_4 describes the elimination rate constant of the drug from blood.

Selection of drug

For successfully developing a transdermal drug delivery system, the drug should be chosen with great care. Drugs which are best suited for transdermal delivery should have molecular weights below 500, solubility greater than 1 mg/ml in water and mineral oil, n-octanol/water partition coefficient of approximately 2, short $t_{1/2}$ and daily parenteral dose of 2–10 mg. Transdermal system is also suitable for drugs which are inactivated by hepatic first pass metabolism or are not completely absorbed from gastro-intestinal tract. Various pharmacokinetic parameters of important cardiovascular drugs, are depicted in Table 1 [12].

Polymers, which control the release of drug from the device, form the backbone of TDS and TMD. Various polymers used for transdermal devices include natural polymers-cellulose derivatives, such as ethyl cellulose (EC) [12,16], hydroxy propyl methyl cellulose phthalate (HPMCP) [12], zein, gelatin, shellac, waxes, or synthetic polymers such as Eudragits, Polyvinyl alcohol (PVA), and polyvinyl pyrrolidone (PVP) [12–15].

Bioadhesive polymers (polymers that can adhere to a biological substrate) have been used in drug delivery system so that it can be retained in a particular region

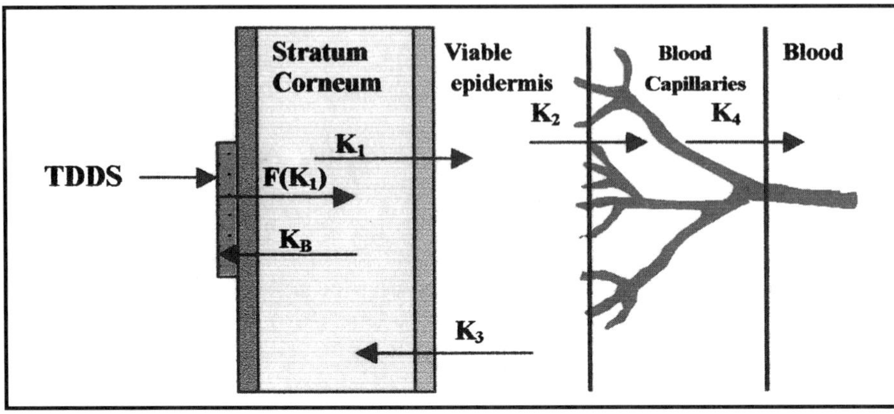

Figure 3. Pharmacokinetic model for TDS.

Table 1. Pharmacokinetic parameters of important cardiovascular drugs studied in our lab and elsewhere

Drug	Oral Availability (%)	Plasma bound (%)	Wt. Distr. (L/Kg)	Half Life ($t^{1/2}$)	Mol. Wt.
Clonidine	100	—	2.1 ± 0.4	8.5 ± 2 min	230
Nitroglycerine	38 ± 26	—	3.3 ± 1.2	2.3 ± 0.6 min	227
Propranolol	36 ± 10	93.3 ± 1	3.9 ± 0.6	3.9 ± 0.4 min	295.8
Verapamil*	22 ± 8	90 ± 2	5 ± 2.1	4 ± 1.5	491.07
Diltiazem*	40	60–75	5.3	4.5	451.0
Atenolol*	56 ± 30	90 ± 2	0.95 ± 0.15	6.1 ± 2	266.33
Carvedilol*	23	95	1.5–2	4–8	406.5

*Studied in our lab.

of body for extended period of time. The various classes of mucoadhesive polymers (these bioadhesive polymers are called so when the substrate adheres to the mucosal tissue) include monomeric α-cyanoacrylate [17] Polyacrylic acid {Carbopol-934P (CP-934P), Carbopol-974P (CP-974P), Carbopol-971P (CP-971P)} [17], hydroxy propyl methyl cellulose (HPMC) [18], polymethacrylate derivatives [19], polyurethanes, epoxy resins, polystyrene, natural product cement [20] as well as naturally occurring polymers such as hyaluronic acid [17] and chitosan [21].

Penetration enhancers viz. *Ocimum sanctum's* fixed oil [22], d-limonene [15], 1,8-cineole [16] benzalkonium chloride (BCL) [14], sodium lauryl sulphate (SLS) [14], polysorbate 80 [14] and dimethyl sulfoxide (DMSO) [14] have been found to increase the permeability of stratum corneum to various drugs in TDS.

The enhancing effects of di- and tri-hydroxy bile salts [23–25], sodium ethylenediamine tetracetic acid (EDTA), aprotinin, sodium lauryl sulphate [26,27], sodium deoxycholate and sodium glycocholate have been reported on drug penetration in TMD.

Penetration enhancers interact with some components of the skin causing stratum corneum to swell and/or leach out some of the structural components and thus increase drug penetration.

Plasticizers like propylene glycol (PG), glycerol, polyethylene glycol 400 (PEG400) [15–17], diethyl phthalate (DEP) [14], dibutyl phthalate (DBP) [12–15] and dimethyl phthalate [12–15] have been found to change the physicochemical properties of the polymer when added to it. They impart flexibility, reduce brittleness and increase resistance of film to cracking due to mechanical stress.

Methodology for fabrication of TDS and TMD uses the drug, polymers, plasticizer, penetration enhancers, blended in the solvent and patches prepared by solvent casting method on Teflon trays. Evaluation of patches is done for drug content, uniformity of thickness, uniformity of weight, aging, stability and relative humidity on storage. In vitro drug diffusion studies are carried out using the Keshary-Chein diffusion cell and modified Keshary-Chein cell of different volumes and surface area. Skin irritation studies were carried out using modified Draize test in rabbits.

III REVIEW OF WORK DONE ON TRANSDERMAL AND BUCCAL DRUG DELIVERY SYSTEMS OF ANTIHYPERTENSIVE AGENTS

Various researchers have studied permeation of various drugs and permeants across skin and other membranes. They have also tried to develop transdermal and buccal drug delivery systems of many drugs. The commercially available transdermal and buccal drug delivery systems are depicted in Table 2.

With this background it was attempted to develop transdermal and transbuccal drug delivery systems for anti-hypertensive agents in our Lab also work done by other workers is revealed.

The transdermal drug delivery systems developed in our lab include diltiazem, verapamil and carvedilol besides the transbuccal studies are being conducted on carvedilol and the results are highly encouraging. Atenolol was also subjected for feasibility studies for TDS. Work on atenolol is in progress.

Nitroglycerine

Keith developed matrix-dispersion type TDS systems of nitroglycerine for once a day medication [29]. Ryden conducted a comparative study on buccal vs. sublingual glyceryl trinitrate administration to patients with angina and found that buccal formulation was more effective as a prophylactic to prevent anginal attacks in 74% compared to 66% for sublingual formulation [30]. Abrams found that both nitroglycerine and isosorbide dinitrate work rapidly via buccal route as well as sublingually [31].

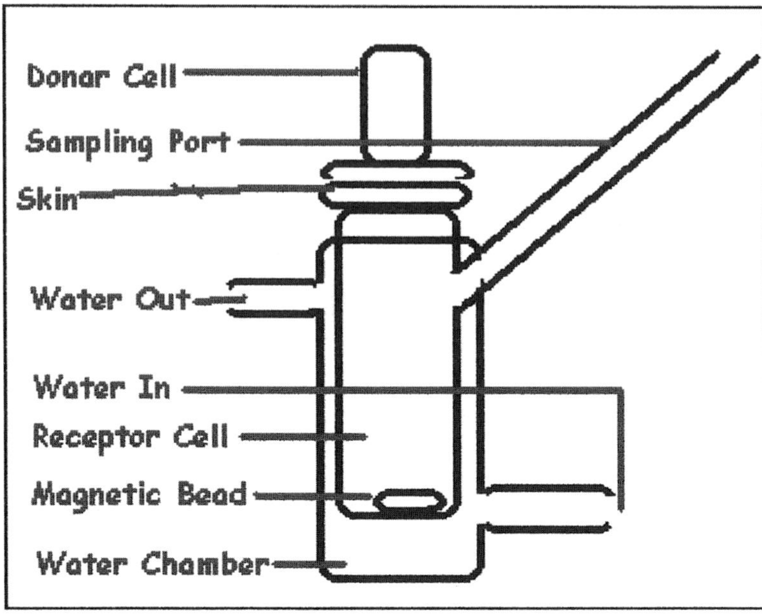

Figure 4. Modified Keshery Chein Diffusion Cell.

Table 2. Commercially available Transdermal and Buccal drug delivery systems (28)

S. No	Active Ingredient	Dosage form	Dose Delivered
1.	Nitroglycerine (glyceryl trinitrate)	B D T	1 mg every 3–5 hrs 1 disc (2.5–15 mg) for 12–24 hrs per day 0.3–0.6 mg as needed
2.	Isosorbide dinitrate	T	2.5–10 mg every 2–3 hrs
3.	Isosorbide 5–mononitrate	T	10–40 mg twice daily
4.	Erithrityl trinitrate	T	5–10 mg as needed
5.	Clonidine	D	3.5, 7.0, and 10.5 cm^2 systems deliver 0.1, 0.2 and 0.3 mgs per day for 7 days.
6.	Propranolol	D	Gives an effective concentration of 20 mg/ml

B: Buccal or Transmucosal Tablet D: Transdermal disc or patch T: Tablet for sublingual use.

Various transdermal preparations of Nitoglycerine which are available in market are: Deponit® Patch, Minitran™ Patch, Nitrek® Patch, Nitrodisc® Patch, Nitro-Dur® Patch, Transdermal-NTG® Patch, Transderm-Nitro® Patch, Cardinit, Nitradisc; Nitroderm-TTS®.

Isosorbide dinitrate

Bhalla et al. formulated transdermal films of isosorbide dinitrate with a 3:2 combination of PVA to PVP and 25% glycerin or 30% PG which gave good permeation profile across guinea pig skin [32]. Nozaki et al. developed a new transmucosal therapeutic system for controlled systemic delivery of isosorbide dinitrate. It consisted of a fast release layer of d-mannitol and PVP which provided a rapid release (20%) of drug in 15 minutes for prompt rise in blood concentration to reach therapeutic level and a sustained release layer of PVP and polyacrylic acid which released the rest of 80% of the drug to maintain therapeutic levels up to 12 hrs [33]. Danjo et al. developed a mucoadhesive film dosage form for isosorbide dinitrate using hydroxy propyl cellulose and hydroxy propyl methyl cellulose phthalate [34]. The film exhibited a sustained release of drug upto 6 hrs. Addition of glycyrrhizic acid increased the in vitro drug dissolution and increased in vivo absorption across the rat oral mucosa.

Clonidine

Zierenberg reported that the average release of clonidine from transdermal films containing acrylic polymers was 40 percent in two days and 90 percent in 6 days [35]. Weber reported that transdermal clonidine produced normal blood pressure in 12 out of 20 patients with mild essential hypertension [36].

Propranolol

Transdermal system of propranolol (a non selective β-blocker) was designed and developed using different polymers HPMC K 4M, K15M and K100M, mixed polymeric grades of Eudragit by Verma et al. [37] and different ratios of EC, PVP by Rao et al. [38]. Further Corbo et al [39] developed a multilaminate adhesive device for transdermal controlled delivery of propranolol and investigated its flexibility by conducting *in vitro* skin permeation studies using rabbit pinna skin. A mixture of hydrophobic polymer carboxy methyl cellulose and hydrophobic polymer Eudragit RS 100 was used by Alhmound et al. [40] to modify the release rate of propranolol HCl and obtain a polymer system that was capable of delivering the drug at a constant rate. Le Brun et al. [41] developed a suitable buccal dosage form for β-blockers i.e. bupranolol, propranolol, oxprenolol (all non selective β-blockers) and acebutalol (selective β-blocker) ranging from lipophilic to hydrophilic drugs. In vitro permeation through porcine buccal mucosa showed that the amount of drug that had penetrated was higher in the case of more lipophilic β blocking agent such as bupranolol. Kislal et al. [42] developed a buccoadhesive tablet formulation of propranolol HCl using poly acrylic acid and hydroxy ethyl cellulose. The release of the drug from tablet was found to be zero order upto 8 hrs. Wen Gang Chen et al. [43] prepared propranolol bioadhesive disc system containing a mixture of hydroxy propyl cellulose and polyacrylic acid, studied their adhesive property and in vitro release characteristics at two different pH (3.5 and 6.8).

Nielson and Rassing [44] related the permeability rates of 10 β-adrenoceptor antagonists (acebutalol, alpenolol, atenolol, labetalol, metoprolol, oxprenolol, pindolol, propranolol, timolol & tertatolol) across the TR146 cell culture model and porcine buccal mucosa to their lipophilicity. Further the permeability enhancement across the TR146 cell culture model in the presence of sodium glycocholate varied between 2.2×10^{-6} cm/sec and 165×10^{-6} cm/sec in case of atenolol.

Atenolol

Atenolol, a β-adrenolytic, cardio selective drug, is incompletely absorbed (about 50%) orally but most of the absorbed dose reaches systemic circulation. The drug is excreted largely in unchanged form in the urine and the elimination half-life varies from 5–8 hrs. Therefore, it requires more frequent administration by oral route.

In vitro percutaneous absorption of atenolol was studied by Kaul et al. [45] in order to assess its feasibility for transdermal development across mouse and guinea pig skins using Keshary-Chien diffusion cell. It was concluded that atenolol had better permeation across skin compared to VHCl and hence indicated that atenolol could be pursued further for TDS.

Metoprolol

Ghosh et al. [46] developed TDS of metoprolol and reported that absolute bioavailability increased to 30.07 ± 4.84% following transdermal delivery. Wong and Yuen [47] reported that incorporation of hydrophilic polymers such as HPMC, sodium CMC and CP of different grades into controlled release buccal patches of metoprolol tartrate using Eudragit NE40D enhanced the bioadhesiveness of the patches but tends to cause non homogeneous distribution of the drug in polymer resulting in unpredictable drug release.

Timolol maleate

Bondi et al. [48] developed a TDS for timolol allowing less than 20 μgm timolol release/cm^2/hr to the skin surface.

Studies on calcium channel blockers

Nifedipine

A study on matrix dispersion system of Nifedipine by Ruan and Zheng [50] showed that steady state plasma levels within therapeutic range were observed between 1.5 and 24.5 hrs after administration.

Save et al. [51] prepared and standardized a novel buccoadhesive erodible carrier consisting of sodium alginate, mannitol and PEG-6000 for the buccal delivery of nifedipine. They also formulated mucoadhesive buccal film of nifedipine consisting of sodium alginate, methyl cellulose (MC), polyvinyl pyrrolidone, mannitol, PEG6000 and glycerol. A comparative evaluation of these two formulations with sublingual capsule of nifedipine in hypertensive patients showed that although these two formulations were comparable in response to the sublingual capsule, they were superior with respect to patient acceptability and provided a fixed dose of the drug.

Remunan-Lopez et al. [52] used nifedipine (slightly water soluble drug) and propranolol HCl (highly water soluble drug) to demonstrate the controlled delivery through bilaminated films and bilayered tablets. The bilaminated films showed a sustained drug release in phosphate buffer (pH 6.4) and the tablets that displayed controlled swelling and drug release and adequate adhesivity was produced by *in situ* cross linking the chitosan with polycarbophil.

Verapamil

VHCl, a calcium channel blocker has low oral bioavailability (about 20%) due to extensive hepatic first pass metabolism which can be avoided by transdermal administration. The drug has a molecular weight of 491.07 and a short half-life, ($t_{1/2} \approx$ 4 hrs) hence requires frequent dosing by oral route. A prolonged duration of action is possible with a single application of transdermal patch.

Chien and Tojo [53] developed a TDS of Verapamil consisting of polymer matrix, mixed with a skin permeation enhancing agent within a space enclosed by an outer backing and a biocompatible adhesive layer in contact with skin and another drug transport enhancing agent. Sawicki [54] reported that sodium glycocholate when used as penetration enhancer in the buccal drug formulation of VHCl, the rate of permeation increased from 1.3 mg/cm^2 of VHCl to 10.35 mg/cm^2 of drug during 6 hrs study.

Jain et al. [13] developed a matrix type monolithic TDS for VHCl using PVA and PVP as polymers, glycerol as plasticizer and d-limonene as penetration enhancer in this lab. Prototype formulations were developed using PVA&PVP and EC&PVP polymers and were evaluated for drug permeation across guinea pig dorsal skin. Since very low permeability coefficient was obtained, d-limonene was used as a penetration enhancer in concentrations of 2, 5, 10 and 20%. However, statistically enhanced permeation was observed with 20% d-limonene only. Propylene glycol in 20% concentration also showed good drug penetration enhancement across guinea pig dorsal skin. The matrices of VHCl showed satisfactory physico-chemical properties except the formulation which contained PVP only.

Matrices stored at 75, 83 and 93% RH showed increase in weight while matrices stored at 20% RH showed decrease in weight. Change in weight of matrices was negligible at 58% RH.

Patches were evaluated *in vitro* using cadaver skin as rate limiting membrane. TDS formulation containing PVA and PVP in a ratio of 3:2 and VHCL (10% w/w), glycerol (30% w/w) and d-limonene (20% w/w) showed best plasma profile (73.94 ng/ml). *In vitro* study using cadaver skin showed that formulation containing propylene glycol did not have significant penetration enhancement. Based on the results of *in vitro* study, optimized formulations were evaluated in vivo in guinea pigs. A positive correlation was observed between the *in vitro* and *in vivo* data. Primary skin irritation studies in rabbits (Modified Draize test) did not show any symptoms of hypersensitivity. Acute toxicity study of the formulation on mice did not show any gross behavioral changes in locomotion i.e autonomic, CNS and other effects. No mortality was seen at a dose of $10\,mg/cm^2$ which showed that the formulation appears to be safe at the dose level tested.

This formulation was subsequently evaluated on human volunteers (Phase I clinical trials) after obtaining permission from Drug Controller General of India. Phase I clinical trials showed mild to severe hypersensitivity reaction in three volunteers. However no drug related systemic effects were observed. This hypersensitivity was attributed to d-limonene. From this study it was concluded that the TDS of VHCl delivers drug at a steady rate of 73.94 ng/ml [below the therapeutic concentration (120 ng/ml)].

This formulation could be further improved by modifications in the system. Hence the next study was undertaken.

Transdermal formulation of VHCl [56] were developed using PVA and PVP as polymers and glycerol as plasticizer, R (+) limonene in 15% w/w and 20% w/w was used as penetration enhancer in place of d-limonene. Drug load was increased from 10% w/w persq. cm to 20% w/w per sq.cm of patch. *In vitro* study showed that statistically enhanced permeation with 20% w/w of R-limonene across guinea pig dorsal skin. It was also observed that decrease in PVA and increase in PVP concentration in the formulation leads to decrease in drug permeation, whereas increase in PVA and decrease in PVP concentration in the formulation leads to enhanced permeation. Modified Draize test indicated that none of the formulations tested had shown any signs of allergy/hypersensitivity reaction.

In vivo evaluation of optimized formulations were carried out in guinea pigs and a positive correlation was seen between *In vitro* & *In vivo* data. Based on in-vitro studies across guinea pig dorsal skin, formulations containing 15% and 20% w/w R (+) limonene were evaluated for permeation across cadaver skin. The permeation of drug across cadaver skin from formulation containing 20% w/w R (+) limonene was 129.34% as compared to formulation containing 15% w/w R (+) limonene. Formulations containing 20% R (+) limonene were further evaluated in albino rabbits for skin irritation by modified Draize Test and did not show signs of allergy/hypersensitivity reaction.

Based on *in vitro* permeation, optimized formulations were further evaluted *in vivo* in guinea pigs. The profile was also compared with oral route (15 mg/Kg body weight). *In vivo* pharmacokinetic evaluation in guinea pig showed that formulation containing PVA and PVP in a ratio of 3:2 and 20% R (+) limonene has C_{max} 41.1 ng/ml, T_{max} 10.00 hrs, AUC 971.7, elimination half life of 112.5 hrs and MRT 14.3 hrs. Formulation containing PVA and PVP in a ratio of 2:1, R (+) limonene showed C_{max} 42.56 ng/ml, T_{max} 10.00 hrs, AUC 1002.8, elimination half-life 112.9 hrs and MRT 124.7 hrs. However oral administration of drug showed C_{max} 17.34 μg/ml, T_{max} 4.00 hrs, AUC 157.11, elimination half-life 7.36 hrs and MRT 9.95 hrs. The in vivo pharmacokinetic data showed that formulations showing higher permeability coefficient have higher AUC. The C_{max} 41.1 and 42.6 μg/ml achieved with optimized patches were compared to C_{max} of 28.3 μg/ml achieved in earlier

Table 3. Optimized formulations of VHCl

COMPOSITION (% w/w)	A[14]	B[13]	C[56]
VHCl	20	10	20
PVA	67	60	67
PVP	33	40	33
Glycerol	30	30	30
(1,8 cineole + R(+) limonene)	20	—	—
d-limonene	—	20	—
R(+) limonene	—	—	20

study. Therefore, the present formulation may be able to achieve the desired level of 120 ng/ml in humans.

These formulation were further modified to improve the drug delivery of VHCl through skin [14] by using 1,8-cineole and d-limonene as skin penetration enhancer. In vitro release profiles across guinea pig dorsal skin showed that formulations containing PVA and PVP in a ratio 2:1, VHCl (20% w/w) and 18 cineole (20% w/w) are the optimum composition. These formulations were further evaluated for in vivo permeation. In vivo pharmacokinetic data of these formulations showed significant increase in plasma concentration, C_{max} increased to 44.47 and 42.04 mcg/ml respectively, which indicates that this formulation might be able to achieve therapeutic plasma concentration of 120 ng/ml.

These formulations were subjected to pharmacodynamic studies using nephrectomized rats (unilateral) for anti-hypertensive activity in rats and a significant fall in systolic blood pressure was observed.

Diltiazem

Diltiazem hydrochloride, a benzothiazepine calcium channel blocker undergoes extensive first pass metabolism be chosen as a model drug for transdermal delivery. It has oral bioavailability of only 36–50%, has short half-life of 4.5 hours and molecular weight of 451.

Rao and Diwan [38] developed and evaluated EC-PVP films containing diltiazem HCl, which reported that release rates increased with increasing drug concentration and polyvinyl pyrrolidone fraction in the film. Miyazaki [57] et al. studied the drug release from oral mucosal adhesive tablets of diltiazem containing chitosan and sodium alginate in the ratio 1:4 which gave a bioavailability of 69.6% when administered sublingually as compared to 30.4% by oral route. Ahuja et al. [58] studied the release of diltiazem HCl from Carbopol 934 P and PVP-K30 (1:4) matrix containing 6% citric acid and 12% PEG 4000. In vitro release of 86% and a 7% release across bovine cheek pouch were observed respectively. A positive correlation was observed between the two release studies.

Studies were conducted on diltiazem hydrochloride in this laboratory as it appeared to be a suitable candidate for transdermal delivery with good *in vitro* and *in vivo* permeation profile. Prototype formulations of diltiazem HCl were developed using PVA and PVP as polymers and glycerol as plasticizer [15]. It was also concluded that increase in PVP concentration in the matrix increased the amount of drug permeated through the skin. Physico chemical evaluation of polymer matrices revealed uniformity of matrices in weight and thickness. The incorporation of 30% glycerol (w/w) resulted in smooth, uniform and flexible films. The drug was distributed uniformly throughout the matrices. Fabricated patches were then evaluated for drug permeation across guinea pig dorsal skin, showed very low flux and permeability coefficient. 1,8 Cineole showed better penetration enhancement across guinea pig skin than R(+)-limonene. Therefore, 1,8-cineole was incorporated as penetration enhancer at concentrations 2, 5, 10, 15 and 20% w/w. However, statistically enhanced permeation was observed with 20% w/w 1,8-cineole. These formulations were further evaluated for permeation across cadaver skin. Statistically significant difference in permeation enhancement was observed with formulations containing 20% w/w 1,8-cineole. The release rate of the drug from the matrices followed Higuchi equation in which the cumulative percent of drug permeated has linear relation to the square root of time. Therefore, the drug release from the matrix was diffusion controlled.

Modified Draize test on formulations did not show any signs of allergy/hypersensitivity reaction. Based on the results of *in vitro* study, optimized formulations were evaluated for *in vivo* study in guinea pigs. Pharmacokinetic evaluation of TDS of diltiazem hydrochloride in guinea pigs showed increase in plasma concentration (Cmax), area under the curve (AUC) and time to achieve maximum concentration (Tmax). This formulation showed best plasma profile (Cmax) and maximum bioavailability (AUC). Thus, formulation containing PVP appeared to be a promising formulation for TDS development of diltiazem hydrochloride based on *in vitro* and *in vivo* data.

Carvedilol

Carvedilol is an aryl ethanol amine beta-adrenoceptor antagonist with vasodilating properties. Carvedilol seemed to be a potential candidate for transdermal drug delivery because of its short half-life (6.4 hrs), extensive hepatic first pass metabolism and consequently low oral bioavailability (about 22%).

In this laboratory matrix type TDS for Carvedilol was fabricated using polymers such as HPMC, HPC, HPMCP, EC, MC, PVP and DEP, DBP, PEG 400, PEG 600 as plasticizers [12]. Carvedilol being a highly lipophilic, several cationic, anionic and nonionic surface active agents were incorporated into the patches to increase the permeation.

Further *in vitro* study indicates that increase in patch thickness caused a decrease in the permeation rate of carvedilol and 0.61 ± 0.03 mm was found to be the optimum patch thickness. Effect of drug load *in vitro* permeation study indicated that increase in drug load increases the cumulative amount released.

This optimized formulation delivers carvedilol across the rat skin at a rate of 18 μgm/cm^2 in a controlled manner for prolonged time.

Survey of literature reveals that permeation by buccal mucosa was **4 to 4,000 times** more than through skin, which prompted us to venture forth and try to develop mucoadhesive buccal patch for carvedilol.

Transbuccal Drug Delivery System of Carvedilol developed in our laboratory [59] includes Carbopol-934P, Carbopol-974P, Carbopol-941P, along with HPMC, HPC, MC and hydroxy propyl cellulose (HPC) as polymers. Parafilm—M® served as a backing layer for the buccal films in order to provide unidirectional drug release. The bioadhesive strength of the formulations was determined using a modified physical beam balance [60]. *In vitro* dissolution rate studies were carried out in a modified version of Woods intrinsic dissolution apparatus, using isotonic phosphate buffer pH 6.6 as the dissolution maintained at 37 ± 1°C. Dissolution media was stirred at 50 r.p.m. A modified version of Franz diffusion medium cell [61] was used (diffusional area of 1 cm^2 and volume of 17.5 ml) to evaluate *in vitro* permeation of drug through mucous membrane.

In vitro dissolution studies conducted on these various films showed that maximum drug release from formulations was found to be between 55.2% to 73.15%.

Accelerated stability studies are being conducted in accordance with WHO/ICH guidelines on stability testing of pharmaceutical products, for a total period of 3 months at a storage temperature of 40 ± 2°C and a relative humidity of 75 ± 5% RH. In vivo studies using rabbits as the model for obtaining the plasma profile and other pharmacokinetic parameters are in progress.

IV CONCLUSION

Transdermal and transmucosal drug delivery systems can deliver drugs in a controlled manner for prolonged time with less side effects & better patient compliance by reducing the total dose required since the hepatic metabolism of drugs is avoided and the bioavailability of the drugs is considerably increased.

Drug delivery using principles of transdermal and transbuccal is a versatile technology that can be used to deliver drugs at a controlled rate. The data from these experiments can be used in the development of optimized drug delivery systems. At the same time, controlled and constant delivery of drugs can be achieved using these systems as drug delivery tools. The various types of transdermal and transbuccal systems were reviewed here. The release of drug (s) from these types of systems is governed by factors such as solubility, type of polymer and permeation enhancer used and skin permeability. By judicious choice of formulation and processing factors, these systems are amnable to deliver the drugs of diverse nature at a preprogrammed rate. In the present scenario, when development of NDDS is looked on as a fruitful business, the development of transdermal and transbuccal drug delivery systems have a strong market potential as shown by the number of marketed products and number of patents granted in the last few years.

V ACKNOWLEDGEMENTS

The author is thankful to Dr. Girish Jain, Mr. D.D Verma, Ms. Nisha Munshi, Ms. Bhawna Gupta, Ms. Kavita Jerath and Ms. Jaspreet Kaur Kochhar for their contributions in this article.

REFERENCES

1. Mishra B, Pandit JK, Bhattacharya SK. 1990. Recent trends in drug delivery systems: Transdermal drug delivery. Indian J Exp Biol 28:1001–1007.
2. Harris D, Robinson JR. 1992. Drug delivery via the mucous membranes of the oral cavity. J Pharm Sci 81:1–10.
3. Gandhi RB, Robinson JR. 1994. Oral cavity as a site for bioadhesive drug delivery. Adv Drug Del Rev 13:43–74.
4. Tabak LA, Levine MJ, Mandel ID, Ellison SA. 1982. Role of salivary mucins in the protection of the oral cavity. J Oral Pathol 11:1–17.
5. Peppas NA, Buri PA. 1985. Surface interfacial and molecular aspects of polymer bioadhesion on soft tissues. J Controlled Release 2:257–275.
6. Shojaei AH. 1998. Buccal mucosa as a route for systemic drug delivery: J Pharm Pharmaceut Sci 1:15–30.
7. Rathbone MJ, Tucker IG. 1993. Mechanisms, barriers and pathways of oral mucosal drug permeation. Adv Drug Del Rev 12:41–60.
8. Ho NFH. 1993. Biophysical kinetic modeling of buccal absorption. Adv Drug Del Rev 12:61–97.
9. Gary RH. 1987. Drug parameters important for transdermal delivery. In: Transdermal Delivery of Drugs Vol III Ed A F Kydonieus, B Berner 3–22 Florida: CRC Press.
10. Guy RH, Hadgraft J. 1985. Kinetic analysis of transdermal Nitroglycerin Delivery Pharm Res 2:206–209.
11. Guy RH, Hadgraft J. 1985. Pharmacokinetic interpretation of plasma levels of clonidine following transdermal delivery J Pharm Sci 74:1016–1021.
12. Jerath K. 2001. Development and evaluation of transdermal drug delivery system of carvedilol. M. Pharm Thesis, University of Delhi, India.
13. Jain G. 1995. Development of transdermal drug delivery system for vasoactive drugs, Ph.D. Thesis, University of Delhi, India.
14. Munshi N. 1997. *In vitro* and *in vivo* evaluation of transdermal therapeutic system of verapamil hydrochloride using terpenes as skin penetration enhancers and its pharmacodynamic study. M. Pharm Thesis, University of Delhi, India.
15. Gupta B. 1999. Development of transdermal therapeutic system of diltiazem hydrochloride using guinea pig dorsal and cadaver skin. M. Pharm Thesis, University of Delhi, India.
16. Misra AN. 1997. Transdermal drug delivery In: Controlled and Novel Drug Delivery. Ed NK Jain, 100–129 New Delhi: CBS Publishers and Distributors.
17. Ch'ng HS, Park H, Kelly P, Robinson JR. 1985. Bioadhesive polymers as platforms for oral controlled drug delivery II: Synthesis and evaluation of some swelling water-insoluble bioadhesive polymers J Pharm Sci 74:399–405.
18. Gandhi RE, Robinson JR. 1988. Bioadhesion in drug delivery. Ind J Pharm Sci 50:145–152.
19. Sanzgiri YD, Topp EM, Beneditti L, Stella VJ. 1994. Evaluation of mucoadhesive properties of hyaluronic acid benzylesters. Int J Pharm 107:91–97.
20. Park K, Robinson JR. 1984. Bioadhesive polymers as platforms for oral controlled drug delivery: Method to study biodhesion. Int J Pharm 19:107–127.
21. Lehr CM, Bouwstra JA, Schact EH, Junginger HE. 1992. In vitro evaluation of mucoadhesive properties of chitosan and some other natural polymers. Int J Pharm 78:43–48.
22. Agrawal SS, Agarwal SP, Goel A. 2001. Transdermal conception control system containing *Ocimum sanctum* oil as penetration enhancer. Indian Patent Appl No 673/Del/2001.
23. Hoogstraate AJ, Verhoef JC, Tuli B, Pypers LAG, Junginger HE, Bodde HE. 1996. In vivo buccal delivery of fluorescent isothiocyanate dextran 4400 with glycodeoxycholate as an absorption enhancer in pigs. J. Pharm Sci 85:457–460.
24. Hoogstraate AJ, Senel S. 1996. Effects of Bile salts on transport rates and routes of FTIC labeled compounds across porcine buccal epithelium *in vitro*. J Controlled Release 40:211–221.

25. Sensel S, Capan Y, Sargon MF. 1997. Enhancement of transbuccal permeation of morpphine sulphare by sodium glycodeoxycholate *in vitro*. J Controlled Release 45:153–162.
26. Aungst BJ. 1988. Comparison of nasal rectal, buccal, sublingual and intramuscular insulin efficacy and the effects of a bile salt absorption promoter. J Pharmacol Exp Ther 244:23–27.
27. Aungst BJ, Rogers NJ. 1988. Site dependance of absorption promoting actions of Laureth-9 Na salicylate Na_2EDTA Aprotinin on rectal, nasal and buccal insulin delivery. Pharm Res 5:305–308.
28. Oates JA, Brown NJ. 2001. Antihypertensive agents and drug therapy of hypertension In: Goodman and Gilman's The Pharmacological Basis of Therapeutics Ed Joel G Hardman, Lee E Limbird, 871–900 USA: McGraw-Hill Medicine Publishing Division.
29. Keith AD. 1983. Polymer matrix consideration for transdermal devices Drug Dev Ind Pharm 9:605–625.
30. Ryden L. 1987. Buccal vs sublingual glyceryl trinitrate administration in treatment of angina pectoris. Drugs 33:96–99.
31. Abrams J. 1984. Nitrate delivery systems in perspective. Am J Med 76:38–46.
32. Bhalla HL, Damle AV, Toddywala RD. 1985. Transdermal films of isosorbide dinitrate. Drug Dev Ind Pharm 14:119–131.
33. Nozaki Y, Kakumato M, Ohta M, Yakimetsu M. 1993. A new transmucosal therapeutic system: An overview of formulation development and *in vitro* clinical performance. Drug Dev Ind Pharm 19:1755–1808.
34. Danjo K, Kitamura Y, Miyagawa Y, Otsuka A. 1994. Release of isosorbide dinitrate from polymer film dosage forms and absorption of this drug through the oral mucosa of rats. Chem Pharm bull 42:2126–2130.
35. Zierenberg B. 1983. Experimental and Theoretical studies on the diffusion of drugs in polymer films. Drug Dev Ind Pharm 9:117–137.
36. Weber MA, Brewer DD, Drayer JI, Lipson JL. 1984. Transdermal continuous antihypertensive therapy. Lancet 1:9–16.
37. Verma PR, Iyer SS. 2000. Controlled transdermal delivery of propranolol using HPMC matrices: Design and *in vitro* and *in vivo* evaluation. J Pharm Pharmacol 52:151–156.
38. Rao PR, Diwan PV. 1997. Permeability studies of cellulose acetate free films for transdermal use: Influence of plasticizers. Pharm Acta Helv 72:47–51.
39. Corbo M, Liu JC, Chien YW. 1989. Transdermal controlled delivery of Propranolol from a multilaminate adhesive device. Pharm Res 6:753–758.
40. Al-Hmound H, Efentakis M, Choulis NH. 1991. A controlled release matrix using a mixture of hydrophilic and hydrophobic polymers. Int J Pharm 68:R1–R3.
41. Le Brun PPH, Fox PLA, De Vries ME, Bodde HE. 1989. *In vitro* penetration of some β adrenoceptor blocking drugs through porcine buccal mucosa. Int J Pharm 49:141–145.
42. Kislal O, Celabi N. 1992, Studies on buccoadhesive tablet formulation of propranol HCl. Proceed of Int Symp on Control Bioact Mat 19:397–398.
43. Chen WG, Hwang GC. 1992. Adhesive and *in vitro* release characteristics of propranolol biodhesive disc system. Int J Pharm 82:61–66.
44. Nielsen HM, Rassing MR. 2000. TR146 cells grown on filter as a model of human buccal epithelium: IV permeability of water, mannitol, testosterone and β adrenoceptor antagonists. Int J Pharm 194:155–167.
45. Kaul JL, Jain GK, Agrawal SS. 1993. *In vitro* transdermal delivery of atenolol using mouse and guinea pig. Ind J Expl Biol 31:691–693.
46. Ghosh TK, Adir J, Xiang SL, Onyilofur S. 1995. Transdermal delivery of metoprolol: *In vitro* skin permeation and bioavailability in hairless rats. J Pharm Sci 84:153–157.
47. Wong CF, Yuen KH, Peh KK. 1999. Formulation and evaluation of controlled release eudragit buccal patches. Int J Pharm 178:11–22.
48. Bondi JV, Loper AE, Cohen EM. 1987. Transdermal system for timolol. Eur Pat Appl EP 186071 through CA 106:23288.
49. Dinsheet, Agarwal SP, Ahuja A. 1997. Preparation of Evaluation of Mucoadhesive buccal Tablets of hydralazine hydrochloride. Indian Journal Pharm. Sci 59:135–141.
50. Ruan LP, Zheng JM. 1991. Research on nifedipine patch. Acta Pharm Sinica 26:286–292. Through IPA: 2902107.
51. Save T, Venkitachalam P. 1994. Buccoadhesive tablets of nifedipine standardization of a novel buccoadhesive erodible carrier. Drug Dev Ind Pharm 20:3005–3014.

52. Remunan LC, Portero A, Vila JJL, Alonso MJ. 1998. Design and evaluation of chitosan/ethylcellulose mucoadhesive bilayered devices for buccal drug delivery. J Controlled Release 55:143–152.
53. Chien YW, Tojo K. 1987. Transdermal Verapamil delivery Device PCT. Int Appl W O 870042 Chem Abstract 107:64932.
54. Sawicki W. 2001. Penetration of Verapamil Hydrochloride in the presence of sodium glycocholate as penetration enhancer through mucous membrane. Pharmazie 56:74–77.
55. Jain GK, Agrawal SS. 1996. *In vitro* percutaneous absorption of Verapamil. Ind J Expl Biol 34: 475–477.
56. Verma DD. 1996. Development and Pharmacokinetic evaluation of Transdermal Drug Delivery System of Verapamil HCl. M. Pharm Thesis, University of Delhi, India.
57. Miyazaki S, Nakayama A, Oda M, Takada M, Attwood D. 1994. Chitosan and sodium alginate based bioadhesive tablet for intraoral drug delivery. Biol Pharm bull 17:745–747.
58. Ahuja A, Dogra M, Agarwal SP. 1995. Development of buccal tablets of Diltiazem hydrochloride. Indian J. Pharm Sci 57:26–30.
59. Kochhar JK. 2002. Develoment and evaluation of Buccal Drug Delivery system of Carvedilol, M Pharm (Thesis work in progress).
60. Gupta A, Garg S, Khar RK. 1992. Measurement of bioadhesive strength of mucoadhesive buccal tablets: Design of *in vitro* assembly. Indian Drugs 30:152–155.
61. Gummer CL, Hinz RS, Maibach HI. 1987. The skin penetration cell: A design update. Int J Pharm 40:101–104.

G.N. Pierce, M. Nagano, P. Zahradka, and N.S. Dhalla (eds.).
ATHEROSCLEROSIS, HYPERTENSION AND DIABETES. Copyright © 2003.
Kluwer Academic Publishers. Boston.

INSULIN RESISTANCE AND EXPERIMENTAL HYPERTENSION

DENISE GALIPEAU and JOHN H. MCNEILL

Faculty of Pharmaceutical Sciences, The University of British Columbia, 2146 East Mall, Vancouver, B.C., Canada V6T 1Z3

Summary. A growing body of evidence suggests a causal role for insulin resistance and hyperinsulinemia in the development of hypertension. This evidence is supported by studies demonstrating that insulin has important, physiologically relevant effects on the cardiovascular system in addition to its effects on metabolism. Several mechanisms have been proposed to mediate the link between insulin and hypertension, indicating that this relationship is intricate and multifactorial in nature. Some of the mechanisms we have extensively investigated in our laboratory include, activation of the SNS, defects in endothelium dependent vasodilation, and enhanced production and activity of endothelium derived vasoconstrictors (ET-1 and TXA_2). Furthermore, we have investigated the intriguing possibility that the relationship between hyperinsulinemia, insulin resistance, and hypertension is dependent upon sex and that the sex hormones may impact this complex interrelationship. Collectively, these data have provided insight into the mechanisms responsible for hypertension, an important first step in improving the treatment of hypertension in a human population.

Key words: Insulin resistance, Hyperinsulinemia, Hypertension, Endothelin, Thromboxane

INTRODUCTION

Hyperinsulinemia and resistance to the glucose lowering effects of insulin (insulin resistance) are often found to be associated with hypertension in both humans and several animal models [1–3]. From this observation, the "insulin hypothesis" was

Corresponding Author: John H. McNeill, PhD, FRSC, Faculty of Pharmaceutical Sciences, The University of British Columbia, 2146 East Mall, Vancouver, B.C., Canada V6T 1Z3. Tel: (604) 822-9373; Fax: (604) 822-8001; email: jmcneill@interchange.ubc.ca

developed, which proposes that these metabolic impairments are directly related to the cause of hypertension in such individuals. This hypothesis was attractive because it helped to explain the apparent inability of conventional antihypertensive drugs to decrease the incidence of coronary ischemic events, since these drugs tended to worsen rather than improve insulin action [4–6]. The term "Syndrome X" has come into use, to represent this commonly found cluster of symptoms: hyperinsulinemia, insulin resistance, glucose intolerance, hypertriglyceridemia, and hypertension. In addition to the studies demonstrating that both obese and lean hypertensive patients exhibit insulin resistance, further evidence for this hypothesis includes the observation that insulin resistance and hyperinsulinemia are also present in normotensive offspring of hypertensive parents [7]. This can be detected as early as the second decade of life and these changes precede any rise in blood pressure. Several hypertensive rodent models also exhibit similar defects in glucose metabolism and insulin action, including the Dahl rat [8], spontaneously hypertensive rat (SHR) [9–11], Milan hypertensive rat [12], and fructose hypertensive rat (FHR) [10,13,14]. As these models are etiologically distinct, the existence of these common defects lends further strength to the hypothesis that they are linked to hypertension.

A central research focus of our laboratory has been to investigate the intriguing relationship between hyperinsulinemia, insulin resistance, and hypertension. It appears that this association is multi-factorial, as we have identified a number of mechanisms that play a role including alterations in sympathetic nervous system activity, impaired endothelium dependent vasorelaxation, and increased release of endothelial contracting factors (endothelin-1 and thromboxane A_2) (Fig. 1). Our most recent work has demonstrated that there are sex differences in the effects of hyperinsulinemia and insulin resistance on blood pressure, indicating that the sex hormones may impact the symptoms of syndrome X. The focus of this paper is to review the studies performed in our laboratory into the mechanisms responsible for hypertension in the presence of hyperinsulinemia and insulin resistance.

INSULIN RESISTANCE AND HYPERINSULINEMIA IN HYPERTENSIVE RAT MODELS

A common animal model used to study the interaction between insulin and hypertension is the fructose hypertensive rat (FHR). This is a form of mild hypertension that also exhibits insulin resistance, hyperinsulinemia, and hypertriglyceridemia [13]. In this model, a simple chronic dietary intervention of substituting high fructose for the normal starch carbohydrate content in laboratory rodent diets has been found by several investigators to increase blood pressure within a period of 3–5 weeks [13–15]. The effects of a fructose diet have been shown to be concentration and duration dependent [14]. The cluster of hypertension, hypertriglyceridemia, hyperinsulinemia, and insulin resistance is also characteristic of other high carbohydrate fed rodent models, including sucrose [16–18] or glucose [18,19]. These models are useful for hypertension studies because feeding with a high fructose diet does not result in any body weight gain, thus enabling one to investigate the relationship between insulin resistance and hypertension independent of obesity. Furthermore,

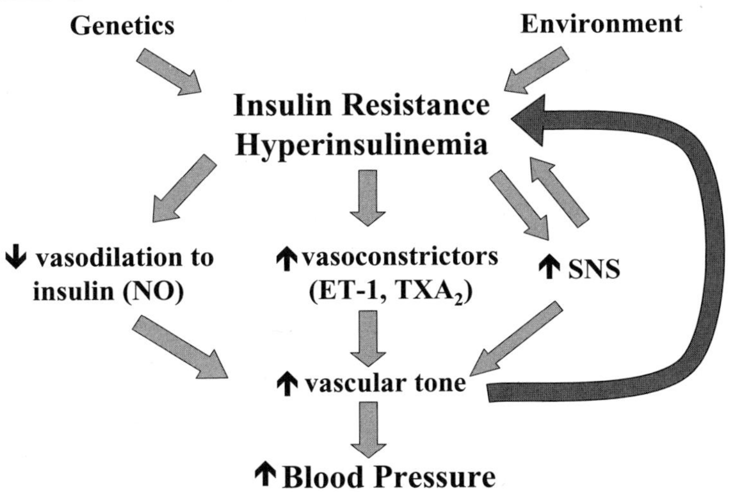

Figure 1. Potential mechanisms linking hyperinsulinemia and insulin resistance to hypertension. In states of hyperinsulinemia and insulin resistance (ie to the glucose lowering effects of insulin), several mechanisms are believed to contribute to the development of hypertension. The key point is that there appears to be tissue-specific loss of insulin action (see text for complete discussion of the mechanisms).

hypertension is acquired simply as a result of a dietary intervention and therefore provides an opportunity to study pathological mechanisms of hypertension that may not have a genetic basis.

It has been shown previously both in our laboratory and elsewhere that several drug interventions which improve insulin sensitivity, including metformin [20], vanadium compounds [10,21], and thiazolidinediones [22–24], can ameliorate the hypertension observed in the FHR. Furthermore, increasing plasma insulin levels to that seen prior to treatment reverses the effects of these drugs [21]. These observations lend support to the hypothesis that insulin resistance/hyperinsulinemia are the primary defect leading to hypertension in the FHR.

As mentioned above, hyperinsulinemia/insulin resistance have been implicated in several other rodent models of hypertension. We have performed the same studies using insulin-sensitizing agents described above in the SHR model as well as FHR [25–28]. These studies have each demonstrated that plasma insulin levels of SHR treated rats are reduced by metformin, vanadium compounds, or pioglitazone with a corresponding decrease in blood pressure, however it is not completely normalized. Despite the fact that the SHR is a genetic model for hypertension, this result indicates that part of the blood pressure increase in this model is also related to insulin resistance and hyperinsulinemia. Indeed, studies using the euglycemic hyperinsulinemic clamp technique have shown that SHR are insulin resistant relative to their control [9,11,26].

MECHANISMS LINKING INSULIN RESISTANCE/ HYPERINSULINEMIA TO HYPERTENSION

Sympathetic nervous system

One of possible links between hyperinsulinemia and hypertension may be related to insulin-induced stimulation of the sympathetic nervous system (SNS). Under hyperinsulinemic conditions, insulin may chronically activate the SNS, thereby leading to increased peripheral vascular tone and elevated blood pressure. In support of this hypothesis, insulin infusion both increases plasma noradrenaline (NA) levels and sympathetic nerve activity in muscle [29–31]. However, studies in humans have shown that although physiological increases in insulin concentration can increase muscle sympathetic nerve firing rate, they result in no overall change in BP [29,32]. The reason why insulin does not increase blood pressure under normal conditions, despite stimulation of the SNS, is that insulin causes vasodilation in the vasculature of skeletal muscle, which consequently leads to a redistribution of cardiac output and therefore no net effect on blood pressure [33,34].

On the other hand, the SNS may be involved in this inter-relationship as the primary defect, causing both insulin resistance and hypertension. Studies have demonstrated that stimulation of β-adrenergic receptors can cause acute insulin resistance [35] and an increase in the ratio of insulin resistant fast-twitch/slow-twitch fibers in skeletal muscle [36]. Elevated SNS activity may also contribute to apparent insulin resistance via vasoconstriction, thereby reducing blood flow and glucose delivery to insulin sensitive tissues [37]. Hyperinsulinemia may occur to compensate for insulin resistance but then serves as a further stimulus for SNS activation, thereby creating a vicious circle that reinforces the insulin resistant state and elevated blood pressure. In our studies of the fructose hypertensive rat (FHR), we have shown that chemical sympathectomy prevents the elevations in both insulin levels and blood pressure [38]. This data is supported by another study in which moxonidine treatment of FHR, an imidazole-1 receptor antagonist which decreases sympathetic discharge, also prevents both hyperinsulinemia and hypertension [39]. Collectively, these data demonstrate that a functional SNS is required for the development of both hyperinsulinemia and hypertension in this model and suggests that SNS activation may be an early defect that preceeds the metabolic defects necessary for hypertension to ensue.

Insulin and endothelium dependent vasodilation

Insulin is a vasodilator and has been shown in many studies to increase blood flow [29,40–44]. Insulin-induced vasodilation is specific to vascular beds in skeletal muscle and occurs at physiologically relevant concentrations [42,45,46]. It is believed that this effect is selective for skeletal muscle because this is the major site of glucose disposal and increases in muscle blood flow will enhance insulin-stimulated glucose disposal [47,48]. In addition to directly increasing blood flow, insulin has also been shown to reduce the pressor response to factors such as NA and angiotensin-II (AII) [49] or to reflex sympathetic discharge [50]. If there is resistance to the vasodilator effects of insulin in subjects who are also resistant to insulin-stimulated glucose disposal then this may contribute to the development of hypertension. It should be noted that although the majority of studies support that insulin has vasodilator effects, a few studies have been unable to demonstrate this response [51–53]. There are several possible reasons for this discrepancy, such as differences in measurement technique or variability in subject age, physical fitness, and basal vascular tone. However, as discussed above, another likely explanation for the lack of an effect by insulin in these studies relates to the simultaneous activation of the SNS, counteracting any direct effects of insulin on vasodilation.

Defects in endothelial function have been proposed to play a role in the "insulin hypothesis" of hypertension [54–57]. The generation of nitric oxide (NO) in the endothelium via the L-arginine-NO pathway appears to be the main determinant of basal vascular tone [58], and defects in this pathway have been linked to the pathogenesis of hypertension [59–61]. Several pieces of evidence indicate that insulin mediated vasodilation in various vascular tissues occurs via the release of endothelium-derived NO. Infusion of a nitric oxide synthase (NOS) antagonist prevents insulin stimulated increases in blood flow in humans [34,41,47]. Furthermore, removal of the endothelium or infusion of a NOS antagonist in isolated arterioles converts insulin induced vasodilation to vasoconstriction [62]. Insulin may affect the NO pathway by several mechanisms. Firstly, insulin has been shown to increase endothelial-NOS (eNOS) mRNA and protein levels in aortic endothelial cells [63,64]. Secondly, insulin may increase NOS activity by increasing the availability of tetrahydrobiopterin (BH_4), a co-factor required for NOS activation. We have studied the vasoreactivity of rat femoral arteries in the presence of 2,4-diamino-6-hydroxypyrimidine (DAHP), an inhibitor of BH_4 synthesis [65]. The results demonstrated an attenuation of the vasodepressor effects of insulin when arteries were pre-incubated with DAHP. This supports the hypothesis that BH_4 is the site of action for endothelium dependent vasodilation mediated by insulin.

In states of insulin resistance, there may also be resistance to the vascular actions of insulin, which in turn could lead to an increase in vascular tone and BP. Indeed, we have examined this hypothesis and shown that arteries from insulin-resistant FHR are resistant to the vasodepressor effects of insulin [66]. This response was observed only in endothelium intact tissues and implies that there are defects in insulin action as an endothelium-dependent vasodilator in the aorta of male FHR. Interestingly, chronic treatment of FHR with the insulin sensitizer metformin restores insulin action with respect to both the vasodepressor and metabolic effects of the hormone [67]. As a result, both the increase in plasma insulin levels and blood pressure were prevented. Taking these investigations further, we subsequently demonstrated a defective endothelium dependent vasodilation to acetylcholine in mesenteric arteries from FHR [68]. Other laboratories have demonstrated similar results and have attributed it to defects in vasodilatory mechanisms associated with NO [69] as well as the endothelium derived hyperpolarizing factor (EDHF) [70,71]. It would follow from our studies on the mechanisms of insulin's vasodepressor effects that the defective endothelium dependent relaxation observed in FHR may be specifically attributed to impairments in the ability of insulin to activate BH_4 and NO synthesis, although other mechanisms cannot be ruled out.

Insulin and endothelium derived vasoconstrictors

Equally important in the pathogenesis of hypertension are defects in the signaling pathways of endothelium derived contracting factors. In our laboratory, we have investigated the role of two potent vasoconstrictors in the development of hypertension in FHR, namely endothelin-1 (ET-1) and thromboxane A_2 (TXA_2).

In addition to its effects on NO, insulin also stimulates the synthesis, secretion, and gene expression of the potent vasoconstrictor endothelin-1 (ET-1) [72–74]. A two fold increase in receptor expression has also been demonstrated in isolated vascular smooth muscle cells (VSMC) treated with insulin [72]. As well as directly stimulating ET-1 release, insulin has been shown to enhance the release of ET-1 from cultured VSMC induced by angiotensin-II and arginine vasopressin [74]. The effects of insulin to activate both the NO and ET-1 pathways appear to occur simultaneously in the same vascular tissue. Cardillo et al. have recently demonstrated that insulin infusion together with an ET-1 antagonist elicits vasodilation in the human forearm and this vasodilation is prevented if a NOS antagonist is added to the insulin + ET-1 antagonist infusion [75]. Insulin did not alter blood flow in the absence of any antagonists, presumably because stimulation of both NO and ET-1 at the same time produces equally opposing responses, and therefore no net effect, on vascular tone. We have supported this with in vitro experiments that show endothelin antagonism will unmask the vasodepressor effects of insulin in tissues which do not demonstrate this effect otherwise [76]. The results of these experiments help to explain some of the discrepancies related to studies of the effects of insulin on vasodilation and blood flow described above.

We have hypothesized that in states of hyperinsulinemia and insulin resistance, the vascular effects of insulin are altered such that the vasoconstrictor effects are favoured over vasodilation, therefore leading to an increase in vascular tone and blood pressure. Since ET-1 release can be stimulated by insulin, hyperinsulinemic conditions would serve as a constant stimulus that would result in elevated levels of this potent vasoconstrictor hormone. To support this, we have demonstrated that treatment of FHR with the ET-1 receptor antagonist bosentan prevents hypertension, but does not correct hyperinsulinemia or insulin resistance, in this model [77]. We have also shown that vascular ET-1 levels are elevated in fructose fed rats [77] and that the reactivity of mesenteric arteries to ET-1 is altered [78]. Furthermore, increased expression of both ET-1 protein and its ET_A receptor subtype (which mediates vascular contraction) has been demonstrated in FHR [79]. Collectively, these data indicate that the ET-1 pathway is enhanced in states of insulin resistance and hyperinsulinemia and that this contributes to the development of hypertension.

Thromboxane A_2 (TxA_2), a metabolite of arachidonic acid, is another potent vasoconstrictor derived from the endothelium that may be important in hypertension.

Insulin, when incubated in vitro with rings of coronary arteries, potentiates the vasoconstrictor actions of TxA_2 [80]. In hyperinsulinemic SHR [81] as well as rats chronically infused with insulin [82], the development of hypertension can be prevented by treatment with a thromboxane synthase inhibitor. Our studies show that hypertension in FHR is accompanied by an increase in plasma TXA_2 levels and both hypertension and the elevation in plasma TXA_2 are prevented by treatment with the thromboxane synthase inhibitor dazmegrel. We have concluded based on this result that hypertension secondary to hyperinsulinemia and insulin resistance is dependent on TxA_2 synthesis [83]. Further data from our laboratory demonstrate that cyclooxygenase (COX) inhibition reduces noradrenaline (NE)–induced contraction in aorta from FHR but not in control rats, suggesting that there is enhanced production of COX-derived vasoconstrictor products, possibly TXA_2, in vascular tissue of FHR (unpublished). Indeed, we have shown that the ET-1 stimulated production of TXA_2 from vascular tissue is increased in FHR [83].

Our findings have demonstrated that both ET-1 and TxA_2 are important in the development of hypertension in the FHR, indicating that there may be an interaction between these two systems. In addition to ours, several studies have shown that ET-1 stimulates the production of TxA_2 [84–86], and that ET-1-induced vasoconstriction in human placenta vessels is dependent on TxA_2 [87]. Hence, it is possible that hyperinsulinemia causes elevations in ET-1, which in turn stimulates TxA_2, and the resulting hypertension may be due to the additive vasoconstrictor effects of both hormones. On the other hand, the interaction between ET-1 and TXA_2 may not be unidirectional. Moreau et al. [88] have demonstrated that bosentan attenuates contractile responses to U46619, a TxA_2 analogue. This suggests that stimulation of the TxA_2 receptor may activate the release of ET-1 and the resulting contractile responses to U46619 are the combined effects of ET and TxA_2 receptor activation. Additionally, administration of dazmegrel to allograft kidney transplanted rats reduces the release of ET-1 from the renal endothelium [89]. Hence in our studies of dazmegrel treated FHR, it is possible that inhibition of thromboxane synthesis altered ET-1 levels and prevented the BP increase by reducing ET-1 as well as TXA_2 concentrations. Furthermore, just as insulin stimulates the expression of ET-1 and its receptor [72,73], insulin may also directly affect TXA_2 synthesis and increase ET-1 levels via this mechanism, but this remains to be investigated. Figure 2 illustrates our proposed model of the interaction between ET-1 and TXA_2 in hyperinsulinemia, insulin resistance, and hypertension.

The influence of sex

Recent evidence has suggested that there may be differences between males and females in the response to feeding with a high carbohydrate diet. It has been shown that female rats do not develop hypertriglyceridemia or insulin resistance after feeding with sucrose [90]. Unfortunately, BP was not measured in this study, nor were male groups included in the experiment. A separate study investigating the effects of high sucrose on development of juvenile rats showed that both male and

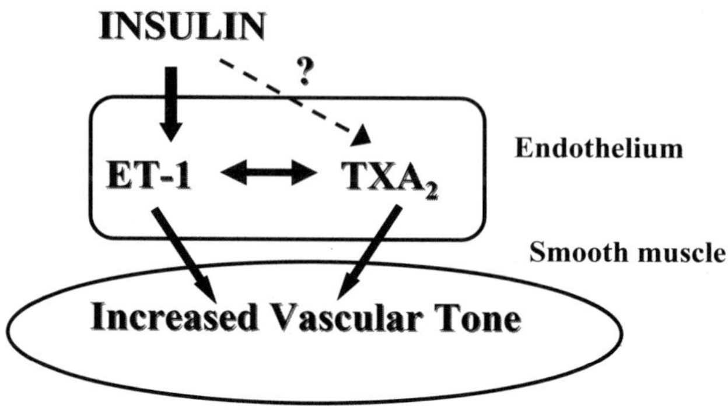

Figure 2. ET-1 and TXA_2 in hyperinsulinemia, insulin resistance, and hypertension. The model we propose is depicted, with insulin activating ET-1 synthesis and secretion, which in turn stimulates TXA_2 activity. In turn, TXA_2 is also known to stimulate ET-1, further increasing ET-1 release. The potent vasoconstrictor actions of both hormones are required for the development of hypertension.

female rats develop hypertension, however, the degree of BP increase was greater in males than in females [91]. The male sucrose fed group was found to be insulin resistant, however, insulin sensitivity was not measured in the female groups. Therefore, it is uncertain if the elevated BP in females is related to impairments in insulin sensitivity or if there were any differences between sexes in this respect.

The studies discussed above appear to provide conflicting results, since if sucrose indeed does not produce hyperinsulinemia and insulin resistance in female rats, then according to our hypothesis, hypertension would also not develop. Given the well documented sex differences in the incidence of cardiovascular disease in humans [92], we hypothesized that the relationship between hyperinsulinemia, insulin resistance, and hypertension may be dependent on sex. To clarify the effects of a fructose diet in female rats, we compared the effects of 9 weeks of fructose diet on BP and metabolism in both male and female Wistar rats. In this experiment, male rats developed significant hypertension and hyperinsulinemia, but females did not [93]. To examine the relationship between insulin and BP in female rats further, we treated both male and female rats chronically with exogenous insulin and measured BP and insulin sensitivity pre- and post-treatment. The results of this experiment demonstrated that chronic hyperinsulinemia produced insulin resistance and hypertension in male rats, but insulin resistance only in females [94]. Based on these studies, we concluded that the link between hyperinsulinemia, insulin resistance, and hypertension depends on sex and we hypothesized that this may be related to the protective effects of estrogen. In support of this hypothesis, we fed female ovariectomized rats with fructose and observed an increase in BP and reductions in insulin sensitivity compared to the ovariectomized control fed group [93].

As a steroid hormone, estrogen acts on nuclear receptors to affect gene expression and regulation, although non-genomic (acute) effects have also been demonstrated in the vasculature [95,96]. The potential protective effects of estrogen have been attributed to a variety of direct and indirect effects on the cardiovascular system. Acute application of estrogen causes relaxation in various vascular tissues [95,97–100]. As this dilation can occur rapidly and in the presence of transcriptional blockade, non-genomic mechanisms appear to be involved. Multiple endothelium dependent and independent pathways have been demonstrated to mediate the vasorelaxation induced by estrogen. The endothelial actions of estrogen include the stimulation of the vasodilators PGI_2 and NO and inhibition of vasoconstrictors such as ET-1 and TXA_2 [101,102]. Basal and stimulated release of NO is greater in female normotensive rats compared to males [103], and this has been suggested to be an important factor in the sex differences in cardiovascular disease incidence. Direct effects of estrogen on VSMC calcium [99,104] and potassium channels [105] have also been demonstrated, leading to reduced intracellular calcium levels and hyperpolarization of VSMC. The effects of estrogen on metabolism have indirect cardiovascular benefits as well. Estrogen can improve insulin action in liver, muscle, and adipose tissue by increasing glycogen deposition, glucose uptake, and lipogenesis [106]. Given the evidence in favour of a link between insulin resistance, hyperinsulinemia and hypertension, such improvements in insulin sensitivity by estrogen may be related to beneficial effects on BP.

We have also examined the vascular actions of insulin in female rats. Since female rats do not develop hypertension after feeding with fructose, we did not expect to observe differences in the vascular actions of insulin between female diet groups. However, we have made the interesting and novel observation that in female rats insulin does not have any significant effect on vascular smooth muscle contraction [93]. Under the same experimental conditions employed in male rats in our laboratory, insulin reduces contraction in control rats, but this response is blunted after fructose feeding [66] (as described above). This sex difference in the vascular effects of insulin may be related to differences in endothelial function. Indeed, sex differences in the insulin-stimulated release of endothelial factors have been reported in human subjects [107]. As well, since insulin causes vasodilation via NO [44] and given that females have greater capacity than males to generate NO under basal conditions [103], insulin may not stimulate the expected NO-mediated vasodepressor response in females because NO synthesis is already so high that it cannot be further increased by insulin. If the hypothesis that hyperinsulinemia/insulin resistance is related to hypertension only in males is true, then it is possible that sex differences in the role and function of insulin as a cardiovascular hormone are another potential explanation.

A collective examination of our studies into the influence of sex on the complex interactions between hyperinsulinemia, insulin resistance and hypertension indicate that several of the pathways we have identified in males may be absent or modified in females (Fig. 3). The exact role of sex and the identity of the key specific hormones remain to be elucidated.

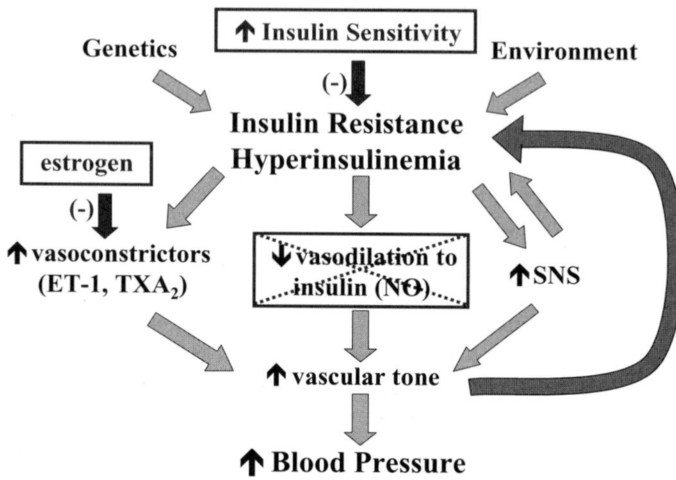

Figure 3. Mechanisms linking hyperinsulinemia and insulin resistance to hypertension which may be dependent upon sex. The pathways illustrated in boxes may be altered in females, which therefore may confer protection against the development of hypertension secondary to hyperinsulinemia and insulin resistance (see text for complete discussion of the mechanisms).

ACKNOWLEDGEMENTS

This work was supported by grants from the Heart and Stroke Foundation of B.C. and Yukon. We thank Sylvia Chan for her secretarial assistance.

REFERENCES

1. Ferrannini E, Natali A. 1991. Essential hypertension, metabolic disorders, and insulin resistance. Am Heart J 121:1274–1282.
2. Reaven GM. 1991. Insulin resistance, hyperinsulinemia, and hypertriglyceridemia in the etiology and clinical course of hypertension. Am J Med 90:7S–12S.
3. Verma S. 2000. Insulin resistance and hypertension: pharmacological and mechanistic studies. Can J Diabetes Care 23:23–42.
4. Goyal RK. 1999. Hyperinsulinemia and insulin resistance in hypertension: differential effects of antihypertensive agents. Clin Exp Hypertens 21:167–179.
5. Lind L, Pollare T, Berne C, Lithell H. 1994. Long-term metabolic effects of antihypertensive drugs. Am Heart J 128:1177–1183.
6. Pollare T, Lithell H, Selinus I, Berne C. 1989. Sensitivity to insulin during treatment with atenolol and metoprolol: a randomised, double blind study of effects on carbohydrate and lipoprotein metabolism in hypertensive patients. Br Med J 298:1152–1157.
7. Grunfeld B, Balzareti M, Romo M, Gimenez M, Gutman R. 1994. Hyperinsulinemia in normotensive offspring of hypertensive parents. Hypertension 23:I12–I15.
8. Kotchen TA, Zhang HY, Covelli M, Blehschmidt N. 1991. Insulin resistance and blood pressure in Dahl rats and in one-kidney, one-clip hypertensive rats. Am J Physiol 261:E692–E697.
9. Hulman S, Falkner B, Chen YQ. 1991. Insulin resistance in the spontaneously hypertensive rat. Metabolism 40:359–361.
10. Bhanot S, Michoulas A, McNeill JH. 1995. Antihypertensive effects of vanadium compounds in hyperinsulinemic, hypertensive rats. Mol Cell Biochem 153:205–209.

11. Qu X, Donnelly R. 1997. Is insulin resistance in the spontaneously hypertensive rat related to changes in protein kinase C in skeletal muscle? Am J Hypertens 10:1053–1057.
12. Dall'Aglio E, Tosini P, Ferrari P, Zavaroni I, Passeri M, Reaven GM. 1991. Abnormalities of insulin and lipid metabolism in Milan hypertensive rats. Am J Hypertens 4:773–775.
13. Hwang IS, Ho H, Hoffman BB, Reaven GM. 1987. Fructose-induced insulin resistance and hypertension in rats. Hypertension 10:512–516.
14. Dai S, McNeill JH. 1995. Fructose-induced hypertension in rats is concentration- and duration-dependent. J Pharmacol Toxicol Methods 33:101–107.
15. Reaven GM, Ho H, Hoffman BB. 1988. Attenuation of fructose-induced hypertension in rats by exercise training. Hypertension 12:129–132.
16. Bunag RD, Tomita T, Sasaki S. 1983. Chronic sucrose ingestion induces mild hypertension and tachycardia in rats. Hypertension 5:218–225.
17. el Zein M, Areas JL, Preuss HG. 1990. Long-term effects of excess sucrose ingestion on three strains of rats. Am J Hypertens 3:560–562.
18. Reaven GM, Ho H. 1991. Sugar-induced hypertension in Sprague-Dawley rats. Am J Hypertens 4:610–614.
19. Claxton CR, Brands MW, Fitzgerald SM, Cameron JA. 2000. Inhibition of nitric oxide synthesis potentiates hypertension during chronic glucose infusion in rats. Hypertension 35:451–456.
20. Verma S, Bhanot S, McNeill JH. 1994. Antihypertensive effects of metformin in fructose-fed hyperinsulinemic, hypertensive rats. J Pharmacol Exp Ther 271:1334–1337.
21. Bhanot S, McNeill JH, Bryer-Ash M. 1994. Vanadyl sulfate prevents fructose-induced hyperinsulinemia and hypertension in rats. Hypertension 23:308–312.
22. Kotchen TA, Reddy S, Zhang HY. 1997. Increasing insulin sensitivity lowers blood pressure in the fructose-fed rat. Am J Hypertens 10:1020–1026.
23. Lee MK, Miles PD, Khoursheed M, Gao KM, Moossa AR, Olefsky JM. 1994. Metabolic effects of troglitazone on fructose-induced insulin resistance in the rat. Diabetes 43:1435–1439.
24. Suzuki M, Nomura C, Odaka H, Ikeda H. 1997. Effect of an insulin sensitizer, pioglitazone, on hypertension in fructose-drinking rats. Jpn J Pharmacol 74:297–302.
25. Bhanot S, McNeill JH. 1994. Vanadyl Sulfate Lowers Plasma Insulin and Blood Pressure in Spontaneously Hypertensive Rats. Hypertension 24:625–632.
26. Bhanot S, Bryer-Ash M, Cheung A, McNeill JH. 1994. Bis(maltolato)oxovanadium(IV) attenuates hyperinsulinemia and hypertension in spontaneously hypertensive rats. Diabetes 43:857–861.
27. Verma S, Bhanot S, McNeill JH. 1994. Metformin decreases plasma insulin levels and systolic blood pressure in spontaneously hypertensive rats. Am J Physiol 267:H1250–H1253.
28. Verma S, Bhanot S, Arikawa E, Yao L, McNeill JH. 1998. Direct vasodepressor effects of pioglitazone in spontaneously hypertensive rats. Pharmacology 56:7–16.
29. Anderson EA, Hoffman RP, Balon TW, Sinkey CA, Mark AL. 1991. Hyperinsulinemia produces both sympathetic neural activation and vasodilation in normal humans. J Clin Invest 87:2246–2252.
30. Lembo G, Napoli R, Capaldo B, Rendina V, Iaccarino G, Volpe M, Trimarco B, Sacca L. 1992. Abnormal sympathetic overactivity evoked by insulin in the skeletal muscle of patients with essential hypertension. J Clin Invest 90:24–29.
31. Liang CS, Doherty JU, Faillace R. 1982. Insulin infusion in conscious dogs: effects on systemic and coronary hemodynamics, regional blood flows, and plasma catecholamines. J Clin Invest 69: 1321–1336.
32. Berne C, Fagius J, Pollare T. 1992. The sympathetic response to euglycemic hyperinsulinemia. Evidence from microelectrode nerve recordings in healthy subjects. Diabetologia 35:873–879.
33. Baron AD. 1993. Cardiovascular actions of insulin in humans. Implications for insulin sensitivity and vascular tone. Baillieres Clin Endocrinol Metab 7:961–987.
34. Sartori C, Trueb L, Nicod P, Scherrer U. 1999. Effects of sympathectomy and nitric oxide synthase inhibition on vascular actions of insulin in humans. Hypertension 34:586–589.
35. Deibert DC, DeFronzo RA. 1980. Epinephrine-induced insulin resistance in man. J Clin Invest 65:717–721.
36. Zeman RJ, Ludemann R, Easton TG, Etlinger JD. 1988. Slow to fast alterations in skeletal muscle fibres caused by clenbuterol, a beta-2-receptor agonist. Am J Physiol 254:E726–E732.
37. Rattigan S, Clark MG, Barrett EJ. 1999. Acute vasoconstriction-induced insulin resistance in rat muscle in-vivo. Diabetes 48:564–569.
38. Verma S, Bhanot S, McNeill JH. 1999. Sympathectomy prevents fructose-induced hyperinsulinemia and hypertension. Eur J Pharmacol 373:R1–R4.

39. Rosen P, Ohly P, Gleichmann H. 1997. Experimental benefit of moxonidine on glucose metabolism and insulin secretion in the fructose-fed rat. J Hypertens Suppl 15:S31–S38.
40. Cleland SJ, Petrie JR, Uedo S, Elliott HL, Connell JMC. 1999. Insulin-mediated vasodilation and glucose uptake are functionally linked in humans. Hypertension 33:554–558.
41. Steinberg HO, Brechtel G, Johnson A, Fineberg N, Baron AD. 1994. Insulin-mediated skeletal muscle vasodilation is nitric oxide dependent. A novel action of insulin to increase nitric oxide release. J Clin Invest 94:1172–1179.
42. Laakso M, Edelman SV, Brechtel G, Baron AD. 1990. Decreased effect of insulin to stimulate skeletal muscle blood flow in obese man. A novel mechanism for insulin resistance. J Clin Invest 85: 1844–1852.
43. Baron AD, Steinberg HO, Chaker H, Leaming R, Johnson A, Brechtel G. 1995. Insulin-mediated skeletal muscle vasodilation contributes to both insulin sensitivity and responsiveness in lean humans. J Clin Invest 96:786–792.
44. Baron AD. 1994. Hemodynamic actions of insulin. Am J Physiol 267:E187–E202.
45. Tack CJJ, Schefman AEP, Willems JL, Thein T, Lutterman JA. 1996. Direct vasodilator effects of physiological hyperinsulinemia in human skeletal muscle. Eur J Clin Invest 26:772–778.
46. Baron AD, Brechtel G. 1993. Insulin differentially regulates systemic and skeletal muscle vascular resistance. Am J Physiol 265:E61–E67.
47. Baron AD. 1996. The coupling of glucose metabolism and perfusion in human skeletal muscle: the potential role of endothelium-derived nitric oxide. Diabetes 45:S105–S109.
48. Cleland SJ, Petrie JR, Schinichiro U, Elliott HL, Connell JM. 1999. Insulin-mediated vasodilation and glucose uptake are functionally linked in humans. Hypertension 33:554–558.
49. Sakai K, Inaizumi T, Masaki H. 1993. Intra-arterial infusion of insulin attenuates vasoreactivity in the human forearm. Hypertension 22:67–73.
50. Lembo G, Rendina V, Iaccarino G. 1993. Insulin reduces reflex forearm sympathetic vasoconstriction in healthy humans. Hypertension 21:1015–1019.
51. DeFronzo RA, Gunnarson R, Bjorkman O. 1985. Effects of insulin on peripheral and splanchnic glucose metabolism in non-insulin dependent (type II) diabete mellitus. J Clin Invest 76:149–155.
52. Jackson RA, Hamling JB, Blix PM, Sim BM, Hawa MI, Jaspan JB, Belin J, Nabarro JD. 1986. The influence of graded hyperglycemia with and without physiological hyperinsulinemia on forearm glucose uptake and other metabolic resposes in man. J Clin Endocrinol Metab 63:594–604.
53. Yki-Jarvinen H, Young AA, Lamkin C. 1987. Kinetics of glucose disposal in whole body and across forearm in man. J Clin Invest 79:1713–1719.
54. Pinkney J, Stehouwer CD, Coppack S, Yudkin J. 1997. Endothelial dysfunction: cause of the insulin resistance syndrome. Diabetes 46:S9–S13.
55. Katakam PV, Ujhelyi MR, Hoenig ME, Miller AW. 1998. Endothelial dysfunction precedes hypertension in diet-induced insulin resistance. Am J Physiol 275:R788–R792.
56. Goodfellow J, Owens D, Henderson A. 1996. Cardiovascular syndromes X, endothelial dysfunction and insulin resistance. Diabetes Res Clin Pract 31 Suppl:S163–S171.
57. Baron AD. 1999. Vascular reactivity. Am J Cardiol 84:25J–27J.
58. Luscher TF, Barton M. 1997. Biology of the endothelium. Clin Cardiol:II-3–II-10.
59. De Meyer G, Herman A. 1997. Vascular endothelial dysfunction. Prog Cardiovasc Dis 39:325–342.
60. Schiffrin EL. 1994. The endothelium and control of blood vessel function in health and disease. Clin Invest Med 17:602–620.
61. Higashi Y, Oshima T, Sasaki S, Ishioka N, Nakano Y, Ozono R, Yoshimura M, Ishibashi K, Matsuura H, Kajiyama G. 1997. Relationship between insulin resistance and endothelium-dependent vascular relaxation in patients with essential hypertension. Hypertension 29:280–285.
62. Schroeder CA, Jr., Chen YL, Messina EJ. 1999. Inhibition of NO synthesis or endothelium removal reveals a vasoconstrictor effect of insulin on isolated arterioles. Am J Physiol 276:H815–H820.
63. Aljada A, Dandona P. 2000. Effect of insulin on human aortic endothelial nitric oxide synthase. Metabolism 49:147–150.
64. Kuboki K, Jiang ZY, Takahara N, Ha SW, Igarashi M, Yamauchi T, Feener EP, Herbert TP, Rhodes CJ, King GL. 2000. Regulation of endothelial constitutive nitric oxide synthase gene expression in endothelial cells and in vivo: a specific vascular action of insulin. Circulation 101:676–681.
65. Verma S, Arikawa E, Yao L, Laher I, McNeill JH. 1998. Insulin-induced vasodilation is dependent on tetrahydrobiopterin synthesis. Metabolism 47:1037–1039.
66. Verma S, Bhanot S, Yao L, McNeill JH. 1997. Vascular insulin resistance in fructose-hypertensive rats. Eur J Pharmacol 322:R1–R2.

67. Verma S, Yao L, Dumont AS, McNeill JH. 2000. Metformin treatment corrects vascular insulin resistance in hypertension. J Hypertens 18:1445–1450.
68. Verma S, Bhanot S, Yao L, McNeill JH. 1996. Defective endothelium-dependent relaxation in fructose-hypertensive rats. Am J Hypertens 9:370–376.
69. Kamata K, Yamashita K. 1999. Insulin resistance and impaired endothelium-dependent renal vasodilatation in fructose-fed hypertensive rats. Res Commun Mol Pathol Pharmacol 103:195–210.
70. Katakam PV, Ujhelyi MR, Miller AW. 1999. EDHF-mediated relaxation is impaired in fructose-fed rats. J Cardiovasc Pharmacol 34:461–467.
71. Miller AW, Katakam PV, Ujhelyi MR. 1999. Impaired endothelium-mediated relaxation in coronary arteries from insulin-resistant rats. J Vasc Res 36:385–392.
72. Frank HJ, Levin ER, Hu RM, Pedram A. 1993. Insulin stimulates endothelin binding and action on cultured vascular smooth muscle cells. Endocrinology 133:1092–1097.
73. Ferri C, Pittoni V, Piccoli A, Laurenti O, Cassone MR, Bellini C, Properzi G, Valesini G, De Mattia G, Santucci A. 1995. Insulin stimulates endothelin-1 secretion from human endothelial cells and modulates its circulating levels in vivo. J Clin Endocrinol Metab 80:829–835.
74. Anfossi G, Cavolot F, Massucco P. 1993. Insulin influences immunoreactive endothelin release by human vascular smooth muscle cells. Metabolism 42:1081–1083.
75. Cardillo C, Nambi SS, Kilcoyne CM, Choucair WK, Katz A, Quon MJ, Panza JA. 1999. Insulin stimulates both endothelin and nitric oxide activity in the human forearm. Circulation 100:820–825.
76. Verma S, Yao L, Stewart DJ, Dumont AS, Anderson TJ, McNeill JH. 2001. Endothelin Antagonism Uncovers Insulin-Mediated Vasorelaxation In Vitro and In Vivo. Hypertension 37:328–333.
77. Verma S, Bhanot S, McNeill JH. 1995. Effect of chronic endothelin blockade in hyperinsulinemic hypertensive rats. Am J Physiol 269:H2017–H2021.
78. Verma S, Skarsgard P, Bhanot S, Yao L, Laher I, McNeill JH. 1997. Reactivity of mesenteric arteries from fructose hypertensive rats to endothelin-1. Am J Hypertens 10:1010–1019.
79. Juan CC, Fang VS, Hsu YP, Huang YJ, Hsia DB, Yu PC, Kwok CF, Ho LT. 1998. Overexpression of vascular endothelin-1 and endothelin-A receptors in a fructose-induced hypertensive rat model. J Hypertens 16:1775–1782.
80. Yanagisawa-Miwa A, Ito H, Sugimoto T. 1990. Effects of insulin on vasoconstriction induced by thromboxane A2 in porcine coronary artery. Circulation 81:1654–1659.
81. Uderman HD, Jackson EK, Puett D, Workman RJ. 1984. Thromboxane synthetase inhibitor UK38,485 lowers blood pressure in the adult spontaneously hypertensive rat. J Cardiovasc Pharmacol 6:969–972.
82. Keen HL, Brands MW, Smith MJ, Jr., Shek EW, Hall JE. 1997. Inhibition of thromboxane synthesis attenuates insulin hypertension in rats. Am J Hypertens 10:1125–1131.
83. Galipeau D, Arikawa E, Sekirov I, McNeill JH. 2001. Chronic thromboxane synthase inhibition prevents fructose induced hypertension. Hypertension 38:877–883.
84. Reynolds E, Mok L. 1990. Role of thromboxane A2/prostaglandin A2 in the vasoconstrictor response of rat aorta to endothelin. J Pharmacol Exp Ther 252:915–921.
85. Zaugg C, Hornstein P, Zhu P, Simper D, Luscher TF, Allegrini P, Buser P. 1996. Endothelin-1 induced release of thromboxane A2 increases the vasoconstrictor effect of endothelin-1 in postischemic rat hearts. Circulation 94:742–747.
86. Muck AO, Seeger H, Korte K, Lippert TH. 1993. The effect of 17 beta-estradiol and endothelin 1 on prostacyclin and thromboxane production in human endothelial cell cultures. Clin Exp Obstet Gynecol 20:203–206.
87. Howarth S, Vallance P, Wilson C. 1995. Role of Thromboxane A2 in the vasoconstrictor response to endothelin-1, angiotensin II, and 5-hydroxytryptamine in human placental vessels. Placenta 16: 679–689.
88. Moreau P, Takase H, Luscher TF. 1996. Effect of endothelin antagonists on the responses to prostanoid endothelium-derived contracting factor. Br J Pharmacol 118:1429–1432.
89. Buyukgebiz O, Aktan A, Haklar G, Bilsel S, Dulger M. 1999. The effects of thromboxane synthase inhibition on reperfusion injury and endothelin-1,2 levels in allograft kidney transplantation in rats. Res Exp Med 198:289–298.
90. Horton TJ, Gayles EC, Prach PA, Koppenhafer TA, Pagliassotti MJ. 1997. Female rats do not develop sucrose-induced insulin resistance. Am J Physiol 272:R1571–R1576.
91. Hulman S, Falkner B. 1994. The effect of excess dietary sucrose on growth, blood pressure, and metabolism in developing Sprague-Dawley rats. Pediatr Res 36:95–101.

92. Gorodeski G, Utian W. 1999. Epidemiology and Risk Factors of Cardiovascular Disease in Postmenopausal Women. In: Treatment of the Postmenopausal Woman: Basic and Clinical Aspects Lobo RA, ed. 331–59. 2 ed. Philadelphia: Lipincott Williams & Wilkins.
93. Galipeau D, Verma S, McNeill JH. 2002. Female rats are protected against fructose induced changes in metabolism and blood pressure. Am J Physiol Heart Circ Physiol. 2002 Dec; 283(6):H2478–H2484.
94. Galipeau D, Yao L, McNeill JH. 2002. The relationship between hyperinsulinemia, insulin resistance, and hypertension is dependent on sex. Am J Physiol Heart Circ Physiol. 2002 Aug; 283(2):H562–H567.
95. Ruehlmann DO, Mann GE. 2000. Rapid non-genomic vasodilator actions of estrogens and sex steroids. Curr Med Chem 7:533–541.
96. Miller VM. 1999. Gender and vascular reactivity. Lupus 8:409–415.
97. Stevenson JC. 1998. Various actions of estrogens on the vascular system. Maturitas 30:5–9.
98. Brosnihan KB, Li P, Ganten D, Ferrario CM. 1997. Estrogen protects transgenic hypertensive rats by shifting the vasoconstrictor-vasodilator balance of RAS. Am J Physiol 273:R1908–R1915.
99. Freay AD, Curtis SW, Korach KS, Rubanyi GM. 1997. Mechanism of vascular smooth muscle relaxation by estrogen in depolarized rat and mouse aorta. Role of nuclear estrogen receptor and Ca2+ uptake. Circ Res 81:242–248.
100. Huang A, Sun D, Kaley G, Koller A. 1998. Estrogen preserves regulation of shear stress by nitric oxide in arterioles of female hypertensive rats. Hypertension 31:309–314.
101. Herrington D. 2000. Role of estrogens, selective estrogen receptor modulators and phytoestrogens in cardiovascular protection. Can J Cardiol 16 Suppl E:5E–9E.
102. Case J, Davison CA. 1999. Estrogen alters relative contributions of nitric oxide and cyclooxygenase products to endothelium-dependent vasodilation. J Pharmacol Exp Ther 291:524–530.
103. Kauser K, Rubanyi GM. 1994. Gender differences in the bioassayable endothelium derived nitric oxed from isolated rat aorta. Am J Physiol 267:H2311–H2317.
104. Browne M, Connolly C, Docherty JR. 1999. Vascular actions of 17beta-oestradiol in rat aorta and mesenteric artery. J Auton Pharmacol 19:291–299.
105. Valverde MA, Rojas P, Amigo J, Cosmelli D, Orio P, Bahamonde MI, Mann GE, Veragara C, Latorre R. 1999. Acute activation of maxi-K channels (hSlo) by estradiol binding to the beta subunit. Science 285:1929–1931.
106. Godsland IF. 1996. The influence of female sex steroids on glucose metabolism and insulin action. J Intern Med Suppl 738:1–60.
107. Polderman KH, Stehouwer CD, van Kamp GJ, Gooren LJ. 1996. Effects of insulin infusion on endothelium-derived vasoactive substances. Diabetologia 39:1284–1292.

III. DIABETES MELLITUS

G.N. Pierce, M. Nagano, P. Zahradka, and N.S. Dhalla (eds.).
ATHEROSCLEROSIS, HYPERTENSION AND DIABETES, Copyright © 2003.
Kluwer Academic Publishers. Boston.

NEW PARADIGM FOR INSULIN RESISTANCE: THE HISS STORY

W. WAYNE LAUTT

Department of Pharmacology & Therapeutics, Faculty of Medicine, University of Manitoba, 753 McDermot Avenue, Winnipeg, Manitoba R3E 0T6, Canada

Summary. There is increasing recognition that the insulin resistance state has its major pathogenic consequences in the post-meal period when the nutrients from the meal are being processed and glucose storage, normally primarily into skeletal muscle, is impaired thus leading to hyperglycemia, hyperinsulinemia, and hypertriglyceridemia. In this review I describe a recently discovered novel mechanism by which postprandial insulin action is potentiated and, when absent, results in severe postprandial insulin resistance. Injection of insulin causes release of HISS (hepatic insulin sensitizing substance) from the liver of fed rats. HISS actions account for 50–60% of the glucose disposal produced by a wide range of insulin doses (5–100 mU/kg). Although the chemical nature of HISS is unknown, precluding pharmacokinetic studies, the pharmacodynamics of HISS has advanced because of the use of a rapid insulin sensitivity test (RIST) which is a transient euglycemic clamp used following a bolus of insulin. HISS action can be blocked by hepatic denervation and restored by intraportal but not intravenous infusion of acetylcholine or nitric oxide donors. HISS release is prevented by blockade of hepatic muscarinic receptors, nitric oxide synthase blockers, indomethacin, and animal models of insulin resistance, including chronic liver disease, sucrose feeding, hypertension, and fetal alcohol exposure. HISS acts on skeletal muscle but liver, gut, or adipose tissue. HISS is released by insulin in the fed state but decreases to insignificance after 24-hour fasting in rats. Lack of HISS action is suggested to be the cause of post-meal hyperglycemia and hyperlipidemia in type 2 diabetes.

Address Correspondence to: W. Wayne Lautt, Department of Pharmacology & Therapeutics, Faculty of Medicine, University of Manitoba, 753 McDermot Avenue, Winnipeg, Manitoba R3E 0T6, Canada. Phone: (204)789-3391; Fax: (204)975-7784; e-mail: wlautt@cc.umanitoba.ca

***Key words*:** Insulin resistance, HISS, Hepatic nerves, Skeletal muscle, Nutrient partitioning, RIST, Obesity, Feeding, Postprandial, Nitric oxide, Cholinergic, Parasympathetic nerves, Glycogen, Glucose uptake

The HISS Story

Insulin levels rise after a meal.
Once thought to act only directly,
it now seems that insulin triggers some nerves
to release HISS to function correctly.

These nerves in the liver squirt Ach out,
to bind to the M_1 receptor.
The efferent pathway is fairly well known.
We do not yet know the detector.

The M_1 receptor makes NO pump out.
Which then causes secretion of HISS.
HISS acts on the muscle, much like insulin.
Insulin action is boosted like this.

When HISS acts on muscle, the glucose is stored
as glycogen rather than fat.
Does HISS add or synergize with insulin?
We still really do not know that.

Diabetics of type 2 have less HISS released —
more insulin must be secreted.
And after a few years of trying to cope —
the pancreas then is depleted.

To treat this condition we've played with some drugs
to mimic the neurotransmitter.
We hope, prior to eating, one might take a pill
to make HISS release so much better.

W. Wayne Lautt
January 1999

INTRODUCTION

The current paradigm for insulin resistance focuses on peripheral defects in insulin signaling with the majority of studies being carried out in the fasted state. While there can be no question that diabetes imparts an enormous risk factor for the development of cardiovascular disease, the continued focus on the fasting state appears misdirected. It has been suggested that hyperglycemia-induced overproduction of superoxide by the mitochondrial electron-transport chain accounts for the four main molecular mechanisms implicated in glucose-mediated vascular damage associated with blindness, renal failure, nerve damage, atherosclerosis, stroke, and hindlimb amputation [1]. The importance of the post-meal, rather than the fasting, metabolic status is amply demonstrated in a number of recent studies.

The relationship between HBA_{1c} and plasma glucose in patients with type 2 diabetes was determined at four time points during the day and found to be significantly predicted by plasma glucose levels measured only at post-lunch and extended post-lunch (5 hours) time points [2]. The strongest age- and sex-adjusted relative risk for all-cause and cardiovascular mortality were associated with 2 hour post-load plasma glucose levels [3]. Increased mortality risk has been associated with 2 hour post-load plasma glucose levels to a much greater extent than with fasting plasma glucose [4,5]. Isolated post-load hyperglycemia is a strong predictor of mortality [4,6,7,8,9,10]. Loss of post-meal glycemic control can account for the postprandial hyperglycemia and elevated insulin secretion known to occur in early stages of type 2 diabetes; the explanation for the post-meal hyperglycemia has generally been based upon observations suggesting that first phase insulin secretion is impaired to varying degrees (reviewed by 11).

The current approach of screening for type 2 diabetes using the fasted metabolic status, while convenient, is not effective. In a recent review evaluating the status of screening for type 2 diabetes, Engelgau et al., [6] stated that one of the criteria for appropriate screening is that the tests should detect the preclinical stage of disease and that the tests be shown to be acceptable and reliable. The conclusion that current screening recommendations are not consistent with available evidence was briefly reviewed. Evidence is accumulating that most people with a 54–67% range of impaired glucose tolerance have fasting glucose in the normal range. Pooled analysis of 20 different European studies showed as many as 31% who were diabetic according to post-challenge plasma glucose but had normal fasting values and therefore would not have been detected by a screening procedure based on fasting glucose measurements.

The recent discovery by our group of a physiological mechanism by which postprandial insulin action is doubled is consistent with recent perceptions that the current paradigm of insulin resistance has sufficient anomalies to require a re-examination and increased focus on the postprandial nutrition partitioning.

The HISS hypothesis

Fifty to sixty percent of the glucose disposal effect of an injection of insulin is actually dependent on the action of a putative hormone, tentatively named the hepatic insulin sensitizing substance (HISS), which is released from the liver and stimulates glucose uptake in skeletal muscle. Blockade of HISS action results in HISS-dependent insulin resistance (HDIR). HDIR may account in whole or in part for insulin resistance in many clinical conditions, including type 2 diabetes, obesity, chronic liver disease, fetal alcohol effects, and chronic hypertension [12]. HISS release and HISS action is maximal in the immediate postprandial period and declines progressively with the duration of fasting [13]. In a manner not yet completely understood, parasympathetic nerves are activated in the liver following a meal to signal the prandial status. In this condition, the insulin which reaches the liver causes pulsatile release of HISS. HISS enters the bloodstream and stimulates glucose uptake primarily into skeletal muscle [14,15]. Thus after a meal, the release of HISS from the liver causes a dramatic stimulation of glucose storage in skeletal muscle and effectively doubles the glucose disposal effect of a pulse of insulin. Insulin resistance thus occurs when HISS action is absent and this condition is referred to as HISS-dependent insulin resistance (HDIR).

Prandial control of HISS release

Insulin release occurs throughout the day in a pulsatile manner with only about 50% of insulin output being meal-regulated [16]. Insulin release occurs in rapid pulses with a period of about 10 minutes, including very large oscillations seen during sleep. Insulin secretion oscillates between 0–600 pmol/min with changes between minimum and maximum levels demonstrated to occur over 30 minute intervals. Even in conditions with continuous enteral nutrition, the mean amplitude of the oscillations reaches 50% of the mean levels for insulin secretion rate. In the postprandial state, the amplitude is maximal immediately after food ingestion and then decreases progressively [9,10].

Insulin is a complex hormone that carries out a number of other growth-related functions and pulsatile insulin release occurs in conditions throughout the day when food is not being absorbed from the intestines. It would be biologically inappropriate for insulin released in the fasting state to produce the same degree of glucose uptake from blood as is required in the absorptive postprandial state. In rats, we demonstrated the ability of insulin to release HISS from the liver at a maximal level immediately after eating and declining progressively with the duration of fasting until it was minor or insignificant after approximately a 24-hour fast in both anesthetized [13] and conscious animals [17]. The glucose disposal effect of a bolus of insulin administered in the postprandial state is double that produced by administration of the same dose of insulin in the fasted state or when the hepatic parasympathetic nerves have been blocked. Regulation of HISS release by insulin is thus an effective means to sensitize the body to insulin released following a meal but not in the fasted state. This suggests a physiological regulation by the hepatic parasympathetic nerves of the ability of insulin to release HISS. In this way the parasympathetic nerves are said to play a permissive regulatory role in HISS release. Thus, in the fasted state, a natural and physiologically regulated state of HDIR exists.

Dysfunction of the hepatic parasympathetic nerves due to any number of causes will also result in HDIR even in the fed state. It is in this condition that the insulin resistance leads to higher blood glucose levels and an increased need for the pancreas to secrete more insulin. As long as the pancreas is able to generate sufficiently large amounts of insulin, the insulin resistant state does not result in a true condition of diabetes. If however the pancreas is unable to rapidly and adequately control the blood glucose levels, the hyperglycemia leads to a wide range of symptoms associated with diabetes.

HDIR may account for the appearance of obesity in type 2 diabetes since HDIR results in a large decrease in the ability of skeletal muscle to store glucose. The elevated insulin levels will stimulate glucose uptake and storage in other tissues, primarily the liver, which has limited capacity. Once the storage capacity for glucose in the form of glycogen is saturated in the liver, excess glucose eventually will be converted to fat for storage in adipose tissues throughout the body.

The effect of HISS on postprandial nutrition partitioning is consistent with HDIR resulting in elevated postprandial levels of circulating triglycerides. Although it is well recognized that high fasting triglyceride levels are associated with the risk of increased coronary heart disease, there is evidence that postprandial rather than fasting triglycerides may be better predictors of coronary heart disease [18,19,20]. Thus atherogenesis could be considered a postprandial phenomenon [21] and may be a consequence of HDIR.

The duration of fasting required to result in HDIR has not been evaluated in humans. As stated previously, a 24-hour fast in rats is sufficient to represent a severe fast with HDIR being virtually complete. In contrast, an 18-hour fast in either cats [22,23,24] or dogs [25] still leaves 25–35% of the glucose disposal action of insulin being accounted for by HISS release.

Methods to detect HISS-dependent insulin action (HDIA)

The insulin tolerance test (ITT)

The ITT is quantitated from the degree of hypoglycemia caused by insulin administered as a pulse, either by rapid injection or a brief (5 minute) infusion. The hypoglycemia can be assessed in a number of ways including from the rate of development of hypoglycemia determined from the slope of the hypoglycemic curve, the nadir, the area under the hypoglycemic curve, or simply the degree of hypoglycemia measured at some convenient time before the counterregulatory hormones and hepatic sympathetic nerve-induced glycogenolysis complicates the test.

The first demonstration that peripheral insulin action was dependent on intact hepatic parasympathetic nerves used the ITT in overnight fasted cats [22]. Although the temporal relationship between fasting and the decrease in HDIA has not been studied in cats, it was serendipitous that we first used the cat model since the cat evolved as a gorge-feeder so that fasting for a cat is much less severe than fasting in the rat. In the overnight fasted cat, approximately 40% of insulin action was HISS-dependent. It was also serendipity that the dose of insulin selected for testing (100 mU/kg) did not produce such a severe hypoglycemia that the counterregulatory systems were activated. A similar dose (150 mU/kg) in the dog tested in the same way caused a considerably larger degree of hypoglycemia, which did cause counterregulation that was impaired by hepatic denervation so that denervation actually led to a greater hypoglycemia [26]. This example illustrates the primary difficulty with the use of the ITT to study HDIA. The ITT is, however, under appropriate conditions, able to demonstrate HDIA in both the cat [22] and rat (unpublished data).

Arterial-venous glucose gradients

The A-V gradient method has been used to detect HDIA in cats where the gradient changes across the extrahepatic splanchnic organs, liver, and hindlimb showed that denervation of the liver, atropine, or combination of the two maneuvers led to similar reductions in hindlimb but not liver or gut glucose uptake [15]. Hepatic denervation in the dog was confirmed to cause reduced hindlimb glucose uptake in response to insulin and reversal of the defect in response to intraportal acetylcholine [25]. Thus the A-V glucose gradient method is capable of detecting HDIA.

The rapid insulin sensitivity test (RIST)

The RIST was developed in 1995 [23] in order to avoid the hypoglycemia caused by the ITT. The RIST is simply a rapidly sampled euglycemic clamp in response to a pulse of insulin. The operating procedures for the RIST have been described [27,28] and the ability of the RIST to detect HDIA in rats has been compared with the ITT and the prolonged hyperinsulinemic euglycemic clamp (unpublished data).

Briefly, the RIST is carried out by establishing the glycemic baseline by taking arterial blood samples at 5 minute intervals until three consecutive measurements are stable. An insulin infusion is commenced (50 mU/kg administered over 5 minutes) and, after 1 minute, glucose samples are taken at 2 minute intervals and glucose is infused at a variable rate to maintain euglycemia. The test is completed when no more glucose is required. At the standard test dose of 50 mU/kg, the RIST is complete within 40 minutes. The RIST index is the amount of glucose that was required to maintain euglycemia.

The primary technical difficulties with this test are related to the need to take multiple rapid arterial blood samples. The solution is the use of a vascular shunt established between the femoral artery or the carotid artery and the femoral vein or jugular vein. The shunt drains blood from the artery, passes it through a segment of silicone catheter and directs it back into the venous compartment. Arterial glucose samples are obtained by needle puncture into the silicone tube and direct transfer of the blood sample (25 μL) to a glucose analyzer capable of providing a reading within 1–2 minutes. The shunt also allows intravenous infusions to be made through the shunt and arterial blood pressure to be monitored through a side branch of the shunt. Continuous monitoring of shunt blood pressure provides early warning of either venous or arterial obstruction. Determination of arterial pressure is obtained by briefly occluding the venous side of the shunt. The construction and use of the shunt is previously described [27]. The A-V shunt, blood sampling and pressure monitoring method has great applicability for many in vivo studies and is well tolerated in the conscious rat.

This method is equally effective in anesthetized or conscious rats and provides similar results related to HDIA and HDIR independent of pentobarbital anesthesia [17]. The impact of other anesthetics has not been assessed.

The RIST is able to be carried out routinely 4 sequential times in the same animal with some tests having been carried out up to 6 times with high reproducibility [27]. The RIST is sufficiently versatile to permit paired experimental designs showing, for example, a control response, development of HDIR following hepatic denervation, reversal of HDIR and restoration of normal HDIA by infusion of the parasympathetic neurotransmitter, acetylcholine, in the same animal on the same day [14]. Both the accuracy and precision of the test can be assessed from determination of the deviation from the ideal euglycemic target [27]. The remainder of this review describes what is known about the pharmacodynamics of HISS based on the RIST.

Quantitation of HISS-dependent insulin action (HDIA)

Because the chemical identity of HISS is not yet available, HDIA is determined entirely from whole body responses in the absence of pharmacokinetic data. The RIST provides two means of quantitating HDIA. The first is simply the use of the RIST index, that is, the total amount of glucose (mg/kg) required to maintain euglycemia after a pulse of insulin. The RIST is carried out in the control state and again after HISS release is blocked. The difference represents the HDIA [14]. HISS blockade by hepatic denervation, nitric oxide synthase antagonism, and atropine in fed rats result in disappearance of the HDIA, causing a reduction of 50–60% in the glucose disposal produced in response to a pulse of insulin.

The second method utilizes the dynamics of the curve of glucose infusion obtained during the RIST. Comparison of the dynamic curves by subtracting the post-blocked curve from the control curve reveals the dynamic pattern of HISS action [13,29].

The difference between the control RIST curve and the blocked RIST curve reveals the dynamic action of the HISS-dependent component. HISS action begins at about 3 minutes after onset of insulin administration at the standard test dose of 50 mU/kg and continues for about 9 minutes after the HISS-independent component of insulin action has ceased. The peak of HISS action occurs around the 15-minute point of the RIST and HISS action is no longer detectable after about 33 minutes. The observation that HDIA continues for 9 minutes after completion of the HISS-independent component suggests that HISS may act directly rather than to sensitize the tissue response to insulin [13].

The proportion of insulin action attributed to HDIA is similar at doses of insulin ranging from 5–100 mU/kg [13]. HDIA appears at similar onsets at all doses, rises at similar rates but reaches earlier and lower peak responses and acts for shorter durations with smaller insulin doses.

Pharmacological induction of HISS-dependent insulin resistance (HDIR)

Studies designed to illuminate the regulatory path of control of HISS release have provided several methods of producing full blockade of HISS release including hepatic denervation, blockade of hepatic muscarinic cholinergic receptors, hepatic nitric oxide (NO) synthase blockade, and hepatic cyclooxygenase (COX) blockade.

Hepatic denervation

The liver receives a rich supply of sympathetic and parasympathetic nerves and relays a wide range of sensory information via afferent nerves that reach the liver through the anterior hepatic plexus along the hepatic artery, the posterior plexus along the portal vein, and some fibers that are reported to exist in the hepatic ligaments and the vena cava. Although reflex sympathetic activation is transmitted through both the anterior and posterior plexus, the parasympathetic nerves of relevance to HISS release appear to pass only through the anterior plexus. Denervation of the anterior plexus of the cat liver resulted in insulin resistance that was not made worse by additional complete denervation of the liver or bilateral vagotomy [22] or by addition of atropine [23]. Denervation of the hepatic anterior plexus in the dog [25] caused HDIR. Anterior plexus denervation in the rat produced HDIR that was similar to that produced by atropine [23] thus showing that the denervation had produced full HDIR. Selective section of the hepatic branch of the vagus nerve or cervical bilateral vagotomy produced a similar degree of HDIR to that achieved by cutting the anterior plexus, demonstrating that the vagus sends nerves to the liver through the anterior plexus [30].

Hepatic muscarinic receptor blockade

We continue to find it surprising that the only effect that atropine appears to have that affects the RIST is to block HDIA. HDIR produced by hepatic denervation and atropine is equal in magnitude and HDIR produced by one procedure is not made worse by the addition of the second procedure [15]. The ED_{50} for atropine in the cat was 1 mg/kg with full HDIR produced at 3 mg/kg [23]. We used the same dose of 3 mg/kg in the initial rat studies and found the dose to be effective at producing a full HDIR with no limiting side effects [14]. Later studies comparing intravenous with intraportal atropine dose-response curves showed that the portal route required a lower dose (0.001 mg/kg) to produce a full block than did the i.v. route (0.01 mg/kg) [31]. Thus, although atropine, by virtue of its long half-life and the high doses used in our routine HISS blockade tests, would have likely blocked muscarinic receptors throughout the body, none of the blocked systems seemed to affect the RIST other than what could be accounted for by the production of HDIR. Similar responses are seen in fed conscious rats [30].

The observation that the selective muscarinic M_1 receptor antagonist, pirenzipine, was ten-fold more potent than the M_2 antagonist, methoctramine, suggests that the hepatic muscarinic receptor involved with HISS release is of the M_1 subtype, although this conclusion is very tentative because of the limited data and testing restricted to the cat.

Hepatic nitric oxide synthase (NOS) antagonism

As with many other systems regulated by parasympathetic nerves, the hepatic parasympathetic regulation of HISS release acts through generation of nitric oxide (NO). The NOS antagonists, L-NMMA and L-NAME, can both produce full HDIR that is not made worse by addition of atropine; the HDIR produced by hepatic denervation is not made worse by addition of NOS antagonists [32]. These data suggest that atropine, hepatic denervation, and NOS antagonism result in HDIR through the blockade of the same hepatic parasympathetic pathway. A submaximal dose of L-NMMA administered into the portal vein causes HDIR whereas the same dose administered intravenously has a minimal effect [32]. This demonstration confirms the hepatic nature of the blockade and also indicates that peripheral NOS blockade does not lead to altered insulin action as detected by the RIST. These conclusions are in contrast to those arrived at by Baron's group [33] who concluded that the insulin resistance produced by administration of NO synthase antagonists was secondary to blockade of NO release in skeletal muscle with a subsequent lack of vasodilator response to insulin accounting for reduced skeletal muscle glucose uptake. However, in our studies, the demonstration that low doses of intraportal but not intravenous NOS antagonists produce insulin resistance and that low doses of NO donors administered intraportally but not intravenously can restore insulin resistance indicates that the site of NO action controlling insulin sensitivity is hepatic and not a direct effect on skeletal muscle. Further, hindlimb blood flow did not change in response to insulin either in the innervated state where HISS action was shown nor in the hepatic denervated state where HISS action was blocked [25]. Full HDIR is achieved in rats using 2.5 mg/kg L-NAME but the duration of blockade is less than 1.5 hours; a dose of 5 mg/kg results in HDIR lasting for at least 2 hours [32]. Recent studies from the Portuguese team of Macedo has added further understanding of this pathway in that the nitric oxide is acting through hepatic cGMP [34].

Hepatic cyclooxygenase (COX) antagonism

As with many systems regulated by NO, prostaglandins also appear to be involved with HISS regulation. The non-selective COX antagonist, indomethacin, causes HDIR and intraportal administration is more effective than intravenous administration [35]. The role and the specific prostaglandin involved remain unknown.

Permissive nature of HISS control

The parasympathetic neural control of HISS release in response to a pulse of insulin is permissive in nature. In the fed state, the parasympathetic nerves permit a large release of HISS which accounts for at least 50% of glucose disposal that occurs in response to insulin. Hepatic denervation prevents HISS release, which can be restored fully to normal levels by intraportal administration of the parasympathetic neural transmitter, acetylcholine in rats [14] and dogs [25], or a NO donor in rats (SIN-1) [13]. The reversal of HDIR is produced by administering acetylcholine by constant infusion for at least 15 minutes prior to the RIST and throughout it, or by bolus administration of SIN-1 at least 15 minutes prior to insulin administration. No notable glucose responses appear during the stabilization period of drug administration but when insulin is administered, the RIST is dramatically potentiated back to normal levels. Thus, HDIA is not caused by cholinergic pulsation but rather a parasympathetic background tone allows insulin to cause release of HISS.

The tone of the parasympathetic permissive effect is physiologically regulated by the feed/fast status of the animal. HDIA progressively decreases with the duration of fasting [13,36]. Placement of food in the stomach of an anesthetized, 18 hour fasted rat results in the fasting-induced HDIR reversing toward levels seen in fed animals [13]. We do not know the signaling pathway that results in feeding leading to the parasympathetic-dependent sensitization of HISS release in response to insulin. Arterial blood glucose levels were not significantly different in fed or 18 hour fasted rats nor does glucose baseline relate to the magnitude of the RIST. Further, the status of glycogen stores is not involved with the signaling process since 4–6 consecutive RISTs can be carried out in the same animal resulting in uptake of 1.5 g glucose/kg body weight with insignificant alteration in the latter RISTs.

Fed anesthetized (pentobarbital) rats show no significant decline in RIST index over an 8 hour period [27], yet a fed rat that is fasted for 6 hours while conscious and is tested under anesthesia shows a significant decline in HDIA [13,36]; consecutive RISTs carried out over 6 hours in a conscious rat show a gradual decline with time with the RIST index decreasing by approximately 10% per hour of fasting over the first 6 hours [17]. The fed rat that is under anesthesia shows gastric paralysis so that the food in the stomach at the start of the experiment remains largely in place for the full duration of the test day. In contrast, rats that are fasted while conscious and tested under anesthesia, or conscious rats that are fasted over the course of the day when 4–6 RISTs are carried out, will show normal gastric emptying and will show a progressive decline in HDIA. Simple gastric distension cannot be eliminated as the feeding signal and would be compatible with these data. Whatever the prandial signal, feeding results in a parasympathetic permissive effect to result in HISS release in response to insulin in the fed but not fasted state. This is an extremely important point since most research and clinical diagnosis is done in the fasted state where HISS action is minimal or absent. While a 24-hour fast is sufficient to prevent significant HISS release in rats, 18-hour fasted cats [22] and dogs [25] still have 25–35% of insulin action accounted for by HISS.

Glucose disposal by IGF-1 is HISS-independent

The pharmacodynamics of the glucose disposal action of IGF-1 is readily quantitated using exactly the same procedure as is used to test insulin sensitivity using the RIST. A dose of 200 μg/kg of IGF-1 results in a similar degree of glucose uptake to that seen in response to 50 mU/kg insulin [37]. The dynamic pattern of glucose uptake of both compounds is similar when administered as a pulse (5 minute infusion). The pharmacodynamics of insulin is regulated by the hepatic parasympathetic-dependent release of HISS. The pharmacodynamics of IGF-1, in contrast, is completely independent of HISS release so that surgical denervation, atropine, or fasting is without effect on IGF-1 glucose disposal action [37]. This dramatic pharmacodynamic difference is important in that it has previously been reported that liver disease results in insulin but not IGF-1 resistance [38] and spontaneously diabetic rats become insulin but not IGF-1 resistant [39]. The comparison of the pharmacodynamics between IGF-1 and insulin is compatible with the presence of HDIR in the disease states, which would not affect the action of IGF-1.

The effect of pathologies on HISS pharmacodynamics

We have previously speculated and provided circumstantial evidence suggesting that insulin resistance seen in several disease states might be accounted for, at least in part, by HDIR [12,40]. This includes many, or most, forms of type 2 diabetes, insulin resistance seen in chronic liver disease, obesity, hypertension, and aging. This hypothesis has not been tested in any of these states in humans or other species and, therefore, pharmacodynamic data are not available.

To create a model of chronic liver disease, rats were subjected to double ligation and section of the bile ducts, which resulted in cholestasis and the eventual development of cirrhosis. When the animals were tested at 10 days post-ligation, they were still in good health and eating and drinking normally and were fully mobile, although showing jaundice. These animals showed severe insulin resistance that was not made worse by the administration of atropine, thereby suggesting that the insulin resistance was HDIR. Intraportal administration of acetylcholine, as done for the previously described denervation studies, resulted in full restoration of insulin action [41]. This observation has important therapeutic implications but, for the present discussion, strongly indicates that the liver was capable of producing and releasing HISS in response to a pulse of insulin if the background tone of parasympathetic nerves was mimicked through the use of infused acetylcholine.

We have also recently demonstrated (42, unpublished data) that alcohol administered to a pregnant rat through the drinking water results in alcohol dose-related insulin resistance in the adult offspring that is attributable to inhibition of HDIA. The HISS-independent component of insulin action was not altered in the adult offspring. When the HDIA dynamics are studied in normal animals by subtracting the post-atropine curve from the control RIST curve, the dynamic action of HISS is revealed. Similarly, when the RIST curves from adult offspring that had been exposed to alcohol in utero are subtracted from the RISTs obtained in the pair-fed control group, the difference is seen to strongly resemble the HDIA.

Further pharmacodynamic comparisons were made in the fetal alcohol exposure study based upon previous studies indicating that methods that block HISS release produce insulin resistance but not resistance to the glucose disposal action of IGF-1. The adult offspring of alcohol fed pregnant dams showed HDIR but normal pharmacodynamic responses to IGF-1 [37].

Sucrose feeding leads to HDIR [43]. After 9 weeks of feeding with normal rat chow and access to both normal water and a 32% sucrose solution, insulin resistance was produced that had the characteristics of HDIR.

HISS as a drug target

In a recent review evaluating new drug targets for type 2 diabetes and the metabolic syndrome, Moller [44] emphasized that current therapies for type 2 diabetes were developed in the absence of defined molecular targets or an understanding of disease pathogenesis. "These therapies have limited efficacy, limited tolerability and significant mechanism-based side effects. Of particular concern is the tendency for most treatments to enhance weight gain. Several current approaches are also associated with episodes of hypoglycemia, and few of the available therapies adequately address underlying defects such as obesity and/or insulin resistance." He further concluded that "Thus, newer approaches are definitely needed. Particular emphasis should be placed on finding and using mechanisms that are dependent on physiological responses and that result in weight loss". With the current, albeit fragmentary, understanding of the physiology and pathology related to HISS, it appears highly likely that targeting of this mechanism offers a novel approach to restoring normal physiological insulin sensitivity in skeletal muscle where the insulin resistance is generally acknowledged to primarily occur in many insulin resistant states.

The approach we are currently exploring is to mimic the hepatic parasympathetic feeding signal by the use of cholinergic agonists or nitric oxide donors so that the permissive signal will restore the ability of a pulse of insulin to release a pulse of HISS. This approach has been successfully demonstrated in the acute model of insulin resistance produced by surgical denervation of the liver in rats [14] and has been recently confirmed in dogs [25]. Insulin resistance produced by HDIR in a chronic liver disease model was also completely reversible by the provision of a cholinergic agonist directly to the liver [41].

ACKNOWLEDGEMENTS

Many trainees, support staff and collaborators have been instrumental in these studies most notably Hongsheng Xie, Dallas Legare, Parissa Sadri, Maria Genovey, and Paula Macedo. Manuscript preparation was greatly assisted by Karen Sanders. Conflict of interest declaration: the author is affiliated with DiaMedica Inc., the licensor of technology to diagnose and treat insulin resistance through the HISS pathway.

REFERENCES

1. Brownlee M. 2001. Biochemistry and molecular cell biology of diabetic complications. Nature 414:813–819.
2. Avignon A, Radauceanu A, Monnier L. 1997. Nonfasting plasma glucose is a better marker of diabetic control than fasting plasma glucose in type 2 diabetes. Diabetes Care 20:1822–1826.
3. de Vegt F, Dekker JM, Ruhé HG, Stehouwer CDA, Nijpels GBLM, Heine RJ. 1999. Hyperglycaemia is associated with all-cause and cardiovascular mortality in the Hoorn population: the Hoorn study. Diabetologia 42:926–931.
4. DECODE Study Group, on behalf of the European Diabetes Epidemiology Group. 1999. Glucose tolerance and mortality: comparison of WHO and American Diabetes Association diagnostic criteria. Lancet 354:617–621.
5. Hanefeld M, Fischer S, Julius U, Schulze J, Schwanebeck U, Schmechel H, Ziegelasch HJ, Lindner J. 1996. Risk factors for myocardial infarction and death in newly detected NIDDM: the Diabetes Intervention Study, 11-year follow-up. Diabetologia 39:1577–1583.
6. Engelgau MM, Narayan KMV, Herman WH. 2000. Screening for type 2 diabetes. Diabetes Care 23:1563–1580.
7. Vaccaro O, Ruffa G, Imperatore G, Iovino V, Rivellese AA, Riccardi G. 1999. Risk of diabetes in the new diagnostic category of impaired fasting glucose. Diabetes Care 22:1490–1493.

8. Shaw JE, Hodge AM, de Courten M, Chitson P, Zimmet PZ 1999. Isolated post-challenge hyperglycemia confirmed as a risk factor for mortality. Diabetologia 42:1050–1054.
9. Simon C, Brandenberger G. 2002. Ultradian oscillations of insulin secretion in humans. Diabetes 51(Suppl 1):S258–S261.
10. Simon C, Follenius M, Brandenberger G. 1987. Postprandial oscillations of plasma glucose insulin and C-peptide in man. Diabetologia 30:769–773.
11. Del Prato S, Tiengo A. 2001. The importance of first-phase insulin secretion: implications for the therapy of type 2 diabetes mellitus. Diabetes Metab Res Rev 17:164–174.
12. Lautt WW. 1999. The HISS story overview: A novel hepatic neurohumoral regulation of peripheral insulin sensitivity in health and diabetes. Can J Physiol Pharmacol 77:553–562.
13. Lautt WW, Macedo MP, Sadri P, Takayama S, Ramos FD, Legare DJ. 2001. Hepatic parasympathetic nerve-dependent control of peripheral insulin sensitivity is determined by feeding and fasting: dynamic control of HISS-dependent insulin action. Am J Physiol Gastrointest Liver Physiol 281:G29–G36.
14. Xie H, Lautt WW. 1996a. Insulin resistance caused by hepatic cholinergic interruption and reversed by acetylcholine administration. Am J Physiol 271:E587–E592.
15. Xie H, Lautt WW. 1996b. Insulin resistance of skeletal muscle produced by hepatic parasympathetic interruption. Am J Physiol 270:E858–E863.
16. Beyer J, Krause U, Dobronz A, Fuchs B, Delver JR, Wagner R. 1990. Assessment of insulin needs in insulin-dependent diabetics and healthy volunteers under fasting conditions. Horm Metab Res Suppl 24:71–77.
17. Latour MG, Lautt WW. 2002b. Insulin sensitivity regulated by feeding in the conscious unrestrained rat. Can J Physiol Pharmacol 80:8–12.
18. Patsch JR, Miesenbock G, Hopferwierser T, Muhlberger V, Knapp E, Dunn JK, Gotto Jr, AM, Patsch W. 1992. Relation of triglycerides metabolism and coronary artery disease. Studies in the postprandial state. Arteroscler Thromb 12:1336–1345.
19. Nikkila M, Solakivi T, Lehtimaki T, Koivula T, Laippala P, Astrom B. 1994. Postprandial plasma lipoprotein changes in relation to apolipoprotein E phenotypes and low density lipoprotein size in men with and without coronary artery disease. Atherosclerosis 106:149–157.
20. Karamanos BG, Thanopoulou AC, Roussi-Penesi DP. 2001. Maximal post-prandial triglyceride increase reflects post-prandial hypertriglyceridaemia and is associated with the insulin resistance syndrome. Diabetic Med 18:32–39.
21. Zilversmit DB. 1979. Atherogenesis. A postprandial phenomenon. Circulation 60:473–485.
22. Xie H, Tsybenko VA, Johnson MV, Lautt WW. 1993. Insulin resistance of glucose response produced by hepatic denervations. Can J Physiol Pharmacol 71:175–178.
23. Xie H, Lautt WW. 1995a. Induction of insulin resistance by cholinergic blockade with atropine in the cat. J Auton Pharmacol 15:361–369.
24. Xie H, Lautt WW. 1995b. M_1 muscarinic receptor blockade causes insulin resistance in the cat. Proc West Pharmacol Soc 38:83–84.
25. Moore MC, Satake S, Baranowski B, Hsieh P-S, Neal DW, Cherrington AD. 2002. Effect of hepatic denervation on peripheral insulin sensitivity in conscious dogs. Am J Physiol Endocrinol Metab 282:E286–E296.
26. Lamarche L, Yamaguchi N, Peronnet F. 1995. Hepatic denervation reduces adrenal catecholamine secretion during insulin-induced hypoglycemia. Am J Physiol 268:R50–R57.
27. Lautt WW, Wang X, Sadri P, Legare DJ, Macedo MP. 1998. Rapid insulin sensitivity test (RIST). Can J Physiol Pharmacol 76:1080–1086.
28. Xie H, Zhu L, Zhang YL, Legare DJ, Lautt WW. 1996. Insulin sensitivity tested with a modified euglycemic technique in cats and rats. J Pharmacol Toxicol Meth 35:77–82.
29. Takayama S, Legare DJ, Lautt WW. 1999. Dynamic control of the release of a hepatic insulin sensitizing substance. Proc West Pharmacol Soc 42:63–64.
30. Latour MG, Lautt WW. 2002a. The hepatic vagus nerve in the control of insulin sensitivity.
31. Takayama S, Legare DJ, Lautt WW. 2000. Dose-related atropine-induced insulin resistance: comparing intraportal versus intravenous administration. Proc West Pharmacol Soc 43:33–34.
32. Sadri P, Lautt WW. 1999. Blockade of hepatic nitric oxide synthase causes insulin resistance. Am J Physiol 277:G101–G108.
33. Baron AD, Zhu JS, Marshall S, Irsula O, Brechtel G, Keech C. 1995. Insulin resistance after hypertension induced by the nitric oxide synthesis inhibitor L-NMMA in rats. Am J Physiol Endocrinol Metab 269:E709–E715.

34. Correia NC, Guarino MP, Raposo J, Macedo MP. 2002. Hepatic guanylyl cyclase inhibition induces HISS dependent insulin resistance. Proc West Pharmacol Soc 45:57–58.
35. Sadri P, Lautt WW. 2000b. Insulin resistance caused by hepatic COX inhibition (abstract). Diabetes 49(Suppl 1):A245.
36. Macedo MP, Legare DJ, Lautt WW. 1998. Insulin sensitivity is reduced by fasting and elevated by feeding (abstract). N-S Arch Pharmacol 358(1)Suppl. 2:R558.
37. Sadri P, Lautt WW. 2000a. Glucose disposal by insulin, but not IGF-1, is dependent on the hepatic parasympathetic nerves. Can J Physiol Pharmacol 78:807–812.
38. Petersen KF, Jacob R, West AB, Sherwin RS, Shulman GI. 1997. Effects on insulin-like growth factor I on glucose metabolism in rats with liver cirrhosis. Am J Physiol 273:E1189–E1193.
39. Jacob R, Barrett E, Sherwin RS, Bowen L, Fryburg D, Fagin KD, Tamborlane WV, Shulman GI. 1991. Metabolic effects of IGF-1 and insulin in spontaneously diabetic BB/w rats. Am J Physiol 260:E262–E268.
40. Lautt WW. 1998. State of the Art 1997: Hepatic parasympathetic nerves and glucose metabolism. In: Liver and Nervous System. Falk Symposium No. 103. Ed. D Haussinger and K Jungermann, 1–14. UK: Kluwer Academic Publishers.
41. Lautt WW, Xie H. 1998. Intraportal acetylcholine reverses insulin resistance caused by chronic bile duct ligation. Proc West Pharmacol Soc 41:35–36.
42. Minuk GY, Meyers AFA, Legare DJ, Sadri P, Lautt WW. 1998. Fetal exposure to alcohol results in adult insulin resistance in the rat. Proc West Pharmacol Soc 41:39–40.
43. Ribeiro RT, Duarte-Ramos F, Macedo MP. 2001. The action of hepatic insulin sensitizing substance is decreased in rats on a high-sucrose diet. Proc West Pharmacol Soc 44:31–32.
44. Moller DE. 2001. New drug targets for type 2 diabetes and the metabolic syndrome. Nature 414:821–827.

G.N. Pierce, M. Nagano, P. Zahradka, and N.S. Dhalla (eds.).
ATHEROSCLEROSIS, HYPERTENSION AND DIABETES.

VANADIUM EFFECTS IN DIABETES

TOD A. CLARK and GRANT N. PIERCE

Cell Biology Laboratory, The National Centre for Agri-food Research in Medicine, And Division of Stroke and Vascular Disease, St. Boniface General Hospital Research Centre, The Department of Physiology, Faculty of Medicine, University of Manitoba, Winnipeg, Manitoba, Canada

Summary. Over the past twenty years vanadium compounds have garnered much attention with respect to the treatment of diabetes. Vanadium's attraction as a hypoglycaemic agent lies in its oral route of administration. Several different vanadium salts have been used to treat both Type 1 and Type 2 diabetes in vivo, including sodium orthovanadate, sodium meta-vanadate and vanadyl sulphate. In addition to the hypoglycaemic action of these agents, several biochemical and cellular changes common in diabetes have been positively affected. However, stepping from the animal model to the human diabetic patient has been hindered by the toxicity of these compounds. Gastrointestinal toxicity has been common while other complications including hepatotoxicity and body weight changes remain controversial. Many approaches are being investigated in attempts to reduce the toxicity of vanadium compounds. These include dosing alterations, combining vanadium with chelating agents, organic modification of the species itself and most recently combining nutraceuticals with the treatment. The anti-diabetic actions of vanadium salts and the toxicity of these substances are reviewed here with mention of the more recent approaches to limiting the toxicity.

***Key words*:** Diabetes mellitus, Insulin, Vanadate, Rat

INTRODUCTION

Diabetes mellitus exists in two different pathophysiologic forms, Type 1 and Type 2. Type 1 diabetes is characterized by a lack of circulating insulin while Type 2

Address for Correspondence: Grant N. Pierce, PhD, FACC, Director, National Centre for Agri-food Research in Medicine, St. Boniface General Hospital Research Centre, 351 Tache Avenue Winnipeg, Manitoba, Canada R2H 2A6. Tel: (204) 235-3414; Fax: (204) 231-1151; e-mail: gpierce@sbrc.ca

diabetes is a state of insulin resistance. Both result in high circulating blood glucose levels and complications to major organ systems. The diabetic patient is predisposed to atherosclerotic disease, retinopathy, peripheral neuropathy and renal failure. Currently, the best treatments available prolong the onset of these complications but do not eliminate them. Furthermore, current diabetic treatment, whether injections or orally dosed, is required daily and often many times each day to maintain normoglycemia. The constantly fluctuating glucose levels found with these treatment regimens are believed to account for many of the complications that persist in diabetes treatment.

For these reasons, the search for alternative therapies continues to grow. One of the more intriguing alternatives is vanadium, an ultratrace element with an unknown biologic function at physiologic doses [1]. For two centuries larger doses have been believed to possess hypoglycaemic potential [2]. Vanadium salts were the first species to be tested in vivo with promising hypoglycemic results compounded by some serious side effects [3]. Peroxovanadium compounds, organically modified vanadium species and the addition of synergistic substances are all currently being tested and will be discussed with respect to their efficacy. Emphasis will be placed on the relative toxicity of each. A limited number of human clinical trials have been completed and these results will be discussed as well.

VANADIUM SALTS AS EFFECTIVE AGENTS IN THE TREATMENT OF DIABETES

The in vivo use of vanadium in the treatment of diabetes stems from a pilot study in 1985. Vanadate administered to Type 1 diabetic rats over a four-week period restored blood glucose to non-diabetic control levels [3]. Subsequently, various vanadate (or vanadium salt) solutions have been exploited for their anti-diabetic properties. Irrespective of the salt solution used, it was shown that sodium orthovanadate, sodium metavanadate and vanadyl sulphate all possess equal hypoglycaemic effects [4]. Urine volume, glycosuria and glucose tolerance were equal in the three vanadate treated diabetic rat groups. Surprisingly, diabetic rats treated with vanadyl sulphate for three weeks remained normoglycemic 13 weeks after termination of the treatment [5].

One of the more common uses in vitro for vanadium compounds are as inhibitors of protein tyrosine phosphatases (PTPases). The role of liver PTPases in vivo is speculated to account for some the insulin mimetic effects of these agents. The enhanced action of protein kinases in the insulin-signalling cascade is a proposed mechanism of vanadate action in diabetes [6]. In fact significant decreases in PTPase activity were found in vanadate treated diabetic animals while markedly increased numbers of hepatic insulin receptors were also apparent [7]. Streptozotocin (STZ) induced Type 1 diabetic rats have reduced islet cell content and insulin secretion. However, with vanadate treatment these diabetic animals responded by increasing islet cell size and insulin content to near control levels [5]. However, the insulin secretion of these same cells was improved only 12% over the untreated diabetic rats. Also, it was shown that other hormones involved in glucose homeostasis including glucagon, corticosterone and noradrenaline are minimally affected by vanadate [8]. The mechanism of vanadium action in diabetes is therefore complex and multifactorial and is reviewed elsewhere [9–11]. Carbohydrate transport is reduced in diabetes primarily through a reduction in GLUT transporter volume and activity. Vanadate treatment has been shown to increase GLUT expression and transcription nearly back to non-diabetic levels [12]. Similarly, cardiac myocyte glucose oxidation and GLUT4 expression are reduced in diabetes. Vanadate treated myocytes responded with normal levels of glucose oxidation and improved GLUT4 expression [13,14]. In addition to the improved glucose response of vanadate treated animals, GLUT-5 expression is also increased and fructose transport is improved [15].

The lipid profile of the diabetic patient is altered drastically from the non-diabetic. The cholesterol and triglyceride changes partially account for the increased rates of atherosclerotic disease and myocardial infarction found in the diabetic population. Ten weeks of vanadate treatment to diabetic mice improved serum total cholesterol and triglyceride levels in combination with their hypoglycaemic actions [16]. Only 21 days of vanadate treatment was necessary to reverse the diabetic lipid profile in Type 1 diabetic rats. This included total lipids, cholesterol and triglycerides [17,18].

The leading cause of death in the diabetic population is cardiac in origin [19,20]. As a result, intense investigation has been placed on the cardiac effects of vanadium compounds. Cardiac performance has been shown to improve with vanadate treatment in diabetes [3]. One study attributed some of this effect to vanadate's ability to reverse diabetic hypothyroidism [21]. The free radical generating enzymes within the heart and vasculature show increased activity in diabetes. With vanadium treatment, diabetic rat levels of glutathione peroxidase, catalase and superoxide dismutase were corrected to near normal, while glycoproteins, plasma lipid peroxide and erythrocyte membrane phospholipids were restored to normal [22,23]. Cardiac lipoprotein lipase, reduced in diabetes and potentially atherogenic has also been restored to normal [24]. Vascular integrity has also been improved with vanadate treatment as evidenced by normalization of endothelin levels in STZ diabetic treated rats [25].

The multisystem effects of diabetes are not limited to the heart, vasculature and serum lipids however. Intestinal alterations in diabetes have also been analysed with respect to vanadium treatment. Increased sodium-dependent glucose transport and Na,K-ATPase activity in Type 1 diabetic rats was corrected with vanadate treatment while the decreased activity of intestinal 6-phosphofructo-1-kinase and 6-phosphofructo-2-kinase were also restored [26–29]. Carbohydrate metabolism relies heavily on the release of pancreatic amylase into the intestine and this is interrupted in diabetes. Vanadate induced normoglycemia was combined with the restoration of amylase transcription and activity in diabetic rats [30,31].

Many biochemical parameters altered in the diabetic state have been assessed to determine the effects of vanadate treatment on general metabolism, liver and renal function. Renal and hepatic glucose-6-phosphatase and fructose-1,6-bisphosphatase activities were returned to normal levels with vanadate [17,32]. Additionally it was found that plasma glutamic pyruvic transaminase, glutamic oxaloacetate transaminase [16], liver arginase activity and expression [33,34], pyruvate kinase expression and tyrosine aminotransferase gene expression [35] were positively affected with vanadium treatment. Increased mRNA synthesis of P-enolpyruvate carboxykinase (PEPCK) and other gluconeogenic enzymes implies improved glucose utilization by the liver [35,36]. Other hepatic indices improved with vanadate include tryptophan-niacin metabolism [37], hexokinase [38], hepatic lipase [24], glucose-6-phosphate [39] and protein C activites [40]. Renal dysfunction and kidney failure are common in diabetes as well. Blood urea nitrogen (BUN), a clinical index of renal disease, increases in diabetes and is reduced in vanadium treated rats [16]. Renal sorbitol, urinary albumin, IgG excretion and kidney size were also reduced with treatment [41,42].

VANADIUM SALTS AS INAPPROPRIATE AGENTS IN THE TREATMENT OF DIABETES

This data suggests vanadium exhibits a remarkable spectrum of anti-diabetic properties, and these are the reasons for its continued interest in the diabetic research community. However, vanadium salts continue to be heavily scrutinized for their toxic side effects [43,44]. These include gastrointestinal toxicity, diarrhea, dehydration and vanadium accumulation in vital organ systems [3,43,45–51]. Indeed, the severity of this toxicity has resulted in vanadate-induced death in animal models. In our laboratory, these results have been demonstrated in both Type 1 and Type 2 diabetic rats. When STZ-induced diabetic Sprague Dawley rats were treated with 2 ml of a 20 mg/ml sodium orthovanadate in water solution, diabetic hyperglycemia was effectively treated (Fig. 1) at the expense of severe toxicity. Over 70% of the diabetic rats orally gavaged with vanadate experienced diarrhea over the 11-week study and greater than 70% of these animals died during the course of the trial (Fig. 2). By comparison, non-diabetic control and diabetic animals gavaged with 2 ml of water alone experienced none of these side effects. In a model of Type 2 diabetes, we found similar results. When treated with sodium orthovanadate, the blood glucose levels of Zucker diabetic fatty rats were returned to near control levels (Fig. 3). The 15 mg vanadate/ml water solution gavaged to these animals produced diarrhea in over one half and resulted in the death of one animal over the 4-month trial (Fig. 4).

Appetite suppression and reduced water intake were some of the first effects noted with vanadium treatment in diabetes. Reduced water intake in diabetic animals is another sign of effective anti-diabetic action. The removal of glucose, an osmotic diuretic from the circulation reduces both polydipsia and polyuria. However, appetite suppression is more of a concern because it will result in reduced body weight gain during vanadate treatment [52,53]. The accumulation of vanadium in various organs has also been documented [50,54]. Although these studies have defined bone as the major reservoir for vanadium, no toxic effects have been found functionally or pathologically to date. While liver and kidney are also sites for vanadium storage, toxic effects on these organs are still debated [18,40].

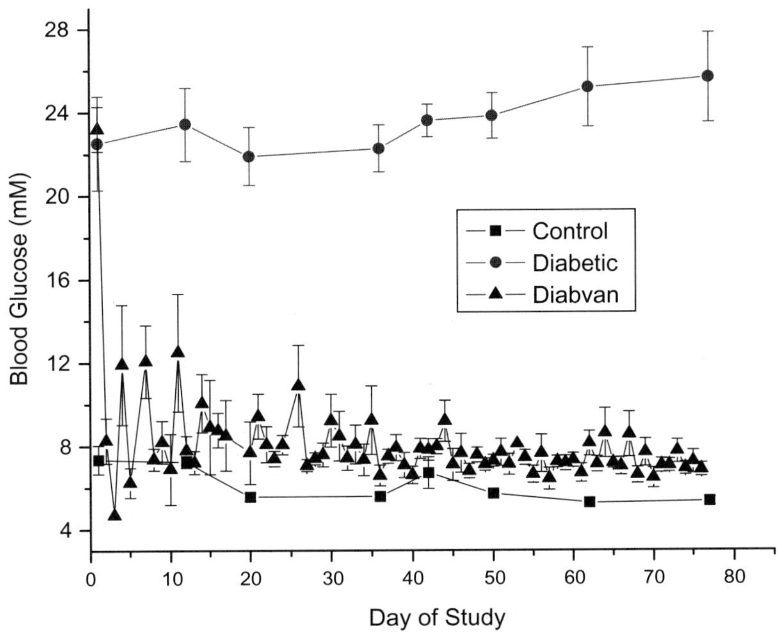

Figure 1. Blood glucose levels in non-diabetic control rats (Control), diabetic rats (Diabetic), and water/vanadate-treated diabetic rats (Diabvan). Values represent mean ± SE of n = 5, 5, and 7 respectively, in each group. *All Diabetic values $P < 0.0001$ vs. Control and Diabvan.

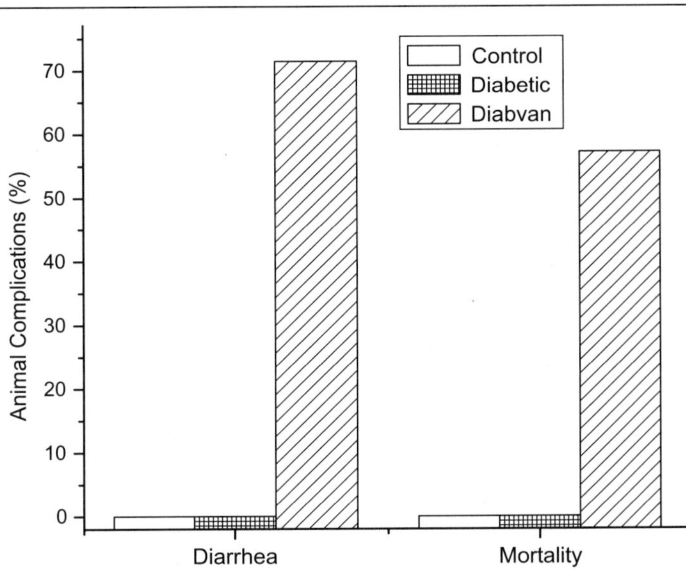

Figure 2. Incidence of diarrhea and death in non-diabetic control rats (Control) diabetic rats (Diabetic) and diabetic rats administered sodium orthovanadate with water (Diabvan). Values represent the % of total number of animals experiencing these parameters; n = 5, 5 and 7 in the Control, Diabetic and Diabvan groups respectively.

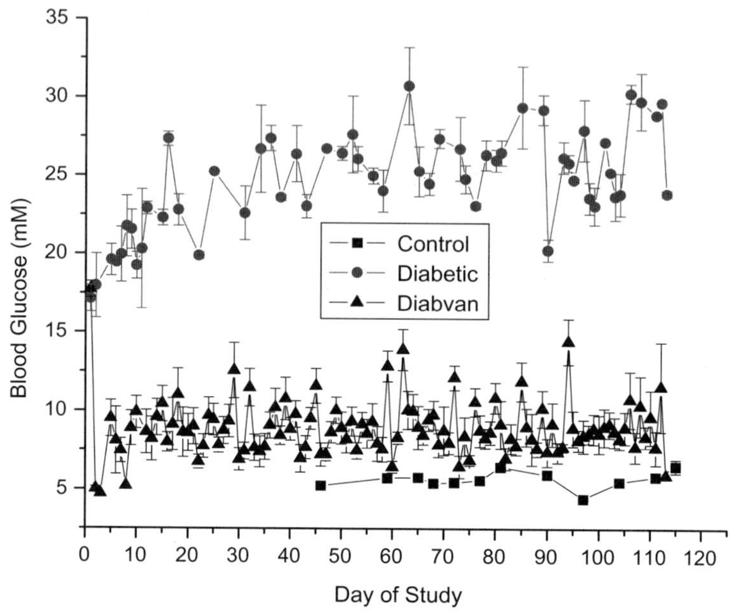

Figure 3. Blood glucose levels in non-diabetic control (Control), diabetic (Diabetic), and water/vanadate-treated (Diabvan) Zucker diabetic fatty rats. Values represent mean ± SE of n = 6, 6, and 9 respectively, in each group.

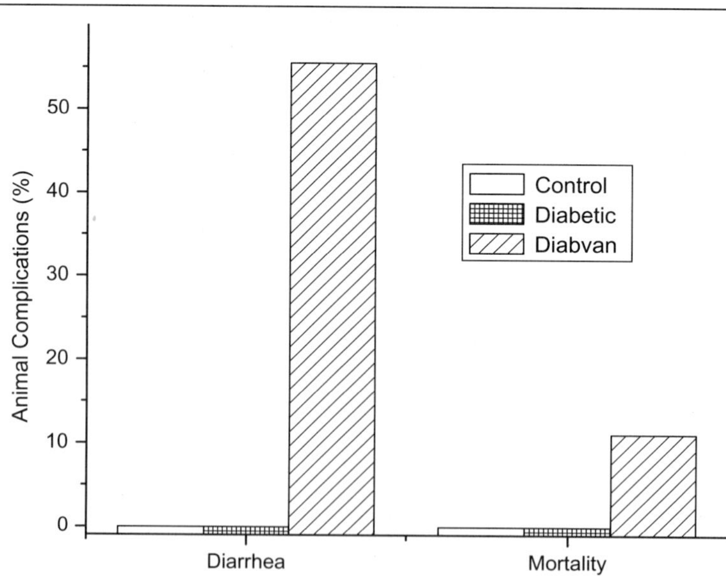

Figure 4. Incidence of diarrhea and death in non-diabetic control (Control), diabetic Zucker fatty (Diabetic) and diabetic Zucker fatty rats administered sodium orthovanadate with water (Diabvan). Values represent the % of total number of animals experiencing these parameters; n = 6, 6 and 9 in the Control, Diabetic and Diabvan groups respectively. *All Diabetic

In diabetic pregnancy, it has been shown that serum vanadium levels are much higher than expected, resulting in nearly 50% mortality in the dams. As well, reproductive capacity was decreased as evidenced by reduced live offspring [55,56]. A complete review of developmental and reproductive effects is cited [44].

In vitro effects of vanadium also point to potential toxicity. Cell culture exposure results in increased proliferation and differentiation of cells and is therefore potentially carcinogenic [57]. The mitogenic effects of the substance include activation of several proteins involved in phosphorylation including c-jun and junB [58,59]. By contrast, vanadium was also shown to possess cytotoxic effects, attributed to the action of vanadate on PTPases. Furthermore vanadium has been shown to inhibit cell adhesion and induce protooncogene expression [57,60].

The role of vanadium salts in the treatment of diabetes has undergone significant advances in the last 20 years. Beneficial effects on the diabetic state range from its hypoglycaemic actions down to effects on specific liver and plasma enzymes as outlined. However, it remains clear that the unknown long-term effects of vanadium accumulation and the known toxic complications of its treatment require further investigation prior to instilling this regimen into the human diabetics drug repertoire.

MODIFICATIONS TO VANADIUM COMPOUNDS

In an attempt to reduce toxicity, several methods of modifying the chemical structure of vanadium have been attempted. Organo-vanadium complexes were synthesized to increase uptake in the intestinal lining, as vanadium salts are poorly ingested [61]. Bis(maltolato)oxovanadium(IV) is one such species found to achieve antidiabetic effects at one half the dosage required of vanadium salts, with minimal toxicity [61]. The same group also found naglivan, another organo-vanadium compound, produced antidiabetic effects without overt signs of toxicity [62]. Vanadyl sulphate administration was directly compared to three newer organic complexes by Reul et al. with success [63]. All three compounds improved glycemic control and restored glycolytic enzyme function greater than vanadium salt therapy alone. Interestingly, this was independent of intestinal uptake as the same results were achieved with an intra-peritoneal route of administration.

The combination of vanadium compounds with hydrogen peroxide produces potent insulin-mimetic agents known as peroxo-vanadium (pV) complexes. While vanadate is known to function independent of the insulin receptor, pV's act on the insulin receptor and insulin receptor substrates [64,65]. By inhibiting the dephosphorylation of the insulin receptor, these substances potentiate the effects of insulin and as such may be useful as insulin adjuvants.

VANADIUM IN COMBINATION

The simplest method of alleviating the toxicity of vanadium compounds in diabetes treatment would appear to be through a reduction in the dosage of vanadate. Recently, it was found that much lower doses than previously used were effective in reducing blood glucose when given in combination with benzylamine [66]. By improving GLUT-4 recruitment and glucose transport in adipose tissue, minimal doses of vanadium incapable of acting as a hypoglycaemic alone possessed substantial effects in combination after as little as two-weeks. The synergistic combination of vanadium and magnesium (MgV) was also tested and found to have beneficial effects [67]. The MgV solution improved insulin sensitivity and glycogen synthesis in treated diabetic rats to a greater degree than V alone. Vanadium's pro-oxidant functions are believed to be detrimental in its use as an anti-diabetic agent. With the administration of the anti-oxidant U-83836E, significantly improved diabetic indices were found after 12 weeks of treatment [68]. Polydipsia, polyuria, glycosuria and hyperglycemia are further decreased with combination treatment while HbA1c and cataract formation were also reduced. The use of chelating agents in synergy with vanadium may also be a route to successful diabetic treatment. Tiron chelation of vanadium produced lower vanadium accumulations in both bone and kidney while not inhibiting the anti-diabetic properties of the agent [69,70]. The recent popularity of nutraceuticals, or functional foods led to another method of delivering vanadium. In combination with Trigonella seed powder, a hypoglycaemic material itself, vanadium restored glycemic control and altered enzymes to normal at a lower dosage [71].

HUMAN TRIALS

The use of vanadium in human diabetic patients is in its early stages. Small studies with Type 2 diabetic patients have been completed with moderate success. Improved cholesterol levels and insulin sensitivity were achieved as assessed by euglycemic, hyperinsulinemic clamp but in the absence of blood glucose control [72,73]. Fasting glucose levels have been reduced but with gastrointestinal complications [74]. These side effects were much less severe than those of animal trials and consisted of mild nausea, abdominal pain, gas, diarrhea and vomiting all of which decreased over time [43]. A comprehensive review of these trials is cited [75].

CONCLUSIONS

Current diabetes therapy involves daily therapy with intramuscular injections of insulin and/or oral hypoglycaemic agents in combination with diet and exercise. The inability of these agents to produce long-lasting normoglycemia requires their administration chronically and even several times daily. The resulting blood glucose fluctuations predispose patients to multi-system complications. As a result, extensive effort is involved in the search for a safe longer-lasting therapy. Vanadium compounds have been the focus of intense investigation over the past twenty years because of their anti-diabetic properties. These include general effects on glucose and specific actions on lipids, hepatic and renal indices as well as cardiac and intestinal function. In spite of toxicity issues, several new methods of administering the drug are being developed. These have lowered the dosage required and improved the actions of vanadium. Whether vanadium substances prove successful as a single diabetic therapy or not, their efficacy as adjuvant treatments in both Type 1 and Type 2 has tremendous potential if the toxic side-effects can be controlled or eliminated.

REFERENCES

1. Nielson F, Uthus E. 1990. The essentiality and metabolism of vanadium. In: N.D. Chasteen (ed.). Vanadium in Biological Systems. Kluwer Academic Publishers, Dordrecht 51–62.
2. Nielson FH. 1998. The nutritional essentiality and physiological metabolism of vanadium in higher animals. In: Vanadium Compounds. American Chemical Society, Washington 297–307.
3. Heyliger CE, Tahiliani AG, McNeill JH. 1985. Effect of vanadate on elevated blood glucose and depressed cardiac performance of diabetic rats. Science Mar 22;227:1474–1477.
4. Becker DJ, Ongemba LN, Henquin JC. 1994. Comparison of the effects of various vanadium salts on glucose homeostasis in streptozotocin-diabetic rats. Eur J Pharmacol 260:169–175.
5. Pederson RA, Ramanadham S, Buchan AM, McNeill JH. 1989. Long-term effects of vanadyl treatment on streptozocin-induced diabetes in rats. Diabetes 38:1390–1395.
6. Fantu IG, Deragon G, Lai R, Tang S. 1996. The insulin-mimetic agent vanadate promotes receptor endocytosis and inhibits intracellular ligand-receptor degradation by a mechanism distinct from the lysosomotropic agents. Diabetes 45:1084–1093.
7. Pugazhenthi S, Hussain A, Yu B, Brownsey RW, Angel JF, Khandelwal. 1995. Vanadate induces normolipidemia and a reduction in the levels of hepatic lipogenic enzymes in obese Zucker rat. Mol Cell Biochem 153:211–215.
8. Brichard SM, Ongemba LN, Kolanowski J, Henquin JC. 1991. The influence of vanadate on insulin counter-regulatory hormones in obese fa/fa rats. J Endocrinol 131:185–191.
9. Fantus IG, Tsiani E. 1998. Multifunctional actions of vanadium compounds on insulin signaling pathways: evidence for preferential enhancement of metabolic versus mitogenic effects. Mol Cell Biochem 182:109–119. Review.
10. Goldfine AB, Simonson DC, Folli F, Patti ME, Kahn CR. 1995. In vivo and in vitro studies of vanadate in human and rodent diabetes mellitus. Mol Cell Biochem 153:217–231. Review.
11. Orvig C, Thompson KH, Battell M, McNeill JH. 1995. Vanadium compounds as insulin mimics. Met Ions Biol Syst 31:575–594. Review.
12. Strout HV, Vicario PP, Biswas C, Saperstein R, Brady EJ, Pilch PF, Berger J. 1990. Vanadate treatment of streptozotocin diabetic rats restores expression of the insulin-responsive glucose transporter in skeletal muscle. Endocrinology 126:2728–2732.
13. Kopp SJ, Daar J, Paulson DJ, Romano FD, Laddaga R. 1997. Effects of oral vanadyl treatment on diabetes-induced alterations in the heart GLUT-4 transporter. J Mol Cell Cardiol 29:2355–2362.
14. Li SH, McNeill JH. 2001. In vivo effects of vanadium on GLUT4 translocation in cardiac tissue of STZ-diabetic rats. Mol Cell Biochem 217:121–129.
15. Hajduch E, Darakhshan F, Hundal HS. 1998. Fructose uptake in rat adipocytes: GLUT5 expression and the effects of streptozotocin-induced diabetes. Diabetologia 41:821–828.
16. Ding W, Hasegawa T, Hosaka H, Peng D, Takahashi K, Seko Y. 2001. Effect of long-term treatment with vanadate in drinking water on KK mice with genetic non-insulin-dependent diabetes mellitus. Biol Trace Elem Res 80:159–174.
17. Gupta D, Raju J, Prakash J, Baquer NZ. 1999. Change in the lipid profile, lipogenic and related enzymes in the livers of experimental diabetic rats: effect of insulin and vanadate. Diabetes Res Clin Pract 46:1–7.
18. Sekar N, Grovindasamy S. 1991. Effects of vanadate on plasma lipoprotein profiles in experimental diabetic rats. Biochem Int 23:935–940.
19. Seranno Rios M. 2001. Epidemiology of cardiovascular disease in type 2 diabetes. Int J Clin Pract Suppl 121:4–7. Review.
20. Janka HU. 1996. Increased cardiovascular morbidity and mortality in diabetes mellitus: identification of the high risk patient. Diabetes Res Clin Pract 30 Suppl:85–88. Review.
21. Ozcelikay AT, Yidizoglu-Ari N, Ozuari A, Ozturk Y, Altan VM. 1993. The effect of vanadate on alloxan-diabetic rat atria. Diabetes Res Clin Pract 19:189–194.
22. Matsubara T, Musat-Marcu S, Misra HP, Dhalla NS. 1995. Protective effect of vanadate on oxyradical-induced changes in isolated perfused heart. Mol Cell Biochem 153:79–85.
23. Sekar N, Kanthasamy A, William S, Balasubramaniyan N, Govindasamy S. 1990. Antioxidant effect of vanadate on experimental diabetic rats. Acta Diabetol Lat 27:285–293.

24. Levy E, Bendayan M. 1991. Lipoprotein lipase in experimental diabetic rats: beneficial effect of vanadate treatment. Diabete Metab 17:44–48.
25. Hopfner RL, Misurski D, Wilson TW, McNeill JR, Gopalakrishnan V. 1998. Insulin and vanadate restore decreased plasma endothelin concentrations and exaggerated vascular responses to normal in the streptozotocin diabetic rat. Diabetologia 41:1233–1240.
26. Madsen KL, Ariano D, Fedorak RN. 1995. Vanadate treatment rapidly improves glucose transport and activates 6-phosphofructo-1-kinase in diabetic rat intestine. Diabetologia 38:403–412.
27. Inoue H, Kaku K, Matsutani A, Tao T, Ayame H, Kaneko T. 1994. Insulin-like effects of vanadate on rat liver 6-phosphofructo-2-kinase/fructose-2,6-bisphosphatase mRNA and protein inductions in diabetic rats. Endocr J 41:75–82.
28. Madsen KL, Porter VM, Fedorak RN. 1993. Oral vanadate reduces Na(+)-dependent glucose transport in rat small intestine. Diabetes 42:1126–1132.
29. Hajjar JJ, Dobish MP, Tomicic TK. 1989. Reversal by vanadate of the effect of diabetes on intestinal growth and transport. Diabetes Res 10:139–141.
30. Johnson TM, Meisler MH, Bennett MI, Willsky GR. 1990. Vanadate induction of pancreatic amylase mRNA in diabetic rats. Diabetes 39:757–759.
31. Bendayan M, Gingras D. 1989. Effect of vanadate administration on blood glucose and insulin levels as well as on the exocrine pancreatic function in streptozotocin-diabetic rats. Diabetologia 32: 561–567.
32. Genet S, Kale RK, Baquer NZ. 1999. Effects of vanadate, insulin and fenugreek (Trigonella foenum graecum) on creatine kinase levels in tissues of diabetic rat. Indian J Exp Biol 37:200–202.
33. Salimuddin, Upadhyaya KC, Raju J, Baquer NZ. 1999. Modulation of mRNA levels of liver arginase by insulin and vanadate in experimental diabetes. Indian J Biochem Biophys 36:125–128.
34. Salimuddin, Upadhyaya KC, Baquer NZ. 1999. Effects of vanadate on expression of liver arginase in experimental diabetic rats. IUBMB Life 48:237–240.
35. Valera A, Rodriguez-Gil JE, Bosch F. 1993. Vanadate treatment restores the expression of genes for key enzymes in the glucose and ketone bodies metabolism in the liver of diabetic rats. J Clin Invest 92:4–11.
36. Miralpeix M, Carballo E, Bartrons R, Crepin K, Hue L, Rousseau GG. 1992. Oral administration of vanadate to diabetic rats restores liver 6-phosphofructo-2-kinase content and mRNA. Diabetologia 35:243–248.
37. Pandharpurkar S, Shastri NV. 1992. Effect of vanadate on tryptophan metabolism in streptozotocin diabetic rats. Indian J Biochem Biophys 29:519–521.
38. Sochor M, Kunjara S, Ali M, McLean P. 1992. Vanadate treatment increases the activity of glycolytic enzymes and raises fructose 2,6-bisphosphate concentration in hearts from diabetic rats. Biochem Int 28:525–531.
39. Sun Q, Sekar N, Goldwaser I, Gershonov E, Fridkin M, Shechter Y. 2000. Vanadate restores glucose 6-phosphate in diabetic rats: a mechanism to enhance glucose metabolism. Am J Physiol Endocrinol Metab 279:E403–E410.
40. Pugazhenthi S, Mantha SV, Khandelwal RL. 1990. Decrease of liver protein kinase C in streptozotocin-induced diabetic rats and restoration by vanadate treatment. Biochem Int 21:651–657.
41. Lohr JW, Bennett MI, Pochal MA, McReynolds J, Acara M, Willsky GR. 1991. Effect of vanadate on renal hypertrophy and sorbitol accumulation in streptozotocin induced diabetes in rats. Res Commun Chem Pathol Pharmacol 72:191–202.
42. Nakazawa A, Igarashi K, Tani N, Momotsu T, Ito S, Shibata A. 1991. Effect of vanadate on renal function in rats with streptozotocin-induced diabetes. J Diabet Complications 5:179–180.
43. Srivastava AK. 2000. Anti-diabetic and toxic effects of vanadium compounds. Mol Cell Biochem 206:177–182. Review.
44. Domingo JL. 1996. Vanadium: a review of the reproductive and developmental toxicity. Reprod Toxicol 10:175–182. Review.
45. Gil J, Miralpeix M, Carreras J, Bartrons R. 1987. Insulin like effects of vanadate on glucoskinase activity and fructose-2,6-bisphosphate levels in the liver of diabetic rats. J Biol Chem 262:6658–6662.
46. Brichard SM, Okitolonda W, Henquin JC. 1998. Long-term improvement of glucose homeostasis by vanadate treatment in diabetic rats. Endocrinology 123:2048–2053.
47. Blondel O, Bailbe D, Portha B. 1989. In vivo insulin resistance in streptozotocin diabetic rats—evidence for reversal following oral vanadate treatment. Diabetologia 32:185–190.

48. Ramanadham S, Mongold JJ, Brownsey RW, Cros GH, McNeill JH. 1989. Oral vanadyl sulphate in treatment of diabetes mellitus in rats. Am J Physiol 257:H904–H911.
49. Sakurai H, Tsuchiya K, Nakatsuka M, Sofue M, Kawada J. 1990. Insulin-like effects of vanadyl ion in streptozotocin induced diabetic rats. J Endocrinol 126:451–459.
50. Dai S, Thompson KH, Vera E, McNeill JH. 1994. Toxicity studies on one-year treatment of non-diabetic and streptozotocin-diabetic rats with vanadyl sulphate. Pharmacol Toxicol 75:265–273.
51. Domingo JL, Gomez M, Sanchez DJ, Llobet JM, Keen CL. 1994. Relationship between reduction in food intake and amelioration of hyperglycemia by oral vanadate in STZ-induced diabetic rats. Diabetes 43:1267, 1269–1270.
52. Malabu UH, Dryden S, McCarthy HD, Kilpatrick A, Williams G. 1994. Effects of chronic vanadate administration in the STZ-induced diabetic rat. The antihyperglycemic action of vanadate is attributable entirely to its suppression of feeding. Diabetes 43:9–15.
53. Wang J, Yuen VG, McNeill JH. 2001. Effect of vanadium on insulin sensitivity and appetite. Metabolism 50:667–673.
54. Mongold JJ, Cros GH, Vian L, Tep A, Ramanadham S, Siou G, Diaz J, McNeill JH, Serrano JJ. 1990. Toxicological aspects of vanadyl sulphate on diabetic rats: effects on vanadium levels and pancreatic B-cell morphology. Pharmacol Toxicol 67:192–198.
55. Ganguli S, Reuland DJ, Franklin LA, Tucker M. 1994. Effect of vanadate on reproductive efficiency in normal and streptozocin-treated diabetic rats. Metabolism 43:1384–1388.
56. Ganguli S, Reuland DJ, Franklin LA, Deakins DD, Johnston WJ, Pasha A. 1994. Effects of maternal vanadate treatment of fetal development. Life Sci 55:1267–1276.
57. Etcheverry SB, Cortizo AM. 1998. Vanadium bioactivity on cells in culture. In: Vanadium Compounds. American Chemical Society, Washington 270–276.
58. Wang H, Wang JY, Johnson LR, Scott RE. 1991. Selective induction of c-jun and jun-B but not c-fos or c-myc during mitogenesis in SV40-transformed cells at the predifferentiation growth arrest state. Cell Growth Differ 2:645–652.
59. Wang H, Scott RE. 1995. Unique and selective mitogenic effects of vanadate on SV40-transformed cells. Mol Cell Biochem 153:59–67. Review.
60. Stern A, Yin X, Tsang SS, Davison A, Moon J. 1993. Biochem Cell Biol 71:103–112. Vanadium as a modulator of cellular regulatory cascades and oncogene expression.
61. McNeill JH, Yuen VG, Dai S, Orvig C. 1995. Increased potency of vanadium using organic ligands. Mol Cell Biochem 153:175–180. Review.
62. Cam MC, Cros GH, Serrano JJ, Lazaro R, McNeill JH. 1993. In vivo antidiabetic actions of naglivan, an organic vanadyl compound in streptozotocin-induced diabetes. Diabetes Res Clin Pract 20:111–121.
63. Reul BA, Amin SS, Buchet JP, Ongemba LN, Crans DC, Brichard SM. 1999. Effects of vanadium complexes with organic ligands on glucose metabolism: a comparison study in diabetic rats. Br J Pharmacol 126:467–477.
64. Posner BI, Faure R, Burgess JW, Bevan AP, Lachance D, Zhang-Sun G, Fantus IG, Ng JB, Hall DA, Lum BS, et al. 1994. Peroxovanadium compounds. A new class of potent phosphotyrosine phosphatase inhibitors which are insulin mimetics. J Biol Chem 269:4596–4604.
65. Bevan AP, Drake PG, Yale JF, Shaver A, Posner BI. 1995. Peroxovanadium compounds: biological actions and mechanism of insulin-mimesis. Mol Cell Biochem 153:49–58. Review.
66. Marti L, Abella A, Carpene C, Palacin M, Testar X, Zorzano A. 2001. Combined treatment with benzylamine and low dosages of vanadate enhances glucose tolerance and reduces hyperglycemia in streptozotocin-induced diabetic rats. Diabetes 50:2061–2068.
67. Matsuda M, Mandarino L, DeFronzo RA. 1999. Synergistic interaction of magnesium and vanadate on glucose metabolism in diabetic rats. Metabolism 48:725–731.
68. Ugazio G, Bosia S, Burdino E, Grignolo F. 1994. Amelioration of diabetes and cataract by Na3VO4 plus U-83836E in streptozotocin treated rats. Res Commun Mol Pathol Pharmacol 85:313–328.
69. Domingo JL, Gomez M, Llobet JM, Corbella J, Keen CL. 1991. Improvement of glucose homeostasis by oral vanadyl or vanadate treatment in diabetic rats is accompanied by negative side effects. Pharmacol Toxicol 68:249–253.
70. Domingo JL, Bosque MA, Luna M, Corbella J. 1993. Prevention by Tiron (sodium 4,5-dihydroxybenzene-1,3-disulfonate) of vanadate-induced developmental toxicity in mice. Teratology 48:133–138.

71. Gupta D, Raju J, Baquer NZ. 1999. Modulation of some gluconeogenic enzyme activities in diabetic rat liver and kidney: effect of antidiabetic compounds. Indian J Exp Biol 37:196–199.
72. Goldfine AB, Simonson DC, Folli, Fpatti ME, Kahn CR. 1995. Metabolic effects of sodium metavanadate in humans with insulin-dependent and noninsulin-dependent diabetes mellitus in vivo and in vitro studies. J Clin Endocrinol Metab 80:3311–3320.
73. Cohen N, Halberstam M, Shlimovich P, Chang CJ, Shamoon H, Rossetti L. 1995. Oral vanadyl sulfate improves hepatic and peripheral insulin sensitivity in patients with non-insulin-dependent diabetes mellitus. J Clin Invest 95:2501–2509.
74. Boden G, Chen Z, Ruiz J, Van Rossum GDV, Turco S. 1996. Effects of vanadyl sulfate on carbohydrate and lipid metabolism in patients with non-insulin-dependent diabetes mellitus. Metabolism 45:1130–1135.
75. Goldfine AB, Willsky G, Kahn CR. 1998. Vanadium salts in the treatment of human diabetes mellitus. In: Vanadium Compounds. American Chemical Society, Washington. 353–368.

G.N. Pierce, M. Nagano, P. Zahradka, and N.S. Dhalla (eds.).
ATHEROSCLEROSIS, HYPERTENSION AND DIABETES.
Kluwer Academic Publishers. Boston.

DYSLIPOPROTEINEMIA AND FIBRINOLYSIS

GARRY X. SHEN

Diabetes Research Group, Department of Internal Medicine, University of Manitoba, Winnipeg, Manitoba, Canada

Summary. Fibrinolysis plays critical roles in the clearance of fibrin clots in vasculature, tissue modeling, embryo development and wound healing. Reduced fibrinolytic activity has been frequently found in patients with ischemic heart disease (IHD) and diabetes mellitus. Dyslipoproteinemia, characterized by increased low density lipoprotein (LDL), very low density lipoprotein (VLDL), lipoprotein(a) [Lp(a)] and decreased high density lipoprotein (HDL), is a common biochemical finding in IHD and diabetes. Previous studies by other groups and ours demonstrated that LDL, VLDL, Lp(a) and their oxidatively modified forms increased the generation of plasminogen activator inhibitor-1 (PAI-1), the major physiological inhibitor for fibrinolysis, from vascular endothelial cells (EC). LDL and Lp(a) reduced the release of tissue plasminogen activator (tPA) from EC. Our group recently demonstrated that glycation enhanced the effects of LDL and Lp(a) on the generation of fibrinolytic regulators from EC. Co-treatment with antixidants or HDL may normalize glycated LDL-induced changes in the fibrinolytic regulators from EC. LDL and VLDL isolated from diabetic patients induced greater increases in PAI-1 generation and further decreased tPA release from EC compared corresponding lipoproteins from healthy subjects. VLDL-responsive element was found in –672/–657 bp region of the PAI-1 promoter. The activation of PKC-β isoform is required for LDL, Lp(a) and their oxidized forms induced PAI-1 production in EC. This review summaries the recent findings on the impact and regulatory mechanism for lipoproteins-induced production of fibrinolytic regulators in vascular cells.

***Key words*:** Lipoproteins, Fibrinolysis, Vascular cells, Ischemic heart disease, Diabetes

Corresponding: Garry X. Shen, MD, PhD, FAHA, Diabetes Research Group, University of Manitoba, Department of Medicine, 835-715 McDermot Ave, Winnipeg, Manitoba, Canada R3E 3P4. Tel: 204-789-3816; Fax: 204-789-3987; e-mail: gshen@ms.umanitoba.ca

INTRODUCTION

Fibrinolysis is essential for maintaining normal blood circulation, tissue remodelling, and wound healing. The abnormalities of fibrinolytic activity have been implicated in a number of common disorders, including atherosclerosis, thrombosis, diabetic vascular complications, inflammation, restenosis and tumor matastasis [1]. The activity of fibrinolysis usually depends on the activities of their activators and inhibitors. The generation of the fibrinolytic regulators is modulated by the a variety of biological activators. The levels of fibrinolytic activity negatively correlated with dyslipoproteinemia, an important biochemical marker for ishemic heart disease (IHD) and diabetes mellitus (DM). This review will summarize the up-to-date information on the impact of plasma lipoproteins on fibrinolytic regulators and the relationship with IHD and DM.

DYSLIPOPROTEINEMIA IN IHD AND DM

Dyslipoproteinemia is characterized by increased levels of low density liprotein (LDL), very low density lipoprotein (VLDL) and decreased level of high density lipoprotein (HDL). Increased levels of LDL-cholesterol in plasma correlate to the incidence of IHD [2]. LDL particle is composed of a cholesterol-rich lipid core and an apolipoprotein (apo)B-100 molecule. LDL is the major cholesterol carrier for individuals with hypercholesterolemia. LDL may be further divided into subclasses based on their particle sizes and lipid composition. The levels of small, dense LDL are associated with high incidence of IHD [3]. Lipoprotein(a) [Lp(a)] differs from LDL with the presence of apo(a) and has been considered as another potent lipoprotein risk factor for premature cardiovascular disease [4]. VLDL, the precursor of LDL in plasma, contains an apoB-100 linked to a larger lipid core which is rich in triglycerides but poor in cholesterol compared to LDL. Increased levels of VLDL were associated with the development of IHD in some studies, but not in others [5,6]. HDL contains apoA-I and A-II, but not apoB. Increased levels of HDL in plasma have been considered as a strong negative risk factor for IHD [7].

The risk for cardiovascular diseases in diabetes is 2-fold or more greater than non-diabetic individuals. The most common lipid disorder in diabetic patients is hypertriglyceridemia with increased levels of VLDL or chylomicrons [8]. Elevated levels of triglycerides, chylomicrons and VLDL are prominent in untreated type 1 DM (insulin-dependent) that is associated with reduced lipoprotein lipase activity. Lipids and lipoproteins abnormalities in type 1 DM are usually normalized by conventional treatment. In untreated type 2 DM (non-insulin-dependent), chylomicronemia and hypertriglyceridemia are not as prominent as in type 1 DM without glucose control. VLDL and LDL concentrations in those patients are usually elevated and associated with reduced HDL-cholesterol. The increase in VLDL levels and the decrease in HDL-cholesterol are only partially related to glucose control in type 2 DM [9–11]. Small, dense LDL has been considered as another lipoprotein risk factor for IHD [12]. Increased proportion of small, dense LDL (LDL_3) has been found in diabetic patients. The sizes of LDL subclasses correlate with triglycerides levels but not with glucose levels in diabetic or normal subjects [13]. Increased triglyceride levels in LDL were found in small, dense LDL from type 2 DM, which were not normalized by insulin treatment [14]. In type 2 DM, high triglycerides and low HDL cholesterol are stronger risk factors for CHD than total or LDL cholesterol [15]. Increased levels of Lp(a) were found in the majority of the studies in type 2 DM and were associated with vascular complications [16–20].

MODIFICATION OF LIPOPROTEINS

Multiple types of residues of the components of lipoproteins, including fatty acids, cholesterol, phospholipids and apolipoproteins, may be oxidized by chemical, physical or long exposure to vascular cells. Numerous studies indicated that oxidation may increase the atherogenicity of lipoproteins, particularly LDL [21]. Oxidized LDL particles are strong ligands for scavenger receptors. Oxidation also enhanced the effects of LDL on thrombosis through stimulating platelet activation and coagulation or inhibiting fibrinolysis [22]. The antigen of oxidized LDL was immunohistochemically detected in human atherosclerotic lesions [23]. Increased levels of autoantibodies against oxidized LDL were detected in patients with IHD [24]. Amino acids and phospholipids containing free N-terminals, such as lysine, arginine, phosphatidylethanolamine and phosphatidylserine, may be non-enzymatically glycated. The levels of glycated LDL were higher in diabetic patients than non-diabetic subjects [25]. Glycation enhances oxidative stress of lipoproteins. The uptake of glyco-oxidized LDL by the classic LDL receptor was reduced but were increased by scavenger receptors in macrophages, which may contribute to the acceleration of the development of atherosclerosis in diabetic patients [26].

FIBRINOLYTIC ACTIVATORS AND INHIBITORS

Plasmin is the biologically active product of the fibrinolytic system. It catalyses the degradation of fibrin in blood or tissue. The precursor of plasmin is plasminogen, which is abundant in most of body fluid and usually serves as a limitless supply. The generation of plasmin is mainly regulated by tissue-type and urokinase-type plasminogen activators (tPA and uPA). tPA is the main PA in blood circulation. uPA is abundant in tissue. The activity of tPA and uPA is modulated by their inhibitors. Plasminogen activator inhibitor-1 (PAI-1) is the major physiological inhibitor for tPA and uPA [27]. Vascular EC and smooth muscle cells synthesize tPA, uPA and PAI-1. The receptors for plasminogen, tPA and uPA were detected on the surface of EC (Fig. 1). The generation of the fibrinolytic regulators in vascular cells may be modulated by a group of biological activators, including thrombin, interleukin-1, angiotensin II (AII), lipopolysacchride, transformation growth factor-β and multiple types of plasma lipoproteins [28].

FIBRINOLYTIC ACTIVITY IN PATIENTS WITH IHD AND DM

Impaired fibrinolytic activity characterized by elevated levels of PAI-1 with or without a reduction in tPA has been frequently found in IHD patients [29,30].

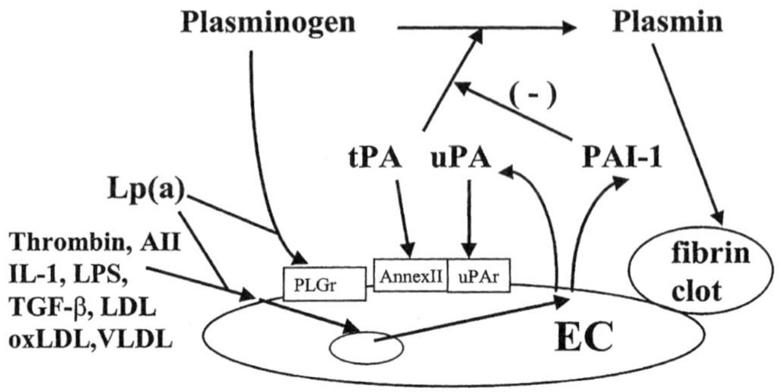

Figure 1. Scheme for fibrinolytic system. tPA: tissue-type plasminogen activator. uPA: urokinase-type plasmingen activator. PAI-1: plasminogen activator inhibitor-1. PLGr: plasminogen receptor. uPAr: uPA receptor. AII: angiotensin II. TGF-β: transforming growth factor-β. IL-1: interleukin-1. LPS: lipopolysacchride. LDL: low density lipoprotein. VLDL: very low density lipoprotein. Lp(a): lipoprotein(a). OxLDL: oxidized LDL.

Increases in PAI-1 protein and mRNA were detected in thrombotic lesions of arteries or veins [31]. Tests of fibrinolytic activity after vascular stimulation found that the release of fibrinolytic activity under stress was impaired in diabetic subjects [32–34]. Elevated plasma levels of PAI-1 were found in diabetic patients [35–39]. Strong correlations were found between PAI-1 and plasma insulin, body mass index, triglycerides or apoB in type 2 DM [40,41]. Immunohistochemical analysis revealed the presence of PAI-1 antigen in human coronary atherosclerotic lesions [42]. Increased plasma PAI activity, which represents the imbalance between PAI-1 and tPA in blood circulation, has been considered as a new risk factor for IHD.

EFFECTS OF LIPOPROTEINS ON PRODUCTION OF FIBRINOLYTIC REGULATORS IN VASCULAR CELLS

The first report for the effect of lipoproteins on the generation of fibrinolytic regulators from EC appeared in 1990. VLDL from hypertriglyceridemic subjects increased PAI-1 antigen from human umbilical vein EC (HUVEC) [43]. LDL or Lp(a) stimulated the transcription and secretion of PAI-1 from EC [44–48]. The effect of Lp(a) on EC-derived PAI-1 was >10-times stronger than LDL [48,49]. The sizes of LDL particles were inversely correlated to PAI-1 levels in a large tri-ethnic population [50]. Addition of LDL and Lp(a) reduced the release of tPA from HUVEC [51]. HDL did not evidently increase the generation of PAI-1 from EC [52]. The findings on the effects of HDL on the generation of tPA from EC were inconsistent [51,52] (Table 1).

IMPACT OF MODIFIED LIPOPROTEINS ON GENERATION OF FIBRINOLYTIC REGULATORS FROM VASCULAR CELLS

Oxidized LDL modified by ultraviolet or copper induced significantly greater production of PAI-1 from EC compared to native LDL [44–48]. Oxidation also enhanced

Table 1. Literatures on the effects and mechanism for lipoproteins-induced generation of fibrinolytic regulators from vascular EC

Authors	Year	Lipoproteins	Fibrinolytic regulators	Ref.
Stiko-Rahm et al.	1990	VLDL	PAI-1 ↑	43
Etingin et al.	1991	Lp(a)	PAI-1 ↑	49
Latron et al.	1991	oxLDL	PAI-1 ↑	45
Tremoli et al.	1993	LDL, oxLDL	PAI-1 ↑	44
Levin et al.	1994	LDL, Lp(a), HDL	tPA ↓, PAI-1 (–)	51
Erickson et al.	1998	VLDL via VLDL-RE	PAI-1 ↑	65
Zhang et al.	1998	glycated LDL	PAI-1 ↑, tPA ↓	56
Ren and Shen	2000	HDL normalizes	glycated LDL-induced PAI-1 ↑, tPA ↓	52
Ren et al.	2000	LDL, Lp(a), oxLDL oxLp(a) via PKC-β	PAI-1 ↑	74
Ren et al.	2002	LDL, VLDL from diabetic patients	PAI-1 ↑, tPA ↓	58

VLDL: very low density lipoprotein. LDL: low density lipoprotein. Lp(a): lipoprotein(a). oxLDL: oxidized LDL. HDL: high density lipoprotein. PAI-1: plasminogen activator inhibitor-1. tPA: tissue-type plasminogen activator. VLDL-RE: VLDL-responsive element. PKC: protein kinase C.

the effect of Lp(a) on the production in EC [48]. Recent studies suggest that O2★-/HO★ free radical oxidized LDL and Lp(a) decreased the release of PAI-1 from EC compared to copper-oxidized LDL and Lp(a). Further observation demonstrated that O2★-/HO★ free radical-oxidized LDL contained lower levels of oxidized lipid components (phosphatidylcholine hydroxyperoxides, lysophosphatidylcholine, 7-ketocholesterol, 7β-hydroxycholesterol, 5,6β-epoxycholesterol compared to copper-oxidized LDL [53]. Lipoproteins may be modified by prolonged incubation with EC, smooth muscle cells or monocytes. Increased PAI-1 production and decreased tPA release in EC induced by LDL was related to EC modification of the lipoprotein. Increased formation of lipid peroxidation products was found in EC-modified LDL. Co-treatment of LDL with antioxidants, butylated hydroxytoluene or vitamin E, normalized the changes in the generation of the fibrinolytic regulators induced by LDL in EC as well as lipid peroxidation products in LDL [52].

The levels of glycated LDL were increased in patients with diabetes [54,55]. Our group originally described the effects of glycated lipoproteins on the generation of fibrinolytic regulators from EC. Glycation of LDL with ≥25 mM of glucose in vitro for ≥2 weeks resulted in significant changes in generation of fibrinolytic regulators from EC compared to native LDL. Glycated LDL stimulated the production of PAI-1 production in EC at mRNA level. Glycated LDL decreased tPA generation without parallel reduction in tPA mRNA, but with the decline of the de novo synthesis of tPA in EC [56]. Glycation also enhanced the effect of Lp(a) on the generation of PAI-1 and tPA from EC [57]. Glycated HDL moderately increased the production of PAI-1 from EC but did not significantly affect tPA release compared to native HDL. Co-treatment with native or glycated HDL prevented glycated LDL-induced changes in the generation of PAI-1 or tPA from EC [52]. Our recent studies demonstrated that LDL from type 1 and type 2 DM patients and VLDL from type 2 DM patients increased the generation of PAI-1, and decreased the release of tPA from cultured EC compared to corresponding lipoproteins from healthy subjects [58]. The findings suggest that atherogenic lipoproteins glycated in vitro or in vivo affect the generation of fibrinolytic regulators from EC, which may contribute to attenuated fibrinolytic activity in diabetic patients.

TRANSCRIPTIONAL AND SIGNAL TRANSDUCTION MECHANISM FOR LIPOPROTEINS-INDUCED FIBRINOLYTIC REGULATORS FROM VASCULAR CELLS

LDL, Lp(a) or VLDL modulated the production of PAI-1 in EC at transcriptional level. The sequence of human PAI-1 promoter was documented in 1988 [59,60]. The proximal region of the PAI-1 promoter contains multiple responsive elements, include a AP-1 binding site-like sequence, for phorbol myristate acetate (PMA), a potent protein kinase C (PKC) agonist, and a homologue for cAMP-responsive element [61]. Responsive elements for transforming growth factor-β, glucocorticoids and VLDL-responsive element (VLDL-RE) locate distal regions of the PAI-1 promoter [62–65]. The VLDL-RE (−672/−657 bp) is adjacent to the region of 4G/5G polymorphism. This polymorphism is characterized by missing or inserting a guanine at −675 bp of the PAI-1 promoter to form GGGG (4G) or GGGGG (5G) [66]. Homozygous 4G allele polymorphism of the PAI-1 promoter is associated with higher plasma levels of PAI-1 compared to 5G/5G or 4G/5G allele. Correlation between 4G allele and IHD was found in some studies, but not in the others [67–69]. The binding site (−682/−675 bp) of a transcription activator (factor A) is adjacent to 4G/5G region and is present in both 4G or 5G alleles. The activation of the factor A is involved in the upregulation of PAI-1 transcription. A transcription repressor (factor B, −676/−670 bp) in the PAI-1 promoter is 5G allele-specific and its sequence is incomplete in 4G allele. VLDL activated the PAI-1 promoter with 4G allele in extents greater than that in 5G allele. This may be due to the lack of a functional transcription repressor in the PAI-1 promoter with 4G-allele. Unsaturated fatty acids, especially 18:3 and 20:5, activated the VLDL-RE in EC [70]. VLDL, Lp(a) and insulin, but not interleukin-1, activated −1106/+1 bp region of the PAI-1 promoter transfected in EC in a genotype-specific pattern [71]. Injection of LDL to rats induced the binding of AP-1 extracted from aortic wall to the proximal AP-1 binding site in the PAI-1 promoter [72]. The preliminary results from our group suggested that oxidized LDL and VLDL activate the PAI-1 promoter through a responsive element distinct from the VLDL-RE [73]. Signal transduction mechanism involved in lipoprotein-induced PAI-1 production has little been known. Phosphatidylinositol turnover may participate oxLDL-induced PAI-1 production in EC [46]. Activation of PKC-β is required for LDL, Lp(a) and their oxidized forms induced PAI-1 production in venous or arterial EC [74].

PHARMACOLOGICAL REGULATION ON THE GENERATION OF FIBRINOLYTIC REGULATORS

Previous studies indicated that fibrinolytic activity in the blood circulation of patients may be improved by various types of medications. Captopril, the first clinically available angiotensin converting enzyme (ACE) inhibitor, did not significantly affect the levels of PAI-1 or tPA in healthy subjects [75], but reduced PAI-1 and tPA levels in uncomplicated myocardial infarction patients [76]. Acute administration of losartan, an AII receptor-1 (AT1) antagonist, reduced PAI-1 and increased tPA in patients with chronic heart failure [77]. However, enalapril or losartan had no significant effect on PAI-1 in patients with essential hypertension [78]. The inhibitory effects of ACE inhibitors and AT1 antagonists on the PAI-1 generation in IHD patients may relate to the stimulating effect of AII on the oxidation of LDL [79].

Pravastatin, a HMG-CoA reductase inhibitor, reduced PAI-1 levels in hypercholesterolemic patients [80]. Our recent studies demonstrated that simvastatin reduced PAI-1 levels in type 2 DM patients. The levels of PAI-1 antigen in plasma of the diabetic patients correlated with total and LDL cholesterol. This suggests the effect of simvastatin on PAI-1 is associated with its effect of reduction of LDL-cholesterol in type 2 DM patients [81]. Estrogen lowered plasma PAI-1 in hypercholesterolemic post-menopausal women [82]. PAI-1 in plasma may come from other sources, such as adipocytes and hepatocytes. Significant increases in PAI-1 antigen and activity were found in obese individuals. Weight loss corrected with the increased level of PAI-1 and the attenuation of fibrinolytic activity in obese subjects [83].

The production of PAI-1 in cultured EC at basal or stimulated conditions may be reduced by the treatment with several types of drugs possibly improving endothelial function, including AT antagonists, statins or antioxidants. AT1 antagonist (DuP 735), but not AT2 antagonist (PD123319), inhibited AII induced overexpression of PAI-1 in vascular EC and smooth muscle cells [84]. Constitutive or tumor necrosis factor-α-induced production of PAI-1, but not tPA, in EC may be reduced by atorvastatin or fluvastatin [85]. Simvastatin reduced platelet-derived growth factor-induced PAI-1 secretion from EC [86]. Antioxidants, BHT and vitamin E, normalized native and glycated LDL-induced increases in PAI-1 production and the decrease in tPA generation from EC [52]. Pre-enrichment of oxidized or glycated LDL with vitamin E reduced PAI-1 production in EC [87]. The results suggest that EC-derived fibrinolytic activity may be safely improved by clinically available medications.

CONCLUSION

Dyslipoproteinemia is common in both IHD and DM. Atherogenic lipoproteins, LDL, Lp(a) and VLDL, may increase the generation of PAI-1 and/or decreased the release of tPA from vascular cells. Oxidation and glycation enhance the hypofibrinolytic effects of the atherogenic lipoproteins. The overproduction of PAI-1 in EC induced by oxLDL is mediated by the activation of PKC-β and the PAI-1 promoter. The generation of fibrinolytic regulators in EC induced by modified atherogenic lipoproteins may be modulated through treatment with clinically available medications, including statins, ACE inhibitors and AT1 antagonists.

ACKNOWLEDGEMENTS

The author would like to appreciate the important contributions from following trainees, including Dr. Kevin Cockell, Song Ren, Jianying Zhang, Lin Lu, Limei Hu, Shalini Shatada, Dr. Donfeng Sun, Dr. Sudharshan Dharmalingham, and collaborators, including Dr. Liam J Murphy, Dr. Harvey Lee and Dr. Sora Ludwig to relevant studies. The studies have been financially supported by Canadian Institute of Health Research, Canadian Diabetes Association, Heart and Stroke Foundation of Manitoba, Manitoba Medical Service Foundation, Manitoba Health Research Council, Health Sciences Centre Foundation, University of Manitoba, Dr. Paul HT Tholakson Foundation and St. James Kawanis Club.

REFERENCES

1. Folsom AR. 2000. Fibrinolytic factors and atherothrombotic events: epidemiological evidence. Ann Med 32 Suppl 1:85–91.
2. Assmann G, Schulte H. 1993. Results and Conclusions of the prospective cardiovascular Munster (PROCAM) study. In Lipid metabolism disorders and coronary heart disease. Ed. G. Assmann. 19–67. Munich. MMV Medizin Verlag.
3. Festa A, Agostino R Jr, Mykkanen L, Tracy R, Howard BV, Haffner SM. 1999. Low density lipoprotein particle sizes is inversely related to plasminogin activator inhibitor-1 levels. The insulin resistance atherosclerosis study. Arterioscler Thromb Vasc Biol 19:605–610.
4. Breckenridge WC. 1990. The role of lipoproteins and apolipoproteins in predication of coronary heart disease risk. Clin Invest Med 13:196–201.
5. Austin MA. 1999. Epidemiology of hypertriglyceridemia and cardiovascular disease. Am J Cardiol 83:13F–16F.
6. Crouse JR III, Furberg CD. 2000. Treatment of dyslipidemia. Room for improvement. Arterioscler Thromb Vasc Biol 20:2333–2335.
7. Kennel WB, Wilson PW. 1997. Efficacy of lipid profiles in prediction of coronary artery disease. Am Heart J 1992;124:768–74. Barter PJ, Rye RA, Clay MA. Anti-atherogenic effects of high density lipoproteins. Atherosclerosis 134:285–291.
8. Ginsberg HN. 1991. Lipoprotein physiology in nondiabetic and diabetic states. Relationship to atherosclerosis. Diabetic Care 14:839–855.
9. Austin MA, Breslow JL, Hennekens CH, Buring JE, Willett WC, Krauss RM. 1987. Low-density lipoprotein subclass patterns and risk of myocardial infraction. JAMA 260:1917–1921.
10. Stewart JM, Kilpatrick ES, Cathcart S, Small M, Domiiniczak MH. 1994. Low-density lipoprotein particle size in type 2 diabetic patients and age matched control. Ann Clin Biochem 31:153–159.
11. Austin MA, Edwards KL. 1996. Small dense low density lipoproteins, the insulin resistance syndrome and noninsulin-dependent diabetes. Curr Opin Lipidol 7:167–171.
12. James RW, Pometta D. 1991. The distribution profiles of very low density and low density lipoproteins in poorly-controlled mail, type 2 (non-insulin-dependent) diabetic patients. Diabetologia 34:246–252.
13. Laakso M. 1997. Dyslipidemia, morbidity, and mortality in non-insulin-dependent diabetes mellitus. Lipoproteins and coronary heart disease in non-insulin-dependent diabetes mellitus. J Diab Complic 11:137–144.
14. Krawczuk-Rybak M, Wojtowicz J, Urban M. 1991. State of lipid metabolism in children and adolescents with insulin-dependent diabetes. I. Evaluation of lipoprotein (A) behavior in children and adolescents with insulin-dependent diabetes. Endokrynol-Pol 42:437–445.
15. Irish AB, Simons LS, Simons J. 1992. Lipoprotein(a) concentration in diabetes: relationship to proteinuria and diabetes control. Aust NZ J Med 22:329–333.
16. Heller FR, Jamart J, Honore P, Derue G, Novik V, Galanti L, Parfonry A, Hondekijn JC, Buysschaert M. 1993. Serum lipoprotein(a) in patients with diabetes mellitus. Diabetes Care 16:819–823.
17. Murakami J, Kumasaka K, Kawano K, Murakami T, Hayashi Y, Arakawa Y. 1994. Lp(a) serum concentrations in diabetes mellitus. Rinsho-Byori 42:1273–1278.

18. Groop PH, Viberti GC, Elliott TG, Firedman R, Mackie A, Ehnholm C, Jauhiainen M, Taskinen MR. 1994. Lipoprotein(a) in type 1 diabetic patients with renal disease. Diabet Med 11:961–967.
19. James RW, Boemi M, Sirolla C, Amadio L, Fumelli P, Pometta P. 1995. Lipoprotein(a) and vascular disease in diabetic patients. Diabetologia 38:711–714.
20. Gall MA, Rossing P, Hommel E, Voldsgaard AI, Andersen P, Nielsen FS, Dyerberg J, Parving HH. 1992. Apolipoprotein(a) in insulin-dependent diabetic patients with and without diabetic nephropathy. Scand J Clin Lab Invest 52:513–521.
21. Steinberg D, Parthasarathy S, Carew TE, Khoo JC, Witztum JL. 1989. Beyond cholesterol. Modifications of low-density lipoprotein that increase its atherogenicity. N Engl J Med 320:915–24.
22. Wada H, Kaneko T, Wakita Y, Minamikawa K, Nagaya S, Tamaki S, Deguchi K, Shirakawa S. 1994. Effect of lipoproteins on tissue factor activity and PAI-II antigen in human monocytes and macrophages. Int J Cardiol 47(1 Suppl):S21–S25.
23. Itabe H, Takeshima E, Iwasaki H, Kimura J, Yoshida Y, Imanaka T, Takano T. 1994. A monoclonal antibody against oxidized lipoprotein recognizes foam cells in atherosclerotic lesions. Complex formation of oxidized phosphatidylcholines and polypeptides. J Biol Chem 269:15274–15279.
24. Erkkila AT, Narvanen O, Lehto S, Uusitupa MI, Yla-Herttuala S. 2000. Autoantibodies against oxidized low-density lipoprotein and cardiolipin in patients with coronary heart disease. Arterioscler Thromb Vasc Biol 20:204–209.
25. Lyons TJ, Baynes JW, Patrick JS, Colwell JA, Lopes-Virella MF. 1986. Glycosylation of low density lipoprotein in patients with type 1 (insulin-dependent) diabetes: correlations with other parameters of glycaemic control. Diabetologia. 29:685–689.
26. Lyons TJ. 1993. Glycation and oxidation: a role in the pathogenesis of atherosclerosis. Am J Cardiol 71:26B–31B.
27. Shen GX. 1998. Vascular cell-derived fibrinolytic regulators and atherothrombotic vascular disorders. Int J Mol Med 1:399–408.
28. Saksela O, Rifkin DB. 1988. Cell-associated plasminogen activation: regulation and physiological functions. Ann Rev Cell Biol 4:93–126.
29. Hamsten A, De Faire U, Walldius G, Dahlen G, Szamosi A, Blomback M, Landou C, Wiman B. 1987. Plasminogen activator inhibitor in plasma: risk factor for recurrent myocardial infarction. Lancet 2:3–9.
30. Cortellaro M, Cafrancesco E, Boschetti C, Mussoni L, Ponati MB, Cardillo M, Garbrielli L, Lombard B, Specchia G. 1993. Increased fibrin turnover and high PAI-1 antigen as predicator of ischemic event in atherosclerotic patients. The PLAT group. Arterioscler Thromb Vasc Biol 13:1412–1417.
31. Arnman V, Nilsson A, Stemme S, Risberg B, Rymo L. 1994. Expression of plasminogen activator inhibitor-1 mRNA in healthy, atherosclerotic and thrombotic arteries and veins. Thromb Res 74:487–499.
32. Geiger M, Binder BR. 1988. Plasminogen activation in diabetes mellitus. Kinetics of plasmin formation with tissue plasminogen activator and plasminogen from individual diabetic donors and with in vitro glycosylated plasminogen. Enzyme 40:149–157.
33. Auwerx J, Bouillon R, Collen D, Geboers J. 1988. Tissue-type plasminogen activator antigen and plasminogen activator inhibitor in diabetes mellitus. Arteriosclerosis 8:68–72.
34. Jokl R, Klein RL, Lopes-Virella MF, Colwell JA. 1995. Release of platelet plasminogen activator inhibitor 1 in whole blood is increased in patients with type II diabetes. Diabetes Care 18:1150–1155.
35. Matsuo T, Kadowaki S, Okada K, Matsuo O. 1990. Activity of tissue plasminogen activator and plasminogen activator inhibitor in noninsulin-dependent diabetes mellitus. J Diabet Complications 4:119–121.
36. Gough SC, Rice PJ, McCormack L, Chapman C, Grant PJ. 1993. The relationship between plasminogen activator inhibitor-1 and insulin resistance in newly diagnosed type 2 diabetes mellitus. Diabet Med 10:638–642.
37. Vicari AM, Vigano-D'Angelo S, Testa S, Comi G, Galardi G, Orsi E, D'Angelo A. 1992. Normal tissue plasminogen activator and plasminogen activator inhibitor activity in plasma from patients with type 1 diabetes mellitus. Horm Metab Res 24:516–519.
38. Ceriello A, Quatraro A, Marchi E, Barbanti M, Giugliano D. 1993. Impaired fibrinolytic response toincreased thrombin activation in type 1 diabetes mellitus: effects of the glycosaminoglycan sulodexide. Diabete Metab 19:225–259.
39. Carmassi F, Morale M, Puccett R, De-Negre F, Monzani F, Navalesi R, Mariani G. 1992. Coagulation and fibrinolytic system impairment in insulin dependent diabetes mellitus. Thromb Res 67: 643–654.

40. Davi G, Violi F, Catalano I, Giammarresi C, Putignano E, Nicolosi G, Barbagallo M, Notarbartolo A. 1991. Increased plasminogen activator inhibitor antigen levels in diabetic patients with stable angina. Blood Coagul Fibrinolysis 2:41–45.
41. Nagi K, Mohamed AV, Jain SK, Walji S, Yudlkin JS. 1996. Plasminogen activator inhibitor (PAI-1) activity is elevated in Asian and Caucasian subjects with non-insulin-dependent (type-2) diabetes but not in those with impaired glucose tolerance (IGT) or non-diabetic Asians. Diabet Med 13: 59–64.
42. Yorimitsu K, Saito T, Toyozaki T, Ishide T, Ohnuma N, Inagaki Y. 1993. Immunohistochemical localization of plasminogen activator inhibitor-1 in human coronary atherosclerosis lesions involved in acute myocardial infarction. Heart Vessels 8:160–162.
43. Stiko-Rahm A, Wiman B, Hamsten A, Nilsson J. 1990. Secretion of plasminogen activator inhibitor-1 from cultured human umbilical vein endothelial cells is induced by very low density lipoprotein. Arteriosclerosis 10:1067–1073.
44. Tremoli E, Camera M, Maderna P, Sironi L, Prati L, Colli S, Piovella F, Bernini F, Corsini A, Mussoni L. 1993. Increased synthesis of plasminogen activator inhibitor-1 by cultured human endothelial cells exposed to native and modified LDLs: An LDL receptor-independent phenomenon. Arterioscler Thromb 13:338–346.
45. Latron Y, Chautan M, Anfosso F, Alessi MC, Lafont H, Juhan-Vague I. 1991. Stimulating effect of oxidized low density lipoprotein on plasminogen activator inhibitor-1 synthesis by endothelial cells. Arterioscler Thromb 11:182–189.
46. Chauton M, Latron Y, Anfosso F, Alessi MC, Lafont H, Juhan-Vague I, Nalbone G. 1993. Phosphatidylinositol turnover during stimulation of plasminogen activator inhibitor-1 secretion induced by oxidized low density lipoproteins in human endothelial cells. J Lipid Res 34:101–110.
47. Kugiyama K, Sakamoto T, Ohgushi M, Ogawa H, Horiguchi M, Yasue H. 1993. Transferable lipids in oxidized low density lipoprotein stimulate plasminogen activator inhibitor-1 and inhibit tissue plasminogen activator release from endothelial cells. Circ Res 73:335–343.
48. Ren S, Man RYK, Angel A, Shen GX. 1997. Oxidative modification enhances lipoprotein(a)-induced overproduction of plasminogen activator inhibitor-1 in cultured vascular endothelial cells. Atherosclerosis 128:1–10.
49. Etingin OR, Hajjar KA, Harpel PC, Nachman RL. 1991. Lipoprotein(a) regulates plasminogen activator inhibitor-1 expression in endothelial cells. J Biol Chem 266:2456–2465.
50. Festa A, D'Agostino R Jr, Mykkanen L, Tracy R, Howard BV, Haffner SM. 1999. Low-density lipoprotein particle size is inversely related to plasminogen activator inhibitor-1 levels. The Insulin Resistance Atherosclersis Study. Arterioscler Thromb Vasc Biol 19:605–610.
51. Levin EG, Miles LA, Fless GM, Scanu AM, Baynhma P, Curtiss LK, Plow EF. 1994. Lipoproteins inhibits the secretion of tissue plasminogen activator from human endothelial cells. Arterioscler Thromb 14:438–442.
52. Ren S, Shen GX. 2000. Impact of antioxidant and HDL on glycated LDL-induced generation of fibrinolytic regulators from vascular endothelial cells. Arterioscler Thromb Vasc Biol 20:1688–1693.
53. Beaudeux JL, Therond P, Bonnefont-Rousselot D, Gardes-Albert M, Legrand A, Delattre J, Peynet J. 2001. Comparison of the effects of O2*-/HO* free radical- and copper-oxidized LDL or lipoprotein(a) on the endothelial cell release of tissue plasminogen activator and plasminogen activator inhibitor-1. Life Sci 69:2371–2382.
54. Bunn HF, Gabbay KH, Gallo PM. 1978. The glycosylation of haemoglobin: relevance to diabetes mellitus. Science 200:21–27.
55. Lyons TJ, Baynes JW, Patrick JS, Colwell JA, Lopes-Virella MF. 1986. Glycosylation of low density lipoprotein in patients with type I (insulin-dependent) diabetes: correlation with other parameters of glycaemic control. Diabetologia 29:685–689.
56. Zhang JY, Ren S, Sun DF, Shen GX. 1998. Influence of Glycation on LDL-induced Generation of Fibrinolytic Regulators in Vascular Endothelial Cells. Arterioscler Thromb Vasc Biol 18:1140–1148.
57. Zhang JY, Ren S, Shen GX. 2000. Glycation Amplifies Lipoprotein(a)-induced Alterations in the Generation of Fibrinolytic Regulators from Human Vascular Endothelial Cells. Atherosclerosis 150:299–308.
58. Ren S, Lee H, Hu L, Lu L, Shen GX. 2002. Impact of diabetes-associated lipoproteins on generation of fibrinolytic regulators from vascular endothelial cells. J Clin Endocr Metab 87:286–291.
59. Bosma PJ, van der Berg E, Kooistra T, Siemieniak DR, Slightom JL. 1988. Human plasminogen activator inhibitor-1. Promoter and structural gene nucleotide sequences. J Biol Chem 263:9129–9141.

60. Strandberg L, Awrence D, Ny T. 1988. The organization of the human-plasminogen-activator-inhibitor-1 gene. Implication on the evolution of the serine-protease inhibitor family. Eur J Biochem 176:609–616.
61. Deschemaeker KA, Wyns S, Nelles L, Auwerx J, Ny T, Collen D. 1992. Interaction of AP-1, AP-2, and Sp1-like proteins with two distinct sites in the upstream regulatory regions of the plasminogen activator inhibitor-1 gene mediates the phorbol 12-myristate 13-acetate response. J Biol Chem 267: 15086–15091.
62. Westrhausen DR Jr, Hopkins WE, Billadello JJ. 1991. Multiple transformation growth factor-β inducible elements regulate expression of the plasminogen activator inhibitor type-1 gene in Hep G2 cells. J Biol Chem 266:1092–1100.
63. Keeton MR, Curriden SA, van Zonneveld AJ, Loskutoff DJ. 1991. Identification of regulatory of sequences in the type-1 plasminogen a gene responsive to transformation growth factor-β. J Biol Chem 266:23048–23052.
64. Bruzdzinski CJ, Johnson MR, Goble CA, Winograd SS, Gelenrter TD. 1993. Mechanism of glucocorticoid induction of the rat plasminogen activator inhibitor-1 gene in HTC Rat hepatoma cells: Identification of cis-acting regulatory elements. Mol Endocrinol 7:1169–1177.
65. Eriksson P, Nilsson L, Karpe F, Hamsten A. 1998. Very-low-density lipoprotein response element in the promoter region of the human plasminogen activator inhibitor-1 gene implicated in the impaired fibrinolysis of hypertriglyceridemia. Arterioscler Thromb Vasc Biol 18:20–26.
66. Dawson S, Wiman B, Hamsten A, Green F, Humphries SE, Hanney AM. 1993. The two allele sequences of a common polymorphism in the promoter of the plasminogen activator inhibitor-1 (gene) respond differently to interleukin-1 in HepG2 cells. J Biol Chem 268:10739–10745.
67. Erikson P, Kallin B, van Hooft FM, Bavenholm P, Hamsten A. 1995. Allele-specific increase in basal transcription of the plasminogen-activator inhibitor-1 gene is associated with myocardial infarction. Proc Natl Acad Sci USA 92:1851–1855.
68. Margaglione M, Cappucci G, Colaizzo D, Giuliani N, Vecchione G, Grandone E, Pennelli O, Minno GD. 1998. The PAI-1 gene locus 4G/5G polymorphism is associated with a faminly history of coronary artery disease. Arterioscler Thromb Vasc Biol 18:152–156.
69. Ye S, Green FR, Scarabin PY, Nicaud V, Bara L, Dawson SJ, Humphries SE, Evans A, Luc G, Cambou JP, Arveiler D, Henney AM, Cambien F. 1995. The 4G/5G genetic polymorphism in the promoter of the plasminogen activator inhibitor-1 (PAI-1) gene is associated with differences in plasma PAI-1 activity but not with risk of myocardial infarction in the ECTIM study. Thromb Haemost 74:837–841.
70. Nilsson L, Banfi C, Diczfalusy U, Tremoli E, Eriksson P. 1998. Unsaturated fatty acids increase plasminogen activator inhibitor-1 expression in endothelial cells. Arteriosc Thromb Vasc Biol 18: 1679–1685.
71. Allison BA, Nilsson L, Karpe F, Hamsten A, Eriksson P. 1999. Effects of native, triglyceride-enriched, and oxidatively modified LDL on plasminogen activator inhibitor-1 expression in human endothelial cells. Arterioscler Thromb Vasc Biol 19:1354–1360.
72. Dichtl W, Stiko A, Eriksson P, Goncalves I, Calara F, Banfi C, Ares MP, Hamsten A, Nilsson J. 1999. Oxidized LDL and lysophosphatidylcholine stimulate plasminogen activator inhibitor-1 expression in vascular smooth muscle cells. Arterioscler Thromb Vasc Biol 19:3025–3032.
73. Lu L, Hu L, Ren S, Shen GX. 2001. Oxidized LDL and VLDL stimulates plasminogen activator inhibitor-1 promoter through a mechanism independent from the VLDL-response element Arterioscler Thromb Vasc Biol 21:641 (abstr).
74. Ren S, Shatadal S, Shen GX. 2000. Protein Kinase C-β Mediates Lipoprotein-induced Generation of PAI-1 from Vascular Endothelial Cells. Am J Physiol: Endocrinol & Metab 278:E656–E662.
75. Lottermiser K, Wostmann B, Weisser B, Hertfelder HJ, Schmitz U, Vetter H, Dusing R. 1999. Effects of catopril on fibrinolytic function in healthy humans. Eur J Med Res 4:31–34.
76. Wright RA, Flapan AD, Alberti KG, Ludlam CA, Fox KA. 1994. Effects of captopril therapy on endogenous fibrinolysis in men with recent, uncomplicated myocardial infarction. J Am Coll Cardiol 24:67–73.
77. Goodfield NE, Newby DE, Ludlam CA, Flapan AD. 1999. Effects of acute angiotension II type 1 receptor antagonism and angiotensin converting enzyme inhibition on plasm fibrinolytic parameters in patients with heart failure. Circ 99:2983–2985.
78. Li-Saw-Hee FL, Beever DG, Lip GY. 2001. Effect of antihypertensive therapy using enalapril or losartan on haemostatic markers in essential hypertension: a pilot prospective randomised double blind parallel group trial. Int J Cardiol 78:241–246.

79. Keidar S, Kaplan M, Hoffman A, Aviram M. 1995. Angiotensin II stimulates macrophage-mediated oxidation of low density lipoproteins. Atherosclerosis 115:201–215.
80. Wada H, Mori Y, Kaneko T, Wakita Y, Nakase T, Minamikawa K, Ohiwa M, Tamaki Tanigawa M, Kageyma S. 1993. Elevated plasma levels of vascular endothelial cell markers in patients with hypercholesterolemia. Am J Hematol 44:112–116.
81. Dharmalingam S, Ludwig S, Ren S, Fenton JW II, Velthius HT, Ofosu FA, Shen G. 2001. Simvastatin reduces plasma levels of plasminogen activator inhibitor-1 in patients with type 2 diabetic patients. Can J Diabetes Care 25:194 (abstr).
82. Koh KK, Cardillo C, Bui MN, Hathaway L, Csalo G, Waclawiw MA, Panza JA, Cannon RO III. 1999. Vascular effects of estrogen and cholesterol lowering therapies in hypercholesterolemic postmenopausal women. Circ 99:354–360.
83. Estelles A, Dalmau J, Falco C, Berbel O, Castello R, Espnan F, Aznar J. 2001. Plasma PAI-1 levels in obese children-effect of weight loss and influence of PAI-1 promoter 4G/5G genetype. Thromb Haemost 86:647–652.
84. Feener EP, Northrup JM, Aiello LP, King GL. 1995. Angiotensin II induces plasminogen activator inhibitor-1 and -2 expression in vascular EC and smooth muscle cells. J Clin Invest 95:1253–1262.
85. Lopez S, Peiretti F, Bonardo B, Juhan-Vague I, Nalbone G. 2000. Effect of atorvastatin and fluvastatin on the expression of plasminogen activator inhibitor type-1 in cultured human endothelial cells. Atherosclerosis 152:359–366.
86. Boucier T, Libby P. 2000. HMG-CoA reductase inhibitors reduce plasminogen activator inhibitor-1 expression by human vascular smooth muscle and endothelial cells. Arterioscler Thromb Vasc Biol 20:556–562.
87. Jenkins AJ, Li W, Moller K, Klein RL, Fu MX, Baynes JW, Thorpe SR, Lyons TJ. 1999. Pre-enrichment of modified low density lipoproteins with alpha toco[herol mitigates adverse effect on cultured retinal capillary cells. Cur Eye Res 19:137–145.

G.N. Pierce, M. Nagano, P. Zahradka, and N.S. Dhalla (eds.).
ATHEROSCLEROSIS, HYPERTENSION AND DIABETES.
Kluwer Academic Publishers. Boston.

ENDOTHELINS AND CARDIOVASCULAR DISEASE IN DIABETES

SUBRATA CHAKRABARTI

Department of pathology, The University of Western Ontario, London, Ontario, Canada

Summary. Cardiovascular affection is a major cause of mortality and morbidity in the diabetic population. Secondary to hyperglycemia, several abnormal metabolic pathways may be activated in diabetes. Some of these pathways may lead to alteration of the endothelins (ETs). ETs, due to their diverse biological action, may act as an effector molecule in the pathogenesis of diabetes associated lesions in the heart and vasculature. This review will discuss the mechanisms and implication of ET alteration in the pathogenesis of cardiovascular complications of diabetes.

***Key words*:** Diabetic complications, Cardiomyopathy, Atherosclerosis, Endothelins

INTRODUCTION

It is estimated that about 6% of the North American population suffers from diabetes mellitus [1–4]. Chronic diabetic complications are responsible for substantial number of morbidity and mortality in this population [1]. Although, due to improved management of glucose homeostasis, diabetics today can have a longer lifespan, most people with this disorder go on to develop chronic complications leading to damage of various organs. Chronic diabetic complications include diabetic neuropathy, nephropathy, retinopathy, cardiomyopathy and macroangiopathic complications like atherosclerosis. The macrovascular complications are not diabetes

Address Correspondences to: Dr. Subrata Chakrabarti, Dept. of Pathology, University of Western Ontario, Dental Sc. Bldg, Room 4011, London, ON, Canada, N6A 5C1. Phone: (519)-661-2111, X85545; Fax: 519-663-2930; e-mail: schakrab@uwo.ca

specific but are more pronounced in diabetics. Cardiovascular complication of diabetes include macrovascular atherosclerosis affecting large and medium sized arteries and cardiomyopathy. In addition cardiac function in diabetics are also affected by autonomic neuropathy. Salient pathologic features of chronic diabetic complications affecting the heart are described below.

CARDIOVASCULAR COMPLICATIONS IN DIABETES

Diabetes may involve the heart in several ways, nemely: coronary artery disease, autonomic neuropathy and diabetic cardiomyopathy. In addition, both atherosclerosis and hypertension occur at a much higher rate in diabetics compared to the non-diabetic counterpart [5–7]. Insulin resistance, if present, may further accelerate atherosclerosis [6].

Diabetic patients develop congestive cardiac failure more readily and have significantly worse prognosis than their non-diabetic counterparts once they develop coronary disease [7,8]. Diabetic individuals are 2 to 4 times more likely to have heart disease compared to their non-diabetic counterparts and 75% of diabetes related deaths are due to heart disease [9]. Primary affection of cardiomyocytes in diabetes, i.e, diabetic cardiomyopathy can act as the independent factor affecting the cardiac structure, function and may also modulate prognosis of other complications such as ischemic heart disease [7–10]. It was demonstrated that diabetics had larger mean diameter of right ventricular myocardial cells and higher percentage of interstitial fibrosis than the control subjects [8,10,11]. Morphological changes in the diabetic cardiomyopathy include myocyte hypertrophy and/or necrosis, interstitial and perivascular fibrosis and capillary basement membrane thickening [8,10,11]. Functional abnormalities involve both the systolic and diastolic properties of the myocardium, such as impaired relaxation, reduced compliance with elevated end diastolic pressure, cardiac hypertrophy and chamber dilatation. Cardiac autonomic neuropathy may manifest as prolongation of R-R interval in the electrocardiogram [8–12].

Atherosclerosis involving medium or large areteries or macroangiopathy is the major cause of mortality in diabetic patients. Although atherosclerosis is not diabetes specific, diabetes mellitus is one independent risk factor for atherosclerosis along with hyperlipidemia, hypertension, and smoking. Coronary atherosclerosis and subsequent myocardial infarction is a leading cause of death in the diabetic population [13,14]. In diabetes, carotid stenosis secondary to an increase intimal and medial wall thickness, has been associated with an increased risk of stroke. Furthermore, a direct relationship of carotid artery wall thickness with blood glucose levels in diabetics has been noted [14]. Lower extremity arterial disease (LEAD) has been considered to be among the major indication for amputation in individuals with diabetes. The progression of LEAD in diabetes is compounded by such co-morbidity as peripheral neuropathy and insensitivity of the feet and lower extremities to pain and trauma [14,15].

ENDOTHELIN(ET)S AND THEIR RECEPTORS

ETs are 21 amino acid vasoactive peptides with widespread tissue distribution. They cause vasodilation at lower concentrations and sustained contraction at high concentrations. Three ET isoforms, namely: ET1, ET2, and ET3 are encoded by three distinct genes [16,17]. The encoded precursor proteins are broken down by endopeptidases to produce big ETs. Endothelin converting enzymes (ECEs) then convert these big ETs into mature ET peptides. Among the two ECEs, ECE1, mainly located on the cell surface, has four isoforms (ECE1a–d) [18–23]. However ECE1b isoform and ECE2 have been localized intracellularly in close proximity to golgi network [22].

ETs act on specific receptors (ET_A and ET_B). ET_A has high affinity for ET-1 and ET-2 but low affinity for ET-3 and is primarily involved in vasoconstriction [24]. ET_B, on the other hand, is equally responsive to all isoforms and is involved in vasodilation as it increases nitric oxide (NO) generation [25]. In some cells these receptors are coupled to voltage gated calcium channels while in others they lead to activation of phospholipase C. The vasoconstrictive property seems to be due to the increase in calcium which results from activation of phospholipase C and production of diacylglycerol and inositol trisphosphate. The differential responsiveness of ET_A receptors to various agonists and antagonists suggests that there exist subtypes of the receptor [26–34]. However, no conclusive study has favored the postulate. Radioligand binding studies conducted in the late 1990s have contradicted the idea of existence of ET_A subtypes [35,36]. This suggests that ET_A responsiveness to various stimulators and inhibitors depends on the intrinsic properties of the ligands. However, similar studies on potencies of ET antagonists on ET_B receptor have suggested the existence of two receptor subtypes, ET_{B1} and ET_{B2} [33,34,37,38].

Hypoxia and ischemia are two important conditions which may lead to ET-upregulation [39,40]. However, at the molecular level several important intracellular molecules may regulate ET mRNA expression in health and disease [41–48].

PATHOGENETIC MECHANISMS LEADING TO ET ALTERATION IN CHRONIC DIABETIC COMPLICATIONS

Hyperglycemia-induced metabolic alterations leading to changes in the structural and functional properties of macromolecules may be one of the major mechanisms in the pathogenesis of chronic diabetic complications [49,50]. Glucose induced abnormal mechanisms, that may participate in the pathogenesis of diabetic complications include protein kinase C (PKC) activation, non-enzymatic glycation, oxidative stress, abnormality in growth factor and vasoactive factor expression, and endothelial damage. Some of these mechanisms and how they may lead to ET alteration in diabetes are outlined below. A diagrammatic representation of these interdependent mechanisms leading to ET alteration in chronic diabetic complications are outlined in Fig. 1.

PKC activation

In diabetes, high glucose concentrations may induce the production of diacylglycerol and activation of PKC in several organs [49–51]. Several hyperglycemia-induced abnormalities such as vascular permeability and flow changes, expansion of extracellular matrix, and the production of various growth factors and cytokines may be mediated via PKC [52–58]. PKCβ, has been shown to be activated in several tissues

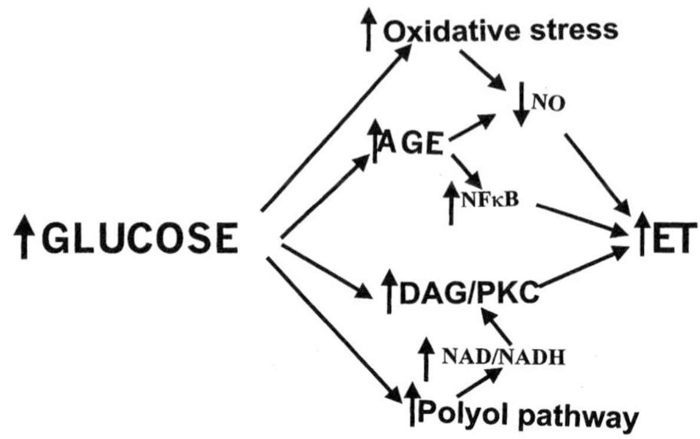

Figure 1. Glucose induced interdependent mechanisms that may lead to increased ET production in diabetes.

that are affected by chronic diabetic complications. PKC activation also leads to activation of phospholipase A and production of arachidonic acid metabolites, impairment of Na^+-K^+-ATPase and endothelial damage [59,60]. Studies on PKC activation and ETs have suggested an interaction between the two factors. We and others have demonstrated that endothelial cells exposed to ET-1 or a PKC activator show similar permeability changes as seen in hyperglycemia [50,52,53]. These changes are prevented when cells are treated with ET receptor antagonists or PKC inhibitors. Furthermore, structural changes such as F-actin microfilament assembly secondary to glucose also occur via PKC activation and ET-1 upregulation [52].

Polyol pathway and redox state

Polyol pathway activation, accumulation of sorbitol and accompanying cellular damage has been extensively studied. Glucose is converted to sorbitol via augmented polyol pathway. Aldose reductase, the enzyme responsible, has been shown to be upregulated in several tissues affected by chronic diabetic complications [53,61]. Increased intracellular concentration of sorbitol can cause osmotic changes, cell swelling, abnormalities in myoinositol metabolism and can lead to impairment of Na^+-K^+-ATPase. Aldose reductase inhibition has been shown to prevent hyperglycemia-induced damage in diabetic cataract, retinopathy, neuropathy, and nephropathy to some extent [53,62,63]. The mechanism by which aldose reductase inhibition prevents development of vascular complications is not fully understood. Aldose reductase requires NADH and NADPH for the conversion of glucose to sorbitol. This suggests that an imbalance in the redox state, i.e. altered NADH : NAD and NADPH : NADP might share some responsibility for endothelial dysfunction secondary to increased aldose reductase activity [53,61]. Interestingly, depleted NADPH may also lead to reduced NO activity [61,64]. As eluded later, decreased NO may lead to ET-1 upregulation.

Non-enzymatic glycation

Non-enzymatic glycation of proteins and generation of advanced glycated end (AGE) products is an important factor in the pathogenesis of chronic diabetic complications. AGEs and the reactive intermediates may have widespread biological actions [53,65–67]. Glucose, fructose, and the product of pentose phosphate pathway may take part in non-enzymatic glycation [53,66–68]. AGEs may lead to oxidative stress and endothelial damage [65–67]. Exogenous administration of superoxide dismutase has been shown to reduce hyperglycemia-induced endothelial permeability and accompanying vascular dysfunction [69–72]. In addition, AGE can form cross-links with collagen in the extracellular matrix and reduce arterial compliance and alter gene expression of several important intracellular molecules [73]. Aminoguanidine, a specific inhibitor of non-enzymatic glycation, has been shown to inhibit the development of retinopathy in diabetic dogs [74].

Both AGEs and their recptors have been localized to the target organs of diabetic complications such as retina [65–67]. These receptors are found on many cells including endothelial and smooth muscle cells. Interaction of AGEs with these receptors leads to MAPK mediated signaling pathway and NF-κB activation [75]. AGE-mediated NF-κB activation has been shown to increase ET-1 expression [76]. Activation of NF-κB secondary to non-enzymatic glycation has also been linked to reduced nitric oxide which would positively effect ET expression [77].

Nitric oxide and oxidative stress

Endothelial dysfunction is characterized by the imbalance between contracting and relaxing factors. NO is a potent vasodilator which is formed from L-arginine by NO synthase (NOS) [78]. This enzyme has two major isoforms, calcium-calmodulin-dependent NOS (also called eNOS) and calcium-calmodulin-independent NOS (also called iNOS). eNOS is expressed constitutively in endothelial cells and some other cells while iNOS is only expressed when the cells are stimulated by various factors [79–81]. NO released from endothelial cells acts on smooth muscle cells to increase intracellular cGMP and cAMP. The result of which is decrease in calcium, probably via efflux, and a dephosphorylation of myosin light chains [82].

The mechanism of glucose-mediated endothelial dysfunction is not fully understood but evidence indicates increased ET production and impaired nitric oxide may contribute significantly in this abnormality [83–87]. There is a negative interaction between NO and ET, thereby, a reduction in NO leads to increased ET expression. Generation of free radicals due to glucose autoxidation may damage proteins [88]. Various lipoxygenase enzymes activated in hyperglycemia may interact with NO forming perxoinitrate and hydroxyl radicals [89,90].

Other factors

One of the characteristic features of endothelial dysfunction in diabetes is Increased vascular permeability. Increased vascular endothelial growth factor (VEGF) which has been demonstrated in diabetes may be of importance in this respect [91–96]. Besides hypertension and hypoxia, various vasoactive peptides can also induce VEGF production [97]. VEGF is a member of a large family of proteins with five isoforms generated by alternative splicing [98–101]. The mechanism by which VEGF carries out the permeability and proliferative changes seems to involve PKC [95]. VEGF is able to activate PI3 Kinase and PLCγ. Activation of PLCγ leads to increase in DAG and activation of PKC α and β. Oral administration of PKC inhibitors, specifically PKCβ, prevent VEGF mediated retinal permeability and endothelial proliferation [95]. ETs are probably also important in mediating glucose induced increased permeability [52]. We have demonstrated that VEGF may further increase ET expression in the endothelial cells as well as in the retina of diabetic rats [52,97].

A large number of studies indicate the role of angiotensin in the development of diabetic micro- and macro-vasculopathy. Angiotensin II has mitogenic effects on smooth muscle cells and can lead to increased ECM protein synthesis by these cells [102]. Recent reports indicate that there might be an interaction between the renin-angiotensin pathway and the ET system [103]. In vitro studies have demonstrated angiotensin II mediated increase in ET expression [104].

PATHOPHYSIOLOGICAL ROLE OF ETs IN DIABETIC HEART DISEASE

ET alteration in diabetes may lead to several functional and structural effects and may be of importance in the development of several chronic complications including diabetic heart disease. Both glucose and insulin, potentially of importance in insulin resistance, are ET-1 upregulators [105–107]. We and others have demonstrated that in the endothelial cells and in several target organs of diabetic complications, ETs are upregulated [107–113]. Studies in human diabetes with respect to serum ET levels have shown widespread variation ranging from increased to unchanged to decreased [114–123]. Several factors may be responsible for such discrepancy. However, as ETs act as aurtocrine and paracrine factors, plasma levels may not be a good indicator of their biological activity [124–126]. Increased ETs may lead to increased vascular permeability and alteration of blood flow [52]. In addition, increased ET levels may contribute greatly to hypertension in diabetics. Studies conducted to determine the role of ETs in essential hypertension have shown inconsistent data. However, there does seem to be a positive association between the two factors [127]. ETs may also lead to increased extracellular matrix protein production in diabetes via activation of transcription factors NF-κB and AP-1 [128,129]. Furthermore, they may potentially play important roles in angiogenesis [130–132]. Major effects of ET alteration in diabetes are outlined in Fig. 2. We would discuss diabetes induced specific lesions affecting the heart and macrovasculature and the role of ETs in the pathogenesis of these changes below.

Macroangiopathy

Alterations of the plasma ET-1 levels have been demonstrated in several diseases associated with endothelial dysfunction, i.e. diabetes, hypertension, and atherosclerosis [107,125]. High levels of plasma ET-1 were also demonstrated in diabetic

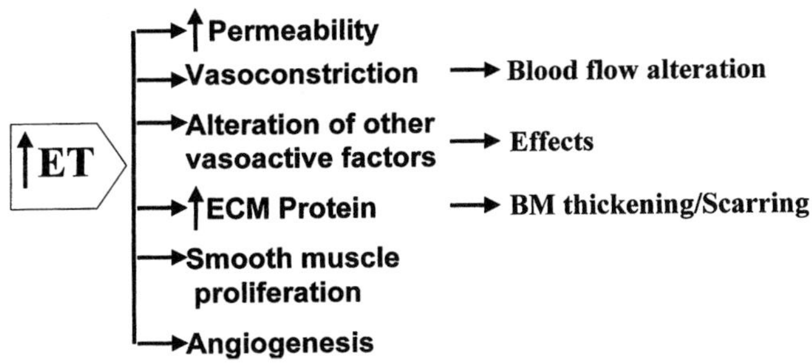

Figure 2. Possible effects of augmented ET production in diabetes.

patients with atherosclerosis [133]. ET-1 is released by endothelial cells and causes phenotypic modulation of the vascular smooth muscle cells from contractile type to synthetic type [134]. ET-1 also causes intimal vasodilation by activation of ET_B receptors on endothelial cells [135]. In addition to its vasoconstrictor properties, ET-1 is a potent mitogen and induces vascular smooth muscle cell proliferation and medial thickening. The importance of ET-1 in diabetes-associated vascular hypertrophy was initially suggested by studies reporting an increased release of this peptide from mesenteric vessels in diabetic rats [136,137] as well as in the type 2 diabetic patients with atherosclerotic macro- and microvascular diseases [138]. Recent studies have demonstrated increased ET-1 expression in the endothelium, adventitia and in the media of diabetic mesenteric vessels in rats and in diabetic patients with macroangiopathy [136,137–139].

Although the expression of prepro ET-1 mRNA was significantly enhanced in aortas from streptozotocin-induced diabetic rats, some investigators demonstrated that, the contractile response of the aorta to ET-1 was weaker in streptozotocin-induced diabetic rats than in the non-diabetic controls in association with a down-regulation of ET receptors. Impaired ET induced signal transduction mechanism have also suggested to be present in these animals [135–139]. In addition to direct effect of ET, there are several interactions between various neurohormonal pathways including the renin-angiotensin system and ET. In a non diabetic model, it has been demostrated that angiotensin II-induced vascular hypertrophy can be attenuated by ET receptor antagonism [104]. ETs may also have roles in mediating increased noradrenaline mediated vasoconstriction in the aorta and mesenteric vessels of diabetic rats [104]. Furthermore, hyperinsulinemia in the context of insulin resistance may further augment action of ET-1, as insulin is a stimulator of ET-1 production, leading to further smooth muscle proliferation [125].

Cardiomyopathy

ETs, cardiovascular peptides with widespread action, play important roles in several cardiovascular diseases including diabetic cardiomyopathy [40,125]. In the heart, both cardiomyocytes and endothelial cells produce ET-1. Cardiac myocytes have high ET-

1 binding affinity sites [140–143]. ET-1 produces pronounced positive inotropic and chronotropic effects on the heart [144,145]. Hypoxia and ischaemia are the two important upregulators of ET-1 expression in heart [40,125]. A duration dependent alteration of chronotropic and inotropic responses of ET-1 was demonstrated in the isolated atria of the diabetic rat [146]. We have demonstrated a significant upregulation of ET-1 and ET_A and ET_B receptor mRNA expression as well as increased ET-immunoreactivity, and ET receptor density in heart of 6 months diabetic rats [109]. These changes were associated with focal apoptosis of cardiomyocytes, scarring of myocardium and increased fibronectin and collagen α1(IV) mRNA expression in heart. Furthermore, such diabetes induced abnormalities were completely prevented by the ET-receptor antagonist, bosentan [109]. In humans, high plasma levels of ET-1 is thought to play an important role in the pathogenesis of diastolic dysfunction in diabetic patients with cardiac autonomic neuropathy [147]. It has further been demonstrated that, reperfusion following cardioplegia during coronary artery bypass grafting procedure can trigger the release of ET-1 in diabetic patients [148], which may further contribute to significant cardiovascular demise in diabetic patients.

Some of the effects of ET-1 on the heart and vasculature could be partially mediated via activation of Na+/H+ exchanger-1 (NHE-1), the major proton pump mechanisms in the heart, through the IP3-DAG pathway [149,150]. We have demonstrated that both ET-1 and NHE-1 play important roles in the pathogenesis of diabetic heart diseases. NHE-1 may act as the downstream mediator in the development of ET-mediated functional and structural changes in diabetic myocardium [151]. PKC activation may be one of the pathways leading to ET upregulation in the heart in diabetes [52–54]. However, several other factors may also be involved in upregulation of ET-1 expression in diabetes. ET-1 interacts with other potent vasoactive substances, nitric oxide (NO) and VEGF [97,152–154]. Increased VEGF in diabetes may also lead to increased ET-1 expression in diabetes [52]. On the other hand, non-enzymatic glycation and oxidative stress may reduces NO production in diabetes, which in turn increases ET-1 expression [152]. We have recently demonstrated that, diabetes induced reduced NOS expression and NO activity in the heart may be corrected by treatment with dual ET receptor antagonist treatment [155].

CONCLUDING REMARKS

Evidences gathered so far indicate that, pathogenetic mechanisms leading to cardiovascular affection in diabetes are indeed complex. Several factors may simultaneously be activated in response to hyperglycemia, and an intricate interplay occurs among such factors. ET, due to their widespread distribution in the cardiovascular system, multiple functional capabilities may play significant roles as effector molecules in diabetic cardiomyopathy and macroangiopathy. Abnormal metabolic pathways secondary to hyperglycemia, such as PKC activation, non-enzymatic glycation, oxidative damage as well as augmented polyol pathway may all in part, directly or indirectly may contribute to the alteration of ETs. ETs may further effect activity of other vasoactive factors. Evidences gathered from multiple animal experiments in several laboratories, indeed, indicate that ETs are of importance in the pathogenesis of diabetic heart disease. ET antagonism may be a potential therapeutic modality in the treatment of cardiovascular complication of diabetes. These data however, have to be further confirmed by additional long term studies in experimental animals and by well designed clinical trials.

ACKNOWLEDGMENT

The cited studies from author's laboratory were supported by grants from Canadian Diabetes Association, in honour of the late Margaret Francis, Canadian Institute of Health Research (MOP43841) and Lawson Health Research Institute.

REFERENCES

1. A Report of the Congressionally-Established Diabetes Research Working Group. 1999. Conquering Diabetes: A Strategic Plan for the 21st Century, Bethesda, Md: National Institutes of Health Publication No. 99-4398.
2. Harris MI. 1998. Diabetes in America: epidemiology and scope of the problem, Diabetes Care 21:C11–C14.
3. Harris MI, Flegal KM, Cowie CC, Eberhardt MS, Goldstein DE, Little RR, Wiedmeyer HM, Byrd-Holt DD. 1998–1994. Prevalence of diabetes, impaired fasting glucose, and impaired glucose tolerance in US adults: the Third National Health and Nutrition Examination Survey, Diabetes Care 21:518–524.
4. American Diabetes Association. Economic consequences of diabetes mellitus in the U.S. in 1997, 1998. Diabetes Care 21:296–309.
5. Epstein M, Sowers Jr. 1992. Diabetes mellitus and hypertension. Hypertension 19:403–418.
6. Hedblad B, Nilsson P, Janzon L, Berglund G. 2000. Relation between insulin resistance and carotid intima-media thickness and stenosis in non-diabetic subjects. Results from a cross-sectional study in Malmo, Sweden. Diabet Med 17:299–307.
7. Savage MP, Krolewski AS, Kenien GG, Lebeis MP, Christlieb AR, Lewis SM. 1988. Acute myocardial infarction in diabetes mellitus and significance of congestive heart failure as a prognostic factor. Am J Cardiol 62:665–669.
8. Lewinter MM. 1996. Diabetic cardiomyopathy: an overview. Coron Artery Dis 7:95–98.
9. International Diabetes Federation Triennial Report 1991–1994. 1994. IDF Brussels.
10. Nunoda S, Genda A, Sekiguchi M, Takeda R. 1985. Left ventricular endomyocardial biopsy findings in patients with essential hypertension and hypertrophic cardiomyopathy with special reference to the incidence of bizarre myocardial hypertrophy with disorganization and biopsy score. Heart Vessels 1:170–175.
11. Shehadeh A, Regan TJ. 1995. Cardiac consequences of diabetes mellitus, Clin. Cardiol 18:301–305.
12. Zhang WX, Chakrabarti S, Green DA, Sima AA. 1990. Diabetic autonomic neuropathy in BB rats and effect of ARI treatment on heart rate variability and vagus structure. Diabetes 39:613–618.
13. Haffner SM, Lehto S, Rönnemaa T, Pyörälä K, Laakso M. 1998. Mortality from Coronary Heart Disease in Subjects with Type 2 Diabetes and in Nondiabetic Subjects with and without Prior Myocardial Infarction. N Engl J Med: 229–234.
14. National Institute of Health, National Institute of Diabetes, Digestive and Kidney Disease. 1995. Diabetes in America 2nd edition, 449–456.
15. Schwartz SM. 1995. The intima. Soil for atherosclerosis and restenosis. Circ Res 77:445–465.
16. Yangisawa M, Kurihara H, Kimura S. 1988. A novel vasoconstrictor peptide produced by the vascular endothelial cells. Nature 332:411–415.
17. Inoue A, Yanagisawa M, Kimura S, Kasuya Y, Miyauchi T, Goto K, Masaki T. 1989. The human endothelin family: three structurally and pharmacologically distinct isopeptides predicted by three separate genes. Proc Natl Acad Sci USA 86:2863–2867.
18. Takahashi M, Matsushita Y, Iijima Y, Tanzawa K. 1993. Purification and characterization of endothelin-converting enzyme from rat lung. J Biol Chem 268:21394–21398.

19. Emoto N, Yanagisawa M. 1995. Endothelin-converting enzyme-2 is a membrane-bound, phosphoramidon-sensitive metalloprotease with acidic pH optimum. J Biol Chem 270:15262–15268.
20. Shimada K, Takahashi M, Ikeda M, Tanzawa K. 1995. Identification and characterization of two isoforms of an endothelin-converting enzyme-1. FEBS Lett 371:140–144.
21. Valdenaire O, Rohrbacher E, Mattei MG. 1995. Organization of the gene encoding the human endothelin-converting enzyme (ECE-1). J Biol Chem 270:29794–29798.
22. Schweizer A, Valdenaire O, Nelbock P, Deuschle U, Dumas Milne Edwards JB, Stumpf JG, Loffler BM. 1997. Human endothelin-converting enzyme (ECE-1): three isoforms with distinct subcellular localizations. Biochem J 328:871–877.
23. Valdenaire O, Lepailleur-Enouf D, Egidy G, Thouard A, Barret A, Vranckx R, Tougard C, Michel JB. 1999. A fourth isoform of endothelin-converting enzyme (ECE-1) is generated from an additional promoter molecular cloning and characterization. Eur J Biochem 264:341–349.
24. Arai H, Hori S, Aramori I, Ohkubo H, Nakanishi S. 1990. Cloning and expression of a cDNA encoding an endothelin receptor. Nature 348:730–732.
25. Sakurai T, Yanagisawa M, Takuwa Y, Miyazaki H, Kimura S, Goto K, Masaki T. 1990. Cloning of a cDNA encoding a non-isopeptide-selective subtype of the endothelin receptor. Nature 348:732–735.
26. Bax WA, Aghai Z, van Tricht CL, Wasenaar C, Saxena PR. 1994. Different endothelin receptors invovled in endothelin-1- and sarafotoxin S6b-induced contractions of the human isolated coronary artery. Br J Pharmacol 113:1471–1479.
27. Clark KL, Pierre L. 1995. Characterization of endothelin receptors in rat renal artery in vitro. Br J Pharmacol 114:785–790.
28. Godfraind T. 1993. Evidence for heterogeneity of endothelin receptor distribution in human coronary artery. Br J Pharmacol 110:1201–1205.
29. Eglazos A, Cucchi P, Patacchini R, Quartara L, Maggi CA, Mizrahi J. 1993. Differential effects of BQ-123 against endothelin-1 and endothelin-3 on the rat vas deferens: evidence of an atypical endothelin receptor. Br J Pharmacol 109:736–738.
30. Ishikawa H, Haruno I, Harada Y, Yoshitomi T, Ishikawa S, Katori M. 1996. Pharmacological characterization of endothelin receptors in rabbit iris sphincter muscle: suggestion for the presence of atypical receptors. Curr Eye Res 15:73–78.
31. Riezebos J, Watts IS, Vallance PJ. 1994. Endothelin receptors mediating functional responses in human small arteries and veins. Br J Pharmacol 111:609–615.
32. Sumner MJ, Cannon TR, Mundin JW, White DG, Watts IS. 1992. Endothelin ETA and ETB receptors mediate vascular smooth muscle contraction. Br J Pharmacol 107:858–860.
33. Warner TD, Allcock GH, Corder R, Vane JR. 1993. Use of endothelin antagonists BQ-123 and PD 142893 to reveal three endothelin receptors mediating smooth muscle contraction and the release of EDRF. Br J Pharmacol 110:777–782.
34. Warner TD, Allcock GH, Mickey EJ, Vane JR. 1993. Characterization of endothelin receptors mediating the effects of endothelin/sarafotoxin peptides on autonomic neurotransmission in the rat vas deferens and guinea-pig ileum. Br J Pharmacol 110:783–789.
35. Devadason PS, Henry PJ. 1997. Comparison of the contractile effects and binding kinetics of endothelin-1 and sarafotoxin S6b in rat isolated renal artery. Br J Pharmacol 121:253–263.
36. Nosaka C, Ishikawa H, Haruno I, Yoshitomi T, Kase H, Ishikawa S, Harada Y. 1998. Radioligand binding characteristics of the endothelin receptor in the rabbit iris. Jpn J Pharmacol 76:289–296.
37. Douglas SA, Beck GRJ, Elliot JD, Ohlstein EH. 1995. Pharmacologic evidence for the presence of three functional endothelin receptor subtypes in rabbit saphenous vein. J Cardiovasc Pharmacol 26:S163–S168.
38. Mizuguchi T, Nishiyama M, Moroi K, Tanaka H, Saito T, Masuda Y, Masaki T, de Wit D, Yanagisawa M, Kimura S. 1997. Analysis of two pharmacologically predicted endothelin B receptor subtypes by using the endothelin receptor B knockout mouse. Br J Pharmacol 120:1427–1430.
39. Blauw GJ, Westendorp RG, Srivistava N, Burggraaf K, Frolich M, Simons R, Cohen AF, Meinders AE. 1995. Hypoxia induced arterial endothelin does not influence peripheral vascular tone. J Cardiovasc Pharmacol 26[Suppl 3]:S242–S243.
40. Karamazyn M. 1996. The role of endothelin in cardiac function in health and disease. In: Myocardial Ischemia, Mechanisms, Reperfusion, Protection. Karamazyn M (Ed.), pp. 209–230. Birkhauser, Basel, Switzerland.

41. Yanagisawa M, Kurihara H, Kimura S, Tomobe Y, Kobayashi M, Mitsui Y, Yazaki Y, Goto K, Masaki T. 1988. A novel potent vasoconstrictor peptide produced by vascular endothelial cells. Nature 332:411–415.
42. Emori T, Hirata Y, Imai T, Ohta K, Kanno K, Eguchi S, Marumo F. 1992. Cellular mechanism of thrombin on endothelin-1 biosynthesis and release in bovine endothelial cell. Biochem Pharmacol 44:2409–2411.
43. Kurihara H, Yoshizumi M, Sugiyama T, Takaku F, Yanagisawa M, Masaki T, Hamaoki M, Kato H, Yazaki Y. 1989. Transforming growth factor-beta stimulates the expression of endothelin mRNA by vascular endothelial cells. Biochem Biophys Res Commun 159:1435–1440.
44. Malek AM, Zhang J, Jiang J, Alper SL, Izumo S. 1999. Endothelin-1 gene suppression by shear stress: pharmacological evaluation of the role of tyrosine kinase, intracellular calcium, cytoskeleton, and mechanosensitive channels. J Mol Cell Cardiol 31:387–399.
45. Yoshimoto S, Ishizaki Y, Sasaki T, Murota S. 1991. Effect of carbon dioxide and oxygen on endothelin production by cultured porcine cerebral endothelial cells. Stroke 22:378–383.
46. Boulanger C, Luscher TF. 1990. Release of endothelin from the porcine aorta. Inhibition by endothelium-derived nitric oxide. J Clin Invest 85:587–590.
47. Prins BA, Hu RM, Nazario B, Pedram A, Frank HJ, Weber MA, Levin ER. 1994. Prostaglandin E2 and prostacyclin inhibit the production and secretion of endothelin from cultured endothelial cells. J Biol Chem 269:11938–11944.
48. Kohno M, Horio T, Yokokawa K, Kurihara N, Takeda T. 1992. C-type natriuretic peptide inhibits thrombin- and angiotensin II-stimulated endothelin release via cyclic guanosine 3′,5′-monophosphate. Hypertension 19:320–325.
49. Okumura K, Nishiura T, Awaji Y, Kondo J, Hashimoto H, Ito T. 1991. 1,2-diacylglycerol content and its composition in thoracic aorta of diabetic rats. Diabetes 40:820–824.
50. Xia P, Inoguchi T, Kern KS, Engerman RL, Oats PJ, King GL. 1994. Characterization of the mechanism for the chronic activation of diacylglycerol-protein kinase C in diabetes and hypergalactosaemia. Diabetes 43:1122–1129.
51. Li W, Wang W, Liu X. 1994. Comparative study of high-glucose effect on phosphatidylcholine hydrolysis of cultured retinal capillary pericytes and endothelial cells, Biochem Biophys Acta 1222:339–347.
52. Chen S, Apostolova MD, Cherian MG, Chakrabarti S. 2000. Interaction of endothelin-1 with vasoactive factors in mediating glucose-induced increased permeability in endothelial cells. Lab Invest 80:1311–1321.
53. King GL, Brownlee M. 1996. The cellular and molecular mechanisms of diabetic complications. Endocrinol Metab Clin North Am 25:255–270.
54. Koya D, King GL. 1998. Protein kinase C activation and the development of diabetic complications. Diabetes 47:859–866.
55. Johannes FJ, Prestle J, Eis S, Oberhagemann P, Pfizenmaier K. 1994. PKC is a novel, atypical member of the protein kinase C family. J Biol Chem 269:6140–6148.
56. Lynch JJ, Ferro TJ, Blumenstock FA, Brockenauer AM, Malik AB. 1990. Increased endothelial albumin permeability mediated by protein kinase C activation. J Clin Invest 85:991–998.
57. Williams B, Gallacher B, Patel H, Orme C. 1997. Glucose-induced protein kinase C activation regulates vascular permeability factor mRNA expression and peptide production by human vascular smooth muscle cells in vitro. Diabetes 46:1497–1503.
58. Kern TS, Engerman RL. 1994. Comparison of retinal lesions in alloxan-diabetic rats and galactose-fed rats. Curr Eye Res 13:863–867.
59. Kowluru RA, Kern TS, Engerman RL, Armstrong D. 1996. Abnormalities of retinal metabolism in diabetes or experimental galactosemia. III. Effects of antioxidants. Diabetes 45:1233–1237.
60. Ishii H, Jirousek MR, Koya D, Takagi C, Xia P, Clermont A, Bursell SE, Kern TS, Ballas LM, Heath WF, Stramm LE, Feener EP, King GL. 1996. Amelioration of vascular dysfunctions in diabetic rats by an oral PKC beta inhibitor. Science 272:728–731.
61. Williamson JR, Chang K, Frangos M, et al. 1993. Perspectives in Diabetes. Hyperglycemic pseudohypoxia and diabetic complications. Diabetes 42:801–813.
62. Costantino L, Rastelli G, Vianello P, Cignarella G, Barlocco D. 1999. Diabetes complications and their potential prevention: aldose reductase inhibition and other approaches. Med Res Rev 19:3–23.
63. Engerman RL, Kern TS, Garment MB. 1993. Capillary basement membrane in retina, kidney, and muscle of diabetic dogs and galactosemic dogs and its response to 5 years aldose reductase inhibition. J Diabetes Complications 7:241–245.

64. Pugliese G, Tilton RG, Williamson JR. 1991. Glucose-induced metabolic imbalances in the pathogenesis of diabetic vascular disease. Diabetes Metab Rev 7:35–59.
65. Vlassara H. 1997. Recent progress in advanced glycation end products and diabetic complications. Diabetes 46(Suppl. 2):S19–S25.
66. Vlassara H. 2001. The AGE-receptor in the pathogenesis of diabetic complications. Diabetes Metab Res Rev 17:436–443.
67. Bierhaus A, Hofmann MA, Ziegler R, Nawroth PP. 1998. AGEs and their interaction with AGE-receptors in vascular disease and diabetes mellitus I. The AGE concept. Cardiovasc Res 37:586–600.
68. Takagi Y, Kashiwagi A, Tanaka Y, Asahian T, Kikkawa R, Shigeta Y. 1995. Significance of fructose-induced protein oxidation and formation of advanced glycation end product. J Diabet Complications 9:89–91.
69. Curcio F, Pegorano I, dello Russo P, Falleti E, Perrilla G, Ceriello A. 1995. SOD and GSH inhibit the high glucose induced oxidative damage and the PDGF increase secretion in cultured endothelial cells. Thromb Haemost 74:969–973.
70. Tesfamariam B, Cohen RA. 1992. Free radicals mediate endothelial cell dysfunction caused by elevated glucose. Am J Phsyiol 263:H321–H326.
71. Ohishi K, Carmines PK. 1995. Superoxide dismutase restores the influence of nitric oxide on renal arterioles in diabetes mellitus. Am J Soc Nephrol 5:1559–1566.
72. Dileepan K, Sharma R, Stechschulte DJ, Savin VJ. 1993. Effect of superoxide exposure on albumin permeability of isolated rat glomeruli. J Lab Clin Med 121:797–804.
73. Vasan S, Foiles PG, Founds HW. 2001. Therapeutic potential of AGE inhibitors and breakers of AGE protein cross-links. Expert Opin Investig Drugs 10:1977–1987.
74. Kern TS, Engerman RL. 2001. Pharmacological inhibition of diabetic retinopathy: aminoguanidine and aspirin. Diabetes 50:1636–1642.
75. Bierhaus A, Chevion S, Chevion M, Hofmann M, Quehenberger P, Illmer T, Luther T, Berentshtein E, Tritschler H, Muller M, Wahl P, Ziegler R, Nawroth PP. 1997. Advanced glycation end product-induced activation of NF-kappaB is suppressed by alpha-lipoic acid in cultured endothelial cells. Diabetes 46:1481–1490.
76. Quehenberger P, Bierhaus A, Fasching P, Muellner C, Klevesath M, Hong M, Stier G, Sattler M, Schleicher E, Speiser W, Nawroth PP. 2000. Endothelin 1 transcription is controlled by nuclear factor-kappaB in AGE-stimulated cultured endothelial cells. Diabetes 49:1561–1570.
77. Hattori Y, Banba N, Gross SS, Kasai K. 1999. Glycated serum albumin-induced nitric oxide production in vascular smooth muscle cells by nuclear factor kappaB-dependent transcriptional activation of inducible nitric oxide synthase. Biochem Biophys Res Commun 259:128–132.
78. Moncada S. 1992. The L-arginine/nitric oxide pathway. Acta Physiol Scand 145:201–227.
79. Bredt DS, Snyder SH. 1990. Isolation of nitric oxide synthetase, a calmodulin-requiring enzyme. Proc Natl Acad Sci USA 87:682–685.
80. Moncada S, Palmer RMJ, Higgs EA. 1991. Nitric oxide, physiology, pathophysiology, and pharmacology. Pharm Rev 43:109–142.
81. Nathan C. 1992. Nitric oxide as a secretory product of mammalian cells. FASEB J 6:3051–3064.
82. Lüüscher TF. 1990. Imbalance of endothelium-derived relaxing and contracting factors. A new concept in hypertension? Am J Hypertens 3:317–330.
83. Cosentino F, Luscher TF. 2001. Effects of blood pressure and glucose on endothelial function. Curr Hypertens Rep 3:79–88.
84. Cosentino F, Luscher TF. 1998. Endothelial dysfunction in diabetes mellitus. J Cardiovasc Pharmacol 32(Suppl 3):S54–S61.
85. Cosentino F, Hishikawa K, Katusic ZS, Luscher TF. 1997. High glucose increases nitric oxide synthase expression and superoxide anion generation in human aortic endothelial cells. Circulation 96:25–28.
86. Van Dam B, Demirci C, Reitsma HJ, van Lambalgen, AA, van den Bos GC, Tangelder GJ, Stehouwer CD. 2000. Alterations in nitric oxide activity and sensitivity in early streptozotocin-induced diabetes depend on arteriolar size. Int J Exp Diabetes Res 1:221–232.
87. Stehouwer CD, Lambert J, Donker AJ, van Hinsbergh VW. 1997. Endothelial dysfunction and pathogenesis of diabetic angiopathy. Cardiovasc Res 34:55–68.
88. Hunt JV, Dean RT, Wolff SP. 1988. Hydroxyl radical production and autoxidative glycosylation. Glucose autoxidation as the cause of protein damage in the experimental glycation model of diabetes mellitus and ageing. Biochem J 256:205–212.

89. Nadler J, Winer L. 1996. Free radicals, nitric oxide and diabetic complications. In Diabetes Mellitus, LeRoith D, Taylor SI, Olefsky M (eds), pp. 840–848. Lippincott-Raven: Philadelphia.
90. Jiang ZY, Woollard AC, Wolff SP. 1990. Hydrogen peroxide production during experimental protein glycation. FEBS Lett 268:69–71.
91. Hammes HP, Lin J, Bretzel RG, Brownlee M, Breier G. 1998. Upregulation of the vascular endothelial growth factor/vascular endothelial growth factor receptor system in experimental background diabetic retinopathy of the rat. Diabetes 47:401–406.
92. Pe'er J, Folberg R, Itin A, Gnessin H, Hemo I, Keshet E. 1996. Upregulated expression of vascular endothelial growth factor in proliferative diabetic retinopathy. Br J Ophthalmol 80:241–245.
93. Joussen AM, Huang S, Poulaki V, Camphausen K, Beecken WD, Kirchhof B, Adamis AP. 2001. In vivo retinal gene expression in early diabetes. Invest Ophthalmol Vis Sci 42:3047–3057.
94. de Vriese AS, Tilton RG, Elger M, Stephan CC, Kriz W, Lameire NH. 2001. Antibodies against vascular endothelial growth factor improve early renal dysfunction in experimental diabetes. J Am Soc Nephrol 12:993–1000.
95. Aiello LP, Bursell SE, Clermont A, Duh E, Ishii H, Takagi C, Mori F, Ciulla TA, Ways K, Jirousek M, Smith LEH, King GL. 1997. Vascular endothelial growth factor-induced retinal permeability is mediated by protein kinase C in vivo and suppressed by an orally effective β-isoform-selective inhibitor. Diabetes 46:1473–1480.
96. Qaum T, Xu Q, Joussen AM, Clemens MW, Qin W, Miyamoto K, Hassessian H, Wiegand SJ, Rudge J, Yancopoulos GD, Adamis AP. 2001. VEGF-initiated blood-retinal barrier breakdown in early diabetes. Invest Ophthalmol Vis Sci 42:2408–2413.
97. Cukiernik M, Hileeto D, Evans T, Mukherjee S, Downey D, Chakrabarti S. 2001. VEGF signal antagonism prevents early microvascular changes in the rat retina in diabetes. Canad. J Diabetes Care 25:192A.
98. Leung DW, Cachianes G, Kuang WJ, Goeddel DV, Ferrara N. 1989. vascular endothelial growth factor is a secreted angiogenic mitogen. Science 246:1306–1309.
99. Tischer E, Gospodarowicz D, Mitchell R, Silva M, Schilling J, Lau K, Crisp T, Fiddes JC, Abraham JA. 1989. Vascular endothelial growth factor: a new member of the platelet-derived growth factor gene family. Biochem Biophys Res Commun 165:1198–1206.
100. Houck KA, Ferrara N, Winer J, Cachianes G, Li B, Leung DW. 1991. The vascular endothelial growth factor family: identification of a fourth molecular species and characterization of alternative splicing of RNA. Mol Endocrinol 5:1806–1814.
101. Tischer E, Mitchell R, Hartman T, Silva M, Gospodarowicz D, Fiddes JC, Abraham JA. 1991. The human gene for vascular endothelial growth factor. Multiple protein forms are encoded through alternative exon splicing. J Biol Chem 266:11947–11954.
102. Kato H, Suzuki H, Tajima S, Ogata Y, Tominaga T, Sato A, Saruta T. 1991. Angiotensin II stimulates collagen synthesis in cultured vascular smooth muscle cells. J Hypertens 9:17–22.
103. Rabelink TJ, Bakris GL. 1998. The renin-angiotensin system in diabetic nephropathy: the endothelial connection. Miner Electrolyte Metab 24:381–388.
104. Moreau P, d'Uscio LV, Shaw S, Takase H, Barton M, Luscher TF. 1997. Angiotensin II increases tissue endothelin and induces vascular hypertrophy: reversal by ET(A)-receptor antagonist. Circulation 96:1593–1597.
105. Oliver FJ, de la Rubia G, Feener EP, Lee ME, Loeken MR, Shiba T, Quertermous T, King GL. 1991. Stimulation of endothelin-1 gene expression by insulin in endothelial cells. J Biol Chem 266:23251–23256.
106. Ferri C, Pittoni V, Piccoli A, Laurenti O, Cassone MR, Bellini C, Properzi G, Valesini G, De Mattia G, Santucci A. 1995. Insulin stimulates endothelin-1 secretion from human endothelial cells and modulates its circulating levels in vivo. J Clin Endocrinol Metab 80:829–835.
107. Hopfner RL, Gopalakrishnan V. 1999. Endothelin: emerging role in diabetic vascular complications. Diabetologia 42:1383–1394.
108. Hargrove GM, Dufresne J, Whiteside C, Muruve DA, Wong NC. 2000. Diabetes mellitus increases endothelin-1 gene transcription in rat kidney. Kidney Int 58:1534–1545.
109. Chen S, Evans T, Mukherjee K, Karmazyn M, Chakrabarti S. 2000. Diabetes-induced myocardial structural changes: role of endothelin-1 and its receptors. J Mol Cell Cardiol 32:1621–1629.
110. Deng D, Evans T, Mukherjee K, Downey D, Chakrabarti S. 1999. Diabetes-induced vascular dysfunction in the retina: role of endothelins. Diabetologia 42:1228–1234.
111. Chakravarthy U, Hayes RG, Stitt AW, Douglas A. 1997. Endothelin expression in ocular tissues of diabetic and insulin-treated rats. Invest Ophthalmol Vis Sci 38:2144–2151.

112. Wu SQ, Tang F. 1998. Impaired paracrine effect of endothelin-1 on vascular smooth muscle in streptozotocin-diabetic rats. Cardiovasc Res 39:651–656.
113. Cameron NE, Dines KC, Cotter MA. 1994. The potential contribution of endothelin-1 to neurovascular abnormalities in streptozotocin-diabetic rats. Diabetologia 37:1209–1215.
114. Letizia C, Iannaccone A, Cerci S, Santi G, Cilli M, Coassin S, Pannarale MR, Scavo D, Iannacone A. 1997. Circulating endothelin-1 in non-insulin-dependent diabetic patients with retinopathy. Horm Metab Res 29:247–251.
115. Laurenti O, Vingolo EM, Desideri GB, Ferri C, Bellini C, Cassone-Faldetta M, Santucci A, De Mattia G. 1997. Increased levels of plasma endothelin-1 in non-insulin dependent diabetic patients with retinopathy but without other diabetes-related organ damage. Exp Clin Endocrinol Diabetes 105(Suppl 2):40–42.
116. De Mattia G, Cassone-Faldetta M, Bellini C, Bravi MC, Laurenti O, Baldoncini R, Santucci A, Ferri C. 1998. Role of plasma and urinary endothelin-1 in early diabetic and hypertensive nephropathy. Am J Hypertens 11:983–988.
117. Takahashi K, Ghatei MA, Lam HC, O'Halloran DJ, Bloom SR. 1990. Elevated plasma endothelin in patients with diabetes mellitus. Diabetologia 33:306–310.
118. Morise T, Takeuchi Y, Kawano M, Koni I, Takeda R. 1995. Increased plasma levels of immunoreactive endothelin and von Willebrand factor in NIDDM patients. Diabetes Care 18:87–89.
119. Kawamura M, Ohgawara H, Naruse M, Suzuki N, Iwasaki N, Naruse K, Hori S, Demura H, Omori Y. 1992. Increased plasma endothelin in NIDDM patients with retinopathy. Diabetes Care 15:1396–1397.
120. Donatelli M, Colletti I, Bucalo ML, Russo V, Verga S. 1994. Plasma endothelin levels in NIDDM patients with macroangiopathy. Diabetes Res 25:159–164.
121. Kamoi K, Ishibashi M, Yamaji T. 1994. Endothelin-1 and big endothelin-1 in NIDDM patients with and without microangiopathy. Diabetes Res Clin Pract 24:125–129.
122. Bertello P, Veglio F, Pinna G, Gurioli L, Molino P, Alban S, Chiandussi L. 1994. Plasma endothelin in NIDDM patients with and without complications. Diabetes Care 17:574–577.
123. Haak T, Jungmann E, Felber A, Hillmann U, Usadel KH. 1992. Increased plasma levels of endothelin in diabetic patients with hypertension. Am J Hypertens 5:161–166.
124. Rubanyi GM, Polokof MA. 1994. Endothelins: Molecular biology, biochemistry, pharmacology, physiology and pathophysiology. Pharmacology Rev 46:326–414.
125. Levin ER. 1995. Endothelins, New Engl J Med 333:356–363.
126. Chakrabarti S, Cukiernik M, Mukherjee S, Chen S. 2000. Therapeutic potentials of endothelin receptor antagonists in diabetes. In: Monthly Focus: Oncologic, Endocrine & Motabolic in Exp Opin Invest Drugs 9(12):2873–2888.
127. Jorkasky DK, Hay DWP, Freed MI. 1995. The role of endothelin in human disease: implications and potential therapeutic intervention. In: Endothelin receptors: from the genes to the human. Ruffolo RR Jr. (Ed.), CRC, Boca Raton, FL, pp. 215–271.
128. Chen S, Mukherjee S, Chakrabarti S. 2001. Hyperglycemia induced, endothelin (ET) mediated, increased extracellular matrix (ECM) protein synthesis is mediated via NFKB activation. Diabetes 50(Suppl 2):A191.
129. Evans T, Deng DX, Chen S, Chakrabarti S. 2000. Endothelin receptor blockade prevents augmented extracellular matrix component mRNA expression and capillary basement membrane thickening in the retina of diabetic and galactose-fed rats. Diabetes 49:662–666.
130. Salani D, Taraboletti G, Rosano L, Di Castro V, Borsotti P, Giavazzi R, Bagnato A. 2000. Endothelin-1 induces an angiogenic phenotype in cultured endothelial cells and stimulates neovascularization in vivo. Am J Pathol 157:1703–1711.
131. Bek EL, McMillen MA. 2000. Endothelins are angiogenic. J Cardiovasc Pharmacol 36(5 Suppl 1):S135–S139.
132. Brennan PA, Zaki GA. 2000. Angiogenesis in cancer: the role of endothelin-1. Ann R Coll Surg Engl 82:363–364.
133. Perfet F, Tarquini R, Tapparini L, Tarquini B. 1998. Influence of non-insulin-dependent diabetes mellitus on plasma endothelin-1 levels in patients with advanced atherosclerosis. J Diabetes Complications 12:187–192.
134. Gilbert RE, Rumber JR, Cao ZM, Cox AJ, van Eeden P, Allen TJ, Kelly DJ, Cooper ME. 2000. Endothelin receptor antagonism ameliorates mast cell infiltration, vascular hypertrophy and epidermal growth factor expression in experimental diabetes. Circ Res 86:158–165.

135. Makino A, Oda S, Kamata K. 2001. Mechanisms underlying increased release of endothelin-1 from aorta in diabetic rats. Peptides 22:639–645.
136. Makino A, Kamata K. 1998. Elevated plasma endothelin-1 levels in streptozotocin induced diabetic rats and responsiveness of the mesenteric arterial bed to endothelin-1. Br J Pharmacol 123:1065–1072.
137. Takeda Y, Miyamori I, Yoneda T, Takeda R. 1991. Production of endothelin-1 from the mesenteric arteries of streptozotocin-induced diabetic rat. Life Sci 48:2553–2556.
138. Migdalis IN, Kalogeropoulou K, Iliopoulou V, Triantafilou P, Charalabides J, Mortzos G, Cordopatis C. 2001. Plasma levels of endothelin, lipid peroxides and prostacyclin in diabetic patients with macroangiopathy. Diab Res Clin Prac 54:129–136.
139. Taylor PD, Graves JE, Bakris GL. 1995. Selective impairment of acetylcholine-mediated endothelium-dependent relaxation in isolated resistance arteries of the streptozotocin-induced diabetic rat. Clin Sci 88:519–524.
140. Suzuki T, Kumazaki T, Mitsui Y. 1993. Endothelin-1 is produced and secreted by neonatal rat cardiac myocytes in vitro. Biochem Biophys Res Commun 191:823–830.
141. Chua BH, Chua CC, Diglio CA, Siu BB. 1993. Regulation of endothelin-1 mRNA by angiotensin II in rat heart endothelial cells. Biochem Biophys Acta 1178:201–206.
142. Fukuchi M, Giaid A. 1998. Expression of endothelin-1 and endothelin-converting enzyme-1 mRNAs and proteins in failing human hearts, J Cardiovasc Pharmacol. 31(Suppl 1):S421–S423.
143. Vesci L, Mattera GG, Tobia P, Corsico N, Calvani M. 1995. Cardiac and renal endothelin-1binding sites in streptozotocin-induced diabetic rats. Pharmacol Res 32:363–367.
144. Hu JR, von Harsdorf R, Lang RE. 1988. Endothelin has potent inotropic effects in rat atria. Eur J Pharmacol 158:275–278.
145. Ishikawa T, Yanagisawa M, Kimura S, Goto K, Masaki T. 1988. Positive chronotropic effects of endothelin, a novel endothelium-derived vasoconstrictor peptide. Pflugers Arch 413:108–110.
146. Lieu AT, Reid JJ. 1994. Changes in the responsiveness to endothelin-1 in isolated atria from diabetic rats. Eur J Pharmacol 261:33–42.
147. Erbas T, Erbas B, Kabakci G, Aksoyek S, Koray Z, Gedik O. 2000. Plasma big-endothelin levels, cardiac autonomic neuropathy, and cardiac functions in patients with insulin-dependent diabetes mellitus. Clin Cardiol 23:259–263.
148. Sharma AC, Fogelson BG, Nawas SI, Vigneswaran WT, Sam AD 2nd, Alden KJ, Ferguson JL, Law WR. 1999. Elevated coronary endothelin-1 but not nitric oxide in diabetics during CABG. Ann Thorac Surg 67:1659–1663.
149. Karmazyn M, Gan XT, Humphreys RA, Yoshida H, Kusumoto K. 1999. The myocardial Na(+)-H(+) exchange: structure, regulation and its role in heart disease. Circ Res 85:777–786.
150. Lazdunski M, Frelin C, Vigne P. 1985. The sodium/hydrogen exchange system in cardiac cells: its biochemical and pharmacological properties and its role in regulating internal concentrations of sodium and internal pH. J Mol Cell Cardiol 17:1029–1042.
151. Hileeto D, Cukiernik M, Evans T, Chen S, Mukherjee S, Downey D, Karmazyn M, Chakrabarti S. 2001. Interaction of endothelin-1 and sodium/hydrogen exchanger-1 in the pathogenesis of diabetes induced changes in the heart. Diabetes 50(Suppl 2):A155.
152. Vanhoutte PM. 1994. Endothelin-1. A matter of life and breath. Nature 368:693–694.
153. Pedram A, Razandi M, Hu RM, Levin ER. (1997). Vasoactive peptides modulate vascular endothelial cell growth factor production and endothelial cell proliferation and invasion. J Biol Chem 27:17097–17103.
154. Matsuura A, Kawashima S, Yamochi W, Hirata K, Yamaguchi T, Emoto N, Yokoyama M. 1997. Vascular endothelial growth factor increases endothelin-converting enzyme expression in vascular endothelial cells. Biochem Biophys Res Commun 235:713–716.
155. Mukherjee S, Evans T, Chen S, Cukiernik M, Hileeto D, Karmazyn M, Chakrabarti S. 2001. Nitric Oxide in diabetic hearts. Canadian Journal of Diabetes Care 25:192.

G.N. Pierce, M. Nagano, P. Zahradka, and N.S. Dhalla (eds.).
ATHEROSCLEROSIS, HYPERTENSION AND DIABETES. Copyright © 2003.
Kluwer Academic Publishers. Boston.

USEFULNESS OF 5-HT$_{2A}$ RECEPTOR ANTAGONISTS FOR THE TREATMENT OF CARDIOVASCULAR COMPLICATIONS IN DIABETES

RAMESH K. GOYAL, DHANANJAY N. UMRANI, DIPALI N. BODIWALA, and NARANJAN S. DHALLA

Department of Pharmacology, L. M. College of Pharmacy, Ahmedabad, India and Institute of Cardiovascular Sciences, St. Boniface General Hospital Research Centre, Winnipeg, Canada

Summary. The elevated level of 5-hydroxytryptamine (5-HT) has been reported to be associated with cardiovascular complications in diabetes. Using different 5-HT receptor agonists and antagonists, 5-HT receptors were found to be involved in glycemic control. Sarpogrelate, 5-HT$_{2A}$ receptor antagonist, was shown to produce beneficial effects in type 1 and type 2 diabetic rats. It not only reduced serum glucose and lipid levels, but was also found to increase serum insulin in type 1 diabetic rats. In view of the antiplatelet aggregation and anti-ischemic effects of 5-HT$_{2A}$ receptor antagonists, as well as of the increased incidence of myocardial infarction, it appears that 5-HT$_{2A}$ antagonists may prove useful in the treatment of diabetes. Accordingly, it is suggested that 5-HT$_{2A}$ receptors may be considered as a novel target to develop anti-diabetic drugs to prevent the cardiovascular complications associated with diabetes.

Key words: 5-Hydroxytryptamine, Sarpogrelate, Cardiovascular System, Diabetes

INTRODUCTION

5-Hydroxytryptamine (5-HT) is one of the earliest autacoids and neurotransmitter reported to be involved in several central and peripheral functions. It plays an important role as a neurotransmitter in the brain mediating sleep, feeding, mood, temperature regulation and sexual behavior [1]. It also serves as a precursor to melatonin in the pineal gland [1]. In the gastrointestinal tract, 5-HT primarily regulates motil-

Address for Correspondence: Prof. Ramesh K. Goyal, Department of Pharmacology, L. M. College of Pharmacy, Ahmedabad-380 009, Gujrat, India. Phone: 91-79-6302746; Fax: 91-79-6304865; e-mail: goyalrk@hotmail.com

ity; 90% in the total 5-HT of the body is found in the enterochromaffin cells of the gastrointestinal tract [2]. 5-HT has revived increasing attention in recent years with the introduction of specific 5-HT receptor agonists (5-HT_{1A} specific buspirone, 5-HT_{1D} specific sumatriptan and 5-HT_4 specific cisapride) and antagonists (5-HT_3 specific ondansetron) in various disorders like anxiety, migraine, reflux esophagitis and chemotherapy induced emesis [3]. Historically, 5-HT was discovered as a substance that produces vasoconstriction and platelet aggregation [4]. With the advent of various receptor subtypes, 5-HT_2 receptors were found to be involved in platelet aggregation and other cardiovascular functions. Application of 5-HT receptor modulators in cardiovascular diseases was not considered seriously until the introduction of sarpogrelate, a specific 5-HT_{2A} receptor antagonist that has been shown to possess significant antiplatelet aggregation activity [5,6]. Sarpogrelate inhibits 5-HT or collagen induced platelet aggregation in diabetes [6]. Since diabetes is also associated with abnormalities of platelet functions such as aggregation, adhesion, and availability of platelet factor-3, sarpogrelate has been suggested as a drug useful in diabetes induced atherothrombotic disease [6]. However, 5-HT levels are reported to be high in diabetes mellitus [7] and as 5-HT_{2A} receptors have been shown to be involved in hyperglycemia in various experimental animals [8–10]. 5-HT causes stimulatory effects on heart that again involves 5-HT_2 receptors present in cardiomyocytes [11]. In addition to cardiac effects, the 5-HT induced vasoconstrictor action is reported to be mediated by 5-HT_2 receptors [12]. 5-HT_{2A} antagonist, sarpogrelate was found to inhibit vascular smooth muscle cell migration and proliferation induced by 5-HT [13]. In diabetic cardiomyopathy myocardial glucose transport is defective [14]. A reduction in the capacity of myocardial glucose transport can be detrimental to the diabetic patient during periods of increased myocardial work or ischemia that is common with diabetes when the demand for glucose uptake is increased [15]. Glucose is carried across the plasma membrane by a family of glucose transporters including GLUT 1 and GLUT 4 and diabetes is reported to produce alterations in the expression of GLUT-1 and GLUT-4 [16,17]. Various stimuli including insulin and 5-HT may recruit these transporters from cytosol to the plasma membrane and alter glucose transport in the heart [18]. The present article will focus on the role of specific 5-HT_{2A} receptors in the prevention of cardiovascular complications in diabetes mellitus.

ROLE OF 5-HYDROXYTRYPTAMINE IN GLUCOSE CONTROL

The association between 5-HT and its role in glucose control has been a subject of controversy for last couple of decades. 5-HT has been shown to have both hyperglycemic and hypoglycemic effects. In mice, it has been demonstrated that 5-hydroxytryptophan (5-HTP), the precursor of 5-HT, produces hypoglycemia, and the effects of 5-HTP are due to the formation of 5-HT [19,20]. In addition, it was reported that the hypoglycemic effect of 5-HTP is accompanied with an increase of serum insulin levels [19–21] and it was suggested that 5-HT may depress blood glucose levels by affecting the mechanisms for insulin release in pancreatic β cells. This action of 5-HT was considered to be via specific 5-HT receptors as pancreatic islets have mechanisms for the uptake of 5-HT and form 5-HT from the precursor 5-HTP [22]. On the other hand, it has also been reported that specific 5-HT receptor agonists induce hyperglycemia in rats. 5-HT_{1A} receptor agonist, 8-hydroxy-2-di-n-(propylamino)tetraline (8-OH-DPAT), as well as the 5-HT_{1A} partial agonists, buspirone or ipsapirone, can induce hyperglycemia in rats [23,24]. Recently, it has been reported that the 5-HT_2 receptor also participates in glucose regulation in rats. It is suggested that a $5\text{-HT}_{2A/2C}$ receptor agonist, 1-(2,5-dimethoxy-4-iodophenyl)-2-aminopropane (DOI), elicits hyperglycemia mediated by centrally located 5-HT_{2A} receptor [25,26]. Furthermore, it is reported that a peripheral 5-HT_2 receptor agonist, α-methyl-5-HT, can cause a hyperglycemic response in rats [9,25,27]. $5\text{-HT}_{2B/2C}$ receptor agonist 1-(3-chlorophenyl) piperazine (mCPP) also produces hyperglycemia in rats [26]. These studies have shown that 5-HT_1 and 5-HT_2 receptor subtypes are involved in hyperglycemic response of 5-HT, whereas the involvement of 5-HT_3 and 5-HT_4 receptor subtypes is ruled out. The 5-HT_{1A} and 5-HT_2 receptor mediated hyperglycemia appears to be associated with adrenaline release as adrenodemedullation or adrenaloctomy was found to suppress the hyperglycemia induced by these receptor agonists. Experiments from our laboratory also supported the hyperglycemic effect of 5-HT. 5-HT (1 and 2 mg/kg) produced dose dependent hyperglycemia in normoglycemic Wistar rats when injected intraperitonealy (Fig. 1). 5-HT-induced hyperglycemia was potentiated by 5-HT uptake blocker, fluoxetine, but not by 5-HT_{1A} receptor agonist buspirone and 5-HT_3 receptor agonist, 1-phenyl-biguanide (Fig. 1). On the other hand, 5-HT-induced hyperglycemia was inhibited by 5-HT_{2A} receptor antagonists, sarpogrelate and mianserin, and 5-HT_3 receptor antagonist ondansetron (Fig. 1) [28,29]. This indicates the involvement of 5-HT2A receptors in role of 5-HT in glycemic control.

5-HT AND STREPTOZOTOCIN-INDUCED DIABETES

Streptozotocin (STZ) injection causes hyperglycemia, hypoinsulinemia, loss of body weight, increased food intake and water intake. Streptozotocin-diabetes is reported to produce a decrease in precursor levels of 5-HT in the brain coupled with a subsequent decrease in synthesis and turn over of 5-HT [30]. Interestingly, depletion of brain 5-HT prior to STZ injection, by pretreatment with 5,7-DHT or parachlorophenyl alanine (PCPA), inhibits effects of STZ [31]. Plasma concentrations of 5-HT are reported to be high in diabetic than in normal subjects [32]. Contractile responses to 5-HT are attenuated in rat aorta [32–35] gastric fundus smooth muscles [36] and blood vessels from diabetic rats [37]. Attenuation of contractile responses to 5-HT in aorta was reportedly due to reduced activation of protein kinase C [38]. In contrast the contractile response to 5-HT was increased in detrusor smooth muscle of STZ-diabetic rat bladder [39]; this effect is related to smooth muscle hypertrophy and/or hyperplasia and is indicated to be mediated by the activation of 5-HT_{2A} receptors.

We studied the effect of 6 week treatment with 5-HT_{2A} receptor antagonist sarpogrelate (1 mg/kg, i.p., daily) on various biochemical parameters of STZ (45 mg/kg,

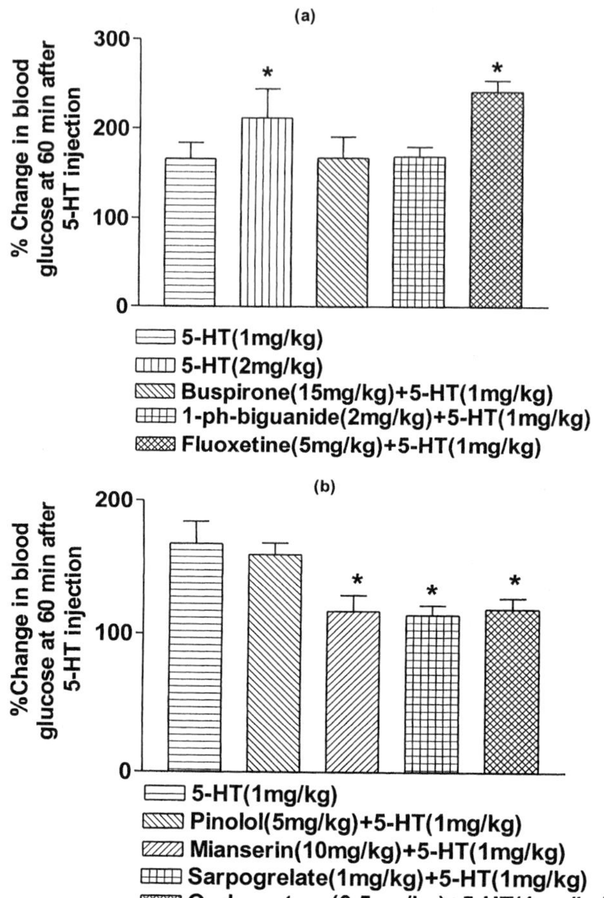

Figure 1. (a) Effect of 5-HT on serum glucose and its interaction with different (a) 5-HT agonists and (b) 5-HT antagonists at 60 min time interval after 5-HT injection. In normoglycemic Wistar rats. Each bar depicts mean ± SEM (n = 6).* significantly different from 5-HT (1 mg/kg) at 60 min. $P < 0.05$, one-way ANOVA followed by Student t-test.

i.v.) type 1 and type 2 diabetic Wistar rats. Sarpogrelate treatment significantly lowered blood glucose, cholesterol, and blood pressure, and insulin levels were significantly elevated in type 1 diabetic rats. Blood triglyceride levels and heart rate remained unaltered (Table 1). During oral glucose tolerance test (OGTT) in type 1 diabetic animals, sarpogrelate treatment showed significant decrease in area under curve (AUC) for glucose while AUC for insulin did not change significantly. In type 2 diabetic rats, sarpogrelate treatment significantly lowered AUC for insulin whereas, all the other above mentioned parameters remained unaltered (Table 1). These results further suggest the involvement of 5-HT_{2A} receptors in glycemic control and

Table 1. Effect of six week treatment with 5-HT2A antagonist sarpogrelate on various biochemical parameters of STZ type 1 and type 2 diabetic Wistar rats

Parameter	Wistar Control (n = 5)	Type 1 Diabetic Control (n = 6)	Type 1 Diabetic Treated (n = 6)	Type 2 Diabetic Control (n = 6)	Type 2 Diabetic Treated (n = 6)
Glucose (mmol/L)	4.3 ± 0.7	14.8 ± 0.6*	6.6 ± 0.9**	7.8 ± 0.2*	6.4 ± 0.3*
Insulin (pmol/L)	514 ± 25	342 ± 29*	595 ± 62**	831 ± 67*	632 ± 50
Cholesterol (mmol/L)	1.84 ± 0.10	4.79 ± 0.14*	3.84 ± 0.09**	2.65 ± 0.54*	2.30 ± 0.42
Triglyceride (mg/dl)	65 ± 10.9	186 ± 4.1*	158 ± 4.5*	124 ± 18.2*	121 ± 8*
$AUC_{glucose}$ (mmMin) × 10^3	18.9 ± 3.3	43.0 ± 2.4*	29.2 ± 3.4**	24.9 ± 1.2*	20.4 ± 3.4*
$AUC_{insulin}$ (mmMin) × 10^3	8.3 ± 0.2	5.2 ± 0.3*	7.8 ± 0.5	11.8 ± 0.8*	8.3 ± 0.9#
Blood Pressure (mm.Hg)	105 ± 10.1	146 ± 3.7*	82 ± 3.2**	140 ± 4.5*	135 ± 1.9*
Heart rate (beats/min)	405 ± 22.6	321 ± 12.3*	378 ± 10.4	393 ± 13.9	368 ± 15.2

*$P < 0.05$, compared with Wistar control; **$P < 0.05$, compared with type 1 diabetic control; #$P < 0.05$, compared with type 2 diabetic control (One way ANOVA followed by Tukey test).

indicate that sarpogrelate or specific 5-HT2A receptor antagonist may be viewed as prospective antidiabetic agent.

5-HT, APPETITE, OBESITY AND LEPTIN

It is well known that 5-HT regulates feeding behavior and decreases food intake in humans and rodents [40]. It has been suggested that 5-HT induced anorexia is mediated by the 5-HT receptors, including the central $5\text{-}HT_{1B}$, $5\text{-}HT_{2A}$, $5\text{-}HT_{2C}$ subtypes, since agonists of these receptors elicit hypophagia in rats [40,41]. Moreover, 5-HT receptors located in the peripheral system relate to the hypophagic effect of 5-HT as the peripheral 5-HT receptor agonists decrease food intake [42]. It has also been observed that male and female $5\text{-}HT_{1B}$ knock out mice have higher body weights than wild type mice [43]. Leptin has been newly identified as the product of ob gene and it is mainly released from adipose tissue [44,45]. Leptin strongly suppresses food intake and is a powerful satiation signal that can reduce body weight [46,47]. It is reported that systemic injection of 5-HT precursor 5-HTP, induces hyperleptinemia in mice [48]. Thus it is likely that the serotonergic mechanism is involved in secretion of leptin and that both leptin and 5-HT may interact for the regulation of food intake.

5-HT, PLATELET AGGREGATION AND DIABETES

Platelets differ from other formed elements of blood in expressing mechanisms for the uptake, storage and endocytotic release of 5-HT. It should be pointed out that

5-HT is not synthesized in platelets but is taken up from the circulation and stored in secretory granules. The main function of platelets is to plug holes in injured endothelial cells. Conversely, the functional integrity of endothelium is critical for the action of platelets [49]. The endothelial surface is exposed to platelets, because the shear forces of the circulating blood favour centrifugal stratification of platelets [50]. Release of endothelium-derived relaxing factor antagonizes the vasoconstrictor action of 5-HT [49]. The net effect of platelet aggregation is critically determined by the functional status of endothelium [51,52]. When platelets make contact with injured endothelium, they release substances including 5-HT that promote platelet adhesion [49]. 5-HT binding to platelet 5-HT_{2A} receptors elicits an aggregation response that is markedly enhanced in the presence of collagen. Diabetes is frequently associated with coronary artery disease. Experimental studies indicate that blood platelets are involved in the development of atherosclerosis [53–55]. Platelets are activated and then aggregate at the sites of coronary artery stenosis and endothelial injury [56–58]. Activated platelets release 5-HT in substantial quantities causing vasoconstriction [57,59]. 5-HT causes platelet aggregation through 5-HT_2 receptors. Increased platelet aggregation is a feature of diabetes and accordingly 5-HT levels are higher in diabetics [60]. 5-HT_{2A} receptor antagonist, sarpogrelate, is reported to inhibit 5-HT induced platelet thrombus formation [61]. In patients with type 1 diabetes, antiplatelet therapy of sarpogrelate is a useful antithrombin therapy as it suppresses the production of intrinsic coagulants by activated platelets and decreases endothelial cell damage via adhesion molecules [62]. Sarpogrelate is equally effective in type 2 diabetes as it is reported to be inhibitory to enhanced platelet aggregability under these conditions [63]. We have found that there is increase in basal platelet aggregation in STZ type 1 diabetic Wistar rats. There was significant reduction in basal as well as 5-HT induced platelet aggregation in these rats with 6 week treatment with 5-HT_{2A} antagonist, sarpogrelate (1 mg/kg, i.p.).

5-HT, GLYCEMIC CONTROL, AND CARDIAC FUNCTIONS

Diabetes co-exists with incidences of heart failure and development of cardiomyopathy [64]. 5-HT regulates cardiovascular function through central [65] as well as peripheral mechanisms [13,66]. 5-HT_{2A} receptor antagonist, sarpogrelate, is reported to inhibit vascular smooth muscle cell migration and proliferation induced by 5-HT [14]. The beneficial effects of 5-HT antagonists, however, have not been studied except for anti-thrombotic effects of sarpogrelate in diabetic situation. In diabetic cardiomyopathy myocardial glucose transport is reported to be defective [15]. A reduction in the capacity of myocardial glucose transport can be detrimental to the diabetic patient during periods of increased myocardial work or ischemia that is common with diabetes when the demand for glucose uptake is increased [67]. Glucose is carried across the plasma membrane by a family of glucose transporters including GLUT 1 and GLUT 4 [18]. Myocardial GLUT 4 and GLUT 1 are also shown to be decreased in diabetes [68]. It is reported that GLUT 1 is recruited to plasma membrane by various types of glucose transport stimuli, including insulin [69] and 5-HT [70]. In view of the importance of glucose carriers in cardiac function and considering critical role of 5-HT_2 receptors in cardiovascular pathophysiology in diabetes, we believe that 5-HT_2 receptor antagonists may produce beneficial effects. Since 5-HT is also reported to have lipolytic action on adipocytes increasing plasma levels of free fatty acids [71], reduction in triglyceride levels may also occur upon blocking the receptor sites for 5-HT.

5-HT plays critical role in the regulation of blood pressure. Activation of 5-HT_2 receptors results in pressor response associated with large increases in sympathetic activity. Circulating levels of 5-HT and catecholamines are increased in the diabetic as well as patients with coronary artery disease as compared to the normal subjects. Earlier studies with sarpogrelate have shown that it exerts cardioprotective action against myocardial infarction induced by coronary occlusion in rats [72]. The protective effect of sarpogrelate in myocardial infarction may be due to its action on blood constituents such as platelets. It is significant to note that platelet aggregability is abnormally increased in diabetes and sarpogrelate is a proven anti platelet aggregation agent. The cardioprotective effect of sarpogrelate may also be due to its direct effect on rat cardiomyocytes via 5-HT_{2A} receptors [73]. The activation of 5-HT_{2A} receptors has been shown to increase phospholipase C mediated hydrolysis of phosphoinositides in mouse ventricular myocytes [74]. It seems that 5-HT mediated deleterious effect on heart may be via 5-HT_{2A} receptor phospholipid linked signal transduction pathway and the protective effect of sarpogrelate against ischemia-reperfusion injury may be occurring at the receptor level.

Recently, Hajduch et al. [75] have reported that both rat and human skeletal muscles express 5-HT_{2A} receptors and specific 5-HT_{2A} receptor agonists can stimulate glucose uptake in skeletal muscles by a mechanism which does not depend upon components that participate in the insulin signaling pathway. Thus, it is possible that the anti-ischemic effects of 5-HT_{2A} antagonists may not be occurring through insulin-mediated signal transduction mechanisms. Nonetheless, in view of the increased incidence of myocardial infarction in diabetics, the anti-ischemic effect of agents such as sarpogrelate may contribute towards the usefulness of 5-HT_{2A} receptor antagonists in the treatment of diabetes-induced cardiovascular complications.

ACKNOWLEDGEMENTS

Authors acknowledge Indian Council of Medical Research (ICMR), New Delhi, India for supporting Mr. D. N. Umrani with senior research fellowship.

REFERENCES

1. Gupta YK, Prakash A. 1994. Therapeutic potential of 5-HT receptor modulators. Ind J Pharmacol 26:94–107.
2. Dhasmana KM, Zhu YN, Cruz SL, Villalon CM. 1993. Gastrointestinal effects of 5-hydroxytryptamine and related drugs. Life Sci 53:1651–1661.
3. Houston DS, Vanhoutte PM. 1986. Serotonin and the vascular system: role in health and disease, and implications for therapy. Drugs 31:149–163.
4. Rapport MM, Green AA, Page IH. 1948. Serum vasoconstrictor (serotonin). IV. Isolation and characterization. J Biol Chem 176:1243–1251.

5. Nakamura K, Kariyazono H, Moriyama Y. 1999. Effects of sarpogrelate hydrochloride on platelet aggregation, and its relation to the release of serotonin and P-selectin. Blood Coagul Fibrinolysis 10:513–519.
6. Shouzu A, Nomura S, Hayakawa T. 2000. Effect of sarpogrelate hydrochloride on platelet derived microparticles and various soluble adhesion molecules in diabetes mellitus. Clin Appl Thromb Hemost 6:139–143.
7. Lackovic Z, Salkovic M. 1990. Streptozotocin and alloxan produce alteration in rat brain monoamines independently of pancreatic beta cell destruction. Life Sci 46:49–54.
8. Yamada J, Sugimoto Y, Yoshikawa T, Kimura I, Horisaka K. 1995. The involvement of the peripheral $5\text{-}HT_{2A}$ receptor in peripherally administered serotonin-induced hyperglycemia in rats. Life Sci 57:819–825.
9. Sugimoto Y, Yamada J, Yoshikawa T, Horisaka K. 1996. The effects of peripheral serotonin2 (5-HT2) and serotonin3 (5-HT3) receptor agonists on blood glucose levels in rats. Biol Pharm Bull 19:1384–1386.
10. Sugimoto Y, Yamada J. 2000. Effects of the 5-HT2A receptor agonist 1-(2,5-dimethoxy-4-iodophenyl)-2-aminopropane (DOI) on plasma glucose and glucagon levels of rats. Biol Pharm Bull 23:1521–1523.
11. Laer S, Remmers F, Scholz H. 1998. Receptor mechanism involved in the 5-HT induced inotropic action in the rat isolated atrium. Br J Pharmacol 123:1182–1188.
12. Saxena PR. 1989. Cardiovascular effects from stimulation of 5-hydroxytryptamine receptors. Fund Clin Pharmacol 3:245–265.
13. Sharma SK, Zahrdka P, Chapman D, Kumamoto H, Takeda N, Dhalla NS. 1999. Inhibition of serotonin induced vascular muscle cell proliferation by sarpogrelate. J Pharmacol Exp Ther 290: 1475–1481.
14. Katz EB, Stenbit AE, Hatton K, DePinho R, Charron MJ. 1995. Cardiac and adipose tissue abnormalities but not diabetes in mice deficient in GLUT 4. Nature 377:151–155.
15. Hall, JL, Sexton WL, Stanley WC. 1995. Exercise training attenuates the reduction in myocardial GLUT-4 in diabetic rats. J Appl Physiol 78:76–81.
16. Badr GA, Tang J, Ismail-Beigi F, Kern TS. 2000. Diabetes downregulates GLUT-1 expression in the retina and its microvessels but not in the cerebral cortex or its microvessels. Diabetes 49:1016–1021.
17. Friedman JE, DeVente JE, Peterson RG, Dohm GL. 1991. Altered expression of muscle glucose transporter GLUT-4 in diabetic fatty Zucker rats (ZDF/Drt-*fa*). Am J Physiol 261:E782–E788.
18. Garvey W, Hardin D, Juhaszova M, Dominguez JH. 1993. Effects of diabetes on myocardial glucose transport system in rats: implications for diabetic cardiomyopathy. Am J Physiol 264:H837–H844.
19. Furman BL, Wilson GA. 1980. Further studies on the effects of 5-hydroxytryptamine on plasma glucose and insulin in mice. Diabetologia 19:386–390.
20. Wilson GA, Furman BL. 1982. Effects of inhibitors on 5-hyroxytryptamine uptake on plasma glucose and their interaction with 5-hydroxytryptophan in producing hypoglycemia in mice. Eur J Pharmacol 78:263–270.
21. Yamada J, Sugimoto Y, Kimura I, Takeuchi N, Horisaka K. 1989. Serotonin-induced hypoglycemia and increased serum insulin levels in mice. Life Sci 45:1931–1936.
22. Sugimoto Y, Kimura I, Yamada J, Watanabe Y, Takeuchi N, Horosaka K. 1990. Effects of serotonin on blood glucose and insulin levels of glucose and streptozotocin treated rats. 54:93–96.
23. Chaouloff F, Laude D, Baudrie V. 1990. Ganglionic transmission is a prerequisite for the adrenaline releaseing and hyperglycemic effects of 8-OH-DPAT. Eur J Pharmacol 185:11–18.
24. Chaouloff F, Baudrie V, Laude D. 1990. Evidence that the $5\text{-}HT_{1A}$ receptor agonists buspirone and ipsapirone activate adrenaline release in the conscious rat. Eur J Pharmacol 177:107–110.
25. Baudrie V, Chaouloff F. 1992. Mechanisms involved in the hyperglycemic effect of the $5\text{-}HT_{1C}/5\text{-}HT_2$ receptor agonist DOI. Eur J Pharmacol 213:41–46.
26. Sugimoto Y, Yamada J, Yoshikawa T, Horisaka K. 1996. Effects of the 5-HT2B/2C receptor agonist 1-(3-chlorophenyl) piperazine on the plasma glucose levels of rats. Eur J Pharmacol 307:75–80.
27. Chaouloff F, Gunn SH, Young JB. 1992. Central 5-hydroxytryptamine2 receptors are involved in the adrenal catecholamine releasing and hyperglycemic effects of the 5-hydroxytryptamine indirect agonist d-fenfluramine in the conscious rat. J Pharmacol Exp Ther 260:1008–1016.
28. Umrani DN, Goyal RK. 2000. Involvement of 5-hydroxytryptamine (5-HT3) receptors in insulin resistance. J Hypertension 18:S138.

29. Umrani DN, Goyal RK. 2001. Effect of sarpogrelate on altered 5-hydroxytryptamine–induced responses in STZ-diabetic rats. J Mol Cell Cardiol 33:A124.
30. Manjarrez-Gutierrez G, Rocio Herrera-Marquez JR, Bueno-Santoyo S, Gonzalez-Ramirez M, Hernandez J. 2000. Changes in brain serotonin biosynthesis in rats with diabetes mellitus induced by streptozotocin: effect of insulin treatment. Rev Invest Clin 52:509–516.
31. Yang YF, Lin MT. 1995. Brain serotonin depletion attenuates diabetogenic effects of streptozotocin. Am J Physiol 268:E839–E844.
32. Martin FJ, Miguez JM, Aldegunde M, Atienza G. 1995. Platelet serotonin transport is altered in streptozotocin-induced diabetic rats. Life Sci 56:1807–1815.
33. Hattori Y, Kawasaki H, Kanno M, Fukao M. 1995. Enhanced 5-HT_2 receptor mediated contractions in diabetic rat aorta: participation of Ca^{2+} channels associated with protein kinase C activity. J Vasc Res 32:220–229.
34. James GM, Hodgson WC, Davis EA, Haynes JM. 1994. Attenuated 5-hydroxytryptamine responses in aortae from streptozotocin-induced diabetic rats. Br J Pharmacol 111:370–376.
35. Sikorski BW, James GM, Glance SD, Hodgson WC, King RG. 1993. Effect of endothelium on diabetes induced changes in constrictor responses mediated by 5-hydroxytryptamine in rat aorta. J Cardiovasc Pharmacol 22:423–430.
36. Zhu BH, Sakai Y. 1996. Alteration of contractile properties to serotonin in gastric fundus smooth muscle isolated from streptozotocin (STZ)-induced diabetic rats. J Smooth Muscle Res 32:165–173.
37. James GM, Hodgson WC. 1995. Attenuated 5-HT_2 receptor-mediated responses in hindquarters of diabetic rats. Eur J Pharmacol 294:109–115.
38. James GM, Hodgson WC. 1997. A role for protein kinase C in the attenuated response to 5-hydroxytryptamine in aortas from streptozotocin-diabetic rats. Eur J Pharmacol 322:55–58.
39. Kodama M, Takimoto Y. 2000. Influence of 5-hydroxytryptamine and the effect of a new serotonin receptor antagonist (sarpogrelate) on detrusor smooth muscle of streptozotocin-induced diabetes mellitus in the rat. Int J Urol 7:231–235.
40. Dourish CT. 1995. Multiple serotonin receptors: opportunities for new treatments for obesity? Obes Res 3:449S–462S.
41. Curzon G. 1990. Serotonin and apetite. Ann N Y Acad Sci 600:521–531.
42. Simansky KJ. 1996. Serotonergic control of the organization of feeding and satiety. Behav Brain Res 73:37–42.
43. Bouwknecht JA, van der Gugten J, Hizen TH, Maes RA, Hen R, Olivier B. 2001. Male and female 5-HT(1B) receptor knock out mice have higher body weights than wild types Physiol Behav 74: 507–516.
44. Flier JS. 1997. Leptin expression and action: new experimental paradigms. Proc Natl Acad Sci 94:4242–4245.
45. Fruhbeck G, Jebb SA, Prentice AM. 1998. Leptin: physiology and pathophysiology. Clin Physiol 18:399–419.
46. Pellymounter MA, Cullen MJ, Baker MBRH, Winters D, Boone T, Collins F. 1995. Effects of the obese gene product on body weight regulation in *ob/ob* mice. Science 269:540–543.
47. Auwerx J, Stales B. 1998. Leptin. Lancet 351:737–742.
48. Yamada J, Ujikawa M, Sugimoto Y. 2000. Serum leptin levels after central and systemic injection of a serotonin precursor, 5-hydroxytryptophan, in mice. Eur J Pharmacol 406:159–162.
49. Furchgott RF, Vanhoutee PM. 1989. Endothelium-derived relaxing factor and constricting factors. FASEB J 3:2007–2018.
50. Gibbons GH, Dzau VJ. 1994. The emerging concept of vascular remodeling. N Eng J Med 330:1431–1438.
51. Hawiger J. 1992. Repertoire of platelet receptors. In, Platelets: Receptors, Adhesion, Secretion. (Hawiger J. ed) Methods in Enzymology 215:131–136.
52. Ware JA, Heistad DD. 1993. Platelet-endothelium interactions. N Eng J Med 328:628–635.
53. Wolf N. 1978. Thrombosis and atherosclerosis. Br Med Bull 34:137–142.
54. Lewis JC, Kottke BA. 1977. Endothelial damage and thrombocyte adhesion in pigeon atherosclerosis. Science 196:1007–1009.
55. Sevitt S. 1986. Platelets and foam cells in the evolution of atherosclerosis: histological nd immunohistological studies in human lesions. Atherosclerosis 61:107–115.
56. Bush LR, Campbell WB, Kern K, Tilton GD, Apprill P, Ashton J, Schmitz J, Buja LM, Willerson JT. 1984. The effects of alpha 2-adrenegic and serotonergic receptor antagonists on cyclic blood flow alterations in stenosed canine coronary arteries. Circ Res 55:642–652.

57. Ashton JH, Benedict CR, Fitzgerald C, Raheja S, Taylor A, Campbell WB, Buja LM, Willerson JT. 1986. Serotonin as a mediator of cyclic flow variations in stenosed canine arteries. Circulation 73: 572–578.
58. Eidt JF, Ashton J, Golino P, McNatt J, Buja LM, Willerson JT. 1989. Thromboxane A_2 and serotonin mediate coronary blood flow reductions in unsedated dogs. Am J Physiol 257:H873–H882.
59. Golino P, Ashton J, Buja LM, Rosolowsky M, Taylor AL, McNatt J, Campbell WB, Willerson JT. 1989. Local platelet activation causes vasoconstriction of large epicardial canine coronay arteries in vivo: Throboxane A_2 and serotonin are possible mediators. Circulation 79:154–166.
60. Barradas MA, Gill DS, Fonseca DP, Mikhailidis DP, Dandona P. 1988. Intraplatelet serotonin in patients with diabetes mellitus and peripheral vascular disease. Eur J Clin Invest 18:399–404.
61. Takano S. 1995. Role of 5-hydroxytryptamine in platelet thrombus formation and mechanisms of inhibition of thrombus formation by 5-hydroxytryptamine 2A antagonists in rabbits. Arch Int Pharmacodyn Ther 330:297–308.
62. Shouzu A, Nomura S, Hayakawa T, Omoto S, Shimizu H, Miyake Y, Yonemoto T, Fukuhara S, Iwasaka T, Nishikawa M, Inada M. 2000. Effect of sarpogrelate hydrochloride on platelet derived microparticles and various soluble adhesion molecules in diabetes mellitus. Clin Appl Thromb Hemost 6:139–143.
63. Pietraszek MH, Takada Y, Taminato A, Yoshimi T, Watanabe I, Takada A. 1993. The effect of MCI-9042 on serotonin-induced platelet aggregation in type 2 diabetes mellitus. Thromb Res 70:131–138.
64. Dhalla NS, Pierce GN, Innes IR, Beamish RE. 1985. Pathogenesis of cardiac dysfunction in diabetes mellitus. Can J Cardiol 1:263–281.
65. McCall RB, Clement ME. 1994. Role of $seretonin_{1A}$ and $serotonin_2$ receptors in the central regulation of the cardiovascular system. Pharm rev 46:231–243.
66. Lee H, Wu C. 1999. Serotonin-stimulated increase in cytosolic Ca^{2+} in cultured rat heart endothelial cells. Eur J Pharmacol 384:60–63.
67. James DE, Strube M, Mueckler M. 1989. Molecular cloning and characterization of an insulin regulatable glucose transporter. Nature 338:83–87.
68. Fischer Y, Thomas J, Rosen P, Kammermeier H. 1995. Action of metformin on glucose transporter GLUT 1 and GLUT 4 in heart muscle cells from healthy and diabetic rats. Endocrinology 136:412–420.
69. Fischer Y, Thomas J, Kamp J, Jungling E, Rose H, Carpene C, Kammermeier H. 1995. 5-Hydroxytryptamine stimulates glucose transport in cardiomyocytes via a monoamine-oxidase dependent reaction. Biochem J 311:575–583.
70. Fischer Y, Thomas J, Holeman GD, Rose H, Kammermeier H. 1996. Contraction independent effects of catecholamines on glucose transport in isolated rat cardiomyocytes. Am J Physiol 270: C1204–C1210.
71. Martinez-Conde A, Mayor de la Torre P, Tamarit-Tores J. 1984. Lipolytic effect of serotonin in vitro. Rev Esp Fisiol 40:213–219.
72. Brasil D, Temsah RM, Kumar K, Kumamoto H, Takeda N, Dhalla NS. 2002. Blockade of $5\text{-}HT_{2A}$ receptors by sarpogrelate protects the heart against myocardial infarction in rats. J Cardiovasc Pharmacol Therapeutic 7:53–59.
73. Temsah RM, Kumamoto H, Takeda N, Dhalla NS. 2001. Sarpogrelate diminishes changes in energy stores and ultrastructure of the ischemic-reperfused rat heart. Can J Physiol Pharmacol 79:761–767.
74. Nebigil CG, Choi DS, Dierich A, Hickel P, Le Meur M, Messaddeq N, Launay JM, Maroteaux L. 2000. Serotonin 2B receptor is required for heart development. Proc Natl Acad Sci 97:9508–9513.
75. Hajduch E, Rencurel F, Balendran A, Batty IH, Downes CP, Hundal HS. 1999. Serotonin (5-hydroxytryptamine), a novel regulator of glucose transporter in rat skeletal muscle. J Biol Chem 274:13563–13568.

G.N. Pierce, M. Nagano, P. Zahradka, and N.S. Dhalla (eds.).
ATHEROSCLEROSIS, HYPERTENSION AND DIABETES. Copyright © 2003.
Kluwer Academic Publishers. Boston.

SELECTIVE ATTENUATION OF ENHANCED ANGIOTENSIN II MEDIATED RESPONSES IN THE STREPTOZOTOCIN DIABETIC RAT THORACIC AORTA BY TEMPOL

BETTADAPURA N. SRIKUMAR, SHAILESH SHASTRI,[1] PODURI RAMARAO, and CHAMAN LAL KAUL[2]

Department of Pharmacology and Toxicology, National Institute of Pharmaceutical Education and Research, Phase-X, Sector 67, S.A.S.Nagar (Mohali)—160 062, Punjab, India

Summary. Previous studies suggest the role of superoxide anion radicals ($O_2^{\cdot -}$) as endothelium derived contractile factor. However, their role in the enhanced responses to angiotensin II (Ang II) or phenylephrine (PE) and diminished relaxation responses to acetylcholine (ACh) in diabetes remain unclear. In the present study, we investigated the possible involvement of $O_2^{\cdot -}$ in the Ang II-, PE- and ACh-mediated responses. Aortic rings were obtained from streptozotocin (STZ)-diabetic rats and contractile responses to Ang II and PE, and relaxation responses to acetylcholine (ACh) were assessed in presence of tempol. The contractile responses to Ang II and PE were significantly increased and the ACh mediated responses were impaired. Ang II and PE mediated responses in control rat aorta were unaffected by the presence of tempol (100 μM). The increase in responses to Ang II in diabetic aorta was decreased in presence of tempol (100 μM) but the PE mediated responses remained unchanged. Further, the impaired ACh mediated relaxation in diabetic aorta were restored by tempol. Removal of the endothelium led to an increase in the maximal response to Ang II and PE in both control and diabetic aorta. Tempol did not alter the responses to Ang II in endothelium-denuded aorta. The present findings indicate that $O_2^{\cdot -}$ may be involved in the increased contractile responses to Ang II but not PE in the diabetic rat thoracic aorta and this is endothelium dependent.

Key words: Streptozotocin-diabetic rat, Aorta, Angiotensin II, Superoxide radicals, Tempol, Endothelium

[1] Deceased before the completion of this work; [2] Corresponding Author. C.L. Kaul, Director, National Institute of Pharmaceutical Education and Research, Phase-X, Sector 67, S.A.S. Nagar—160 062 (Pb), India. NIPER Communication No: _; Tel: +91-172-214682; Fax: +91-172-214692; e-mail: kaulniper@yahoo.com

1. INTRODUCTION

Vascular complications persist to be the main cause of morbidity and mortality in the diabetic population [1]. The mechanisms involved in the development of diabetic vascular disease remain poorly understood despite numerous investigations [2]. Reports regarding vascular reactivity to alpha-adrenergic agonists and angiotensin II (Ang II) are inconsistent. Responses were found to be increased [3], decreased [4] or unchanged [5]. However, there are consistent reports that endothelial dependent vasodilatation (EDV) responses are impaired [6]. Reactive oxygen species (ROS), superoxides ($O_2^{\cdot-}$) in particular have been implicated to be responsible for the impaired vasorelaxation. In this context, increased generation of $O_2^{\cdot-}$ and other ROS [6] and decreased plasma or tissue concentrations of superoxide dismutase (SOD), catalase, glutathione and ascorbic acid in both clinical and experimental diabetes are reported [7]. The role of ROS has been established in most of the vascular beds like aorta [8], mesenteric artery [9], renal afferent arterioles [2] and basilar artery [10]. Amongst the ROS, $O_2^{\cdot-}$ [11], hydoxyl radical ($OH^{\cdot-}$) [12] and hydrogen peroxide (H_2O_2) [13] have been found responsible for the impaired relaxation responses to ACh. Therefore, the studies thus far have established the role of ROS in the impaired vasorelaxation. However, there are no reports indicating the involvement of $O_2^{\cdot-}$ in the evoked contractile responses to agonists in diabetes.

Ang II has been implicated in the diabetic vascular complications [14]. Ang II has been shown to produce $O_2^{\cdot-}$ by vascular smooth cells [15]. Ang II mediated hypertension in rats has been shown to be increase $O_2^{\cdot-}$ production in vascular smooth muscle and endothelium [16]. Increased levels of Ang II in rats [17] and decreased levels of Ang II in swine [18] and rats [19] have been found to cause oxidative stress. Recently, we have shown that the involvement of superoxides in the contractile response to acute addition of Ang II in aortic rings obtained from SHR [20]. Thus, although a link has been established for Ang II-stimulation of superoxide generation and superoxide involvement in the diabetic vascular complications, no systematic study has been undertaken to examine the involvement of $O_2^{\cdot-}$ in the contractile responses to Ang II in diabetes. The likelihood of $O_2^{\cdot-}$ role in the contractile response to Ang II may vary between the normal and diabetic rats. In this study, we have examined this possibility.

Tempol, a membrane-permeable, water-soluble SOD mimetic [21], was used in this study. Tempol has been shown to normalize mean arterial pressure in both short-term infusion and 7-day intraperitoneal administration [22]. The same authors reported that long-term oral administration of tempol ameliorated hypertension and renal excretion of $PGF_{2\alpha}$, a marker of oxidative stress in vivo [23]. Furthermore, tempol has been found valuable in demonstrating the role of $O_2^{\cdot-}$ in most models of hypertension like long-term infusion of Ang II [24], low levels of Ang II [19], renal hypertension [25], DOCA-salt hypertension [26], salt hypertensive Dahl rats [27] and lead-induced hypertension [28]. Hence, in order to evaluate the role of $O_2^{\cdot-}$ in the contractile responses to Ang II and PE in the diabetic rat aorta, we studied the Ang II- and PE-mediated responses in presence of tempol. ACh has been suggested to cause the release of $O_2^{\cdot -}$ in afferent renal arterioles of diabetic rabbits [2]. Hence, to examine the role of $O_2^{\cdot -}$ in the ACh mediated responses in the rat aorta, we studied the Ach induced relaxation in pre-contracted aorta in presence of tempol.

2. MATERIALS AND METHODS

All the experiments were approved by the Institutional Animals Ethics Committee (IAEC, NIPER).

2.1 Animals

Experiments were performed on male Sprague-Dawley rats weighing 180–200 g (Central Animal Facility, India), housed four per cage in a room with controlled ambient temperature (23 ± 1°C), humidity (50 ± 10%), 12 h light/dark cycle and free access to food and water through out the study.

2.2 Drugs

STZ (Calbiochem, U.S.A.) L-PE, tempol (both from Sigma Chemical Co., St. Louis, MO, U.S.A.), glucose GOD-POD kit (Glaxo Qualigens, Mumbai, India) and Ang II (Bachem, Basel, Switzerland) were used in the study. All other chemicals were of reagent grade obtained from Loba chemicals, India. All the drugs except STZ were dissolved in distilled water.

2.3 Induction of diabetes

Rats were made diabetic as described earlier [29]. Briefly, STZ (65 mg/kg, i.p.; dissolved in cold 0.01 M citrate buffer, pH 4.4) was injected to rats. Age-matched control rats were injected with citrate buffer. After 48 h of the STZ injection, blood samples were taken from the retro-orbital plexus and the plasma was analyzed for glucose using the GOD-POD kit (Glaxo-Qualigens, Mumbai, India). Rats with a blood glucose level >250 mg/dl were selected for the study.

2.4 Vascular tissue experiments

8 weeks after the STZ injection, rats were killed by cervical dislocation; the thoracic aorta was quickly excised and placed in cold oxygenated (95% O2–5% CO2) Kreb's-Henseleit buffer (KHB). The aorta was cleaned of adhering fat and adventitial tissues and 5 mm segments were cut. Care was taken not to stretch the tissue or damage the endothelium. In some preparations, the endothelium was deliberately removed by passing a steel wire of suitable diameter through the lumen and gently rubbed using the finger. The composition (mM) of KHB was NaCl: 2.6, KCl: 4.7, $MgCl_2.2H_2O$: 1.2, $CaCl_2$: 2.6, KH_2PO_4: 1.2, $NaHCO_3$: 25 and glucose: 11.1 per liter for the depolarizing solution, 90 mM KCl was added with corresponding decreases in NaCl.

2.5 Experimental design

Aortic ring was suspended by a pair of stainless steel hooks in water-jacketed organ bath, filled with 10 ml of oxygenated KHB maintained at 37°C. A resting tension of 2 g was applied to the aortic rings, which were then allowed to equilibrate for 2 h and the buffer was changed every 15 min. Isometric tension responses were measured on a student's physiograph chart recorder (BioDevices, Ambala, India) using an isometric force transducer (T-305, BioDevices, Ambala, India). The tissues were exposed to 90 mM KCl buffer (depolarizing solution). After two such challenges, contractile responses to increasing concentrations of Ang II (10 nM–30 μM) were recorded. Further concentrations were not used because tissues responses underwent rapid desensitization. Similarly, PE (1 nM to 10 μM) responses were obtained. In case of ACh, after the equilibration for 2 h, tissues were pre-contracted with 10 μM PE and responses to increasing concentrations of ACh (1 nM 10 μM) were obtained.

2.6 Effect of tempol on vascular responses

To evaluate the role of O_2^{-} in the enhanced contraction to Ang II and PE or impaired relaxation to ACh, the responses were evaluated in presence of tempol (100 μM). The tissues were incubated either in presence of tempol dissolved in Kreb's buffer (tempol treated) or Kreb's buffer alone (vehicle treated) for half an hour before the obtaining the responses. At the end of all the experiments, the rings were blotted dry, their lengths measured and weighed to calculate tension as normalized for cross-sectional area by the formula:

$$\text{Cross} - \text{sectional area}\ (\text{mm}^2) = \frac{\text{wieght (mg)}}{[\text{Length (mm)} \times \text{density}]}$$

with the density of vascular smooth muscle being 1.05 mg/mm^3. The KCl, PE and Ang II responses are expressed as mg/mm^2.

2.7 Statistical analysis

Cumulative concentration response curves were analyzed for pD_2 value (the negative log concentration required to produce 50% of the maximal response) and E_{max}. E_{max} is expressed as mg/mm^2 for the tension responses for Ang II, PE and KCl. ACh responses are expressed as percentage of maximum PE responses. All experimental values are expressed as mean ± S.E.M. Data analysis was done by Student's t test at 5% level of significance using GraphPad Prism version 3.00 for Windows, GraphPad Software, San Diego California USA.

3. RESULTS

3.1 Features of experimental animals

All the STZ treated animals marked showed hyperglycemia (blood sugar levels >400 mg/dl) and other characteristics like polyphagia, polydypsia and polyuria.

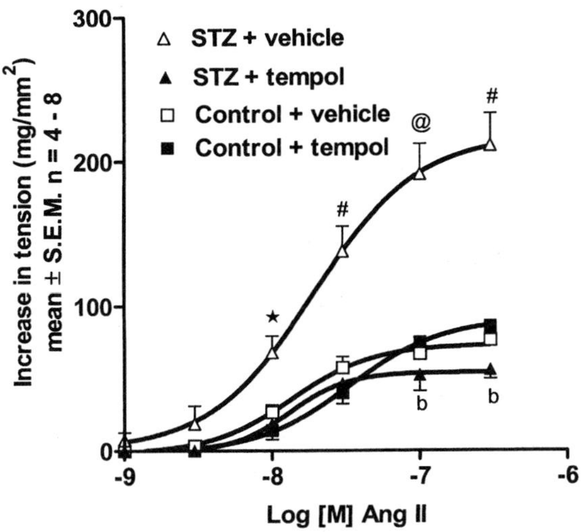

Figure 1. Cumulative Concentration Response Curves to Ang II in endothelium intact aortic ring preparations obtained from control and STZ-diabetic (STZ) rats in either absence (+ vehicle) or in presence (+ tempol) of tempol (100 μM). Tissues were incubated in presence of tempol (100 μM) or vehicle for half an hour prior to and during the exposure to Ang II. Each point is represented as mean ± S.E.M., n = tissues obtained from 4–8 rats. ★$P < 0.05$ vs respective control, #$P < 0.01$ vs respective control, @$P < 0.001$ vs respective control; b$P < 0.01$ vs respective + vehicle group.

3.2 Agonist induced contraction

The log dose response curves for Ang II and PE are shown in Figs. 1 and 2, respectively. The maximal contractile responses (E_{max}) were significantly increased to Ang II (Fig. 1) and PE (Fig. 2) in STZ-rats as compared to age matched control rats. But there was no difference in the E_{max} of the aorta from STZ diabetic and control rats to 90 mM KCl (KCl E_{max} for control and diabetic rats were 2,538.7 ± 209.8 and 2,782 ± 65.3, respectively). There was no change in the sensitivity (pD_2) of the aortas from STZ diabetic rats to KCl and Ang II. The increase in the Ang II response was blocked by tempol (100 μM).

3.3 ACh induced relaxation

The maximum relaxation response to ACh in pre-contracted aorta was decreased in STZ diabetic rats (Fig. 3). There was no change in the pD_2 in the ACh responses between control and diabetic rats. Tempol reversed the impaired ACh mediated responses to near control values (Fig. 3).

3.4 Effect of endothelium denudation on tempol effect

Removal of the endothelium led to an increase in the maximal responses to Ang II (Fig. 4) in both normal and STZ rats. There was no difference in the pD_2 values

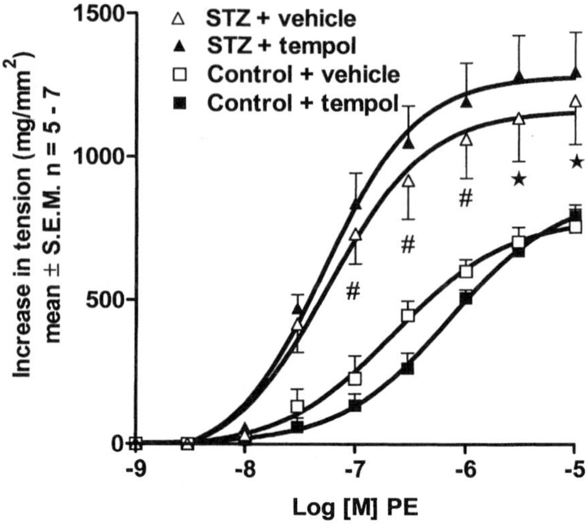

Figure 2. Cumulative Concentration Response Curves to PE in endothelium intact aortic ring preparations obtained from control and STZ-diabetic (STZ) rats in either absence (+ vehicle) or in presence (+ tempol) of tempol (100 μM). Tissues were incubated in presence of tempol (100 μM) or vehicle for half an hour prior to and during the exposure to PE. Each point is represented as mean ± S.E.M., n = tissues obtained from 5–7 rats. ⋆P < 0.05 vs respective control, #P < 0.01 vs respective control.

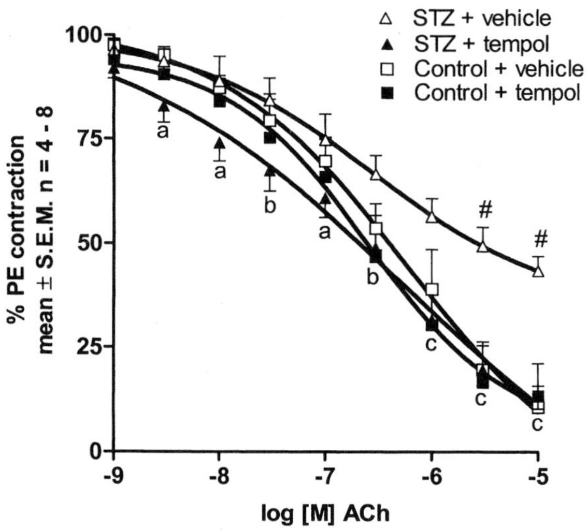

Figure 3. Cumulative Concentration Response Curves to ACh in endothelium intact aortic ring preparations obtained from control and STZ diabetic (STZ) rats in either absence (+ vehicle) or in presence (+ tempol) of tempol (100 μM). Rings were pre-contracted with 10^{-5} M PE. Tissues were incubated in presence of tempol (100 μM) or vehicle for half an hour prior to and during the exposure to PE and ACh Each point is represented as mean ± S.E.M., n = tissues obtained from 4–8 rats. #P < 0 .01 vs respective control, [a]P < 0.05 vs respective + vehicle group, [b]P < 0.01 vs respective + vehicle group, [c]P < 0.001 vs respective + vehicle group.

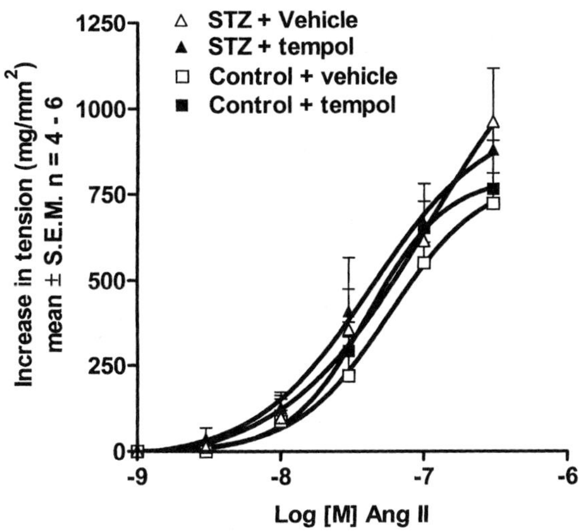

Figure 4. Cumulative Concentration Response Curves to Ang II in endothelium denuded aortic ring preparations obtained from control rats and STZ diabetic (STZ) rats in either absence (+ vehicle) or in presence (+ tempol) of tempol (100 μM). Tissues were incubated in presence of tempol (100 μM) or vehicle for half an hour prior to and during the exposure to Ang II. Each point is represented as mean ± S.E.M., n = tissues obtained from 4–6 rats.

between endothelium intact and endothelium denuded aortic rings. The KCl responses were unaffected by the removal of the endothelium. The E_{max} of KCl are 2,018 ± 117 and 2,372 ± 321.4, in intact and denuded, respectively). To evaluate the role of endothelium in the tempol-mediated effects, the vascular responses of Ang II were studied in endothelium-denuded preparations. Tempol did not affect the vascular responses to Ang II in the endothelium denuded aortic preparations (Fig. 4).

4. DISCUSSION

In this study, we report that the probable involvement of $O_2^{\cdot -}$ in the enhanced contractile responses to Ang II in diabetic rat aorta. In addition, O_2^- may not be involved in the enhanced responses to PE in STZ diabetic aorta. Furthermore ACh mediated responses may recruit O_2^-, which may be escalated in the STZ diabetic rat aorta. Our data also indicates that the vascular endothelium might have a role in the superoxide-mediated responses.

Studies indicate that the responses to Ang II are elevated in STZ-diabetes [30,31]. Our studies show that contractile responses to Ang II are elevated in STZ-diabetic rat aorta also. In good accordance with earlier reports [3,32], contractile responses to PE were increased in the STZ diabetic rat aorta. Further, the ACh mediated responses were impaired in the STZ diabetic rat thoracic aorta, which supports results from other studies [33,34]. This indicates that the vascular complications in diabetes may be having a dual component, which includes enhanced contraction to vasoconstrictor agonists and impaired relaxation to vasodilators.

The mechanisms, which contribute to these alterations in the responses, are multifarious. They may be changes in the receptor status or change in the post-receptor signal transduction mechanisms. Some of the mechanisms may be changes in PLC activity and altered subcellular calcium [35]. The present study demonstrates that $O_2^{\cdot -}$ might contribute to the exaggerated responses to Ang II. How $O_2^{\cdot -}$ cause the increase in the contractile response has been a investigated by several authors. $O_2^{\cdot -}$ is known to stimulate IP_3-induced Ca^{2+} release by inhibiting the degradation of IP_3 [36]. Changes in the carrier-mediated transport, passive diffusion and ligand-receptor interaction may occur as a consequence of $O_2^{\cdot -}$ reaction with the lipids in the cell membrane [37]. Most importantly, $O_2^{\cdot -}$ cause the degradation of NO which has a modulatory effect on the contractile responses of the blood vessels [38]. Tempol, which is a SOD mimetic, scavenges the superoxide radicals and restores the enhanced vascular responses to Ang II.

Tempol, in addition to restoring the enhanced Ang II mediated responses to control values, brought it beyond it. This may not be due to the concentration of tempol used because the vascular responses to Ang II were unaffected by lower concentrations (<100 μM) of tempol. Hence other mechanisms may be involved. H_2O_2 has been shown to cause direct vasorelaxation [39]. Studies have shown that this H_2O_2-induced relaxation is more in the diabetic aorta than in control vessels [13]. Superoxide radical levels are increased in diabetes [6] and in this study, we have shown that Ang II might induce the production of superoxide radicals in diabetic aorta. Tempol, a SOD mimetic causes the dismutation of $O_2^{\cdot -}$ and leads to the formation of H_2O_2. The H_2O_2, thus produced might cause vasorelaxation. This could possibly explain the tempol induced decrease in the Ang II induced contraction in diabetic aorta beyond the control response. Whether catalase prevents this decrease remains to be investigated. Further, spontaneous release of EDRF might be more in diabetic vessels [40]. But due to the presence or generation of superoxide radicals, such release might not be obvious. Scavenging of $O_2^{\cdot -}$ by tempol could cause more vasorelaxation or decreased contractile response to agonists like Ang II. Tempol at concentrations lower than 100 μM failed to produce any change in the responses to Ang II.

There are many enzymes, which act as the source of superoxides in the vasculature, including xanthine oxidase, NADH/NADPH oxidase and eNOS. Ang II is thought to cause the generation of superoxides through the NADH/NADPH oxidase [16]. Whether Ang II produces superoxides in diabetes through this enzyme needs further investigation.

Kawazoe and others [41] have demonstrated in rat aortic rings that superoxide radicals are involved in the contractile response to Ang II but not norepinephrine and epinephrine. Further, it has been shown that superoxide anions are involved in Ang II induced hypertension but not in catecholamine induced hypertension [17]. To determine whether superoxide radicals are involved in the enhanced contractile response to PE in diabetes, responses to PE were studied in presence of tempol. Similar to the report [41], tempol failed to alter the PE responses in diabetic rat aorta implicating that superoxide radicals are not involved in the enhanced vascular responses to PE. But in contrast to the same study, tempol did not alter Ang II induced contraction in control rat aorta. This may be attributed to the species difference as they used WKY rats and we in our study used SD rats. Investigators have shown that SOD reduces norepinephrine-induced contraction in the diabetic rat aorta [12]. Norepinephrine, a dihydroxyphenyl derivative that is subject to autooxidation in oxygenated buffer might be a source of superoxide radicals. Where as phenylephrine, which we used in our study is a synthetic monohydroxyphenyl derivative and is not prone to autooxidation. The reduction in the norepinephrine-induced contraction with pretreatment of SOD might have been in reality due to an improved EDV [12].

Superoxide radicals may be present both intracellularly and extracellularly implied by the physiological presence of different isoforms of SOD like Cu/ZnSOD, MnSOD and ecSOD [42]. Exogenously administered SOD is presumably confined to the extracellular space because of its large molecular weight. In the present study, tempol, a water soluble, membrane permeable, SOD mimetic [21] was used which is capable of scavenging both intracellular and extracellular O_2^{-}.

There are numerous studies, which emphasize the role of superoxide radicals in the impaired EDV in diabetes. Recently, Schnackenberg and Wilcox proposed that ACh per se can lead to the generation of superoxide radicals in the diabetic rabbit afferent renal arterioles [2]. Whether this is true in the aorta is not known. In this study, we have demonstrated that tempol improves the impaired EDV in response to ACh in diabetic rat aorta. How ACh causes the release of superoxides is not yet clear. As studies have shown, eNOS could be a possible source of superoxides [43].

Superoxides are found to be produced by both VSMCs and endothelial cells [44]. Many studies have implicated the endothelium as the source of superoxide radicals in the vasculature in diabetes. SOD pretreatment failed to alter the endothelium independent relaxation [13,12]. Hence, we evaluated the responses to Ang II in endothelium denuded aortic preparations. Similar to other reports [32], the removal of endothelium led to a drastic increase in the maximal responses to Ang II and PE [45]. Tempol did not alter the vascular responses to Ang II in endothelium denuded diabetic rat aorta. This indicates that the source of Ang II induced superoxide production may be the endothelium. NO is known to migrate to the VSMC from the endothelium, where it is produced. It is also possible that the superoxides released from the VSMC by Ang II may modulate the vascular tone by scavenging the NO and that modulation is lost on removal of endothelium. If endothelium is a source of superoxide radicals, how Ang II produces the superoxides in the endothelium is not known. eNOS has been shown to be a source of superoxide radicals and Ang II stimulates this to produce superoxide radicals in some vascular beds [44].

In conclusion, this study demonstrates the role of O_2^{-} in the enhanced contractile responses to Ang II and impaired relaxation responses to ACh in the STZ-diabetic rat aorta. Vascular complication associated with diabetes mellitus is of multifactorial origin and it is very unlikely that only one class of drug will produce tremendous change in the course of the disease. The results of this study lead to the speculation that SOD mimetics may prove to be a valuable therapeutic option in the treatment of diabetic vasculopathy in the future.

ACKNOWLEDGEMENTS

BNS was supported by a NIPER funding. The authors acknowledge NIPER for providing the necessary facilities.

REFERENCES

1. Cooper ME, Bonnet F, Oldfield M, Jandeleit-Dahm K. 2001. Mechanisms of diabetic vasculopathy: an overview. Am J Hypertens 14:475–486.
2. Schnackenberg CG, Wilcox CS. 2001. The SOD mimetic tempol restores vasodilation in afferent arterioles of experimental diabetes. Kidney Int 59:1859–1864.
3. Chang KS, Stevens WC. 1992. Endothelium-dependent increase in vascular sensitivity to phenylephrine in long-term streptozotocin diabetic rat aorta. Br J Pharmacol 107:983–990.
4. Head RJ, Longhurst PA, Panek RL, Stitzel RE. 1987. A contrasting effect of the diabetic state upon the contractile responses of aortic preparations from the rat and rabbit. Br J Pharmacol 91:275–286.
5. MacLeod KM, McNeill JH. 1985. The influence of chronic experimental diabetes on contractile responses of rat isolated blood vessels. Can J Physiol Pharmacol 63:52–57.
6. De Vriese AS, Verbeuren TJ, Van de Voorde J, Lameire NH, Vanhoutte PM. 2000. Endothelial dysfunction in diabetes. Br J Pharmacol 130:963–974.
7. Giugliano D, Ceriello A, Paolisso G. 1996. Oxidative stress and diabetic vascular complications. Diabetes Care 19:257–267.
8. Chang KC, Chung SY, Chong WS, Suh JS, Kim SH, Noh HK, Seong BW, Ko HJ, Chun KW. 1993. Possible superoxide radical-induced alteration of vascular reactivity in aortas from streptozotocin-treated rats. J Pharmacol Exp Ther 266:992–1000.
9. Diederich D, Skopec J, Diederich A, Dai FX. 1994. Endothelial dysfunction in mesenteric resistance arteries of diabetic rats: role of free radicals. Am J Physiol 266:H1153–H1161.
10. Mayhan WG. 1997. Superoxide dismutase partially restores impaired dilatation of the basilar artery during diabetes mellitus. Brain Res 760:204–209.
11. Hattori Y, Kawasaki H, Abe K, Kanno M. 1991. Superoxide dismutase recovers altered endothelium-dependent relaxation in diabetic rat aorta. Am J Physiol 261:H1086–H1094.
12. Pieper GM, Langenstroer P, Siebeneich W. 1997. Diabetic-induced endothelial dysfunction in rat aorta: role of hydroxyl radicals. Cardiovasc Res 34:145–156.
13. Pieper GM, Gross GJ. 1988. Oxygen free radicals abolish endothelium-dependent relaxation in diabetic rat aorta. Am J Physiol 255:H825–H833.
14. Komers R, Komersova K. 2000. Therapeutic potential of ACE inhibitors for the treatment of hypertension in Type 2 diabetes. Expert Opin Investig Drugs 9:2601–2617.
15. Griendling KK, Minieri CA, Ollerenshaw JD, Alexander RW. 1994. Angiotensin II stimulates NADH and NADPH oxidase activity in cultured vascular smooth muscle cells. Circ Res 74:1141–1148.
16. Rajagopalan S, Kurz S, Munzel T, Tarpey M, Freeman BA, Griendling KK, Harrison DG. 1996. Angiotensin II-mediated hypertension in the rat increases vascular superoxide production via membrane NADH/NADPH oxidase activation. Contribution to alterations of vasomotor tone. J Clin Invest 97:1916–1923.
17. Laursen JB, Rajagopalan S, Galis Z, Tarpey M, Freeman BA, Harrison DG. 1997. Role of superoxide in angiotensin II-induced but not catecholamine-induced hypertension. Circulation 95:588–593.
18. Haas JA, Krier JD, Bolterman RJ, Juncos LA, Romero JC. 1999. Low-dose angiotensin II increases free isoprostane levels in plasma. Hypertension 34:983–986.
19. Ortiz MC, Sanabria E, Manriquez MC, Romero JC, Juncos LA. 2001. Role of endothelin and isoprostanes in slow pressor responses to angiotensin II. Hypertension 37:505–510.
20. Shastri S, Ramarao P, Kaul CL, McNeill JR, Gopalakrishnan V. Tempol selectively attenuates vasoconstrictor responses to Ang II in aorta and perfused mesenteric vascular bed of spontaneously hypertensive rats (SHR). *Annual Conference of Ind. Pharmacol. Soc., 2000.* Gandhinagar, India; 2000.

21. Samuni A, Krishna CM, Mitchell JB, Collins CR, Russo A. 1990. Superoxide reaction with nitroxides. Free Radic Res Commun 9:241–249.
22. Schnackenberg CG, Welch WJ, Wilcox CS. 1998. Normalization of blood pressure and renal vascular resistance in SHR with a membrane-permeable superoxide dismutase mimetic: role of nitric oxide. Hypertension 32:59–64.
23. Schnackenberg CG, Wilcox CS. 1999. Two-week administration of tempol attenuates both hypertension and renal excretion of 8-Iso prostaglandin f2alpha. Hypertension 33:424–428.
24. Nishiyama A, Fukui T, Fujisawa Y, Rahman M, Tian RX, Kimura S, Abe Y. 2001. Systemic and Regional Hemodynamic Responses to Tempol in Angiotensin II- Infused Hypertensive Rats. Hypertension 37:77–83.
25. Dobrian AD, Schriver SD, Prewitt RL. 2001. Role of angiotensin II and free radicals in blood pressure regulation in a rat model of renal hypertension. Hypertension 38:361–366.
26. Beswick RA, Zhang H, Marable D, Catravas JD, Hill WD, Webb RC. 2001. Long-term antioxidant administration attenuates mineralocorticoid hypertension and renal inflammatory response. Hypertension 37:781–786.
27. Zicha J, Dobesova Z, Kunes J. 2001. Relative deficiency of nitric oxide-dependent vasodilation in salt-hypertensive Dahl rats: the possible role of superoxide anions. J Hypertens 19:247–254.
28. Vaziri ND, Ding Y, Ni Z. 2001. Compensatory up-regulation of nitric-oxide synthase isoforms in lead-induced hypertension; reversal by a superoxide dismutase-mimetic drug. J Pharmacol Exp Ther 298:679–685.
29. Gullapalli S, Gurumoorthy K, Kaul CL, Ramarao P. In Press. Role of L-type Ca^{2+} channels in attenuated morphine antinociception in streptozotocin-diabetic rats. Eur J Pharmacol 435:187–194.
30. Kaul CL, Grewal RS. 1980. Vascular reactivity in streptozotocin induced diabetic rat. Pharmacol Res Commun 12:945–958.
31. Schoonmaker GC, Fallet RW, Carmines PK. 2000. Superoxide anion curbs nitric oxide modulation of afferent arteriolar ANG II responsiveness in diabetes mellitus. Am J Physiol Renal Physiol 278: F302–F309.
32. Cinar MG, Ulker S, Alper G, Evinc A. 2001. Effect of dietary vitamin E supplementation on vascular reactivity of thoracic aorta in streptozotocin-diabetic rats. Pharmacology 62:56–64.
33. Oyama Y, Kawasaki H, Hattori Y, Kannon M. 1986. Attenuation of endothelium-dependent relaxation in aorta from diabetic rats. Eur J Pharmacol 132:75–78.
34. Pieper GM, Siebeneich W. 2000. Temocapril, an angiotensin converting enzyme inhibitor, protects against diabetes-induced endothelial dysfunction. Eur J Pharmacol 403:129–132.
35. Fleischhacker E, Esenabhalu VE, Spitaler M, Holzmann S, Skrabal F, Koidl B, Kostner GM, Graier WF. 1999. Human diabetes is associated with hyperreactivity of vascular smooth muscle cells due to altered subcellular Ca2+ distribution. Diabetes 48:1323–1330.
36. Freeman BA, Rosen GM, Barber MJ. 1986. Superoxide perturbation of the organization of vascular endothelial cell membranes. J Biol Chem 261:6590–6593.
37. Suzuki YJ, Ford GD. 1992. Superoxide stimulates IP3-induced Ca2+ release from vascular smooth muscle sarcoplasmic reticulum. Am J Physiol 262:H114–H116.
38. Rubanyi GM, Vanhoutte PM. 1986. Superoxide anions and hyperoxia inactivate endothelium-derived relaxing factor. Am J Physiol 250:H822–H827.
39. Rubanyi GM, Vanhoutte PM. 1986. Oxygen-derived free radicals, endothelium, and responsiveness of vascular smooth muscle. Am J Physiol 250:H815–H821.
40. Langenstroer P, Pieper GM. 1992. Regulation of spontaneous EDRF release in diabetic rat aorta by oxygen free radicals. Am J Physiol 263:H257–H265.
41. Kawazoe T, Kosaka H, Yoneyama H, Hata Y. 2000. Acute production of vascular superoxide by angiotensin II but not by catecholamines. J Hypertens 18:179–185.
42. Fridovich I. 1995. Superoxide radical and superoxide dismutases. Annu Rev Biochem 64:97–112.
43. Kojda G, Harrison D. 1999. Interactions between NO and reactive oxygen species: pathophysiological importance in atherosclerosis, hypertension, diabetes and heart failure. Cardiovasc Res 43: 562–571.
44. Griendling KK, Ushio-Fukai M. 2000. Reactive oxygen species as mediators of angiotensin II signaling. Regul Pept 91:21–27.
45. Carrier GO, White RE. 1985. Enhancement of alpha-1 and alpha-2 adrenergic agonist-induced vasoconstriction by removal of endothelium in rat aorta. J Pharmacol Exp Ther 232:682–687.

G.N. Pierce, M. Nagano, P. Zahradka, and N.S. Dhalla (eds.).
ATHEROSCLEROSIS, HYPERTENSION AND DIABETES. Copyright © 2003.
Kluwer Academic Publishers. Boston.

ROLE OF RENIN-ANGIOTENSIN SYSTEM IN DIABETIC HEART DYSFUNCTION AND CHANGES IN PHOSPHOLIPASE C ACTIVITY

PARAMJIT S. TAPPIA, SUSHMA A. MENGI, and NARANJAN S. DHALLA

Institute of Cardiovascular Sciences, St. Boniface General Hospital Research Centre, Departments of Human Nutritional Sciences and Physiology, Faculties of Human Ecology and Medicine, University of Manitoba, Winnipeg, Canada

Summary. The incidence of heart disease is greater in the diabetic population as compared to nondiabetics. Although cardiac abnormalities in diabetics are independent of coronary artery disease, hypertension and valvular disease, the molecular events underlying the contractile dysfunction of the heart during diabetes are incompletely defined. Since renin-angiotensin system is activated in diabetes, an accelerated generation of angiotensin II may be involved in the pathophysiological chain of events leading to diabetic cardiomyopathy. This article deals with the potential role of changes in phospholipase C-mediated signaling mechanisms induced by activation of the renin-angiotensin system in diabetes. Such information will extend our knowledge in the field of heart disease due to diabetes and help in the development of new therapy for its treatment.

***Key words*:** Diabetic cardiomyopathy, Cardiac sarcolemma, Phospholipase C, Renin-angiotensin system, Signal transduction mechanisms

INTRODUCTION

It is known that patients with diabetes mellitus have an increased risk of mortality from cardiac dysfunction that cannot simply be explained in terms of atherosclerosis, microangiopathy or autonomic neuropathy [1–7]. Pathological and physiological studies have provided evidence for a cardiomyopathy in clinical diabetes mellitus

Address for Correspondence: Dr. Paramjit S. Tappia, Institute of Cardiovascular Sciences, St. Boniface General Hospital Research Centre (R3020), 351 Tache Avenue, Winnipeg, Manitoba, Canada R2H 2A6. Tel: 204-235-3681; Fax: 204-233-6723; e-mail: ptappia@sbrc.ca

[8,9] that may manifest as impaired ventricular function even before clinical signs of cardiac failure develop [10]. There is also direct evidence obtained from diabetic animals for changes in cardiomyocytes [11–16]. Apart from cases of diabetic patients developing congestive heart failure (CHF), the most important clinical consequences of diabetic cardiomyopathy are its complications, which include enhanced susceptibility to hypertension-mediated damage, increased mortality rate associated with acute myocardial infarction, blunted mechanical response to myocardial stress, and increased incidence of post-infarction CHF [17]; however, the mechanisms for such complications as well as for heart dysfunction in diabetes are not fully understood. This article is intended to deal with the role of renin-angiotensin system (RAS) in diabetes-induced cardiac dysfunction because RAS is known to be activated in this condition. Furthermore, in view of the participation of phospholipase C (PLC)-mediated signal transduction mechanisms in the regulation of heart function, it is planned to discuss the significance of the changes in PLC activity in relation to heart dysfunction in diabetes.

STREPTOZOTOCIN-INDUCED RAT MODEL OF INSULIN-DEPENDENT DIABETES MELLITUS

Diabetic cardiomyopathy is present in experimental animal models of insulin-dependent diabetes mellitus (IDDM), like [streptozotocin (STZ)-induced diabetic rats, alloxan-induced diabetic rats and insulin-dependent BioBreeding (BB) rats that spontaneously develops diabetes [18]. Because it is virtually impossible to examine the etiopathological changes that lead to cardiomyopathy in diabetic patients, valuable information has been obtained by using animal models [4,18]. In particular, young adult rats injected with intermediate doses of STZ (55–65 mg/kg body wt., i.v.) display many features seen in human subjects with uncontrolled IDDM [6]. Severe insulin deficiency results in hyperglycemia (with reduced glucose transport into the cell), glycosuria, polydipsia, polyuria and weight loss. Increased hepatic gluconeogenesis and glucose release are also prominent whereas nitrogen balance is negative due to enhanced proteolysis coupled with impaired protein synthesis [4]. STZ-diabetic rats mobilize stored triglycerides, as evident from the rise in the intracellular lipase activity in adipose tissue, which is followed by a pronounced outflow and increased oxidation of free fatty acids (FFA) [19]. Although present, ketosis and ketonuria do not usually progress to lethal ketoacidosis. This is a significant distinction from the insulin-dependent BioBreeding (BB) rats and indicates that a residual insulin secretion persists in STZ-treated rats. An elevation in plasma triglycerides, cholesterol and phospholipids carried by the very low-density and low-density lipoprotein fractions is evident in the diabetic animals, which also are hypothyroid [4,20]. Some studies in patients with diabetes mellitus have shown reduced conversion of L-thyroxine (T_4) to triiodothyronine (T_3) [21] and an increased incidence of subclinical thyroid failure [22]. Hypothyroidism is known to have effects on the myocardium [4,6,23,24]. Therefore, it is important to be aware of the role that hypothyroidism may play in the development of diabetic cardiomyopathy.

ROLE OF RENIN-ANGIOTENSIN SYSTEM IN THE DIABETIC HEART DYSFUNCTION

Clinical and experimental investigations have suggested that increased sympathetic activity [25], activated cardiac RAS [26,27], myocardial ischemia/functional hypoxia [28] and elevated glucose levels [29–31] due to insulin deficiency, result in oxidative stress [4]. Since cellular defense mechanisms, such as antioxidants and antioxidant enzymes (superoxide dismutase, catalase and glutathione peroxidase), play a fundamental role in protecting the cell against reactive free radical and other oxidant species [32], it is possible that a loss of these factors will promote the occurrence of oxidative stress during the development of diabetic cardiomyopathy. However, increases in CuZn superoxide dismutase, catalase and glutathione peroxidase activities have been observed in the diabetic rat heart [33–35]. Although increased levels of tissue antioxidants may serve as an adaptive mechanism during the early stages of diabetes, this antioxidant reserve may get depleted with time and shift the balance towards oxidative stress and subsequent heart dysfunction. In fact, increases in myocardial lipid hydroperoxide, an index of oxidative stress, have been detected in chronic diabetes stage [36]. The impairment of the endothelium may also promote oxidative stress activity. Although a direct relationship between endothelial changes and the development of diabetic cardiomyopathy has not been examined, a defective endothelium has been shown to produce an imbalance, due to reduced formation of nitric oxide and increased production of oxyradicals [37]. Furthermore, an excessive amount of nitric oxide produced due to endothelial dysfunction and superoxide radicals formed as a consequence of increased auto-oxidation of glucose and protein glycation [38–40] can also be seen to react with each other to result in the formation of a potent oxidant, peroxynitrite and therefore promote the occurrence of oxidative stress in diabetes [41,42]. It should be noted that the role of oxidative stress in diabetic cardiomyopathy is indicated by the observations that vitamin E treatment has been shown to increase tissue antioxidant concentration, improve the action of insulin, promote endothelial function, prevent oxidation of serum lipids, suppress protein glycation and reduce oxidative load [43–48]. Furthermore, epidemiological observations and clinical studies underlie the impact of oxidative stress for the development of heart disease in diabetes and suggest that an antioxidant treatment could prove to be of benefit; however, a direct relationship between oxidative stress and the development of cardiomyopathy in chronic diabetes remains to be established. It should be noted that a significant increase in myocardial AT_1 receptor density and mRNA level in STZ-induced diabetic rats has been reported [26,49–51], while the AT_2 receptor density remains constant [26]. Recent evidence has indicated that angiotensin II can mediate reactive oxygen species formation via membrane-bound NAD(P)H-oxisases [52,53] and may lead to oxidative damage [54]. Studies with angiotensin II type 1 receptor antagonist, losartan, have demonstrated a reduction in reactive oxygen species production in diabetic cardiomyocytes [55]. The role of activated RAS and oxidative stress is further supported by observations the angiotensin converting enzyme (ACE) inhibitors increase both the enzymatic and nonenzymatic antioxidant defense

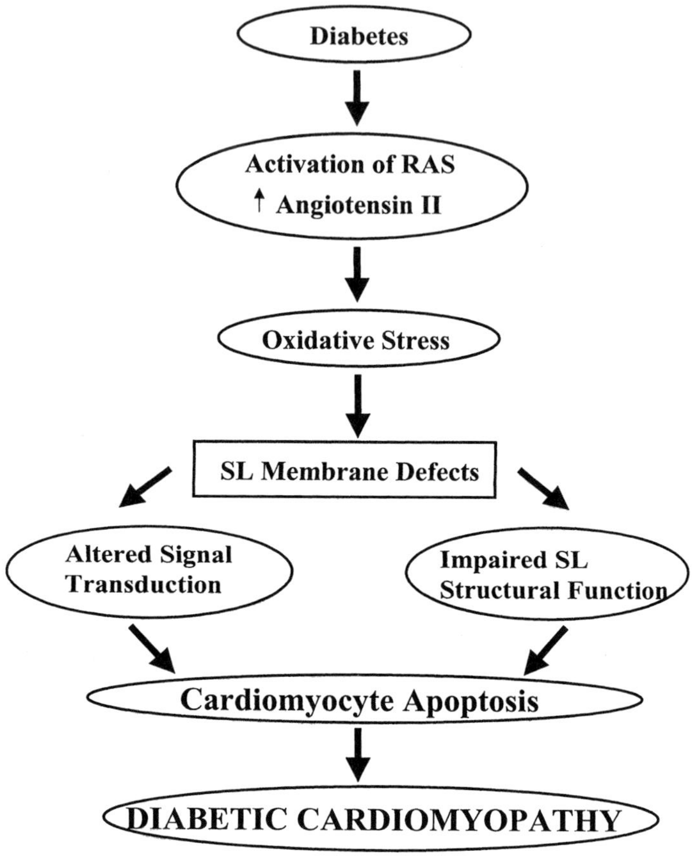

Figure 1. Role of renin-angiotensin system in the pathogenesis of ventricular dysfunction due to diabetes.

mechanisms in the heart [56–58]. Therefore, RAS seems to be involved in the pathogenesis of diabetic cardiomyopathy and promoting oxidative stress and activating cell death (Fig. 1); this view is confirmed by the demonstration that losartan prevents cardiac cell death in the STZ-induced diabetes model [26]. However, the cellular and molecular mechanisms involved in this beneficial effect have yet to be clearly defined.

SARCOLEMMAL DEFECTS IN DIABETIC CARDIOMYOPATHY

The cardiac sarcolemma (SL) membrane is considered to play an important role in the cardiomyocyte Ca^{2+} homeostasis and maintaining the contractile status [59,60]. Extensive studies have been conducted to identify defects in SL functional activities during the development of cardiomyopathy in rats with STZ-induced diabetes. Depressed SL Ca^{2+} pump [61,62] and Na^{+}-Ca^{2+} exchange [16,62] activities were reported. Since the two Ca^{2+} transport systems are believed to remove Ca^{2+} from the myocardial cell under normal conditions [59], their abnormalities may lead to intracellular Ca^{2+} overload and subsequent cell damage [4]. Of note, the intracellular Ca^{2+} overload referred here should not be confused with the intracellular concentration of free Ca^{2+} which may not change in diabetes [63], as free Ca^{2+} in the cytoplasm may become accumulated in the intracellular organelles of cardiomyocytes. In fact, elevated levels of myocardial Ca^{2+} have been reported in diabetes [64,65], although some investigators have suggested a decrease [66] or even no change [67]. Interestingly, the diabetic heart has been suggested to adapt to Ca^{2+} overload [68,69]. Superficial SL Ca^{2+} stores, which linearly correlate with contractile force generation [70], are reduced [71]. This would suggest a decreased Ca^{2+} entry into the diabetic cardiomyocyte and may contribute to the depressed mechanical function seen in humans [21,22] and STZ experimental animals [10]. On the other hand, binding studies have shown either no change [72] or increase [73] in voltage-sensitive Ca^{2+} channels in crude membrane extracts from diabetic hearts. Alteration of Na^{+}, K^{+} ATPase [74,75] and Na^{+}, H^{+} exchange [76] activities indicates imbalance of Na^{+} transport across SL, and this may affect the Na^{+}-Ca^{2+} exchanger which depends on the Na^{+} gradient.

Changes in membrane phospholipid composition are considered to change the activities of various membrane-bound enzymes and subsequently heart function under pathophysiological conditions [77]. Alterations in molecular species of the major SL phospholipid classes have been observed in STZ-induced diabetes [78]. Although insulin treatment was able to restore these changes, diabetes-induced changes in the membrane composition may be responsible for alterations in the function of integral membrane proteins, contributing to some of the changes observed in the diabetic myocardium. Elevations in total myocardial DAG content have been reported in STZ-injected diabetic rats and in diabetic BB rats [79]. It is interesting to note that insulin therapy did not normalize DAG content and its fatty acid composition [80]. Taken together, sustained elevations in DAG may be a contributory factor for the development of diabetic cardiomyopathy. Accumulation of lysophosphatidylcholine (LPC) has also been reported in diabetic cardiomyopathy [71], due to an increase in phospholipase A_2 activity [81]. A decrease in the SL phosphatidic acid levels has also been detected in the diabetic heart, which is only partially normalized by insulin [20]. Plasma and cardiac levels of norepinephrine are elevated in diabetes [82] and are accompanied by a decreased density and mRNA expression of myocardial β-adrenoceptors, reduced expression and concomitant G_i functional uncoupling with post-receptor activities, and reduced responsiveness to agonists [18,83]. The α_1-adrenoceptors, that are associated to positive inotropic effect via phosphoinositide pathway [84], are reduced in density [18]. Nonetheless, the diabetic heart showed augmented α_1-mediated biochemical and mechanical responses [14,85,86]. Decreased receptor number and α_1-adrenergic supersensitivity may indicate abnormalities in the post-receptor functional activities

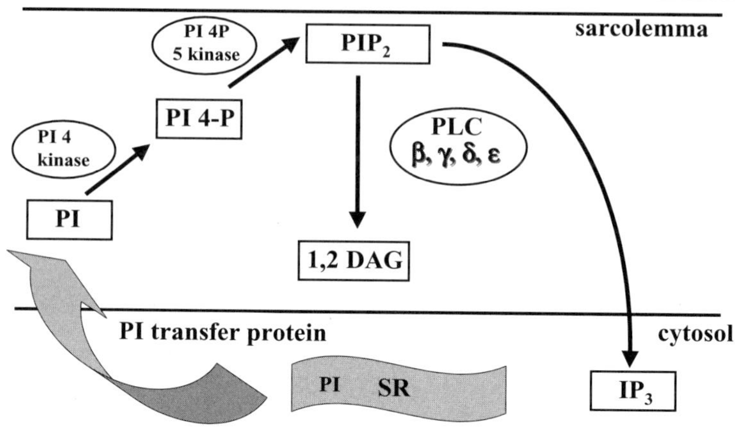

Figure 2. Phosphoinositide-signaling pathway in cardiac sarcolemma. Phospholipase C (PLC) hydrolyzes its most common physiological substrate, phosphatidylinositol 4,5-bisphosphate (PIP_2) to produce two messenger molecules, inositol 1,4,5- trisphosphate (IP_3) and 1,2 diacylglycerol (1,2 DAG). PIP_2 is synthesized in the SL membrane by the coordinated and successive action of phosphatidylinositol 4 kinase (PI 4 kinase) to produce phosphatidylinositol 4-phosphate (PI 4-P) and phosphatidylinositol 4-phosphate 5 kinase (PI 4-P 5 kinase). Newly synthesized phosphatidylinositol (PI) in sarcoplasmic reticulum (SR) is transported to the SL membrane from SR via PI transfer protein.

involved in the cell response to the adrenergic agonist. At any rate, these results suggest that the α_1-adrenoceptors may subserve as a source of positive inotropy in diabetic cardiomyopathy.

PHOSPHOINOSITIDE-SPECIFIC PLC

The phosphoinositide-signaling pathway is shown in Fig. 2. The phosphoinositide-specific PLC is involved in numerous transmembranal signals [87]. The four known classes of mammalian PLC (β, γ, δ and ε) comprise at least eleven isoforms [87] and display differences in structure, function and activation mechanisms in response to stimulation of specific cell-surface receptors [85,88–101]. Although little is known about the number and characteristics of PLC isoforms in normal cardiac cells, β_1, β_2, β_3, δ_1, γ_1 and two forms of ε are expressed in adult ventricular cardiomyocytes [88,102–105]. It is pointed out that PLC δ_1 is the predominant SL PLC isoenzyme [88,102]. The distinct functions of each PLC isoenzyme in the cardiomyocytes, and the extent of their overlap has yet to be established. However, recently by using adenovirus infection, the α_1-adrenoceptor mediated IP_3 generation in rat neonatal cardiomyocytes has been shown to be mediated by PLC β_1 [106]. Binding sites for IP_3 and its phosphorylated derivative inositol 1,3,4,5-tetrakisphosphate have been found at the cardiac sarcoplasmic reticulum (SR) level [107,108] and may serve to enhance the SR Ca^{2+}—release and uptake, activities [109–111]. These messenger-mediated

SR Ca^{2+}—movements (in addition to phosphorylation- induced increase in Ca^{2+}—entry through the slow inward Ca^{2+}—current or via the Na^+–Ca^{2+} exchange; [109,112] may modulate the inotropic response of the cardiac muscle to agonists [84,109]. Immunolocalizaton of IP_3 receptors at the fascia adherens of the intercalated discs may suggest a possible role of these receptors in local Ca^{2+}-entry or in intercellular signaling between cardiomyocytes [113]. Among the biological functions of DAG, one of the most significant is the activation of most protein kinase C (PKC) isoenzymes which phosphorylate several cardiac ion channels and are involved in myocyte hypertrophy via downstream signaling mechanisms [84,112,114,115]. However, different DAG species may originate from the hydrolysis of PIP_2 by PLC or from that of phosphatidylcholine by phospholipase D [116], and there are multiple forms of PKC with diverse biochemical and functional characteristics [84,112,114,115]. Accordingly, DAG species derived from PC or PIP_2 may activate different PKC isoforms, thus inducing PKC-dependent phosphorylation of different proteins and different physiological responses [116–118]. It should be noted that angiotensin II and PKC has been implicated in cardiac dysfunction during diabetes [119–123]; however, virtually nothing is known about the status of PLC in the diabetic heart. In acute diabetes (3 days, after the induction) the enhanced inotropic response to methoxamine, an α_1-adrenoceptor agonist, was ascribed to an increased PLC activity [86]. *In vitro studies* have demonstrated that LPC inhibits both SL PI 4 kinase and PI 4-P 5 kinase activities [124]. This is of particular relevance as LPC accumulates in SL during diabetic cardiomyopathy [71], suggestive of a diminished synthesis of PIP_2 substrate for PLC. Furthermore, nonradical oxidants have also been shown to inhibit both SL phosphatidylinositol 4 kinase and phosphatidylinositol 4-phosphate 5 kinase activities [125] as well as SL total PLC activity [126].

CONCLUDING REMARKS

Although the role of changes in PLC in the development of cardiac dysfunction during diabetes remains to be established, it is conceivable from the evidence presented that changes in the PLC-mediated signal transduction mechanisms may constitute an important factor for the altered cardiac contractile performance during diabetes. Given the implicit relationship between activation of the RAS and PLC, interventions with ACE inhibitors and angiotensin II receptor antagonists could prove to be of benefit in the prevention of the development of diabetic cardiomyopathy.

ACKNOWLEDGMENTS

The work reported in this article was supported by the Heart and Stroke Foundation of Manitoba. NSD hold a Canadian Institutes of Health Research/Pharmaceutical Research Development Chair in Cardiovascular Research supported by Merck Frosst Canada. SAM was a visiting scientist from the CU Shah College of Pharmacy, S.N.D.T. Women's University, Santacruz, Mumbai, India.

REFERENCES

1. Gargiulo P, Jacobellis G, Vaccari V, Andreani D. 1998. Diabetic cardiomyopathy: pathophysiological and clinical aspects. Diab Nutr Metab 11:336–346.
2. Mahgoub MA, Abd-Elfattah AS. 1998. Diabetes mellitus and cardiac function. Mol Cell Biochem 180:59–64.
3. Schaffer SW, Mozaffari M. 1996. Abnormal mechanical function in diabetes: relation to myocardial calcium handling. Coronary Artery Disease 7:109–115.
4. Pierce GN, Beamish RE, Dhalla NS. 1988. Heart dysfunction in diabetes. 1–245. Boca Raton: CRC Press.
5. Dhalla NS, Liu X, Panagia V, Takeda N. 1998. Subcellular remodeling and heart dysfunction in chronic diabetes. Cardiovasc Res 40:239–247.
6. Tomlison KC, Gardiner SM, Herdes RA, Bennet T. 1992. Functional consequences of streptozotocin-induced diabetes mellitus, with particular reference to the cardiovascular system. Pharmacol Rev 44:103–150.
7. Fein FS, Sonnenblick EH. Diabetic cardiomyopathy. 1994. Cardiovasc Drug Ther 8:65–73.
8. Fein FS, Sonnenblick EH. 1985. Diabetic cardiomyopathy. Progr Cardiovasc Dis 27:255–270.
9. Crepaldi G, Nosadini R. 1988. Diabetic cardiomyopathy: Is it a real entity. Diabetes Metab Rev 4: 273–288.
10. Ren J, Davidoff AJ. 1997. Diabetes rapidly induces cardiac dysfunction in isolated ventricular myocytes. Am J Physiol 272:H148–H158.
11. Yu Z, Tibbits GF, McNeill JH. 1994. Cellular functions of diabetic cardiomyocytes: contractility, rapid-cooling contracture and ryanodine binding. Am J Physiol 266:H2082–H2089.
12. Yu JZ, Quamme GA, McNeill JH. 1995. Altered $[Ca^{2+}]i$ mobilization in diabetic cardiomyocytes: responses to caffeine, KCl, ouabain, and ATP. Diabetes Res Clin Pract 30:9–20.
13. Tamada A, Hattori Y, Houzen H, Yamada Y, Sakuma I, Kitabatake A, Kanno M. 1998. Effect of β-adrenoceptor stimulation on contractility, $[Ca^{2+}]i$ and Ca^{2+} current in diabetic rat cardiomyocytes. Am J Physiol 274:H1849–H1857.
14. Ha T, Kotsanas G, Wendt I. 1999. Intracellular Ca^{2+} and adrenergic responsiveness of cardiac myocytes in streptozotocin-induced diabetes. Clin Exp Pharmacol Physiol 26:347–353.
15. Kotsanas G, Delbridge LM, Wendt IR. 2000. Stimulus interval-dependent differences in Ca^{2+} transients and contractile responses of diabetic rat cardiomyocytes. Cardiovasc Res 46:450–462.
16. Hattori Y, Matsuda N, Kimura J, Ishitani T, Tamada A, Gando S, Kemmotsu O, Kanno M. 2000. Diminished function and expression of the cardiac Na^{+}-Ca^{2+} exchange in diabetic rats: implications in Ca^{2+} overload. J Physiol 527:85–94.
17. Schaffer SW. 1991. Defective calcium homeostasis in noninsulin-dependent diabetic cardiomyopathy. In: The Diabetic Heart. Ed. M Nagano and NS Dhalla, 183–197. New York: Raven Press.
18. Black SC McNeil JH. 1991. Functional status of the cardiac sympathetic system in diabetes. In: Catecholamines and Heart Disease. Ed. PK Ganguly, 145–161. Boca Raton: CRC Press.
19. Schafrir E. 1997. Diabetes in animals: contribution to the understanding of diabetes by study of its etiopathology in animal models. In: Ellenberg & Rifkins Diabetes Mellitus. Ed. D Porte Jr. and RS Sherwin, 301–348. Stamford: Appleton and Lange.
20. Williams SA, Tappia PS, Yu C-H, Bibeau M, Panagia V. 1998. Impaiment of the sarcolemmal phospholipase D-phosphatidate phosphohydrolase pathway in diabetic cardiomyopathy. J Mol Cell Cardiol 30:109–118.
21. Pittman CS, Suda AK, Chambers JB Jr., McDaniel HG, Ray GY, Preston BK. 1989. Abnormalities of thyroid hormone turnover in patients with diabetes mellitus before and after insulin therapy. J Clin Endocrinol Metab 48:854–860.
22. Gray RS, Borsey DO, Seth J, Herd R, Brown NS, Clarke BF. 1980. Prevalence of subclinical thyroid failure in insulin-dependent diabetes. J Clin Endocrinol Metab 50:1034–1037.
23. Kahaly G, Mohr-Kahaly S, Beyer J, Meyer J. 1995. Left ventricular function analyzed by Doppler and echocardiographic methods in short-term hypothyroidism. Am J Cardiol 75:645–648.
24. Gay RG, Raya TE, Lancaster LD, Lee RW, Morkin E, Goldman S. 1988. Effects of thyroid state on venous compliance and left ventricular performance in rats. Am J Physiol 254:H81–H88.
25. Dhalla NS, Pierce GN, Innes IR, Beamish RE. 1985. Pathogenesis of cardiac dysfunction in diabetes mellitus. Can J Cardiol 1:263–281.
26. Fiordaliso F, Li B, Latini R, Sonnenblick EH, Anversa P, Leri A, Kajstura J. 2000. Myocyte death in streptozotocin-induced diabetes in rats is angiotensin II-dependent. Lab Invest 80:513–527.

27. Flack JM, Hamaty M, Staffileno BA. 1998. Renin-angiotensin-aldosterone-kinin system influences on diabetic vascular disease and cardiomyopathy. Miner Electrolyte Metab 24:412–422.
28. Feuvray D, Idell-Wenger JA, Neely JR. 1979. Effects of ischemia on rat myocardial function and metabolism in diabetes. Circ Res 44:322–329.
29. Duckworth WC. 2002. Hyperglycemia and cardiovascular disease. Curr Atheroscler Rep 3:383–391.
30. Kikkawa R. 2000. Chronic complications in diabetes mellitus. Br J Nutr 84:Suppl. 2:S183–S185.
31. Singh JP, Larson MG, O'Donnell CJ, Wilson PF, Tsuji H, Lloyd-Jones DM, Levy D. 2000. Association of hyperglycemia with reduced heart rate variability (The Framingham Heart Study). Am J Cardiol 86:309–312.
32. Freeman BA, Crapo JD. 1982. Biology of disease. Free radicals and tissue injury. Lab Invest 47: 412–426.
33. Kakkar R, Kalra J, Mantha V, Prasad K. 1995. Lipid peroxidation and activity of antioxidant enzymes in diabetic rats. Mol Cell Biochem 151:113–119.
34. Kakkar R, Mantha V, Kalra J, Prasad K. 1996. Time course study of oxidative stress in aorta and heart of diabetic rat. Clin Sci 91:441–448.
35. Mak DHF, Ip SP, Li PC, Poon MKT, Ko MN. 1996. Alterations in tissue glutathione antioxidant system in streptozotocin-induced diabetic rats. Mol Cell Biochem 162:153–158.
36. Sun F, Iwaguchi K, Shudo R, Nagaki Y, Tanaka K, Ikeda K, Tokumaru S, Kojo S. 1999. Change in tissue concentrations of lipid hydroperoxides, vitamin C and vitamin E in rats with streptozotocin-induced diabetes. Clin Sci 96:185–190.
37. Giugliano D, Cariello A, Paolisso G. 1995. Diabetes mellitus, hypertension and cardiovascular disease: Which role for oxidative stress? Metabolism 44:363–368.
38. Gillery P, Monboisse JC, Maquart FX, Borel JP. 1988. Glycation of proteins as a source of superoxide. Diabetes Metab 14:25–30.
39. Wolff SP, Dean RT. 1987. Glucose auto-oxidation and protein modification. The potential role of "autooxidative glycosylation" in diabetes. Biochem J 245:243–250.
40. Rosen P, Ballhausen T, Bloch W, Addicks K. 1995. Endothelial relaxation is disturbed by oxidative stress in the diabetic rat heart: influence of tocopherol as antioxidant. Diabetologia 38:1157–1168.
41. Ceriello A, Mercuri F, Quagliaro L, Assaloni R, Motz E, Tonutti L, Taboga C. 2001. Detection of nitrotyrosine in the diabetic plasma: evidence of oxidative stress. Diabetologia 44:834–838.
42. Suarez-Pinzon WL, Mabley JG, Strynadka K, Power RF, Szabo C, Rabinovitch A. 2001. An inhibitor of inducible nitric oxide synthase and scavenger of peroxynitrite prevents diabetes development in NOD mice. J Autoimmun 16:449–455.
43. Yadav P, Sarkar S, Bhatnagar D. 1997. Action of capparis deciduas against alloxan-induced oxidative stress and diabetes in rat tissues. Pharmacol Res 36:221–228.
44. Sivian E, Recce EA, Wu YK, Homko CJ, Polansky M, Borenstein M. 1996. Dietary vitamin E prophylaxis and diabetic embryopathy: Morphological and biochemical analysis. Am J Obstet Gynecol 175:793–799.
45. Douillet C, Chancerelle Y, Cruz C, Maroncles C, Kergonou JF, Renaud S, Ciavatti M. 1993. High dosage vitamin E effect on oxidative stress and serum lipids distribution in streptozotocin-induced diabetic rats. Biochem Med Metab Biol 50:265–276.
46. Paolisso G, D'Armore A, Giugliano D, Ceriello A, Varricchio M, D'Onofrio F. 1993. Pharmacologic doses of vitamin E improve insulin action in healthy subjects and non-insulin-dependent diabetic patients. Am J Clin Nutr 57:650–656.
47. Ting HH, Timimi FK, Boles KS, Creager SJ, Ganz P, Creager MA. 1996. Vitamin C improves endothelium-dependent vasodilation in patients with non-insulin-dependent diabetes mellitus. J Clin Invest 97:22–28.
48. Bierhaus A, Chevion S, Chevion M, Hofman M, Quehenberger P, Illmer T, Luther T, Berentshtein E, Tritschler H, Muller M, Wahl P, Ziegler R, Nawroth PP. 1997. Advanced glycation end-product induced activation of NF κB is suppressed by alpha-lipoic acid in cultured endothelial cells. Diabetes 46:1481–1490.
49. Sechi A, Griffin CA, Shambelan M. 1994. The cardiac renin-angiotensin system in STZ-induced diabetes. Diabetes 43:1180–1184.
50. Khatter JC, Sadi P, Zhang M, Hoeschen RJ. 1996. Myocardial angiotensin II (Ang II) receptors in diabetic rats. Ann NY Acad Sci 793:466–472.

51. Brown L, Sernia C. 1994. Angiotensin receptors in cardiovascular diseases. Clin Exp Pharmacol Physiol 21:811–818.
52. Wolf A. Free radical production, angiotensin. 2000. Curr Hypertens Rep 2:167–173.
53. Rey FE, Cifuentes ME, Kiarash A, Quinn MT, Pagano PJ. 2001. Novel competitive inhibitor of NAD(P)H oxidase assembly attenuates vascular O_2^- and systolic blood pressure in mice. Circ Res 89:408–414.
54. Frustaci A, Kajstura J, Chimenti C, Jakoniuk I, Leri A, MAseri A, Nadal-Ginard B, Anversa P. 2000. Myocardial cell death in human diabetes. Circ Res 87:1123–1132.
55. Kajstura J, Fiordaliso F, Andreoli AM, Li B, Chimenti S, Medow MS, Limana F, Nadal-Ginard, Leri A, Anversa P. 2001. IGF-1 overexpression inhibits the development of diabetic cardiomyopathy and angiotensin II-mediated oxidative stress. Diabetes 50:1414–1424.
56. de-Cavanagh EM, Fraga CG, Ferder L, Inserra F. 1997. Enalapril and captopril enhance antioxidant defenses in mouse tissues. Am J Physiol 272:R514–R518.
57. de-Cavanagh EM, Inserra F, Toblli J, Stella I, Fraga CG, Ferder L. 2001. Enalapril attenuates oxidative stress in diabetic rats. Hypertension 38:1130–1136.
58. Sand C, Peters SLM, Pfaffendorf M, van Zwieten PA. 2001. Oxidative stress impairs the haemodynamic activity of cardiovascular agents with antioxidant properties. Naunyn-Schmiedeberg's Arch Pharmacol 364:454–461.
59. Langer GA. 1997. Excitation-contraction coupling and calcium compartmentation. In: The Myocardium. 2nd Edition. Ed. GA Langer, 181–233. San Diego: Academic Press.
60. Pierce GN, Russell JC. 1997. Regulation of intracellular Ca^{2+} in the heart during diabetes. Cardiovasc Res 34:41–47.
61. Heyliger CE, Prakash A, McNeill JH. 1987. Alterations in cardiac sarcolemmal Ca^{2+} pump activity during diabetes mellitus. Am J Physiol 253:H540–H544.
62. Makino N, Dhalla KS, Elimban V, Dhalla NS. 1987. Sarcolemmal Ca^{2+} transport in streptozotocin-induced diabetic cardiomyopathy in rats. Am J Physiol 253:E202–E207.
63. Xu Y-J, Botsford MW, Panagia V, Dhalla NS. 1996. Responses of heart function and intracellular free Ca^{2+} to phosphatidic acid in chronic diabetes. Can J Cardiol 12:1092–1098.
64. Regan TJ, Wu CF, Yeh CK, Oldewurtel HA, Haider B. 1981. Myocardial composition and function in diabetes. The effects of chronic insulin use. Circ Res 49:1268.
65. Afzal N, Ganguly PK, Dhalla KS, Pierce GN, Singal PK, Dhalla NS. 1988. Beneficial effects of verapamil in diabetic cardiomyopathy. Diabetes 37:936–942.
66. Hayashi H, Noda N. 1997. Cytosolic Ca^{2+} concentration decreases in diabetic rat myocytes. Cardiovasc Res 34:99–103.
67. Yu JZ, Rodrigues B, McNeill JH. 1997. Intracellular calcium levels are unchanged in the diabetic heart. Cardiovasc Res 34:91–98.
68. Ziegelhoffer A, Ravingerova T, Styk J, Dzurba A, Volkovova K, Carsky J, Waczulikova I. 1998. Hearts with diabetic cardiomyopathy: adaptation to calcium overload. Wxp Clin Cardiol 3:158–160.
69. Ziegelhoffer A, Ravingerova T, Styk J, Sebokova J, Waczulikova I, Breier A, Dzurba A, Volkovova K, Carsky J, Turecky L. 1997. Mechanisms that may be involved in calcium tolerance of the diabetic heart. Mol Cell Biochem 176:191–198.
70. Dhalla NS, Pierce GN, Panagia V, Singal PK, Beamish RE. 1982. Calcium movements in relation to heart function. Basic Res Cardiol 77:117–139.
71. Pierce GN, Kutryk MJ, Dhalla NS. 1983. Alterations in Ca^{2+} binding by and composition of the cardiac sarcolemmal membrane in chronic diabetes. Proc Natl Acad Sci USA 80:5412–5416.
72. Yu Z, McNeill JH. 1991. Altered inotropic responses in diabetic cardiomyopathy and hypertensive-diabetic cardiomyopathy. J Pharmacol Exp Ther 257:64–71.
73. Nishio Y, Kashiwagi A, Ogawa T, Asahina T, Ikebuchi M, Kodama M, Shigeta Y. 1990. Increase in $[^3H]$ PN 200–110 binding to cardiac muscle membrane in streptozotocin-induced diabetic rats. Diabetes 39:1064–1069.
74. Pierce GN, Dhalla NS. 1983. Sarcolemmal Na^+-K^+-ATPase activity in diabetic rat heart. Am J Physiol 245:C241–C247.
75. Kuwahara Y, Yanagishita T, Konno N, Katagiri T. 1997. Changes in microsomal membrane phospholipids and fatty acids and in activities of membrane-bound enzyme in diabetic rat heart. Basic Res Cardiol 92:214–222.
76. Pierce GN, Ramjiawan B, Dhalla NS, Ferrari R. 1990. Na^+-H^+ exchange in cardiac sarcolemmal vesicles isolated from diabetic rats. Am J Physiol 258:H255–H261.

77. Dhalla NS, Elimban V, Rupp H. 1992. Paradoxical role of lipid metabolism in heart function and dysfunction. Mol Cell Biochem 116:3–9.
78. Vecchini A, Del Rosso F, Binaglia L, Dhalla NS, Panagia V. 2000. Molecular defects in sarcolemmal glycerophospholipids subclasses in diabetic cardiomyopathy. J Mol Cell Cardiol 32:1061–1074.
79. Okumura K, Akiyama N, Hashimoto H, Ogawa K, Satake T. 1988. Alteration of 1,2-diacylglycerol content in myocardium from diabetic rats. Diabetes 37:1168–1172.
80. Okumura K, Nishiura T, Shimizu K, Iwama Y, Kondo J, Hashimoto H, Ito T. 1991. Jpn Heart J 32: 667–673.
81. McHowat J, Creer MH, Hicks KK, Jones JH, McCrory R, Kennedy RH. 2000. Induction of Ca-independent PLA_2 and conservation of plasmalogen polyunsaturated fatty acids in diabetic heart. Am J Physiol 279:E25–E32.
82. Ganguly PK, Beamish RE, Dhalla KS, Innes IR, Dhalla NS. 1987. Norepinephrine storage, distribution, and release in diabetic cardiomyopathy. Am J Physiol 252:E734–E739.
83. Wichelhaus A, Russ M, Petersen S, Eckel J. 1994. G protein expression and adenylate cyclase regulation in ventricular cardiomyocytes from STZ-diabetic rats. Am J Physiol 267:H548–H555.
84. De Jonge HW, van Heugten HA, LAmers JMJ. 1995. Signal transduction by the phosphatidylinositol cycle in myocardium. J Mol Cell Cardiol 27:93–106.
85. Xiang H, McNeill JH. 1991. α_1-adrenoceptor-mediated phosphoinositide breakdown and inotropic responses in diabetic hearts. Am J Physiol 260:H557–H562.
86. Wald M, Borda ES, Sterin-Borda L. 1988. α-adrenergic supersensitivity and decreased number of α-adrenoceptors in heart from acute diabetic rats. Can J Physiol Pharmacol 66:1154–1160.
87. Rhee SG. 2001. Regulation of phosphoinositide-specific phospholipase C. Annu Rev Biochem 70: 281–312.
88. Tappia PS, Liu S-Y, Shatadal S, Takeda N, Dhalla NS, Panagia V. 1999. Changes in sarcolemmal PLC isoenzymes in postinfarct congestive heart failure: partial correction by imidapril. Am J Physiol 272:H40–H49.
89. Ji QS, Winnier GE, Niswender KD, Hortsman D, Wisdom R, Magnuson MA, Carpenter G. 1997. Essential role of the tyrosine kinase substrate phospholipase C-γ1 in mammalian growth and development. Proc Natl Acad Sci USA 94:2999–3003.
90. Singer WD, Brown HA, Sternweis PC. 1997. Regulation of eukaryotic phosphatidylinositol-specific phospholipase C and phospholipase D. Annu Rev Biochem 66:475–509.
91. Yagisawa H, Sakuma K, Paterson HE, Cheung R, Allen V, Hirata H, Watanabe Y, Hirata M, Williams RL, Katan M. 1998. Replacements of single basic amino acids in the pleckstrin homology domain of phospholipase C-δ_1 alter the ligand binding, phospholipase activity and interaction with the plasma membrane. J Biol Chem 273:417–424.
92. James SR, Downes CP. 1997. Structural and mechanistic features of phospholipase C: effectors of inositol phospholipid-mediated signal transduction. Cell Signal 9:329–336.
93. Katan M. Biochim. Biophys. Acta 1998. Families of phosphoinositide-specific phospholipase C: structure and function 1436:5–17.
94. Rhee SG, Bae YS. 1997. Regulation of phosphoinositide-specific phospholipase C isoenzymes. J Biol Chem 272:15045–15048.
95. Lee CW, Lee KH, Lee SB, Park D, Rhee SG. 1994. Regulation of phospholipase C-β_4 by ribonucleotides and the α subunit of Gq. J Biol Chem 269:25335–25338.
96. van Bilsen M. 1997. Signal transduction revisited: recent developments in angiotensin II signaling in the cardiovascular system. Cardiovasc Res 36:310–322.
97. Tappia PS, Padua RR, Panagia V, Kardami K. 1999. Fibroblast growth factor-2 stimulates phospholipase C β in adult cardiomyocytes. Biochem Cell Biol 77:569–575.
98. Sekiya F, Bae Y-S, Rhee SG. 1999. Regulation of phospholipase C isoenzymes: activation of phospholipase C-γ in the absence of tyrosine-phosphorylation. Chem Phys Lipids 98:3–11.
99. Im H-J, Russell MA, Feng J-F. 1997. Transglutaminase II: a new class of GTP-binding protein with new biological functions. Cell Signal 9:477–482.
100. Park H, Park ES, Lee HS, Yun HY, Kwon NS, Baek KJ. 2001. Distinct characteristic of Gαh (transglutaminase II) by compartment: GTPase and transglutaminase activities. Biochem Biophys Res Commun 284:496–500.
101. Lopez I, Mak EJ, Ding J, Hamm HE, Lomasney JW. 2001. A novel bifunctional phopsholipase C that is regulated by Gα12 and stimulates the Ras/mitogen-activated protein kinase pathway. J Biol Chem 276:2758–2765.

102. Wolf RA. 1993. Specific expression of phospholipase C-δ_1 and γ_1 by adult cardiac ventricular myocytes (Abstract) Circulation 88 Suppl. 1:I–241.
103. Wolf RA. 1992. Association of phospholipase C-δ with a highly enriched preparation of canine sarcolemma. Am J Physiol 263:C1021–C1028.
104. Gonzalez-Yanes C, Santos-Alvarez J, Sanchez-Margalet V. 2001. Pancreastatin, a chromogranin A-derived peptide, activates $G\alpha_{16}$ and phospholipase C-β2 by interacting with specific receptors in rat heart membranes. Cell Signal 13:43–49.
105. Song C, Hu CD, Masago M, Kariyai K, Yamawaki-Kataoka Y, Shibatohge M, Wu D, Satoh T, Kataoka T. 2001. Regulation of a novel human phospholipase C, PLCε, through membrane targeting by Ras. J Biol Chem 276:2752–2757.
106. Arthur JF, Matkovich SJ, Mitchell CJ, Biden TJ, Woodcock EA. 2001. Evidence for selective coupling of α_1- adrenergic receptors to phospholipase C-β_1 in rat neonatal cardiomyocytes. J Biol Chem 276:37341–37346.
107. Huisamen B, Mouton R, Opie LH, Lochner A. 1994. Demonstration of a specific [^{3}H]Ins(1,4,5)P_3 binding site in rat heart sarcoplasmic reticulum. J Mol Cell Cardiol 26:341–349.
108. Kijima Y, Fleischer S. 1992. Two types of inositol trisphosphate binding in cardiac microsomes. Biochem Biophys Res Commun 189:728–735.
109. Gilbert JC, Shirayama T, Pappano AJ. 1991. Inositol trisphosphate promotes Na-Ca exchange current by releasing calcium from sarcoplasmic reticulum in cardiac myocytes. Circ Res 69:1632–1639.
110. Jaconi M, Bony C, Richards SM, Terzic A, Arnaudeau, Vassort G, Pucéat M. 2000. Inositol 1,4,5-trisphosphate directs Ca^{2+} flow between mitochondria and the endoplasmic/sarcoplasmic reticulum: a role in regulating cardiac autonomic Ca^{2+} spiking. Mol Biol Cell 11:1845–1858.
111. Quist EE, Foresman BH, Vasan R, Quist CW. 1994. Inositol tetrakisphosphate stimulates a novel ATP-dependent Ca^{2+} uptake mechanism in cardiac junctional sarcoplasmic reticulum. Biochem Biophys Res Commun 204:69–75.
112. Pucéat M, Vassort G. 1996. Signalling by protein kinase C isoforms in the heart. Mol Cell Biochem 157:65–72.
113. Kijima Y, Saito A, Jetton JL, Magnuson MA, Fleischer S. 1993. Different intracellular localization of inositol 1,4,5-trisphosphate and ryanodine receptors in cardiomyocytes. J Biol Chem 268: 3499–3506.
114. Jalili T, Takeishi Y, Song G, Ball NA, Howles G, Walsh RA. 1999. PKC translocation without changes in $G\alpha q$ and PLC-β protein abundance in cardiac hypertrophy and failure. Am J Physiol 277: H2298–H22304.
115. Jalili T, Takeishi Y, Walsh RA. 1999. Signal transduction during cardiac hypertrophy: the role of $G\alpha q$, PLC-β1, and PKC. Cardiovasc Res 44:5–9.
116. Quest AFG, Raben DM, Bell RM. 1996. Diacylglycerols-biosynthetic intermediates and lipid second messengers. In: Handbook of Lipid Research. Lipid Second Messengers. Ed. RM Bell, JH Exton and SE Prescott, Vol 8, 1–58. New York: Plenum Press.
117. Billah MM. Phospholipase D and cell signaling. 1993. Curr Opin Immunol 5:114–123.
118. Hodgkin MN, Pettitt TR, Martin A, Michell RH, Pemberton AJ, Wakelam MJ. 1998. Diacylglycerols and phosphatidates: which molecular species are intracellular messengers? Trends Biochem Sci 23:200–204.
119. Malhotra A, Reich D, Reich D, Nakouzi A, Sanghi V, Geenen DL, Buttrick PM. 1997. Experimental diabetes is associated with functional activation of protein kinase Cε and phosphorylation of troponin I in the heart, which are prevented by angiotensin II receptor blockade. Circ Res 81:1027–1033.
120. Malhotra A, Kang BP, Cheung S, Opawumi D, Meggs LG. 2001. Angiotensin II promotes glucose-induced activation of cardiac protein kinase C isozymes and phosphorylation of troponin I. Diabetes 50:1918–1926.
121. Xiang H, McNeill JH. 1992. Protein kinase C activity is altered in diabetic rat hearts. Biochem Biophys Res Commun 187:703–710.
122. Tanaka Y, Kashiwagi T, Ogawa T, Abe T, Asahina M, Ikebuchi Y, Takagi Y, Shigeta Y. 1991. Effect of verapamil on cardiac protein kinase C activity in diabetic hearts. Eur J Pharmacol 200:353–356.
123. Liu X, Wang J, Takeda N, Binaglia L, Panagia V, Dhalla NS. 1999. Changes in cardiac protein kinase C activities and isozymes in streptozotocin-induced diabetes. Am J Physiol 277:E798–E804.

124. Liu S-Y, Yu C-H, Hays J-A, Panagia V, Dhalla NS. 1997. Modification of heart sarcolemmal phosphoinositide pathway by lysophosphatidylcholine. Biochim Biophys Acta 1349:264–274.
125. Mesaeli N, Tappia PS, Suzuki S, Dhalla NS, Panagia V. 2000. Oxidants depress the synthesis of phosphatidylinositol 4,5-bisphosphate in heart sarcolemma. Arch Biochem Biophys 382:48–56.
126. Meij JTA, Suzuki S, Panagia V, Dhalla NS. 1994. Oxidative stress modifies the activity of cardiac sarcolemmal phospholipase C. Biochim Biophys Acta 1199:6–12.

G.N. Pierce, M. Nagano, P. Zahradka, and N.S. Dhalla (eds.).
ATHEROSCLEROSIS, HYPERTENSION AND DIABETES.
Kluwer Academic Publishers. Boston.

REGULATION OF CARDIAC FUNCTION IN DIABETES

THOMAS NETTICADAN, SHARAD RASTOGI, PUNAM K. CHOHAN, RAMESH K. GOYAL, and NARANJAN S. DHALLA

Institute of Cardiovascular Sciences St. Boniface General Hospital Research Centre & Department of Physiology, Faculty of Medicine University of Manitoba, Winnipeg, Canada

Summary. Phosphorylation and dephosphorylation of various subcellular target sites are known to regulate heart function, metabolism and cation homeostasis. Since cardiac function, sarcoplasmic reticulum Ca^{2+}-pump and myofibrillar ATPase activities in chronic diabetes are depressed, it is likely that changes in phosphorylation and/or dephosphorylation processes may explain the abnormalities in the diabetic heart. It is now well known that the phosphorylation-dephosphorylation system plays a major role in determining the activities of subcellular organelles in the myocardium. In view of the involvement of protein kinases and protein phosphatases in phosphorylation and dephosphorylation, it is possible that changes in subcellular activities in the diabetic heart are associated with alterations in the activities of these enzymes. This review describes the regulation of Ca^{2+}-movement and cardiac dysfunction in diabetes mellitus, and how protein kinases and protein phosphatases are involved in the regulation of cardiac function.

Key words: Diabetic cardiomyopathy, Cardiac dysfunction

INTRODUCTION

Diabetes mellitus is a chronic disorder characterized by impaired metabolism of glucose involving distinct pathogenic mechanisms with hyperglycemia as the common denominator [1]. This disease is associated with deficiency of insulin

Address Correspondence to: Dr. Naranjan S. Dhalla, Institute of Cardiovascular Sciences, St. Boniface General Hospital Research Centre, 351 Tache Avenue, Winnipeg, MB R2H 2A6, Canada. Tel: (204) 235-3417; Fax: (204) 233-6723; e-mail: cvso@sbrc.ca

and/or insulin resistance. Hyperglycemia in turn plays a major role in the complications of the disease [2]. In North America diabetes is the fourth major cause of premature disability and mortality. Chronic diabetes increases the risk of cardiac, cerebral and peripheral vascular disease two- to seven-fold [2]. It causes blindness, renal disease, neuropathic complication, impaired peripheral artery circulation, coronary artery disease leading to myocardial infarction and cerebral vascular disease resulting in stroke [3]. The Chinese recognized this disease as a syndrome of polyphagia, polyuria, and polydipsia whereas Indians noted the sweet taste of the urine and called it "honey urine" [4]. Indian physicians also suggested the hereditary and environmental factors causing diabetes. However, the name diabetes was first given by Aretaeus of Cappodocia (200–130 B.C), which in Greek means "to run through" or siphon. Avicenna (980–1037), a Persian physician and author of "Canon Medicinae", noted the sweet taste of urine in diabetics and found an association between gangrene of limbs and diabetes [5]. In the sixteenth century, Paraclesus (1493–1541), a Swiss physician and pioneer of chemical therapeutics, studied the urine of diabetics and mistook the residue of boiled urine for salt instead of sugar, it was later proven to be glucose which led to a more rational dietary treatment [3]. In 1859, Claude Bernard, a French physiologist, recognized hyperglycemia as a cardinal feature and the glycogenic effect of the liver. Mering and Minkowski in 1889 demonstrated that pancreatectomy in dogs caused diabetes. A solution to test urine for glucose was introduced by an American physician Staneley Benedict (1884–1936). A Romanian physiologist, Nicholae Paulescu (1869–1931), demonstrated in 1921 that hypoglycemia could be introduced in dogs by injecting pancreatic extract and he named the substance "pancrein". Frederick Banting (1891–1941), a Canadian surgeon, and John Macleod (1876–1935), a physiologist at the University of Toronto, won the Nobel prize in Biochemistry in 1923 for their discovery of insulin in 1921; the prize money was shared with co-workers Charles Best (1899–1978) and James Collip (1892–1965) [6]. Although, discovery of insulin has totally changed and revolutionized the treatment of diabetes and has saved countless lives worldwide, cardiovascular dysfunction still remains the major cause of death in patients with diabetes. Since force generation by the heart is a cellular event, it is believed that subcellular defects are involved in the pathogenesis of heart dysfunction. Studies carried out in the past 25 years have focused on the role of Ca^{2+} in the contraction-relaxation coupling process for muscle contraction. A major role is also played by protein kinases and phosphatases in the regulation of cardiac function.

CLASSIFICATION OF DIABETES MELLITUS

Diabetes mellitus (DM) has been known for many centuries. In fact, the ancient people from India were first to characterize the urine of diabetic patients to be "honeyed" in approximately 400 B.C. [7]. It is a serious disease that seems to make afflicted individuals more susceptible to heart dysfunction, independent of atherosclerosis and hypertension. Diabetes mellitus involves defects in protein, carbohydrate and fat metabolism; these abnormalities are associated with the deficiency in systemic insulin or inability of insulin to act on the cell and thus create a hyperglycemic status in the body. According to the National Diabetes Data Group [8] and the World Health Organization [9], diabetes mellitus can be divided in two groups, namely the insulin dependent diabetes mellitus (IDDM) and non-insulin dependent diabetes mellitus (NIDDM). The IDDM (Type 1 diabetes) or juvenile-onset diabetes involves the destruction of β-cells of the pancreas and their inability to produce insulin. The IDDM patients are required to take exogenous insulin to control their blood glucose levels and prevent ketoacidosis. Ketoacidosis occurs when the ketone levels in the body are high enough that it leads to metabolic acidosis, diabetic coma and sometimes death. Symptoms that accompany IDDM are excessive thirst, unexplained weight loss, polyuria and ketosis. The NIDDM (Type II diabetes) or Adult-onset diabetes involves the body's inability to utilize insulin due to receptor defects or genetic predisposition, and therefore individuals are usually hyperinsulinemic. The NIDDM patients are not required to take exogenous insulin, and their risk of ketosis is rare in comparison to IDDM. It is estimated that approximately 80–85% of all diabetics are NIDDM [10]; the majority of these patients are also obese.

COMPLICATIONS OF DIABETES MELLITUS

Complications of diabetes can be divided into two groups: a) Microvascular complications, which include retinopathy, neuropathy and nephropathy, b) Macrovascular complications, which include atherosclerosis, stroke, myocardial infarction and gangrene. Even with the discovery of insulin by Banting and Best for the treatment of diabetes, the diabetic patients still suffer a higher mortality than the general population. Insulin has increased the life expectancy of diabetic patients, but the question remains why about 80% of deaths in diabetic patients are related to cardiovascular disease [11,12]. Even in the absence of hypertension, atherosclerosis and vascular complications, diabetics still suffer cardiovascular dysfunction. The following are some of the cardiovascular complications which are commonly associated with diabetes:

a. Hypertension

Elevated blood pressure seems to be quite common in diabetes and in fact, hypertension precedes the microvascular and macrovascular changes seen in diabetics and is considered to exacerbate the increased mortality. Hypertension in diabetics makes these individuals more susceptible to the occurrence of renal, stroke, coronary artery disease, retinal and cardiovascular dysfunction. Studies conducted in the past have estimated that diabetics with hypertension are twice that of non-diabetics [13]. Factor et al. [14] have confirmed that hypertensive-diabetics suffer increased myocellular damage which may account for their higher mortality than non-diabetics. Hyperinsulinemia may provide an answer for the increased sodium retention seen in diabetics since increased endogenous insulin was shown to increase sodium reabsorption [15]. An increase in intracellular sodium poses a threat, because it can lead to increased vasoconstriction. The use of anti-hypertensive therapy such as α- and β-adrenoceptor blockers, angiotensin converting enzyme (ACE) inhibitors, calcium channel blockers, vasodilators and diuretics may provide some benefit in reducing blood pressure and coronary artery disease. However, these agents are also known to cause some adverse effect on glucose and lipid metabolism and may accelerate vascular disease in some [16–18]. Nonetheless, hypertension is of great concern to health practitioners searching for the reason why diabetics show increased mortality and cardiovascular disease than non-diabetics.

b. Myocardial infarction

Diabetic patients have been shown to suffer from more frequent (2.5–5 times) and severe myocardial infarction (MI) versus non-diabetics [19–21]. Studies conducted in the past demonstrated that male diabetics have an increased likelihood of cardiovascular problems by 2 times, whereas female diabetics have an increased chance of cardiovascular problems by 3–5 times the normal risk [22]. Dhalla et al. [22] have indicated three risk factors that may account for the increased incidence of cardiovascular dysfunction in diabetics: atherosclerosis, microvascular alterations and primary myopathic disorder in cardiac muscle. Studies in the past have demonstrated that two months after an MI the mortality in diabetic patients was approximately 41% in comparison to 15% in non-diabetics [23]. Even more alarming is the evidence that regardless of infarct size, diabetics still suffer a higher mortality than non-diabetics [24]. The increased incidence of MI in diabetics has been linked to glycemic status. It has been shown that when the hyperglycemic state of diabetics was stringently controlled the incidence of MI fell significantly [25]. Hyperglycemia has also been linked to endothelial dysfunction and hypertension. Another danger that increases the mortality in diabetics is the occurrence of a silent MI which has been suggested to be due to the damage of cardiac nerves and the inability of afferent nerves to transmit information as a result of visceral neuropathy [26]. Silent MI was shown to be more common in the diabetic population [27,28] and is of great concern because the patients are unaware that they have suffered an MI and thus may not summon the proper medical attention [29]. The survival of diabetic patients with MI after 1, 2 and 5 years is 82%, 78% and 58% whereas that for non-diabetic patients with MI is 94%, 92% and 82% respectively. Thrombolytic therapy with aspirin and/or heparin seems to be the standard treatment for diabetic patients with MI [30]. The poor outcome in diabetics is the result of advanced coronary artery disease present in the diabetic population; however, β-adrenoceptor blockers have proven to provide long-term benefit to diabetics with MI [30]. Nonetheless, it has been shown that diabetes mellitus increases the prevalence of coronary artery disease [31]. It has been suggested that factors such as age, cholesterol and hypertension amplify the affect of diabetes on the prevalence of coronary artery disease. It has also been established that diabetics suffer from 4–5 times more incidences of congestive heart failure following MI independent of age, weight, cholesterol level, blood pressure and coronary artery disease [20,32–35].

c. Coronary thrombosis and stroke

Atherosclerosis involves dysfunction of cerebral arteries and peripheral vasculature. As a result of poor lipoprotein metabolism and hypercholesterolemia, plaque formation or thrombosis has been shown to occur. It has been recognized that high level of LDL (low-density lipoprotein) and low level of HDL (high-density lipoprotein) lead to the initiation and progression of arterial lesions. It has been suggested that the atherosclerotic process is similar in the general population; however, in diabetic patient it proceeds at a faster pace [36]. Thrombosis seems to be initiated by injury to the arterial wall; this will result in alterations in platelet coagulation and fibrin activity in the diabetic patient. It is now believed that thrombosis may occur prior to vascular injury and endothelial cell dysfunction in the diabetic patient. One possible explanation for the increased prevalence of thrombosis in diabetics could be due to the increased platelet hyperaggregability seen in patients with IDDM and NIDDM [37]. Some studies have confirmed that if patients do not control their diabetes, their platelets release more vascular growth factors and this results in increased progression of lesion via smooth muscle cell proliferation [38]. It has been suggested that the production of thromboxane (a potent vasoconstrictor) is increased in the insulin deficient diabetic and this may hasten the thrombolytic process [39]. Treatment of diabetic patients with coronary thrombosis as well as stroke may involve proper glycemic status via insulin regulation, diet and weight reduction, exercise, use of antiaggregant agents such as aspirin, and also use of anticoagulants. Postmortem studies have shown stroke to be a major cause of death in diabetic patient [40–42]. It has been estimated that 7% of deaths in diabetics are related to stroke and 25% to cerebrovascular disease [43]. Women diabetics have also shown to be at more risk than their male counterparts [44].

REGULATION OF Ca^{2+}-MOVEMENTS AND HEART DYSFUNCTION IN DIABETES

Depolarization of cardiomyocytes (normally by an action potential) leads to a voltage dependent opening of L-type Ca^{2+} channels in the membrane, resulting in entry of a small amount of Ca^{2+} [45–58]. A small amount of Ca^{2+} may also enter via the Na^+/Ca^{2+} exchange operating in the reverse mode [50]. This small amount of Ca^{2+} triggers a much larger release of Ca^{2+} from the main intracellular store, the SR [45,51,54,56]. When the SR is triggered to release Ca^{2+}, there is a transient rise in the cytoplasmic concentration of Ca^{2+} from a resting level of 100 nM to a peak between 1 and 2 μM within 20 to 40 msec after depolarization [48,57]. The rise in Ca^{2+} concentration activates the myofilaments and produces cardiac contraction. This process of Ca^{2+}-induced Ca^{2+}-release is widely accepted as the major mechanism of SR Ca^{2+}-release in the heart [58–60]. After the initial release of Ca^{2+} there is a period of recovery during which Ca^{2+} is pumped back into the SR by the SR Ca^{2+}-stimulated ATPase and extruded from the cell primarily by the Na^+/Ca^{2+} exchanger, which is present in the sarcolemmal membrane in addition to Ca^{2+} ATPase [61,62]. Although activation of the sympathetic nervous system has been shown to increase the activities of sarcolemmal L-type Ca^{2+}-channels and Ca^{2+}-pump

ATPase, no conclusive information with respect to sarcolemmal Na^+/Ca^{2+} exchanger is available. Nonetheless, activation of the sympathetic nervous system is now well known to increase the SR Ca^{2+}-pump and Ca^{2+}-release activities in the heart.

The SR in the cardiac muscle is an important intracellular membrane system which is involved in the relaxation process in the cardiac muscle. When Ca^{2+}-pump ATPase transports Ca^{2+} from the cytosol to the intraluminal side of the sarcoplasmic reticulum the relaxation of cardiac muscle occurs. A phosphoprotein called phospholamban regulates the Ca^{2+}-pump. Phosphorylation of phospholamban takes place at distinct sites by protein kinases such as cAMP-dependent protein kinase, Ca^{2+}-calmodulin-dependent protein kinase, and Ca^{2+}-phospholipid-dependent protein kinase resulting in an increase in the transport of Ca^{2+} by SR [63–68]. Protein phosphatase activity associated with SR can reverse the stimulatory effect of protein kinases on Ca^{2+} transport [69]. In fact the endogenous protein phosphatase is present in cardiac SR membrane, and this phosphatase activity has been shown to dephosphorylate phospholamban and regulate calcium transport [70,71]. One study has shown that the phosphatase which dephosphorylates phospholamban in the cardiac muscle had type 2A phosphatase characteristics [72] whereas in other studies there is evidence that type 1 enzyme is the SR-membrane bound phosphatase and is responsible for the dephosphorylation of phospholamban [70]. Thus phosphorylation of SR by different protein kinases and dephosphorylation by different protein phosphatases are considered to regulate SR Ca^{2+}-uptake and Ca^{2+}-release activities and play a crucial role in processes involved in determining the status of heart function.

Studies conducted around the world have concluded that the heart is indeed compromised in diabetic patients. The diabetic heart has been shown to have lower ejection fractions and stroke volume [44,73,74]. It has also been suggested that the compromised heart is due to decreased compliance of the left ventricle [44] and a slower relaxation process [75]. It has also been suggested that a lack of systemic insulin may result in loss of membrane integrity. This may alter membrane permeability, allowing for increased entry of cations such as calcium and resulting in dysfunction of contractile units; this eventually leads to arrythmias and heart failure. Factors such as isovolumic contraction or relaxation time and left ventricular ejection time have been shown to increase in diabetics, a clear indication of cardiac dysfunction [76,77]. A larger ejection fraction than normal indicates contractile dysfunction whereas a lower ejection fraction indicates the presence of heart disease [78]. Experimental data has pinpointed a direct linear relationship between serum glucose levels and ejection fraction levels [79]. Since diabetes mellitus has been linked to other vascular complications such as hypertension and atherosclerosis, these factors may attenuate the afterload on the heart resulting in higher filling pressures [44]. It has been indicated that if the hyperglycemic state of these patients was regulated with insulin to approximately control levels, their cardiac performance also improved to control levels [80]. When myocardial shortening was examined it was also found to be subnormal in diabetics [81,82]. Systolic and diastolic dysfunction have been discussed in the past in correlation with diabetes. Some studies have also shown that in most cases diastolic dysfunction or impaired isovolumic relaxation, preceded systolic dysfunction or impaired isovolumic contraction [82–84], this is important clinically, because it allows for the early detection of cardiac disease in diabetic patients. A study on isolated diabetic ventricular tissue has shown that diabetes mellitus itself results in compromised cardiac function [32]. Experiments on animal models of diabetes mellitus have shown decreased force generation, as well as decrease in cardiac output and other hemodynamic factors [84–95]. The duration of diabetes may also have a bearing on the recovery of contractile function once insulin is administered. It has been indicated that in the chronically diabetic rat, insulin treatment only led to partial recovery of function to normal levels but contractile dysfunction was still observed [86,96,97].

Treatment of diabetics in general has been mostly centered around correcting the hyperglycemic state of diabetics with insulin. It has been shown that if insulin treatment is given immediately after induction of diabetes, insulin will allow recovery of cardiac function to normal levels, as well as the restoration of physical attributes such as heart and body weight [95,98]. While assessing the effectiveness of insulin treatment, it has been concluded that factors such as dosage of insulin, severity and duration of diabetes should be taken into account since insulin did not reverse dysfunction in trials conducted over longer periods of time [99]. It has been suggested that insulin itself and not the systemic glucose level may play a role in recovery of contractile dysfunction [100]. Various investigators have also examined the possible role of depressed thyroid hormone levels in diabetics [85,101,102]. Restoration of thyroid hormone levels did not result in correction of contractile dysfunction to control values but in fact cardiac dysfunction was still evident [85,87,100,101,103]. Therefore, the possible role of hypothyroidism in generation of cardiac dysfunction in diabetics has not been validated.

SUBCELLULAR DEFECTS IN DIABETES MELLITUS

It has been noted that heart function in the diabetic population is compromised but the question still remains on exactly what causes this dysfunction. Some investigators have concentrated on the excitation-contraction coupling mechanism because the force generation by the heart is a cellular event. Other researchers have focused solely on the importance of Ca^{2+} in the contraction process. Intracellular Ca^{2+} homeostasis is crucial to the viability of the heart as a pump, as concentrations of Ca^{2+} are seen to fluctuate from 10^{-5} M in contraction to 10^{-7} M in relaxation. Investigators have also focused their attention on the subcellular organelles such as the sarcoplasmic reticulum (SR), sarcolemmal membrane (SL) and the mitochondria (Mt), since these organelles regulate cations such as Ca^{2+} and play a vital role in the process of excitation-contraction coupling. The process of excitation-contraction coupling involves the binding of Ca^{2+} to troponin C, allowing the release of tropomyosin and the crossbridge cycling of myosin with actin. The activity of the myofibrillar Ca^{2+}-stimulated ATPase which mediates crossbridge cycling [104,105] was found to be decreased in the diabetic myocardium in comparison to control values [106–109]. Depressed actomyosin ATPase and myosin ATPase activities in the diabetic heart [110,111] have been reported to be improved upon treatment with insulin [107]. It has been suggested that the most likely explanation for a decrease in myofibrillar ATPase activity may be the conformational modification at or in the vicinity of the enzymatic activity [106,107]. The deficiency in circulating thyroid hormones was also examined but ruled out as a primary cause for the decrease in ATPase activity [110,112]. This defect was considered to be of importance clinically because ATPase activity is associated with force generation in the heart, and a decrease in its activity is indicative of heart dysfunction in diabetes [104,113].

a. Changes in the sarcoplasmic reticulum in diabetes

The sarcoplasmic reticulum (SR) is the major source of Ca^{2+} storage in the heart, and is primarily responsible for the release and subsequent uptake of Ca^{2+} for the cardiac contraction and relaxation phases. Ca^{2+}-pump ATPase protein (SERCA2a) accounts for approximately 75–90% of the SR proteins [114] and Ca^{2+}-uptake is an energy dependent process. It has been postulated that a slower relaxation time in the diabetic heart may be due to the slower removal of cytosolic Ca^{2+}. Since the SR is the major storage site of Ca^{2+} in the myocardium, it was speculated that the depressed Ca^{2+}-uptake may be due to an abnormality in the SR in the diabetic condition. Penpargkul et al. [115] were the first to confirm that indeed the ability of SR to accumulate Ca^{2+} was decreased in the diabetic heart. Other investigators over the years have confirmed these findings and also have found that SR Ca^{2+} binding is also depressed in the diabetic heart [85,116,117]. It was found that the Mg^{2+}-dependent ATPase activity was unaffected [85]; treatment of diabetic animals with insulin corrected the depression in SR Ca^{2+}-pump ATPase and Ca^{2+}-uptake activities [85,117]. In search of an answer for the depressed function of the SR in diabetes, it was suggested that hypothyroidism may cause defect in cardiac SR Ca^{2+}-transport [118], however, treatment of diabetic animals with thyroxine did not alter the depressed SR Ca^{2+}-transport [85]. It has also been suggested that the defect in SR Ca^{2+}-transport could be due to a change in lipid accumulation, especially long-chain acyl-carnitines observed in the diabetic hearts [119]. Chronic treatment with carnitine prevented the accumulation of long-chain acyl-carnitines and allowed for recovery of SR function but not cardiac function in diabetics [117].

The contractile state of the myocardium is regulated via protein phosphorylation and dephosphorylation [120,121]. This process includes phosphorylation and dephosphorylation of various intracellular proteins and it is when these regulatory mechanisms fail cardiac dysfunction occurs. Initially researchers only focused on the cAMP-dependent processes mediated by the cAMP-dependent protein kinase (PKA) [122–124], but now they have expanded to include Ca^{2+}-calmodulin dependent protein kinase (CAMK) [125,126], protein kinase C (PKC) [127,128], cGMP-dependent protein kinase (PKG) [129], tryosine protein kinases [130], extracellularly signal-regulated kinases [131], mitogen-activated protein kinases [130,132] and c-jun N-terminal protein kinases [133]. It should be pointed out that the cardiac SR is involved in the regulation of intracellular Ca^{2+} and therefore it affects contraction and relaxation through the phosphorylation of various Ca^{2+} cycling proteins such as SERCA2a, Ca^{2+}-release channel or ryanodine receptor (RyR) and phospholamban (PLB) [123,125,134].

It is believed that in the unphosphorylated state PLB interacts with SERCA2a inhibiting SR Ca^{2+}-uptake [135]. This view is substantiated in PLB deficient SR hearts which show increased Ca^{2+}-uptake activity [136]. It has been suggested that phosphorylation is a key factor in the mechanism of Ca^{2+}-uptake. It has been proposed that upon phosphorylation PLB undergoes a conformational change allowing for the activation of SERCA2a pump [137,138]. Kirchberger et al. [139] were the first to show that PKA-dependent phosphorylation of cardiac SR resulted in an increase in Ca^{2+}-transport activity. It has been suggested that PKA may accomplish this by increasing the affinity of the SERCA2a pump for Ca^{2+} [140]. The increase in SERCA2a pump activity by PKA-dependent phosphorylation of PLB [139–141] could also be due to the increased coupling ratio of SERCA2a for Ca^{2+} or an increased turnover of SERCA2a [142]. Numerous studies have also confirmed the role of phospholamban as a regulator of cardiac relaxation in response to catecholamine or sympathetic stimulation. For example, β-adrenergic stimulation increased PLB phosphorylation and SR Ca^{2+}-transport in addition to shortening the myocardial relaxation [122,123,143–145]. In order to confirm the effects of β-adrenergic stimulation, some researchers inhibited this stimulation via muscarinic and cholinergic mediated processes and found that the parasympathetic stimulation can reverse the effects of β-adrenergic stimulation on PLB phosphorylation [145–149].

CAMK has also been shown to phosphorylate PLB, and increase Ca^{2+}-uptake [140,150,151]. The increase in SR Ca^{2+}-uptake activity seems to be due to the increase in affinity of SERCA2a pump for Ca^{2+} [150,151]. It is speculated that both PKA and CAMK are involved in the phosphorylation of PLB and seem to act independently of each other, but when these regulatory mechanisms operate together their effect is additive [140,150,152]. It is estimated that approximately 50% of PLB phosphorylation is accounted for by CAMK [153]. It has also been observed that PKG can also increase the phosphorylation of PLB but the significance of this mechanism is not clearly understood [154]. PKC has also been observed to increase PLB phosphorylation, and therefore Ca^{2+}-uptake activity [155,156]. Protein phosphatases dephosphorylate proteins and regulate a variety of signal transduction pathways [157]. Some researchers have suggested the presence of a "PLB-specific" phosphatase that can dephosphorylate PKA and CAMK phosphorylation sites thus resulting in a decrease in Ca^{2+}-uptake activity [70,71,158]. It has been recently shown that CAMK also directly phosphorylates SERCA2a resulting in enhanced V_{max} of SR Ca^{2+}-transport [134].

SR Ca^{2+}-release occurs through the RyRs. The influx of Ca^{2+} from voltage-gated Ca^{2+}-channels in the sarcolemmal membrane leads to further release of Ca^{2+} from the SR (via RyR) by a process called calcium-induced calcium-release [159]. RyR has been suggested to be regulated by PKA, CAMK and Ca^{2+} [160–163]; PKA and CAMK phosphorylation of RyR promote SR Ca^{2+}-release. Calsequestrin is a

Ca^{2+}-binding protein involved in the binding of large amount of Ca^{2+} that is sequestered by the SERCA2a pump. It is believed that this phosphoprotein is phosphorylated by casein kinase II, but its effect on calsequestrin has yet to be identified [164,165]. PKA and CAMK have also been implicated in the phosphorylation of phospholipids present in cardiac muscle [166].

b. Changes in the sarcolemmal membrane in diabetes

The sarcolemmal membrane plays a crucial role in the regulation of membrane potential and thus excitation-contraction coupling. Ca^{2+} enters the cytoplasm through the voltage-gated Ca^{2+} channels in the SL membrane. Upon entry, a small amount of Ca^{2+} can act as trigger and allow the release of more Ca^{2+} from the SR through calcium-induced calcium release [167,168]. Any alterations of the SL may therefore result in cardiac dysfunction in diabetic animals. A decrease in α- and β-adrenergic receptor number rather than changes in the receptor affinity has been reported in the diabetic hearts [169]. The result would be a decrease in adrenergic stimulation of cardiac function in the diabetic heart. If the density of α- and β-adrenergic receptors on the SL membrane is decreased in the diabetic animal, then it must follow that the ability of catecholamines to bind these receptors and initiate adenylate cyclase to produce cyclic AMP (cAMP) to further activate PKA to release more SR Ca^{2+} for force generation will also be compromised. It is believed that diabetes itself is responsible for the depression in adrenergic receptor density; the severity of depression is dependent upon the duration of diabetes in animals [170]. Also in support of this hypothesis is the fact that insulin treatment was able to rectify this defect in the diabetic animal [171]. Lastly, the weight loss experienced by these animals was not a factor, because food restrictions had no bearing on the receptor density [172]. It has been suggested that the hypothyroid state of the diabetic may be a causal factor in the occurrence of adrenergic receptor depression [171].

The Na^+-K^+ pump allows for the exchange of 3 Na^+ for 2 K^+ against their concentration gradients. The Na^+-K^+ pump of the cardiac sarcolemmal membrane plays a critical role in the regulation of membrane depolarization and repolarization. Ion homeostasis is essential for the maintenance of proper cardiac function. Schwartz et al. [173] have indicated that if the Na^+-K^+ pump was inhibited the intracellular concentration of Na^+ will rise. This would activate the Na^+-Ca^{2+} exchanger, increase the intracellular Ca^{2+} and thus result in the contractile dysfunction observed in diabetes. Experiments conducted on diabetic dog hearts by Onji and Liu [174], provided the first data that the Na^+-K^+ ATPase enzyme system was significantly decreased in comparison to control values. Other studies have also confirmed this depression in Na^+-K^+ ATPase in the diabetic animals [175–177]. By using the purified cardiac SL from diabetic animals, Pierce and Dhalla [178] showed that the Na^+-K^+ ATPase activity and K^+-pNPPase activity were significantly decreased. The decrease in enzyme activity and subsequent Na^+-pump activity was reversed by the administration of insulin to diabetic animals [179]. Some investigators focused on the Na^+-Ca^+ exchanger as a possible mechanism to explain contractile dysfunction observed in diabetics. This exchanger is of importance because Ca^{2+} is directly involved in the contraction and relaxation of cardiac function and the Na^+-Ca^{2+} exchanger is involved in the influx and efflux of Ca^{2+} [180,181]. It was demonstrated that the Na^+-Ca^{2+} exchanger and Ca^{2+}-pump activities are decreased in the diabetic heart SL but were normalized with insulin administration [174–177,182]. The role of the Na^+-H^+ exchanger in the cardiac SL has also been examined as the mechanism for influx of Na^+ and efflux of H^+. If there is a depression in Na^+-H^+ exchange, as confirmed by Pierce et al. [177], then the diabetic heart will show a marked depression in recovery due to acidosis; the combined effect of sodium concentration and intracellular pH will clearly result in an altered myocardium.

c. Changes in the mitochondria in diabetes

The mitochondria is an important storage site for calcium. Although the SR is considered the primary source of calcium, the mitochondria is a secondary source of Ca^{2+}-uptake when a surplus of Ca^{2+} is present in the cytoplasm under pathological conditions [183]. This defense mechanism of the mitochondria will act to prevent any cardiac contractile dysfunction that may occur [183]. It was found that the Ca^{2+}-uptake activity in the mitochondria of diabetic hearts was decreased in comparison to control animals, and administration of insulin reversed the decrease in activity observed in diabetics [184,185]. This may be indicative of cardiac dysfunction present in diabetes, especially since insulin treatment corrected the defect. Mitochondrial oxidative metabolism has been found to be depressed in the hearts of diabetic animals; this change was corrected with insulin treatment [186,187]. It should be noted that these studies were conducted on acute diabetic animals, and thus their relevance to the chronic diabetic animal is questionable. Studies on strepzotocin (STZ)-induced diabetic rats by Pierce and Dhalla [184] demonstrated decreased oxidative phosphorylation, Mg^{2+}-dependent ATPase and respiratory control index activities. Insulin treatment reversed the decrease in activities observed in diabetic animals. Examination of other variables to find the solution to the decreased activity of the mitochondria in diabetes, uncovered the decrease in ATP content and ATP synthesis observed in diabetic animals [184]. ATP and phosphocreatine play a vital role in the energy production and utilization by cardiac muscle; a defect in ATP synthesis could manifest itself as a dysfunction in contractility and thus lead to the occurrence of heart dysfunction. If insulin treatment was administered, then these alterations were reversible.

PERSPECTIVES

All aspects of cellular regulation have the involvement of protein kinases and protein phosphatases. Protein kinases and phosphatases are divided into various classes based on biochemical characteristics. It is predicted that mammalian genome encodes about 1,000 protein phosphatases and a bigger number of protein kinases. For many years protein phosphatases were considered to be enzymes without any use, but studies done recently have demonstrated that protein phosphatases are comparable in sophistication to their counterparts "Protein kinases". Regulation of both protein kinases and protein phosphatases is similar in nature.

The future challenge will be to discover and identify other members of protein kinase and protein phosphatase family, and to study how they react to different signals which induce phosphorylation and dephosphorylation of various proteins. Another important aspect of future will be to study how kinases and phosphatases are altered in a variety of diseases in various systems of the body. This in turn may pave a path for the development of new drugs which will benefit man.

ACKNOWLEDGMENTS

This work was supported by a grant from the Canadian Institutes of Health Research (CIHR Group in Experimental Cardiology). NSD holds CIHR/ Pharmaceutical Research and Development Chair in Cardiovascular Research supported by Merck Frosst, Canada. RG was a Visiting Scientist from Department of Pharmacology, L.M. College of Pharmacy, Ahmedabad, India.

REFERENCES

1. Sherwin RS. 2000. Diabetes mellitus. In: Cecil Textbook of Medicine, 21st ed. Ed. JC Bennet and L Goldman. Philadelphia, PA: W.B. Saunders, pp. 1263–1285.
2. Unger RH, Foster DW. 1998. Diabetes mellitus. In: Williams Textbook of Endocrinology, 9th ed. Ed. JD Wilson, DW Foster, HM Kronenberg and P Reed Larsen. Philadelphia, PA: W.B. Saunders, pp. 973–1058.
3. Chudley AE. 1999. Genetic landmarks through philately—a brief history of diabetes mellitus. Clin Genet 55:231–233.
4. Onat T. 1997. The history of endocrinology in philately. J Pediatr Endocrinol Metab 10:371–377.
5. Wilson T. 1997. Diabetes in philately. American Philately 44–46.
6. Bliss M. 1982. Banting's, Best's, and Collip's accounts of the discovery of insulin. Bull Hist Med 56:554–568.
7. Schadewaldt H. The history of diabetes mellitus. In: Diabetes: Its Medical and Cultural History. Ed. D Van Engelhardt. Berlin, Germany: Springer Verlag, pp. 43–100.
8. National Diabetes Data Group. 1979. Classification and diagnosis of diabetes mellitus and other categories of glucose intolerance. Diabetes 28:1039–1057.
9. WHO Expert Committee on Diabetes Mellitus. 1980. Second Report. WHO Tech Rep Ser 68:122–133.
10. Craig JW. 1980. Clinical implications of the new diabetes classification. Postgrad Med 68:122–133.
11. Klassen GA, Tanser PH, Marpole D, Agarwal JB. 1973. Adaptation of the coronary circulation to primary myocardial disease. Rec Adv Cardiac Struct Metab 3:497–506.
12. Christlieb AR. 1973. Diabetes and hypertensive vascular disease. Am J Cardiol 32:592–606.
13. Christlieb AR, Warram JH, Krolewsky AS, Busick EJ, Ganda OP, Asmal AC, Soeldner JS, Bradley RF. 1981. Hypertension: the major risk factor in juvenile-onset insulin dependent diabetics. Diabetes 30 (Suppl. 2):90–96.
14. Factor SM, Borczuk A, Charron MJ, Fein FS, van Hoeven KH, Sonnenblick EH. 1996. Myocardial alterations in diabetes and hypertension. Diabetes Res Clin Pract 31 (Suppl.):S133–S142.
15. Semplicini A, Ceolotto G, Massimino M, Valle R, Serena L, De Toni R, Pessina AC, Dal Palu C. 1994. Interactions between insulin and sodium homeostasis in essential hypertension. Am J Med Sci 307 (Suppl. 1):S43–S46.
16. Pollare T, Lithell H, Berne C. 1989. A comparison of the effects of hydrochlorothiazide and captopril on glucose and lipid metabolism in patients with hypertension. N Engl J Med 321:868–873.
17. Kodama J, Katayama S, Tanaka K, Itabashi A, Kawazu S, Ishii J. 1990. Effect of captopril on glucose concentration: Possible role of augmented postprandial forearm blood flow. Diabetes Care 13:1109–1111.
18. Talseth T, Westlie L, Daae L. 1991. Doxazosin and atenolol as monotherapy in mild and moderate hypertension: A randomized, parallel study with a three-year follow-up. Am Heart J 121:280–285.

19. Pell S, D'Alonzo CA. 1963. Acute myocardial infarction in a large industrial population. JAMA 185:831–838.
20. Goldenberg S, Alex M, Blumenthal HT. 1958. Sequelae of arteriosclerosis of the aorta and coronary arteries. Diabetes 7:98–108.
21. Herlitz J, Malmberg K, Karlson BW, Ryden L, Hjalmarson A. 1988. Mortality and morbidity during a five-year follow-up of diabetics with myocardial infarction. Acta Med Scand 224:31–38.
22. Dhalla NS, Pierce GN, Innes IR, Beamish RE. 1985. Pathogenesis of cardiac dysfunction in diabetes mellitus. Can J Cardiol 1:263–281.
23. Partamian JO, Bradley RF. 1965. Acute myocardial infarction in 258 cases of diabetes. Immediate mortality and 5 year survival. N Engl J Med 273:455–461.
24. Stone PH, Muller JE, Hartwell T, York BJ, Rutherford JD, Parker CB, Turi ZG, Strauss HW, Willerson JT, Robertson T, et al. 1989. The effect of diabetes mellitus on prognosis and serial left ventricular function after acute myocardial infarction: Contribution of both coronary disease and diastolic left ventricular dysfunction to the adverse prognosis. The MILIS Study Group. J Am Coll Cardiol 14:49–57.
25. Clark RS, English M, McNeill GP, Newton RW. 1985. Effect of intravenous infusion of insulin in diabetics with acute myocardial infarction. Br Med J 291:303–305.
26. Faerman I, Faccio E, Milei J, Nunez R, Jadzinsky M, Fox D, Rapaport M. 1977. Autonomic neuropathy and painless myocardial infarction in diabetic patients. Histologic evidence of their relationship. Diabetes 26:1147–1158.
27. Niakan E, Harati Y, Rolak LA, Comstock JP, Rokey R. 1986. Silent myocardial infarction and diabetic cardiovascular autonomic neuropathy. Arch Intern Med 146:2229–2230.
28. Theron HD, Steyn AF, du Raan HE, Bennett JM, de Wet JI. 1987. Autonomic neuropathy and atypical myocardial infarction in a diabetic clinic population. S Afr Med J 72:253–254.
29. Soler NG, Bennett MA, Pentecost BL, Fitzgerald MG, Malins JM. 1975. Myocardial infarction in diabetes. Q J Med 44:125–132.
30. Robinson JW. 1952. Coronary thrombosis in diabetes mellitus. New Engl J Med 246:332–335.
31. Shortleff D. 1974. Some characteristics related to the incidence of cardiovascular disease and death: Framingham study 18-year follow up. Washington, DC: Government Printing Office, Section 30.
32. Kannel WB, McGee DL. 1979. Diabetes and cardiovascular disease. JAMA 241:2035–2038.
33. Kannel WB, Hjortland M, Castelli WP. 1974. Role of diabetes in congestive heart failure: The Framingham study. Am J Cardiol 34:29–34.
34. Abbott RD, Donahue RP, Kannel WB, Wilson PW. 1988. The impact of diabetes on survival following myocardial infarction in men and women. The Framingham study. JAMA 260:3456–3460.
35. Savage MP, Krolewski AS, Kenien GC, Lebeis MP, Christlieb AR, Lewis SM. 1988. Acute myocardial infarction in diabetes mellitus and significance of congestive heart failure as a prognostic factor. Am J Cardiol 62:665–669.
36. Sternby NH. 1968. Atherosclerosis and diabetes mellitus. Acta Pathol Microbial Scand 194 (Suppl):152–164.
37. Winocour PD, Halushka PV, Colwell JA. 1985. Platelet involvement in diabetes mellitus. In: The Platelets: Physiology and Pharmacology. Ed. GL Longenecker. Orlando, FL: Academic Press, pp. 341–366.
38. Sugimoto H, Franks DJ, Lecavalier L, Chiasson JL, Hamet P. 1987. Therapeutic modulation of growth promoting activity in platelets from diabetics. Diabetes 36:667–672.
39. Jokl R, Laimins M, Klein RL, Lyons TJ, Lopes-Virella MF, Colwell JA. 1994. Platelet plasminogen activator inhibitor-1 in patients with type II diabetes mellitus. Diabetes Care 17:818–823.
40. Garcia MJ, McNamara PM, Gordon T, Kannel WB. 1974. Morbidity and mortality in diabetes in the Framingham study. Diabetes 23:105–111.
41. Pulsinelli WA, Levey DE, Sigsbee B, Sherer P, Plum F. 1983. Increased damage after ischemic stroke in patients with hyperglycemia with or without established diabetes mellitus. Am J Med 74:540–544.
42. Weinberger J, Biscarra V, Weisberg MK, Jacobson JH. 1983. Factors contributing to stroke in patients with atherosclerotic disease of the great vessels: the role of diabetes. Stroke 14:709–714.
43. McCall AL. 1990. The impact of diabetes on the CNS. Diabetes 41:557–570.
44. Regan TJ, Lyons MM, Ahmed SS, Levinson GE, Oldewurtel HA, Ahmed MR, Haider B. 1977. Evidence for cardiomyopathy in familial diabetes mellitus. J Clin Invest 60:885–899.
45. Beuckelmann DJ, Wier WG. 1988. Mechanism of release of calcium from sarcoplasmic reticulum of guinea-pig cardiac cells. J Physiol (Lond) 405:233–255.

46. du Bell WH, Houser SR. 1989. Voltage and beat dependence of Ca^{2+} transient in feline ventricular myocytes. Am J Physiol 257:H746–H759.
47. London B, Krueger JW. 1986. Contraction in voltage-clamped, internally perfused single heart cells. J Gen Physiol 88:475–505.
48. Niggli E, Lederer WJ. 1990. Voltage-independent calcium release in heart muscle. Science 250:565–568.
49. Hobai IA, Bates JA, Howarth FC, Levi AJ. 1997. Inhibition by external Cd^{2+} of Na/Ca exchange and L-type Ca channel in rabbit ventricular myocytes. Am J Physiol 272:H2164–H2172.
50. Leblanc N, Hume JR. 1990. Sodium current-induced release of calcium from cardiac sarcoplasmic reticulum. Science 248:372–376.
51. Levi AJ, Brooksby P, Hancox JC. 1993. One hump or two? The triggering of calcium release from the sarcoplasmic reticulum and the voltage dependence of contraction in mammalian cardiac muscle. Cardiovasc Res 27:1743–1757.
52. Levi AJ, Li J, Spitzer KW, Bridge JH. 1996. Effect on the indo-1 transient of applying Ca^{2+} channel blocker for a single beat in voltage-clamped guinea-pig cardiac myocytes. J Physiol (Lond) 494:653–673.
53. Lipp P, Niggli E. 1994. Sodium current-induced calcium signals in isolated guinea-pig ventricular myocytes. J Physiol (Lond) 474:439–446.
54. Bers DM. 1985. Ca influx and sarcoplasmic reticulum Ca release in cardiac muscle activation during postrest recovery. Am J Physiol 248:H366–H381.
55. Fabiato A, Fabiato F. 1977. Calcium release from the sarcoplasmic reticulum. Circ Res 40:119–129.
56. Cannell MB, Berlin JR, Lederer WJ. 1987. Effect of membrane potential changes on the calcium transient in single rat cardiac muscle cells. Science 238:1419–1423.
57. Nabauer M, Callewaert G, Cleemann L, Morad M. 1989. Regulation of calcium release is gated by calcium current, not gating charge, in cardiac myocytes. Science 244:800–803.
58. Balke CW, Egan TM, Wier WG. 1994. Processes that remove calcium from the cytoplasm during excitation-contraction coupling in intact rat heart cells. J Physiol (Lond) 474:447–462.
59. Bassani JW, Bassani RA, Bers DM. 1993. Ca^{2+} cycling between sarcoplasmic reticulum and mitochondria in rabbit cardiac myocytes. J Physiol (Lond) 460:603–621.
60. Bers DM, Bassani JW, Bassani RA. 1993. Competition and redistribution among calcium transport systems in rabbit cardiac myocytes. Cardiovasc Res 27:1772–1777.
61. Barcenas-Ruiz L, Beuckelmann DJ, Wier WG. 1987. Sodium-calcium exchange in heart: membrane currents and changes in $[Ca^{2+}]_i$. Science 238:1720–1722.
62. Hobai IA, Howarth FC, Pabbathi VK, Dalton GR, Hancox JC, Zhu JQ, Howlett SE, Ferrier GR, Levi AJ. 1997. "Voltage-activated Ca release" in rabbit, rat and guinea-pig cardiac myocytes, and modulation by internal cAMP. Pflugers Arch 435:164–173.
63. Simmerman HK, Collins JH, Theibert JL, Wegener AD, Jones LR. 1986. Sequence analysis of phospholamban. Identification of phosphorylation sites and two major structural domains. J Biol Chem 261:13333–13341.
64. Davis BA, Schwartz A, Samaha FJ, Kranias EG. 1983. Regulation of cardiac sarcoplasmic reticulum calcium transport by calcium-calmodulin-dependent phosphorylation. J Biol Chem 258:13587–13591.
65. Kirchberger MA, Antonetz T. 1982. Calmodulin-mediated regulation of calcium transport and (Ca^{2+} + Mg^{2+})-activated ATPase activity in isolated cardiac sarcoplasmic reticulum. J Biol Chem 257:5685–5691.
66. Kranias EG, Mandel F, Wang T, Schwartz A. 1980. Mechanism of the stimulation of calcium ion dependent adenosine triphosphatase of cardiac sarcoplasmic reticulum by adenosine 3′,5′-monophosphate dependent protein kinase. Biochemistry 19:5434–5439.
67. Movsesian MA, Nishikawa M, Adelstein RS. 1984. Phosphorylation of phospholamban by calcium-activated, phospholipid-dependent protein kinase. Stimulation of cardiac sarcoplasmic reticulum calcium uptake. J Biol Chem 259:8029–8032.
68. Tada M, Inui M. 1983. Regulation of calcium transport by the ATPase-phospholamban system. J Mol Cell Cardiol 15:565–575.
69. Kranias EG. 1985. Regulation of calcium transport by protein phosphatase activity associated with cardiac sarcoplasmic reticulum. J Biol Chem 260:11006–11010.
70. Steenaart NA, Ganim JR, Di Salvo J, Kranias EG. 1992. The phospholamban phosphatase associated with cardiac sarcoplasmic reticulum is a type 1 enzyme. Arch Biochem Biophys 293:17–24.

71. Kranias EG, Di Salvo J. 1986. A phospholamban protein phosphatase activity associated with cardiac sarcoplasmic reticulum. J Biol Chem 261:10029–10032.
72. Kranias EG, Steenaart NA, Di Salvo J. 1988. Purification and characterization of phospholamban phosphatase from cardiac muscle. J Biol Chem 263:15681–15687.
73. Hamby RI, Zoneraich S, Sherman L. 1974. Diabetic cardiomyopathy. JAMA 229:1749–1754.
74. D'Elia JA, Weinrauch LA, Healy RW, Libertino RW, Bradley RF, Leland OS. 1979. Myocardial dysfunction without coronary artery disease in diabetic renal failure. Am J Cardiol 43:193–199.
75. Shapiro LM, Leatherdale BA, Coyne ME, Fletcher RF, Mackinnon J. 1980. Prospective study of heart disease in untreated maturity onset diabetics. Br Heart J 44:342–348.
76. Rubler S, Sajadi MRM, Araoye MA, Holford MD. 1978. Noninvasive estimation of myocardial performance in patients with diabetes. Diabetes 27:127–134.
77. Shapiro LM, Howat AP, Calter MM. 1981. Left ventricular function in diabetes mellitus. I. Methodology and prevalence and spectrum of abnormalities. Br Heart J 45:122–128.
78. Garrard CL, Weissler AM, Dodge HT. 1970. The relationship of alterations in systolic time intervals to ejection fraction in patients with cardiac disease. Circulation 42:455–462.
79. Goldweit RS, Borer JS, Jovanovic LG, Drexler AJ, Hochreiter CA, Devereux RB, Peterson CM. 1985. Relation of hemogloblin A1 and blood to cardiac function in diabetes mellitus. Am J Cardiol 56:642–650.
80. Uusitupa M, Siitonen O, Aro A, Korhonen T, Pyorala K. 1983. Effect of correction of hyperglycemia on left ventricular function in non-insulin-dependent (Type 2) diabetics. Acta Med Scand 213: 363–368.
81. Abenavoli T, Rubler S, Fisher VJ, Axelrod H, Zuckerman KP. 1981. Exercise testing with myocardial scintigraphy in asymptomatic diabetic males. Circulation 63:54–64.
82. Zarich SW, Arbuckle BE, Cohen LR, Roberts M, Nesto RW. 1988. Diastolic abnormalities in young asymptomatic diabetic patients assessed by pulsed doppler echocardiography. J Am Coll Cardiol 12:114–120.
83. Raev DC. 1994. Which left ventricular function is impaired earlier in the evolution of diabetic cardiomyopathy? An echocardiographic study of young type I diabetic patients. Diabetes Care 17:633–639.
84. Ruddy TD, Shumak SL, Liu PP, Barme AN, Seawright SJ, McLaughlin PR, Zinman B. 1988. The relationship of cardiac diastolic dysfunction to concurrent hormonal and metabolic status in type I diabetes mellitus. J Clin Endocrinol Metab 66:113–118.
85. Ganguly PK, Pierce GN, Dhalla KS, Dhalla NS. 1983. Defective sarcoplasmic reticular calcium transport in diabetic cardiomopathy. Am J Physiol 244:E528–E535.
86. Fein FS, Kornstein LB, Strobeck JE, Capasso JM, Sonnenblick EH. 1980. Altered myocardial mechanics in diabetes rats. Circ Res 47:922–933.
87. Bhimji S, Godin DV, McNeill JH. 1985. Biochemical and functional changes in hearts from rabbits with diabetes. Diabetologia 28:452–457.
88. Biebfeld DR, Pace CS, Boshell BR. 1983. Altered sensitivity of chronic diabetic rat heart to calcium. Am J Physiol 245:E560–E567.
89. Fein FS, Miller-Green B, Sonnenblick EH. 1985. Altered myocardial mechanics in diabetic rabbits. Am J Physiol 248:H729–H736.
90. Heyliger CE, Pierce GN, Singal PK, Beamish RE, Dhalla NS. 1982. Cardiac alpha- and beta-adrenergic receptor alterations in diabetic cardiomyopathy. Basic Res Cardiol 77:610–618.
91. Afzal N, Ganguly PK, Dhalla KS, Pierce GN, Singal PK, Dhalla NS. 1988. Beneficial effects of verapamil in diabetic cardiomyopathy. Diabetes 37:936–942.
92. Haider B, Ahmed SS, Moschos CB, Oldewurtel HA, Regan TJ. 1977. Myocardial function and coronary blood flow response to acute ischemia in chronic canine diabetes. Circ Res 40:577–583.
93. Ku DD, Sellers BM. 1982. Effects of streptozotocin diabetes and insulin treatment on myocardial sodium pump and contractility of the rat heart. J Pharmacol Exp Ther 222:395–400.
94. Ingebretsen CG, Moreau P, Hawelu-Johnson C, Ingebretsen WR. 1980. Performance of diabetic rat hearts: Effects of anoxia and increased work. Am J Physiol 239:H614–H620.
95. Tahliani AG, Vadlamudi RVSV, McNeill JH. 1983. Prevention and reversal of altered myocardial function in diabetic rats by insulin treatment. Can J Physiol Pharmacol 61:516–523.
96. Vadlamudi RVSV, Rodgers RL, McNeill JH. 1982. The effect of chronic alloxan- and streptozotocin-induced diabetes on isolated rat heart performance. Can J Physiol Pharmacol 60:902–911.

97. Penpargkul S, Schaible T, Yipintsoi T, Scheuer J. 1980. The effect of diabetes on performance and metabolism of rat hearts. Circ Res 47:911–921.
98. Fein FS, Strobeck JE, Malhotra A, Scheuer J, Sonnenblick EH. 1981. Reversibility of diabetic cardiomyopathy with insulin in rats. Circ Res 49:1251–1261.
99. Reagan TJ, Wu CF, Yeh CK, Oldewurtel HA, Haider B. 1981. Myocardial composition and function in diabetes: The effects of chronic insulin use. Circ Res 49:1268–1277.
100. Schaible TF, Malhotra A, Bauman WA, Scheuer J. 1983. Left ventricular function after chronic insulin treatment in diabetic and normal rats. J Mol Cell Cardiol 15:445–458.
101. Dillmann WH. 1982. Influence of thyroid hormone administration on myosin ATPase activity and myosin isoenzyme distribution in the heart of diabetic rats. Metabolism 31:199–204.
102. Saunders J, Hall SEH, Sonksen PH. 1978. Thyroid hormones in insulin requiring diabetes before and after treatment. Diabetologia 15:29–35.
103. Malhotra A, Mordes JP, McDermot L, Schaible TF. 1985. Abnormal cardiac biochemistry in spontaneously diabetic Bio-Breeding/Worcester rat. Am J Physiol 249:H1051–H1055.
104. Scheuer J, Bhan AK. 1979. Cardiac contractile proteins: adenosine triphosphatase activity and physiological function. Circ Res 45:1–12.
105. Gergely J. 1974. Some aspects of the role of the sarcoplasmic reticulum and the tropomyosin-troponin system in the control of muscle contraction by calcium ions. Circ Res 34/35 (Suppl III):74–82.
106. Pierce GN, Dhalla NS. 1981. Cardiac myofibrillar ATPase activity in diabetic rats. J Mol Cell Cardiol 13:1063–1069.
107. Pierce GN, Dhalla NS. 1985. Mechanisms of the defect in cardiac myofibrillar function during diabetes. Am J Physiol 248:E170–E175.
108. Afzal N, Pierce GN, Elimban V, Beamish RE, Dhalla NS. 1989. Influence of verapamil on some subcellular defects in diabetic cardiomyopathy. Am J Physiol 256:E453–E458.
109. Pollack PS, Malhotra A, Fein FS, Scheuer J. 1986. Effects of diabetes on cardiac contractile proteins in rabbits and reversal with insulin. Am J Physiol 251:H448–H454.
110. Malhotra A, Penpargkul S, Fein FS, Sonnenblick EH, Scheuer J. 1981. The effect of streptozotocin-induced diabetes in rats on cardiac contractile proteins. Circ Res 49:1243–1250.
111. Garber DW, Neely JR. 1983. Decreased myocardial function and myosin ATPase in hearts from diabetic rats. Am J Physiol 244:H586–H591.
112. Garber DW, Everett AW, Neely JR. 1983. Cardiac function and myosin ATPase in diabetic rats treated with insulin, T_3 and T_4. Am J Physiol 244:H592–H599.
113. Solaro RJ, Wise RM, Shiner JS, Briggs FN. 1974. Calcium requirements for cardiac myofibrillar activation. Circ Res 34:525–530.
114. Carafoli E. 1987. Intracellular Ca^{2+} homeostasis. Ann Rev Biochem 56:395–433.
115. Penpargkul S, Fein F, Sonnenblick EH, Scheuer J. 1981. Depressed sacroplasmic reticular function for diabetic rats. J Mol Cell Cardiol 13:303–309.
116. Lopaschuk GD, Katz S, McNeill JH. 1983. The effect of alloxan- and streptozotocin-induced diabetes on calcium transport in rat cardiac sarcoplasmic reticulum. The possible involvement of long chain acyl-carnitines. Can J Physiol Pharmacol 61:439–448.
117. Lopaschuk GD, Thahiliani AG, Vadlamudi RVSV, Katz S, McNeill JH. 1983. Cardiac sarcoplasmic reticulum function in insulin- or carnitine-treated diabetic rats. Am J Physiol 245:H969–H976.
118. Pierce GN, Ganguly PK, Dzurba A, Dhalla NS. 1985. Modification of the function of cardiac subcellular organelles by insulin. Adv Myocardiol 6:113–125.
119. Feuvray D, Idell-Wenger JA, Neely JR. 1979. Effects of ischemia on rat myocardial function and metabolism in diabetes. Circ Res 44:322–329.
120. Solaro RJ, ed. 1986. Protein Phosphorylation in Heart Muscle. Boca Raton, FL: CRC Press.
121. Raju RVS, Kakkar R, Sharma RK. 1997. Biological significance of phosphorylation and myristoylation in the regulation of cardiac muscle proteins. Mol Cell Biochem 176:135–143.
122. Rapundalo ST, Solaro RJ, Kranias EG. 1989. Inotropic responses to isoproterenol and phosphodiesterase inhibitors in intact guinea pig hearts: comparison of cyclic AMP levels and phosphorylation of sarcoplasmic reticulum and myofibrillar proteins. Circ Res 64:104–111.
123. Lindemann JP, Jones LR, Hathaway DR, Henry BG, Watanabe AM. 1983. β-Adrenergic stimulation of phospholamban phosphorylation and Ca^{2+}-ATPase activity in guinea pig ventricles. J Biol Chem 258:464–471.
124. Kranias EG, Solaro RJ. 1982. Phosphorylation of troponin I and phospholamban during catecholamine stimulation of rabbit heart. Nature 298:182–184.

125. Lindemann JP, Watanabe AM. 1985. Phosphorylation of phospholamban in intact myocardium. Role of Ca^{2+}-calmodulin-dependent mechanisms. J Biol Chem 260:4516–4525.
126. Vittone L, Mundina C, Chiappe de Cingolani G, Mattiazi A. 1993. Role of Ca^{2+}-calmodulin dependent phopholamban phosphorylation on the relaxant effect of beta-adrenergic agonists. Mol Cell Biochem 124:33–42.
127. Talosi L, Kranias EG. 1992. Effect of alpha-adrenergic stimulation on activation of protein kinase C and phosphorylation of proteins in intact rabbit hearts. Circ Res 70:670–678.
128. Venema RC, Kuo JF. 1993. Protein kinase C-mediated phosphorylation of troponin I and C-protein in isolated myocardial cells is associated with inhibition of myofibrillar actomyosin MgATPase. J Biol Chem 268:2705–2711.
129. Sabine B, Willlenbrock R, Haase H, Karczewski P, Wallukat G, Dietz R, Krause EG. 1995. Cyclic GMP-mediated phospholamban phosphorylation in intact cardiomyocytes. Biochem Biophys Res Commun 214:75–80.
130. Srivastava AK. 1995. Protein tyrosine phosphorylation in cardiovascular system. Mol Cell Biochem 149/150:87–94.
131. Foncea R, Andersson M, Ketterman A, Blakesley V, Sapag-Hagar M, Sugden PH, Le Roith D, Lavandero S. 1997. Insulin-like growth factor-I rapidly activates multiple signal transduction pathways in cultured rat cardiac myocytes. J Biol Chem 272:19115–19124.
132. Clerk A, Gillespie-Brown J, Fuller SJ, Sugden PH. 1996. Stimulation of phosphatidylinositol hydrolysis, protein kinase C translocation and mitogen-activated protein kinase activity by bradykinin in rat ventricular myocytes: dissociation from the hypertrophic response. Biochem J 317:109–118.
133. Clerk A, Sugden PH. 1997. Cell stress-induced phosphorylation of ATF2 and c-jun transcription factors in rat ventricular myocytes. Biochem J 325:801–810.
134. Xu H, Hawkins C, Narayanan N. 1993. Phosphorylation and activation of the Ca^{2+}-pumping ATPase of cardiac sarcoplasmic reticulum by Ca^{2+}/calmodulin-dependent protein kinase. J Biol Chem 268:8394–8397.
135. James P, Inui M, Tada M, Chiesi M, Carafoli E. 1989. Nature and site of phospholamban regulation of the Ca^{2+} pump of sarcoplasmic reticulum. Nature 342:90–92.
136. Luo W, Grupp IL, Harrer J, Ponniah S, Grupp G, Duffy JJ, Doetschman T, Kranias EG. 1994. Targeted ablation of the phospholamban gene is associated with markedly enhanced myocardial contractility and loss of β-agonist stimulation. Circ Res 75:401–409.
137. Colyer J, Wang JH. 1991. Dependence of cardiac sarcoplasmic reticulum calcium pump activity on the phosphorylation status of phospholamban. J Biol Chem 266:17486–17493.
138. Huggins JP, England PJ. 1987. Evidence for a phosphorylation-induced conformational change in phospholamban from the effects of three proteases. FEBS Lett 217:32–36.
139. Kirchberger MA, Tada M, Katz AM. 1974. Adenosine 3′:5′-monophosphate-dependent protein kinase-catalyzed phosphorylation reaction and its relationship to calcium transport in cardiac sarcoplasmic reticulum. J Biol Chem 249:6166–6173.
140. Kranias EG. 1985. Regulation of Ca^{2+} transport by cyclic 3′,5′-AMP-dependent and calcium-calmodulin-dependent phosphorylation of cardiac sarcoplasmic reticulum. Biochim Biophys Acta 844:193–199.
141. Tada M, Kirchberger MA, Katz AM. 1975. Phosphorylation of a 22,000 dalton component of the cardiac sarcoplasmic reticulum by adenosine 3′:5′-monophosphate-dependent protein kinase. J Biol Chem 250:2640–2647.
142. Tada M, Yamada M, Ohmori F, Kuzuya T, Inui M, Abe H. 1980. Transient state kinetic studies of Ca^{2+}-dependant ATPase and calcium transport by cardiac sarcoplasmic reticulum. Effect of cyclic AMP-dependent protein kinase-catalyzed phosphorylation of phopholamban. J Biol Chem 255: 1985–1992.
143. Miyakoda G, Yoshida A, Takisawa H, Nakamura T. 1987. Beta-adrenergic regulation of contractility and protein phosphorylation in spontaneously beating isolated rat myocardial cells. J Biochem Tokyo 102:211–224.
144. Kaumann AJ, Sanders L, Lynham JA, Bartel S, Kuschel M, Karczewski P, Krause EG. 1996. β_2-adrenoceptor activation by zinterol causes protein phosphorylation, contractile effects and relaxant effects through a cAMP pathway in human atrium. Mol Cell Biochem 163/164:113–123.
145. Sulakhe PV, Vo XT. 1995. Regulation of phospholamban and troponin-I phosphorylation in the intact rat cardiomyocytes by adrenergic and cholinergic stimuli: roles of cyclic nucleotides, calcium, protein kinases and phosphatases and depolarization. Mol Cell Biochem 149/150:103–126.

146. Gupta RC, Neumann J, Watanabe AM. 1993. Comparison of adenosine and muscarinic receptor-mediated effects on protein phosphatase inhibitor-1 activity in the heart. J Pharmacol Exp Ther 266:16–22.
147. Iwasa Y, Hosey MM. 1983. Cholinergic antagonism of beta-adrenergic stimulation of cardiac membrane protein phosphorylation in situ. J Biol Chem 258:4571–4575.
148. Lindemann JP, Watanabe AM. 1985. Muscarinic cholinergic inhibition of beta-adrenergic stimulation of phospholamban phosphorylation and Ca^{2+} transport in guinea pig ventricles. J Biol Chem 260:13122–13129.
149. Gupta RC, Neumann J, Boknik P, Watanabe AM. 1994. M_2-specific muscarinic cholinergic recepor-mediated inhibition of cardiac regulatory protein phosphorylation. Am J Physiol 266:H1138–H1144.
150. Davis BA, Schwartz A, Samaha FJ, Kranias EG. 1983. Regulation of cardiac sarcoplasmic reticulum calcium transport by calcium-calmodulin-dependent phosphorylation. J Biol Chem 258:13587–13591.
151. Gupta RC, Davis BA, Kranias EG. 1987. Mechanism of the stimulation of cardiac sarcoplasmic reticulum calcium pump by calmodulin. Membr Biochem 7:73–86.
152. Tada M, Inui M, Yamada M, Kadoma M, Kuzuya T, Abe H, Kakiuchi S. 1983. Effects of phospholamban phosporylation catalyzed by adenosine 3′:5′-monophosphate- and calmodulin-dependent protein kinases on calcium transport ATPase of cardiac sarcoplasmic reticulum. J Mol Cell Cardiol 15:335–346.
153. Baltas LG, Karozweski P, Bartel S, Krause EG. 1997. The endogenous cardiac sarcoplasmic reticulum Ca^{2+}/calmodulin-dependent kinase is activated in response to β-adrenergic stimulation and becomes Ca^{2+}-dependent in intact beating hearts. FEBS Lett 409:131–136.
154. Huggins JP, Cook EA, Piggott JR, Mattinsley TJ, England PJ. 1989. Phopholamban is a good substrate for cyclic GMP-dependent protein kinase in vitro, but not in intact cardiac or smooth muscle. Biochem J 260:829–835.
155. Movesesian MA, Nishikawa M, Adelstein RS. 1984. Phosphorylation of phospholamban by calcium-activated, phopholipid-dependent protein kinase. Stimulation of cardiac sarcoplasmic reticulum calcium uptake. J Biol Chem 259:8029–8032.
156. Allen BG, Katz S. 1996. Phosphorylation of cardiac junctional and free sarcoplasmic reticulum by PKC α, PKC β, PKA and the Ca^{2+}/calmodulin-dependent protein kinase. Mol Cell Biochem 155:91–103.
157. Cohen P. 1989. The structure and regulation of protein phosphatases. Annu Rev Biochem 58:453–508.
158. Kranias EG. 1985. Regulation of calcium transport by protein phosphatase activity associated with cardiac sarcoplasmic reticulum. J Biol Chem 260:11006–11010.
159. Fabiato A. 1983. Calcium-induced release of calcium from the cardiac sarcoplasmic reticulum. Am J Physiol 245:C1–C14.
160. Hohenegger M, Suko J. 1993. Phosphorylation of the purified cardiac ryanodine receptor by exogenous and endogenous protein kinases. Biochem J 296:303–308.
161. Witcher DR, Kovacs RJ, Schulman H, Cepali DC, Jones LR. 1991. Unique phosphorylation site on the cardiac ryanodine receptor regulates calcium channel activity. J Biol Chem 266:11144–11152.
162. Marx SO, Reiken S, Hisamatsu Y, Jayaraman T, Burkhoff D, Rosemblit N, Marks AR. 2000. PKA phosphorylation dissociates FKBP 12.6 from the calcium release channel (ryanodine receptor) defection regulation in failing hearts. Cell 101:365–376.
163. Li L, Satoh H, Ginsburg KS, Bers DM. 1997. The effect of Ca^{2+}-calmodulin dependent protein kinase II on cardiac excitation-contraction coupling in ferret ventricular myocytes. J Physiol 501:17–31.
164. Scott BT, Simmerman HKB, Collins JH, Nadal-Ginard B, Jones LR. 1988. Complete amino acid sequence of canine cardiac calsequestrin deduced by cDNA cloning. J Biol Chem 263:8958–8964.
165. Cala SE, Miles K. 1992. Phosphorylation of the cardiac isoform of calsequestrin in cultured rat myotubes and rat skeletal muscle. Biochim Biophys Acta 1118:277–287.
166. Enyedi A, Farago A, Sarkadi B, Gardos G. 1984. Cyclic AMP-dependent protein kinase and Ca^{2+}-calmodulin stimulate the formation of polyphosphoinositides in a sarcoplasmic reticulum preparation of rabbit heart. FEBS Lett 176:235–238.
167. Fabiato A. 1985. Time and calcium dependence of activation and inactivation of calcium-induced release of calcium from the sarcoplasmic reticulum of a skinned canine cardiac purkinje cell. J Gen Physiol 85:247–289.

168. Cleemann L, Morad M. 1991. Role of Ca^{2+} channel in cardiac excitation contraction in rat: Evidence from Ca^{2+} transients and contraction. J Physiol (Lond) 432:283–312.
169. Heyliger CE, Pierce GN, Singal PK, Beamish RE, Dhalla NS. 1982. Cardiac alpha- and beta-adrenergic receptor alterations in diabetic cardiomyopathy. Basic Res Cardiol 77:610–618.
170. Latifpour J, McNeill JH. 1984. Cardiac autonomic receptors: effect of long term experimental diabetes. J Pharmacol Exp Ther 230:230–242.
171. Sundaresan PR, Sharma VK, Gingold SI, Banerjee SP. 1984. Decrease β-adrenergic receptors in rat heart in streptozotocin-induced diabetes: role of thyroid hormones. Endocrinology 114:1358–1363.
172. Williams RS, Schaible TF, Scheuer J, Kennedy R. 1983. Effects of experimental diabetes on adrenergic and cholinergic receptors for rat myocardium. Diabetes 32:881–886.
173. Schwartz A, Lindemayer GE, Allen JC. 1975. The sodium-potassium, adenosine triphosphatase: Pharmacological, physiological and biochemical aspects. Pharmacol Rev 27:3–134.
174. Onji T, Liu M-S. 1980. Effects of alloxan-diabetes on the sodium potassium adenosine triphosphate enzyme system in dog hearts. Biochem Biophys Res Commun 96:799–804.
175. Heyliger CE, Prakash A, McNeill JH. 1987. Alterations in cardiac sarcolemmal Ca^{2+} pump activity during diabetes mellitus. Am J Physiol 252:H540–H544.
176. Makino N, Dhalla KS, Elimban V, Dhalla NS. 1987. Sarcolemmal Ca^{2+} transport in streptozotocin-induced diabetic cardiomyopathy in rats. Am J Physiol 253:E202–E207.
177. Pierce GN, Ramjiawan B, Dhalla NS, Ferrari R. 1990. Na^+-H^+ exchanger in cardiac sarcolemmal vesicles isolated from diabetic rats. Am J Physiol 258:H255–H261.
178. Pierce GN, Dhalla NS. 1983. Sarcolemmal Na^+-K^+-ATPase activity in diabetic rat heart. Am J Physiol 245:C241–C247.
179. Ku DD, Sellers BM. 1982. Effects of streptozotocin diabetes and insulin treatment on myocardial sodium pump and contractility of the rat heart. J Pharmacol Exp Ther 222:395–400.
180. LeBlanc N, Hume JR. 1990. Sodium current-induced release of calcium from cardiac sarcoplasmic reticulum. Science 248:372–376.
181. Bridge JHB, Smoley JR, Spitzer KW. 1990. The relationship between charge movements associated with ICa^{2+} and INa^+-Ca^{2+} in cardiac myocytes. Science 248:370–376.
182. Borda E, Pascual J, Wald M, Sterin-Borda L. 1988. Hypersensitivity to calcium associated with an increased sarcolemmal Ca^{2+}-ATPase activity in diabetic rat heart. Can J Cardiol 4:97–101.
183. Dhalla NS, Pierce GN, Panagia V, Singal PK, Beamish RE. 1982. Calcium movements in relation to heart function. Basic Res Cardiol 77:117–139.
184. Pierce GN, Dhalla NS. 1985. Heart mitochondrial function in chronic experimental diabetes in rats. Can J Cardiol 1:48–54.
185. Tanaka Y, Konno N, Kako KJ. 1992. Mitochondrial dysfunction observed in situ in cardiomyocytes of rats in experimental diabetes. Cardiovasc Res 26:409–414.
186. Puckett SW, Reddy WJ. 1979. A decrease in the malate-aspartate shuttle and glutamate translocase activity in heart mitochondria from alloxan-diabetic rats. J Mol Cell Cardiol 11:173–187.
187. Flutson NJ, Kerbey AL, Randle PJ, Sugden PH. 1978. Conversion of inactive (phosphorylated) pyruvate dehydrogenase complex into active complex by the phosphate reaction in heart mitochondria is inhibited by alloxan-diabetes or starvation in the rat. Biochem J 173:669–675.

G.N. Pierce, M. Nagano, P. Zahradka, and N.S. Dhalla (eds.).
ATHEROSCLEROSIS, HYPERTENSION AND DIABETES.
Kluwer Academic Publishers. Boston.

DIABETES AND CARDIAC DYSFUNCTION

DAVID L. SEVERSON,[1] ELLEN AASUM,[3] DARRELL D. BELKE,[1] TERJE S. LARSEN,[3] LISA M. SEMENIUK,[1] and YAKHIN SHIMONI[2]

[1] *Departments of Pharmacology & Therapeutics and* [2] *Physiology & Biophysics, Faculty of Medicine, University of Calgary, Calgary, AB, Canada, and* [3] *Department of Medical Physiology, Institute of Medical Biology, University of Tromsø, Tromsø, Norway*

Summary. Type 2 diabetes is associated with a marked increase in cardiovascular disease. This review summarizes some of the experimental evidence supporting the existence of a diabetic cardiomyopathy, defined as ventricular dysfunction in the absence of coronary artery disease, in three rodent models of type 2 diabetes produced by leptin receptor mutations: diabetic *db/db* mice, diabetic ZDF *fa/fa* rats, and corpulent JCR:LA-*cp/cp* rats. Results showing cardiac dysfunction in type 2 diabetic hearts have been obtained from studies using: (i) in vivo echocardiography; (ii) ex vivo perfused hearts; and (iii) isolated cardiomyocytes. The most complete assessment of cardiac dysfunction in type 2 diabetic hearts has come from investigations with *db/db* mice. Diabetic *db/db* hearts exhibit a distinct cardiomyopathy, with both systolic and diastolic dysfunction from echocardiographic measurements. Perfused *db/db* hearts also have reduced contractile performance and altered metabolism, with decreased glucose utilization and increased fatty acid oxidation. Finally, isolated cardiomyocytes from *db/db* hearts have altered electrophysiology with reduced potassium currents producing a prolongation of the action potential. A key objective for future studies will be to establish the mechanistic basis for this cardiac dysfunction, so that therapeutic interventions can be developed to improve the function of type 2 diabetic hearts.

***Key words*:** Diabetic cardiomyopathy, Type 2 diabetes

Corresponding Author: Dr. D.L. Severson, Department of Pharmacology & Therapeutics, University of Calgary, Faculty of Medicine, 3330 Hospital Drive NW, Calgary, AB T2N 4N1. Telephone: 403-220-3020; Fax: 403-270-2211; e-mail: severson@ucalgary.ca

INTRODUCTION

Diabetes mellitus is a very prevalent disease. The number of people diagnosed as diabetic has increased substantially over the past two decades, and the incidence of diabetes is predicted to increase explosively in the future [1]. Diabetes mellitus has been classified into two forms. Type 1 diabetes is caused by the autoimmune destruction of pancreatic beta cells, producing insulin deficiency that requires insulin replacement therapy (insulin-dependent diabetes mellitus, IDDM). This type 1 form accounts for about 10% of all cases of diabetes. The most prevalent form (90%) is type 2 (non-insulin-dependent) diabetes (NIDDM), resulting from the combination of insulin resistance plus a beta-cell secretory defect [2,3]. The diabetes epidemic [1] relates particularly to type 2 diabetes.

An increased incidence of cardiovascular disease is the most common complication of diabetes [4]. Manifestations of diabetes-induced cardiovascular disease include myocardial infarction, congestive heart failure, peripheral vascular disease, and stroke. The cardiac complications associated with type 2 diabetes [5] are due to two pathophysiological processes. First, coronary (ischemic) heart disease is increased as a consequence of accelerated atherosclerosis because of associated risk factors such as visceral obesity, hypertension, dyslipidemia (elevated triglycerides, reduced HDL, and the presence of small dense LDL) and pro-thrombotic factors such as elevated fibrinogen and PAI-1 [6–8]. Second, a diabetic cardiomyopathy also exists, defined as ventricular dysfunction in the absence of coronary heart disease or hypertension [9–13]. In diabetic cardiomyopathy, diastolic dysfunction often precedes impairment of systolic function in subjects with type 2 diabetes.

Experimental studies with rodent models of diabetes allow assessment of direct deleterious effects of a diabetic cardiomyopathy without complications of concomitant atherosclerotic coronary heart disease because rodents are typically atherosclerosis-resistant. However, most reports of diabetes-induced cardiac dysfunction have used type 1 diabetic models, using chemical induction of insulin deficiency with agents like streptozotocin that produce selective necrosis of pancreatic beta cells [14]. By comparison, relatively few studies on cardiac function have been conducted with type 2 diabetic animal models exhibiting insulin resistance [15]. Therefore, this review will focus on assessment of cardiac function in animal models of type 2 diabetes.

GENETIC ANIMAL MODELS OF TYPE 2 DIABETES

There are a number of monogenic models of obesity and type 2 diabetes, characterized by mutations in the leptin receptor (Table 1). Leptin is a polypeptide that is secreted by adipose tissue in response to an increase in fat cell size [16,17]. Leptin then acts on the hypothalamus to decrease food intake and increase energy expenditure, providing a feedback mechanism to reduce adipose tissue mass. Leptin also has direct actions on other targets; pancreatic beta-cell insulin secretion is enhanced [18] along with altered lipid metabolism in skeletal muscle [19,20] and other tissues [21]. These effects of leptin are mediated by the leptin receptor, a member of the

Table 1. Characteristics of monogenic animal models of obesity and type 2 diabetes, caused by leptin receptor mutations

		Characteristics		
Animal model	Mutation	Obesity	Hyperinsulinemia	Hyperglycemia
1. Diabetic *db/db* Mouse	*Lepr*^{db}: selective loss of "long" form of leptin receptors	+++	+++	+++
2. Zucker Diabetic Fatty (ZDF-drt) *fa/fa* Rat	*Lepr*^{fa}: decreased cell surface binding of leptin	++	+++	+
3. Corpulent JCR:LA *cp/cp* Rat	*Lepr*^{faf}: receptor-null	+++	+++	+/−

class I cytokine receptor superfamily. It follows that mutations in the leptin receptor producing leptin resistance will result in the characteristics of type 2 diabetes: obesity, insulin resistance (absence of direct leptin action on skeletal muscle and indirect consequences of altered secretions from expanded adipose tissue mass), and impaired insulin secretion from pancreatic beta cells [22].

Diabetic *db/db* mice were discovered at Jackson Laboratory, as the consequence of a spontaneous mutation [23,24]. The natural history of *db/db* mice follows a distinct pattern [25,26]. Initially, peripheral insulin resistance is accompanied by increased pancreatic beta-cell insulin secretion; thus, hyperinsulinemia is a compensatory mechanism to counter-act insulin resistance, allowing normoglycemia. Increased levels of plasma insulin are the earliest feature of *db/db* mice, evident as soon as 10–12 days of age. Hyperglycemia eventually develops when enhanced beta-cell insulin secretion can no longer compensate for peripheral and hepatic insulin resistance. The maximal extent of hyperinsulinemia occurs at 2–3 months of age; insulin levels then fall rapidly as beta-cells exhibit a severe secretory defect. Body weights of *db/db* mice increase progressively and plateau at about 2 months of age (40–50 g), almost double the weight of control mice. There is a marked influence of strain in terms of severity of diabetic features [27]. Thus, the general metabolic features of *db/db* mice [24], with initial insulin resistance followed by an insulin secretion defect, are very similar to the pathogenesis of type 2 diabetes in humans [2,3].

The *db* mutation (*Lepr*^{db}) was subsequently identified as a G→T point mutation in mouse chromosome 4 that produces a frameshift which selectively eliminates the "long" isoform of the leptin receptor (Table 1), one of five differentially spliced mRNA transcripts, resulting in defective leptin signaling [28]. Interestingly, *db/+* heterozygotes with one mutant copy of the leptin receptor are phenotypically normal with respect to body weight, and blood concentrations of glucose and lipids. Despite substantial dyslipidemia [29], *db/db* mice actually exhibit less atherosclerosis on a high fat diet [30] compared to lean *db/+* heterozygotes on both C57BL/6 and

C57BL/Ks genetic backgrounds. Therefore, *db/db* mice provide an excellent model to examine the manifestation of a diabetic cardiomyopathy without confounding coronary heart disease. An early ultrastructural study by Giacomelli and Weiner [31] provided evidence for damage to myocardial cells in *db/db* hearts without any coronary artery disease.

The diabetic ZDF rat has a point mutation (*Lepr*^{fa}) on chromosome 5 that does not alter expression of the leptin receptor [28]. Rather, this mutation in the extracellular domain may affect folding and/or transport of the receptor to the cell surface, resulting in decreased binding of leptin to the plasma membrane (Table 1). Although ZDF rats are obese with hyperinsulinemia, their degree of hyperglycemia (about 12 mM glucose) [32] is much less than that observed with *db/db* mice which develop plasma glucose concentrations >30 mM.

The corpulent JCR:LA-*cp/cp* rat has a point mutation (*Lepr*^{faf}) that produces a premature stop codon (Table 1), eliminating all leptin receptor isoforms to produce a receptor-null model [28]. Corpulent rats exhibit severe obesity and marked hyperinsulinemia with little or no elevation in plasma glucose concentrations [33–35]. In other words, the corpulent *cp/cp* rat provides a model of obesity and insulin resistance without overt signs of diabetes such as hyperglycemia.

ASSESSMENT OF FUNCTION IN HEARTS FROM TYPE 2 DIABETIC ANIMALS

This review of techniques used for phenotypic analysis of cardiac function in hearts from type 2 diabetic animals (Table 1) will follow a reductionist approach (Table 2), with progression from in vivo analysis of intact animals to the use of ex vivo perfused hearts and finally isolated cardiomyocytes [36].

1. In vivo assessment of cardiac function by echocardiography

Trans-thoracic echocardiography can assess cardiac function, using the principles of ultrasound with high-frequency transducers to obtain echocardiograms [37–39]. Since echocardiography is non-invasive, this technique is particularly well suited for serial studies such as age-dependent changes in cardiac function. M-mode measurements of left ventricular (LV) dimensions in end-systole and end-diastole allow calculation of systolic function (fractional shortening, FS%; velocity of circum-

Table 2. Type 2 diabetic animals: Assessment of cardiac function

(1) *In Vivo*: Echocardiography-conscious and anesthetized animals
- Morphology (LV mass)
- Systolic and diastolic function

(2) *Ex Vivo*: Isolated Perfused Hearts
- Contractile function (normoxic perfusions and recovery after ischemia-reperfusion)
- Metabolism of exogenous substrates

(3) Isolated Cardiomyocytes: Electrophysiology
- Ionic currents
- Action potential configuration

ferential fiber shortening, V_{cf}) and LV mass, therefore the onset and progression of cardiac hypertrophy can be monitored in addition to assessment of systolic (contractile) function (Table 2). Doppler measurements of trans-mitral flows (early E wave and late atrial A wave) provide information on diastolic function (LV diastolic filling); in particular, the ratio of E and A waves can be used as an index of impaired LV relaxation. Another advantage of echocardiography is that cardiac function can be assessed in conscious animals, thus avoiding the cardiodepressant effects of anesthetics [40–42]. The chief disadvantage of echocardiography is an extension of its in vivo advantage, namely analysis of a complex whole animal as the model system. Many echocardiographic parameters are heart rate- and load-dependent, therefore differences in afterload, preload and heart rates in different animal models can complicate the interpretation of results.

Cardiac function of *db/db* mice in vivo has been examined by echocardiography (Table 3). Both systolic dysfunction (decreased FS% indicating reduced contractility) and diastolic dysfunction (decreased E/A ratio of trans-mitral flows indicating impaired relaxation) was evident, with unchanged LV mass (no cardiac hypertrophy). [42a]. Similar results were obtained with diabetic ZDF rats [32], who exhibited reduced contractility (decreased FS%) but unchanged LV mass. Heart function in corpulent JCR:LA-*cp/cp* rats has not been assessed by echocardiography.

2. Ex vivo assessment of cardiac function with isolated perfused hearts

Isolated perfused hearts provide an ex vivo preparation (Table 2) that permits phenotypic analysis of cardiac contractile function and metabolism under experimental conditions where heart rate and supply of metabolic substrates can be carefully controlled without neurohormonal influences, in contrast to the complex in vivo situation. In the case of working perfused hearts, afterload and preload can also be controlled [43]. The considerable advantage provided by control over experimental conditions must be balanced by concerns over the physiological relevance of an isolated heart model, particularly given the possibility of damage to the heart

Table 3. Echocardiographic assessment of cardiac function in control *db/+* and diabetic *db/db* mice

	Control *db/+*	Diabetic *db/db*
LV mass (mg)	81 ± 2	79 ± 4
Systolic function: FS (%)	60 ± 2	44 ± 3*
Diastolic function: E/A ratio	3.6 ± 0.3	2.4 ± 0.2*

Results are mean ± SE for 10–12 mice (12 weeks of age). M-mode measurements for calculation of left ventricular (LV) mass and systolic function (percentage fractional shortening, FS%) were obtained from conscious mice. Diastolic function, the ratio of E and A waves from Doppler measurements of trans-mitral flows, was assessed with anesthetized mice. *, significantly different ($p < 0.05$) compared to control.

during isolation and perfusion. In addition, the typical use of a blood-free perfusate requires care to ensure that oxygen supply to the isolated heart is adequate.

Two different perfused heart preparations can be used for ex vivo assessments of cardiac function [43]. The simpler Langendorff heart preparation involves cannulation of the aorta and retrograde perfusion of coronary arteries, but this is a non-working preparation. The more complex working (LV ejecting) heart preparation is more physiological, requiring cannulation of the left atrium *via* the pulmonary vein for inflow of perfusate with control over preload (left atrial filling pressure), in addition to aortic cannulation. Perfusate is ejected in the normal direction into the aorta and then to an afterload column. A variety of methods can be used to measure contractile performance with both non-working Langendorff and working perfused hearts that are either beating at their intrinsic rates or are paced [43–45]. Isolated hearts are typically perfused under normoxic conditions, but the recovery of contractile function can also be monitored during reperfusion after an ischemic perfusion period produced by reducing coronary flow (no-flow or low-flow). In addition to monitoring contractile function, the ability to control the supply of metabolic substrates in the perfusate means that metabolic rates can also be measured (Table 2) with isolated hearts perfused with radiolabelled substrates [46].

The function of hearts from diabetic *db/db* mice has been evaluated with a working perfusion system [47]. Diabetic *db/db* hearts had reduced cardiac output, due entirely to decreased aortic flow, and reduced cardiac power (Table 4), consistent with evidence for systolic dysfunction by echocardiography with *db/db* mice in vivo (Table 3). In addition, the recovery of contractile function after an ischemia-reperfusion protocol was reduced in perfused *db/db* hearts (Table 4), indicating

Table 4. Cardiac function in *ex vivo* working perfused hearts from control *db/+* and diabetic *db/db* mice

	Control *db/+*	Diabetic *db/db*
A. Contractile performance (normoxia)		
Coronary flow (ml/min)	2.3 ± 0.3	1.7 ± 0.3
Aortic flow (ml/min)	4.6 ± 0.6	2.1 ± 0.7*
Cardiac output (ml/min)	6.9 ± 0.8	3.9 ± 0.9*
Cardiac power (mW/g)	30 ± 5	12 ± 5*
B. Recovery of contractile function after ischemia-reperfusion (% of pre-ischemic cardiac output)	49 ± 12	22 ± 3*
C. Metabolism		
Glycolysis (μmol/min/g)	3.2 ± 0.3	1.6 ± 0.3*
Glucose oxidation (μmol/min/g)	0.49 ± 0.07	0.08 ± 0.03*
Palmitate oxidation (μmol/min/g)	0.35 ± 0.07	0.74 ± 0.13*

Results in A and C are from Belke et al. (47), using perfused working hearts from control *db/+* and diabetic *db/db* mice (10–14 weeks of age). Preliminary results shown in B are from Aasum and Larsen (63), for recovery of cardiac output during reperfusion after 15 minutes of global no-flow ischemia. *, significantly different ($p < 0.05$) from control hearts.

enhanced susceptibility of the type 2 diabetic heart to ischemic injury. Metabolism of exogenous substrates was altered in perfused working *db/db* hearts; glucose utilization (glycolysis and glucose oxidation) was reduced whereas fatty acid (palmitate) oxidation was almost doubled [47]. Thus, perfused *db/db* hearts rely almost exclusively on lipid metabolism for their energy source.

The function of perfused hearts from diabetic ZDF rats has not been reported. Interpretation of results obtained with perfused hearts from insulin resistant corpulent JCR:LA *cp/cp* rats is complicated because ex vivo perfusions required modification of the perfusate, with addition of a high concentration of insulin and reduction in calcium concentration, in order to obtain a stable ex vivo preparation [33]. With this modified perfusion condition, contractile function was not reduced and metabolism of exogenous substrates was not altered [33,34,48]. Interestingly, perfused hearts from corpulent JCR:LA *cp/cp* rats did show enhanced sensitivity to an ischemia-reperfusion challenge, even though normoxic (pre-ischemic) function was not compromised [34]. These results suggest reduced recovery of contractile performance during reperfusion of ex vivo perfused hearts from type 2 diabetic animals after a period of ischemia provides a sensitive index of cardiac dysfunction. The increased susceptibility of *db/db* and JCR:LA-*cp/cp* hearts to ischemic injury is consistent with observations that type 2 diabetes is associated with an increase in ischemic heart disease in humans [4,5].

3. Electrophysiological measurements with isolated cardiomyocytes

Individual cardiomyocytes can be isolated after perfusion of hearts with collagenase. The chief advantage of this approach is the ability to conduct experiments with a homogenous cell population, eliminating any issue caused by the cellular heterogeneity of the whole heart. In addition, cardiomyocytes can be isolated from specific heart regions (e.g., epicardium and endocardium) for analysis of regional differences in heart function. The principal disadvantage of conducting experiments with isolated cardiomyocytes is the use of cells in isolation, a situation that is far removed from the functional syncytium of the heart.

Isolated cardiomyocytes are particularly well suited for electrophysiological studies. Application of the patch clamp technique to isolated cardiomyocytes can reveal information on whole cell currents as well as single channel recordings. Shimoni [49] has measured repolarizing outward potassium currents in isolated ventricular cardiomyocytes from control *db*/+ and diabetic *db/db* mouse hearts, using whole cell voltage-clamp methodology (Table 5). Both peak and sustained steady-state potassium currents were reduced in *db/db* cardiomyocytes. Action potentials were recorded in current-clamp mode. The action potential duration was prolonged markedly in *db/db* cardiomyocytes, consistent with reduced repolarizing potassium currents. These electrophysiological changes in *db/db* hearts could have implications in terms of both contractile performance and arrhythmogenesis. First, prolongation of the mouse heart action potential by administration of 4-aminopyridine to reduce potassium currents resulted in a positive inotropic response with perfused mouse hearts [50], perhaps by increasing the time for calcium influx through L-type

Table 5. Electrophysiological measurements in isolated cardiomyocytes from control *db/+* and diabetic *db/db* mice

	Control *db/+*	Diabetic *db/db*
A. K^+ currents		
Peak (pA/pF)	47 ± 4	25 ± 3★
Steady state (pA/pF)	32 ± 4	15 ± 2★
B. Action potential duration (ms)	13 ± 1	45 ± 7★

Results are from Shimoni (49). Action potential duration was recorded at −60 mV. ★, significantly different ($p < 0.05$) from control *db/+* cardiomyocytes.

calcium channels into cardiomyocytes. Therefore, the increased action potential duration noted in cardiomyocytes from *db/db* hearts (Table 5) could be a compensatory mechanism to counter-act the reduction in contractile performance seen by echocardiography (Table 3) and in perfused working hearts (Table 4). On the other hand, if the potassium current changes show regional differences with a greater reduction in the epicardium compared to the endocardium, as shown with cardiomyocytes from an insulin-deficient rat heart [51], the resulting change in repolarization could increase the incidence of arrhythmias in the diabetic heart. An increased dispersion of repolarization time can initiate re-entrant arrhythmias [52].

Electrophysiological measurements have not been reported for cardiomyocytes from diabetic ZDF rat hearts. In contrast to the results shown in Table 5, potassium currents were unchanged in ventricular cells from JCR:LA-*cp/cp* rat hearts [53]. Interestingly, insulin no longer augmented the sustained potassium current in cardiomyocytes from corpulent *cp/cp* rat hearts, indicating that insulin resistance is also manifested at the level of ion channel function. Treatment of corpulent *cp/cp* rats with metformin, a drug that improves insulin sensitivity, restored the ability of insulin to stimulate potassium currents [53].

SUMMARY AND FUTURE DIRECTIONS FOR RESEARCH

A summary of the experimental evidence for alterations in cardiac phenotype (diabetic cardiomyopathy) in hearts from three animal models of type 2 diabetes is shown in Table 6. Diabetic *db/db* mice exhibit a severe degree of diabetes (Table 1) and show marked signs of cardiac dysfunction (Table 6). Reduced contractility is evident from in vivo echocardiographic measurements and from indices of contractile performance with ex vivo perfused hearts [47]. In addition, *db/db* hearts have an altered pattern of metabolism with increased reliance on fatty acid oxidation as an energy source. Isolated cardiomyocytes from *db/db* hearts show electrophysiological changes that could predispose to cardiac arrhythmias [49].

Zhou et al. [32] reported that diabetic ZDF rats had reduced systolic function in vivo by echocardiography (Table 6). Clearly, additional studies with ex vivo perfused hearts and with isolated cardiomyocytes from ZDF rats must be performed to further establish the degree of cardiac dysfunction in this type 2 model of diabetes.

Table 6. Summary of experimental evidence for diabetic cardiomyopathy in animal models of type 2 diabetes

Animal Model	Cardiac Function		
	In Vivo Echocardiography	Ex Vivo Perfused Heart	Isolated Cardiomyocytes
1. Diabetic *db/db* Mice	↓ Systolic function ↓ Diastolic function No change LV mass	↓ Contractility (normoxia and after ischemia-reperfusion) Altered metabolism	↓ K^+ currents ↑ Action potential duration
2. Zucker Diabetic Fatty (ZDF) rat	↓ Systolic function No change LV mass		
3. Corpulent JRC:LA-*cp/cp* rat		Altered perfusate conditions required for beating Reduced recovery after ischemia	No change in K^+ currents

Corpulent JCR: LA-*cp/cp* rats have severe insulin resistance but are not hyperglycemic (Table 1). The requirement for altered perfusate conditions with high insulin and decreased calcium concentrations to permit assessment of function in ex vivo perfused hearts is a confounding factor [33]. Under these conditions, however, normoxic contractile function was not reduced but *cp/cp* hearts did show reduced recovery after ischemia-reperfusion [34]. In contrast to the *db/db* model [49], isolated cardiomyocytes from *cp/cp* rat hearts did not exhibit any changes in potassium currents [53]. It will be very important to evaluate cardiac function in corpulent JCR:LA-*cp/cp* rats by echocardiography, since this in vivo assessment will eliminate the issue of altered perfusate requirements for ex vivo perfusion experiments.

A number of additional experimental approaches will need to be applied to these type 2 diabetic models in the future. Invasive in vivo experiments with cardiac catheterization will allow determination of additional hemodynamic parameters [36,41,54]. In vivo electrophysiological measurements [55,56] will be necessary to supplement information on potassium current changes obtained with isolated cardiomyocytes, although the rapid beating frequency and rapid repolarization in mouse hearts makes it difficult to detect a distinct T wave in the electrocardiogram. Optical mapping with voltage-sensitive dyes and a CCD camera can measure repolarization time with ex vivo whole tissue preparations [52]. Finally, surgically-implanted telemetry transducers could be used for analysis of heart rate variability and carotid and femoral pressures [39].

Ex vivo perfused heart preparations could be used to obtain further information on metabolic changes in type 2 diabetic hearts. In particular, the metabolism of lactate and ketone bodies, along with lipoproteins as an alternate source of fatty acids, should be investigated. The nearly exclusive use of fatty acids as an energy source by the type 2 diabetic heart may have important implications with respect to oxygen consumption and cardiac efficiency.

Finally, a key objective for future investigations will be to establish the mechanistic basis for the cardiac dysfunction (diabetic cardiomyopathy) observed in type 2 diabetic hearts (Table 6). Studies with isolated cardiomyocytes could give insight into the mechanism of contractile dysfunction, using the combination of video edge detection as an index of contractility along with fluorescent detection of calcium transients [36,57]. Alterations in calcium transients could be linked to changes in expression of key proteins (phospholamban, sarco/endoplasmic reticulum Ca^{2+}-ATPase) that can be detected in whole hearts [58].

Other mechanistic studies should investigate if the altered metabolism in type 2 diabetic hearts, with decreased glucose utilization and increased fatty acid oxidation [47], has a causative role in the contractile dysfunction [59]. Zhou et al. [32] have obtained evidence for lipotoxicity in ZDF rat hearts; increased triglyceride and ceramide content plus evidence for increased apoptosis was associated with contractile dysfunction by echocardiography [22]. In this regard, it is interesting that normalization of cardiac metabolism in perfused hearts from transgenic *db/db* mice that over-express the insulin-regulatable hGLUT4 glucose transporter was associated with complete normalization of contractility in experiments with ex vivo perfused working hearts [47] and echocardiography in vivo [42a].

An additional mechanism that needs further study involves alterations in the cardiac renin-angiotensin system, which is activated in diabetes. Incubation of isolated cardiomyocytes from *db/db* mouse hearts with an angiotensin receptor antagonist (Valsartan®) increased the depressed potassium currents [49]. The potential beneficial effects of inhibiting the formation or action of angiotensin II on other aspects of cardiac function in diabetic hearts should be studied in the future. By understanding the mechanistic basis for diabetic cardiomyopathy, it should be possible to develop improved pharmacological interventions [60] that will reduce the substantial cardiac dysfunction in diabetics [4,5].

This review has been restricted to monogenic models of type 2 diabetes (Table 1). The creation of genetically engineered mice with manipulations in the insulin signalling cascade to explore mechanisms of insulin resistance [61] will be used increasingly in the future. For example, the creation of a cardiac-specific insulin receptor knock-out mouse using cre/loxP recombination [62] permitted analysis of the direct role of insulin signalling on post-natal heart development and cardiac function, without the confounding effects of diabetes produced by alterations in systemic metabolism (hyperglycemia and hyperlipidemia).

REFERENCES

1. Zimmet P, Alberti GMM, Shaw J. 2001. Global and societal implications of the diabetes epidemic. Nature 414:782–787.
2. Cavaghan MK, Ehrmann DA, Polonsky KS. 2000. Interactions between insulin resistance and insulin secretion in the development of glucose intolerance. J Clin Invest 106:329–333.

3. Saltiel AR. 2001. New perspectives into the molecular pathogenesis and treatment of type 2 diabetes. Cell 104:517–529.
4. Grundy SM, Benjamin IJ, Burke GL, Chait A, Eckel RH, Howard BV, Mitch W, Smith SC Jr, Sowers JR. 1999. Diabetes and cardiovascular disease. A statement for healthcare professionals from the American Heart Association. Circulation 100:1134–1146.
5. Haffner SM, Lehto S, Ronnemaa T, Pyörälä K, Laakso M. 1998. Mortality from coronary heart disease in subjects with type 2 diabetes and in nondiabetic subjects with and without prior myocardial infarction. N Engl J Med 339:229–234.
6. Taskinen M. 1997. Triglyceride is the major atherogenic lipid in NIDDM. Diabet Met Rev 13:93–98.
7. Hayden JM, Reaven PD. 2000. Cardiovascular disease in diabetes mellitus type 2: a potential role for novel cardiovascular risk factors. Curr Opin Lipidol 11:519–528.
8. James RW. 2001 Diabetes and other coronary heart disease risk equivalents. Curr Opin Lipidol 12:425–431.
9. Regan TJ, Lyons MM, Ahmed SS, Levinson GE, Oldewurtel HA, Ahmad MR, Haider B. 1977. Evidence for cardiomyopathy in familial diabetes mellitus. J Clin Invest 60:885–899.
10. Fein FS. 1990. Diabetic cardiomyopathy. Diabetes Care 13:1169–1179.
11. Shehadeh A, Regan TJ. 1995. Cardiac consequences of diabetes mellitus. Clin Cardiol 18:301–305.
12. Mahgoub MA, Abd-Elfattah AS. 1998. Diabetes mellitus and cardiac function. Mol Cell Biochem 180:59–64.
13. Frustaci A, Kajstura J, Chimenti C, Jakoniuk I, Leri A, Maseri A, Nadal-Ginard B, Anversa P. 2000. Myocardial cell death in human diabetes. Circ Res 87:1123–1132.
14. Tomlinson KC, Gardiner SM, Hebden RA, Bennett T. 1992. Functional consequences of streptozotocin-induced diabetes mellitus, with particular reference to the cardiovascular system. Pharmacol Rev 44:103–179.
15. Pierce GN, Maddaford TG, Russell JC. 1997. Cardiovascular dysfunction in insulin-dependent and non-insulin-dependent animal models of diabetes mellitus. Can J Physiol Pharmacol 75:343–350.
16. Ahima RS, Flier JS. 2000. Leptin. Annu Rev Physiol 62:413–437.
17. Frühbeck G, Gómez-Ambrosi J, Muruzábal FJ, Burrell MA. 2001. The adipocyte: a model for integration of endocrine and metabolic signaling in energy metabolism regulation. Am J Physiol 280:E827–E847.
18. Unger RH, Zhou Y-T, Orci L. 1999. Regulation of fatty acid homeostasis in cells: novel role of leptin. Proc Natl Acad Sci USA 96:2327–2332.
19. Muoio DM, Dohm GL, Tapscott EB, Coleman RA. 1999. Leptin opposes insulin's effects on fatty acid partitioning in muscles isolated from obese *ob/ob* mice. Am J Physiol 276:E913–E921.
20. Lau R, Blinn WD, Bonen A, Dyck DJ. 2001. Stimulatory effects of leptin and muscle contraction on fatty acid metabolism are not additive. Am J Physiol 281:E122–E129.
21. Lee Y, Wang M-Y, Kakuma T, Wang Z-W, Babcock E, McCorkle K, Higa M, Zhou Y-T, Unger RH. 2001. Liporegulation in diet-induced obesity. The antisteatotic role of hyperleptinemia. J Biol Chem 23:5629–5635.
22. Unger RH, Orci L. 2001. Diseases of liporegulation: new perspective on obesity and related disorders. FASEB J 15:312–321.
23. Hummel KP, Dickie MM, Coleman DL. 1966. Diabetes, a new mutation in the mouse. Science 153:1127–1128.
24. Coleman DL. 1982. Diabetes-obesity syndromes in mice. Diabetes 31:1–6.
25. Wyse BM, Dulin WE. 1970. The influence of age and dietary conditions on diabetes in the db mouse. Diabetologia 6:268–273.
26. Coleman DL, Hummel KP. 1974. Hyperinsulinemia in pre-weaning diabetes (*db*) mice. Diabetologia 10:607–610.
27. Hummel KP, Coleman DL, Lane PW. 1972. The influence of genetic background on expression of mutations at the diabetes locus in the mouse. I. C57BL/KsJ and C57BL/6J strains. Biochem Genet 7:1–13
28. Leibel RL, Chung WK, Chua SC Jr. 1997. The molecular genetics of rodent single gene obesities. J Biol Chem 272:31937–31940.
29. Kobayashi Y, Fortre TM, Taniguchi S, Ishida BY, Oka K, Chan L. 2000. The *db/db* mouse, a model for diabetic dyslipidemia: molecular characterization and effects of Western diet feeding. Metabolism 49:22–31.
30. Nishina PM, Naggert JK, Verstuyft J, Paigen B. 1994. Atherosclerosis in genetically obese mice: the mutants obese, diabetes, fat, tubby, and lethal yellow. Metabolism 43:554–558.

31. Giacomelli F, Wiener J. 1979. Primary myocardial disease in the diabetic mouse. An ultrastructural study. Lab Invest 40:460–473.
32. Zhou Y-T, Grayburn P, Karim A, Shimabukuro M, Higa M, Baetens D, Orci L, Unger RH. 2000. Lipotoxic heart disease in obese rats: implications for human obesity. Proc Natl Acad Sci USA 97:1784–1789.
33. Lopaschuk GD, Russell JC. 1991. Myocardial function and energy substrate metabolism in the insulin-resistant JCR:LA corpulent rat. J Appl Physiol 71:1302–1308.
34. Maddaford TG, Russell JC, Pierce GN. 1997. Postischemic cardiac performance in the insulin-resistant JCR:LA-*cp* rat. Am J Physiol 273:H1187–H1192.
35. Misra T, Gilchrist JS, Russell JC, Pierce GN. 1999. Cardiac myofibrillar and sarcoplasmic reticulum function are not depressed in insulin-resistant JCR:LA-*cp* rat. Am J Physiol 276:H1811–H1817.
36. Christensen G, Wang Y, Chien KR. 1997. Physiological assessment of complex cardiac phenotypes in genetically engineered mice. Am J Physiol 272:H2513–H2524.
37. Hoit BD, Walsh RA. 1997. In vivo echocardiographic assessment of left ventricular function in transgenic and gene-targeted mice. Trends Cardiovasc Med 7:129–134.
38. Hoit BD. 2001. New approaches to phenotypic analysis in adult mice. J Mol Cell Cardiol 33:27–35.
39. Hoit BD, Nadeau JH. 2001. Phenotype-driven genetic approaches in mice. High-throughput phenotyping for discovering new models of cardiovascular disease. Trends Cardiovasc Med 11:82–89.
40. Yang X-P, Liu Y-H, Rhaleb N-E, Kurihara N, Kim HE, Carretero OA. 1999. Echocardiographic assessment of cardiac function in conscious and anesthetized mice. Am J Physiol 277:H1967–H1974.
41. Hart CYT, Burnett Jr., JC, Redfield MM. 2001. Effects of avertin versus xylazine-ketamine anesthesia on cardiac function in normal mice. Am J Physiol 281:H1938–H1945.
42. Takuma S, Suehiro K, Cardinale C, Hozumi T, Yano H, Shimizu J, Mullis-Jansson S, Sciacca R, Wang J, Burkhoff D, Di Tullio MR, Homma S. 2001. Anesthetic inhibition in ischemic and nonischemic murine heart: comparison with conscious echocardiographic approach. Am J Physiol 280:H2364–H2370.
42a. Semeniuk LM, Kryski AJ, Severson DL. 2002. Echocardiographic assessment of cardiac function in diabetic db/db and transgenic db/db-hGLUT4 mice. Am J Physiol 283:H976–H982.
43. Sutherland FJ, Hearse DJ. 2000. The isolated blood and perfusion fluid perfused heart. Pharmacol Res 41:613–627.
44. Larsen TS, Belke DD, Sas R, Giles WR, Severson DL, Lopaschuk G, Tyberg JV. 1999. The isolated working mouse heart: methodological considerations. Pflügers Arch 437:979–985.
45. De Windt LJ, Willems J, Reneman RS, Van der Vusse GJ, Arts T, Van Bilsen M. 1999. An improved isolated, left ventricular ejecting, murine heart model. Functional and metabolic evaluation. Pflügers Arch 437:182–190.
46. Belke DD, Larsen TS, Lopaschuk GD, Severson DL. 1999. Glucose and fatty acid metabolism in the isolated working mouse heart. Am J Physiol 277:R1210–R1217.
47. Belke DD, Larsen TS, Gibbs EM, Severson DL. 2000. Altered metabolism causes cardiac dysfunction in perfused hearts from diabetic (*db/db*) mice. Am J Physiol 279:E1104–E1113.
48. Brunner F, Wölkart G, Pfeiffer S, Russell JC, Eascher TC. 2000. Vascular dysfunction and myocardial contractility in the JCR-:LA-corpulent rat. Cardiovasc Res 47:150–158.
49. Shimoni Y. 2001. Inhibition of the formation or action of angiotensin II reverses attenuated K^+ currents in type 1 and type 2 diabetes. J Physiol 537:83–92.
50. Fiset C, Clark RB, Larsen TS, Giles WR. 1997. A rapidly activating sustained K^+ current modulates repolarization and excitation-contraction coupling in adult mouse ventricle. J Physiol 504:557–563.
51. Shimoni Y, Severson D, Giles WR. 1995. Thyroid status and diabetes modulate regional differences in potassium current in rat ventricle. J Physiol 488:673–688.
52. Burton FL, Cobbe SM. 2001. Dispersion of ventricular repolarization and refractory period. Cardiovasc Res 50:10–23.
53. Shimoni Y, Severson D, Ewart HS. 2000. Insulin resistance and the modulation of rat cardiac K^+ currents. Am J Physiol 279:H639–H649.
54. Georgakopoulos D, Mitzner WA, Chen C-H, Byrne BJ, Millar HD, Hare JM, Kass DA. 1998. In vivo murine left ventricular pressure-volume relations by miniaturized conductance micromanometry. Am J Physiol 274:H1416–H1422.
55. Saba S, Wang PJ, Estes III NAM. 2000. Invasive cardiac electrophysiology in the mouse: techniques and applications. Trends Cardiovasc Med 10:122–132.
56. Wehrens ZHT, Kirchhoff S, Doevendans PA. 2000. Mouse electrocardiography: an interval of thirty years. Cardiovasc Res 45:231–237.

57. Sande JB, Sjaastad I, Hoen IB, Bøkenes J, Tønnessen T, Holt E, Lunde PK, Christensen G. 2002. Reduced level of serine[16] phosphorylated phospholamban in the failing rat myocardium: a major contributor to reduced SERCA2 activity. Cardiovasc Res 53:382–391.
58. Zhong Y, Ahmed S, Grupp II, Matlib MA. 2001. Altered SR protein expression associated with contractile dysfunction in diabetic rat hearts. Am J Physiol 281:H1137–H1147.
59. Lopaschuk GD. 1996. Abnormal mechanical function in diabetes: relationship to altered myocardial carbohydrate/lipid metabolism. Coronary Artery Dis 7:116–123.
60. Moller DE. 2001. New drug targets for type 2 diabetes and the metabolic syndrome. Nature 414:821–827.
61. Gannon M. 2001. Molecular genetic analysis of diabetes in mice. Trends Genetics 17:S23–S28.
62. Belke DD, Betuing S, Tuttle MJ, Pham M, Young ME, Graveleau C, Zhang D, Litwin SE, Taegtmeyer H, Severson D, Kahn CR, Abel ED. 2002. Central role of insulin signalling in the coordinate regulation of size, metabolism and contractile protein isoform expression in the mammalian heart. J Clin Invest 109:629–639.
63. Aasum E, Larsen TS. 2001. Changes in cardiac metabolism in ischemic-reperfused isolated mouse hearts. J Mol Cell Cardiol 33:A161.

G.N. Pierce, M. Nagano, P. Zahradka, and N.S. Dhalla (eds.).
ATHEROSCLEROSIS, HYPERTENSION AND DIABETES.
Kluwer Academic Publishers. Boston.

MECHANISMS UNDERLYING CONTRACTILE DYSFUNCTION IN STREPTOZOTOCIN-INDUCED TYPE 1 AND TYPE 2 DIABETIC CARDIOMYOPATHY

NICOLAS K. BRACKEN, JAIPAUL SINGH, WILLIAM WINLOW, and FRANK C. HOWARTH[1]

Department of Biological Sciences, University of Central Lancashire, Preston, PR1 2HE, Lancashire, England and Department of Physiology, Faculty of Medicine & Health Sciences, United Arab Emirates University, PO Box 1766, Al Ain, United Arab Emirates[1]

Summary. Diabetes Mellitus is characterised by fasting hyperglycaemia and glucose intolerance, due to insulin deficiency, impaired effectiveness of insulin action or both. There is clear evidence of the negative influence of both type 1 diabetes and type 2 diabetes on the prevalence, severity and prognosis of cardiovascular disease. Cardiovascular disease represents the commonest cause of morbidity and mortality within diabetic patients. Human and animal studies have shown that the excess risk of cardiovascular complications cannot be explained by conventional cardiovascular risk factors alone and therefore, the diabetic state itself is likely to account for this alteration in cardiac function. The cellular mechanisms associated with contractile dysfunction and calcium mobilisation will be reviewed with respects to the streptozotocin-induced model of type 1 and type 2 diabetes mellitus.

***Key words*:** Diabetes mellitus, Streptozotocin, Contractility, Calcium and dysfunction

INTRODUCTION

Diabetes has been recognised as a diseased state since ancient times. The Ebers papyrus discovered by a German Egyptologist in 1862, dates from 1550 BC and describes a state of polyuria resembling diabetes. For thousands of years, no one knew how to live with the diabetes, let alone correct the disease. Children with the disease died quickly, often within days of onset, and older people struggled with devastating complications [1].

All Correspondence to: Professor Jaipaul Singh, Department of Biological Sciences, University of Central Lancashire, Preston, PR1 2HE, Lancashire, England. Tel: 01772-893515; Fax: 01772-892929; e-mail: jsingh3@uclan.ac.uk

Diabetes Mellitus is recognised as a group of heterogeneous population disorders characterised by fasting hyperglycaemia and glucose intolerance, due to insulin deficiency, impaired effectiveness of insulin action or both [2]. It is classified on the basis of aetiology, natural history and clinical presentation of the disease. In 1997 the American Diabetes Association (ADA) classified diabetes in terms of aetiology and not by treatment, and to date, diabetes is classified into two main types; type 1 diabetes mellitus (previously known as insulin-dependent diabetes mellitus (IDDM) or juvenile onset) and type 2 diabetes mellitus (previously known as non-insulin-dependent diabetes mellitus (NIDDM) and maturity onset) [1].

Diabetes is a global problem. In 1997, an estimated 124 million people worldwide had diabetes, 97% of these having type 2 diabetes [3]. This figure has now increased to an estimated 150 million today and expected to reach a level of 221 million in 2010 [3] and 300 million worldwide by 2025 [4].

TYPE 1 DIABETES

Type 1 diabetes can occur at all ages but is predominant in children and young adults, with a peak incidence before school age [1]. The exact cause of the disease is multiple in nature and still imperfectively understood, but is thought to be a consequence of the cellular mediated autoimmune degeneration of pancreatic islet-beta (β) cells and/or environmental factors [5]. The commonest cause of type 1 diabetes is the autoimmune destruction of the pancreatic β-cells in the islets of Langerhans. The exact aetiology is complex and not thoroughly understood. It is thought, however, that environmental factors trigger the response in people who have an inherent genetic predisposition for the disease. Inherited susceptibility to type 1 diabetes depends on several genes at different loci. A major component of the genetic predisposition is encoded within the human leukocyte antigen (HLA) genes lying within the region of the short arm chromosome 6 (Newly called the "type 1 diabetes locus"). HLA antigens are cell surface glycoproteins and certain HLA-DR [3,4] and DQ alleles encoding antigen-presenting molecules have been established to be involved in the susceptibility of type 1 diabetes [6].

Type 1 diabetes is characterised by the loss of insulin production, resulting in a decrease in circulating plasma insulin. This insulin deficiency in the presence of catabolic counter-regulatory hormones such as catecholamines, cortisol, glucagon and growth hormones increase lipolysis within the adipose tissue. The consequence of this is the release of non-esterified fatty acids (NEFA) into the circulation. Within the liver the fatty acids (FA) are partially oxidised to produce ketone bodies, acetoacetic acid and 3-hydroxybutyric acid. All of these contribute to the state of acidosis [1]. The symptoms of ketoacidosis include polydipsia, polyuria, weight loss, leg cramps and weakness, and if not dealt with, can soon lead to diabetic coma and eventual death [3]. Therefore, type 1 diabetic patients have an absolute requirement for insulin, to prevent the life threatening consequences of hyperglycaemia and ketoacidosis [5].

TYPE 2 DIABETES

Type 2 diabetes is by far the commonest type of diabetes. This form of diabetes is polygenic, and although affected by genes, the environment is also important. The disease is commonly associated with a number of clinical risk factors including obesity, increasing age, strong familial links and ethnic and geographical variations [1]. The disease is characterised by insulin resistance and relative insulin deficiency. These patients usually have normal insulin levels, which require little therapy. The defect associated with this disease does not originate in the pancreas, but is typified by a cellular resistance at the insulin receptor and the post receptor level [7].

DIABETIC CARDIOMYOPATHY AND CARDIOVASCULAR DISEASE

There is clear evidence of the negative influence of both type 1 diabetes and type 2 diabetes on the prevalence, severity and prognosis of cardiovascular disease (coronary heart disease, stroke, peripheral vascular disease) [8]. Cardiovascular disease represents the commonest cause of morbidity and mortality within diabetic patients [5,9–12]. Human and animal studies have shown that the excess risk of cardiovascular complications cannot be explained by conventional cardiovascular risk factors alone and therefore, the diabetic state itself is likely to account for this alteration in cardiac function [12,13]. This lesion developing in the absence of any manifest cardiovascular disease is termed diabetic cardiomyopathy [14] and is defined as a decrease in cardiac contractile performance (involving a defect in diastolic and systolic function) leading to congestive heart failure [5]. Many invasive and non-invasive clinical studies on human diabetic patients have reported alterations in cardiac performance [15].

Studies in type 1 diabetes patients have reported an increase in atrial contraction, impaired diastolic function of left ventricle and reduced rapid filling rate [13,14,16,17]. While patients with type 2 diabetes have reported faster heart rates (HR), elevated end diastolic pressure to volume ratios, low diminished stroke volume (SV), reduced diastolic filling rate, prolonged isovolumteric relaxation period, mitral diastolic closure rate and decreased shortening [5,16,18–20]. It is thought to be the diastolic dysfunction in the diabetic heart, which is responsible for increased morbidity and mortality [21,22].

ANIMAL MODEL OF DIABETES

Most of the experimental data about the pathogenesis of diabetic complications have been accumulated using animal models of diabetes, which can be characterised into two main types: experimentally-induced diabetes and spontaneous, genetically determined diabetes [7].

Type 1

Experimental-induction of diabetes frequently involves the administration of an agent, which will induce β-cell necrosis of the pancreas. Two widely used diabetogenic agents are alloxan and streptozotocin (STZ). STZ (2-deoxy-2-[[(methylnitrosamino)carbonyl]amino]-D-lucopyranose) appears to be highly specific to β-cells whereas alloxan has been shown to elicit non-specific necrotic effects [23]. When administered to young adult rats, STZ (60 mg/kg) destroys the insulin producing β-cells of the pancreas and produces symptoms, which include severe insulinopaenia, hyperglycaemia, glycosuria, polydipsia and muscle wasting (features associated with type 1 diabetes) [24].

Type 2

Despite the much higher prevalence, far fewer studies have been performed in type 2 animal models of diabetes because of the complex aetiology and lack of understanding of the disease. Many of the animal models have a genetic predisposition to spontaneously develop type 2 diabetes. The most frequently employed models with this predisposition are the Goto-Kakizaki (GT) rat [25], the obese mouse (C57BL/6J ob/ob) [26], the obese Zucker fatty rat [27], the Otsuka Long-Evans Tokushima fatty rat [28], the BioBreed (BB) spontaneously diabetic-prone (BB/DP) rat [29], the BHE rat [30] and the Israeli dessert sand rat (*Psammomys obesus*) [31]. Unfortunately, many models of type 2 diabetes are problematic and develop complications, which are independent of diabetes mellitus [7].

To overcome some of the complications associated with genetic models of type 2 diabetes, a chemically-induced model has been developed. STZ (90 mg/kg), administered by intraperitoneal (i.p.) injection to neonatal rats (0–2 days old) produces some symptoms which resemble clinical type 2 diabetes [32,33]. In both type 1 and type 2 models of diabetes, STZ-induced β-cell degeneration is accompanied, within a few days, by transient hyperglycaemia and a severe decrease in pancreatic insulin release [32]. However, unlike the condition produced in young adult rats exposed to STZ, in neonatal rats, normalisations of plasma and glucose levels are seen within a few days. This may be due to partial regeneration of the β-cells in the neonatal rat [5]. Following a period of normal basal glucose levels, glucose levels start to rise. At 6 months, these animals become severely glucose intolerant (see Fig. 1) and insulin-resistant, demonstrating severe hyperglycaemia and hyperinsulinaemia following a glucose challenge [34].

Comparable to human patients with type 2 diabetes [35], the STZ rat model of type 2 diabetes develops a deficiency in the first phase of insulin release in response to a glucose challenge. Following 6 to 14 months of treatment the insulin secretory response of the type 2 diabetic rat undergoes a transition from hyper to hyposecretion [36]. These chemically-induced diabetic animals serve as an excellent model to study the effects of the modulating factors involved in the appearance and/or deterioration of type 2 diabetes [32].

The cellular mechanisms, which may be responsible for abnormal contraction in the diabetic heart, are examined in this review. In particular, attention is focussed on the mechanisms of calcium (Ca^{2+}) transport, which are fundamental to the normal process of excitation-contraction coupling in ventricular myocytes.

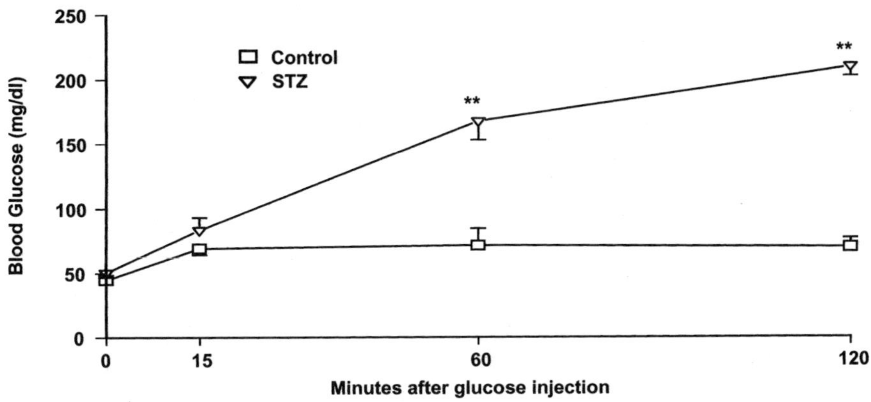

Figure 1. Whole blood glucose concentrations in response to an intraperitoneal glucose challenge test (2 g glucose/kg body weight) in six-month-old STZ-treated and control (n = 6) Wistar rats following a 16 hour fast. Values represent the mean ± SEM (**P < 0.01).

EXCITATION-CONTRACTION COUPLING IN THE NORMAL HEART

Excitation-contraction coupling is the highly organised process of signal transduction pathways that overrides contractile force and function in the heart. The process is initiated by the depolarisation of the cardiac cell membrane, during the cardiac action potential, which leads to Ca^{2+} entry via the voltage-gated L-type channels as inward Ca^{2+} current (I_{Ca}) [37]. The sodium/calcium (Na^+/Ca^{2+}) exchanger operating in reverse mode has also been proposed as a candidate mechanism of Ca^{2+} entry into the myocyte [38,39], however, the magnitude and potency of this mechanism are still controversial [40,41]. This small influx of Ca^{2+} triggers a much larger release of Ca^{2+} from ryanodine receptors (CaRyR) on the surface of the sarcoplasmic reticulum (SR). Following the activation of the SR and Ca^{2+} release, there is a transient rise in the cytosolic free Ca^{2+} concentration $[Ca^{2+}]_i$ typically from a diastolic level of 100 nM to a peak systolic level of around 1 µM within a period of 20 to 40 msec after depolarisation [42–44]. This process is referred to as "Ca^{2+}-induced Ca^{2+}-release" (CICR) and is the widely accepted main mechanism of Ca^{2+} release from the SR [45–47]. Other mechanisms leading to the release of Ca^{2+} from the SR have been proposed, and include voltage-activated Ca^{2+} release [48] and inositol [1,4,5] trisphosphate ($InsP_3$) triggered Ca^{2+} release through ($InsP_3$) receptors [49]. The process of contraction is initiated when Ca^{2+} binds to the myofilament troponin-C, which in turn switches on the contractile machinery [50] (Fig. 2a). Relaxation occurs when the Ca^{2+} transient decays and Ca^{2+} dissociates from troponin-C leading to the re-uptake of Ca^{2+} into the SR by a SR Ca^{2+}-ATPase- dependent pump (SERCA) [50,51] and the extrusion of Ca^{2+} from the cell by the Na^+/Ca^{2+} exchanger [37,52,53] (Fig. 2b).

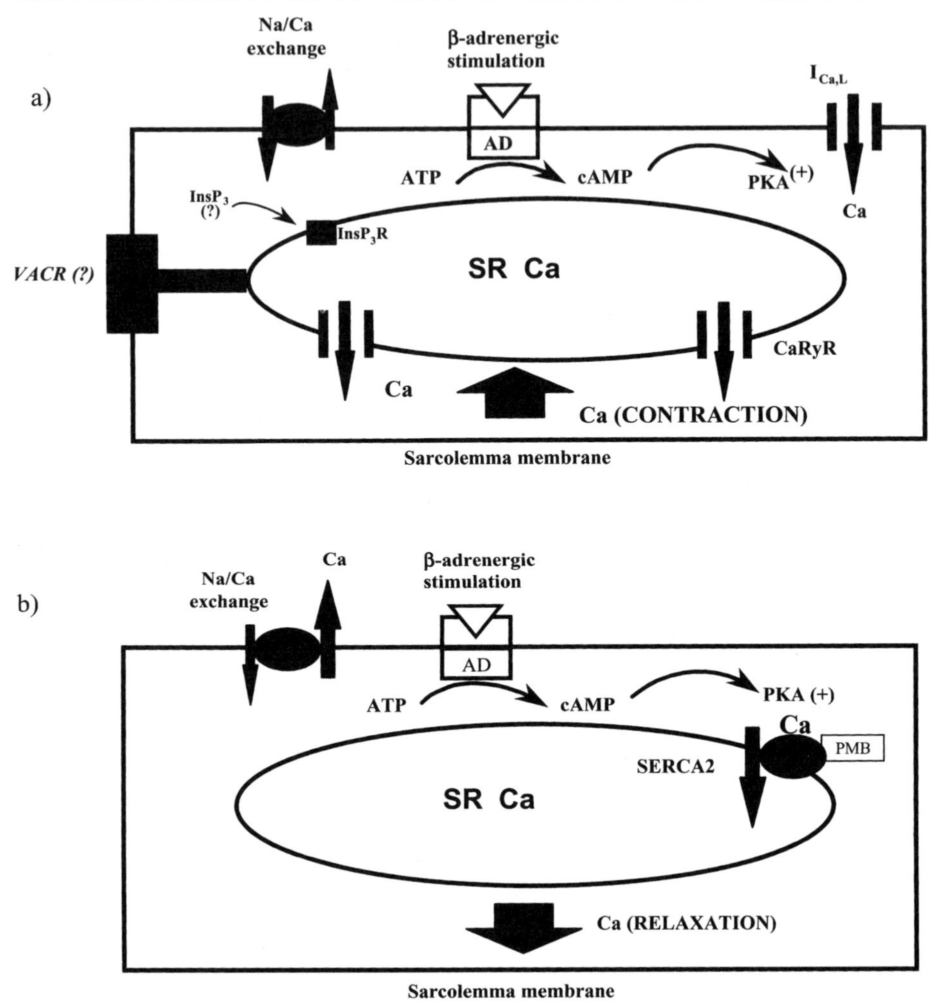

Figure 2. Schematic model of E-C coupling in a normal ventricular cell, showing mechanisms that underpin Ca^{2+} transport following membrane depolarisation and contraction (a) and during relaxation (b). Also shown are the effects of β-adrenergic stimulation on L-type Ca current and SERCA. (AD, adenylate cyclase; PKA, protein kinase A; PMB, phospholamban).

CONTRACTILE FUNCTION IN THE DIABETIC HEART

Many workers have reported contractile dysfunctions in experimentally-induced diabetic heart muscle. Depressed stroke volume (SV), AO, positive (+dP/dt) and negative (−dP/dt) left ventricular developed pressure have all been reported in various type 1 induced diabetic heart preparations [54]. More significantly, perhaps, are

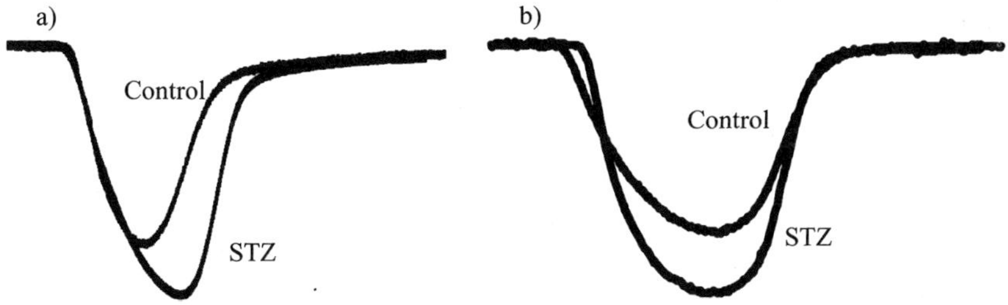

Figure 3. Fast time base records of twitch contractions in (a) 2 month and (b) 10 month STZ treated ventricular myocytes stimulated at 1 Hz.

reports suggesting that type 1 induced-diabetic papillary muscles show a decrease in the speed of contraction, a prolongation in the contraction, and a delay in relaxation [21,55–59]. There is, however, some controversy in the reports regarding mechanical dysfunction in cardiac myocytes isolated from STZ-induced type 1 diabetic hearts. Yu et al. [60] reported that myocytes from diabetic rats showed a reduction (44%) in peak shortening (PS), reduced maximum rates of shortening and relenghtening (58 and 56% decrease, respectively), and a prolonged time to peak shortening (tpk) (47% increase) [60] which was in agreement with Ren and Davidoff [61] who showed markedly prolonged contraction and relaxation phases in the diabetic myocyte [61]. Moreover, the normalized maximal velocity of shortening, and relenghtening of myocytes from diabetic rats were significantly lower than those in myocytes from control rats [62]. Howarth et al. [63] reported a time-dependent alteration in mechanical function between 2 and 10 months STZ-treatment (Fig. 3). In both treatment times, the amplitude of contraction was larger in diabetic compared to control myocytes.

The tpk of contraction was significantly longer at 2 months but appeared to normalise at 10 months after STZ treatment. In contrast, the time from the peak of contraction to half relaxation ($t_{1/2}$) was not significantly different after 2 months STZ-treatment but was significantly reduced at 10 months after STZ treatment compared to control. An enhanced PS was and prolonged tpk shortening and time from the peak of contraction to 90% relaxation (TR90) were also reported in STZ myocytes compared to the age-matched controls [64]. Changes in contractility have also been reported in BB/DP hearts which display similar characteristics to a type 1 diabetes were rats displayed increased PS, prolonged TPS and TR(90) compared to the control group [65]. However, it has been reported that the contractile responses were similar in myocytes from diabetic and age-matched control rats [66]. A progressive mechanical dysfunction has also been reported in the neonatal type 2 model of diabetes [5]. Contractile abnormalities were characterized by reductions in aortic output (AO), ventricular pressure, and cardiac work. After 4 months of treatment with STZ, the diabetic rats presented no detectable signs of mechanical dysfunction or metabolic abnormalities, however, after 8–12 months, cardiac function was significantly depressed [67,68]. Recently, Howarth and Qureshi [69] have reported that the amplitude and kinetics of myocyte shortening were not significantly altered following 10-month STZ treatment of the type 2 neonatal rat model. Moreovr, non-fasting blood glucose and plasma insulin were not significantly different, but glucose mobilisation was impaired, suggesting that a partial recovery of β-cells within the pancreas contributes to the normalised amplitude of kinetics [69]. Therefore, it would appear that the degree of mechanical dysfunction which has been reported in STZ-induced diabetic myocardium may be associated with alterations in experimental protocol including dose and treatment times of the experimental animals.

CONSEQUENCES OF SYMPATHETIC RESPONSE IN THE DIABETIC HEART

The stimulation of myocardial-adrenoceptors results in the activation of a guanine nucleotide-binding protein (G protein), known as Gs. This in turn triggers the activation of adenylate cyclase (AC), which culminates in an increased level of adenosine 3′,5′-cyclic-monophosphate (cAMP). Elevated levels of cAMP lead to the dissociation of the regulatory and catalytic sub units of cAMP-dependent protein kinase A (PKA). The activated PKA phosphorylates a number, and variety of regulatory proteins, including the sarcolemmal L-type Ca^{2+} channel [70] and the phospholamban protein in the SR [71]. Phosphorylation of the L-type Ca^{2+} channels leads to their opening and results in a Ca^{2+} influx into the cell during the cardiac action potential [70]. Phosphorylation of phospholamban causes an in increase in the rate of Ca^{2+} uptake by SERCA [72]. An increase in Ca^{2+} uptake within the SR results in an increased accumulation of Ca^{2+} within the SR. Moreover, increasing the available Ca^{2+} to be released from the SR. Therefore, the process of myocardial-adrenoceptor stimulation coincides with a systolic increase in cytoplasmic $[Ca^{2+}]_i$ which is associated with increase in contractility [73].

The mechanism associated with increased sympathetic drive represents an important contribution associated in maintaining cardiac output (CO), not just to meet the need of an increased functional demand but also in the malfunctioning heart [74]. There is a great deal of controversy and contradiction in the literature regarding the effects of experimentally-induced diabetes on cardiac adrenoceptor responses [75]. Many workers have reported that the increases in responsiveness produced by the β-adrenoceptor agonist, isoprenaline are markedly diminished in experimental-induced type 1 STZ-diabetic hearts in whole heart preparations [76], in 4–6 week [77] and 8 week [78] STZ-treated papillary muscles and in isolated cardiomyocytes from 4–6 [73] week and 8–10 week [79] compared to control preparations. In contrast, other workers have reported an increase in β-adrenoceptor-mediated functional responses to sub maximal doses of isoprenaline from STZ-induced type 1 diabetic rats [75].

Schaffer et al. [34] reported that stimulation of the type 2 diabetic heart with isoprenaline resulted in a concentration-dependent attenuation in both the (+dP/dt), a measure of contraction and (–dP/dt), a measure of the rate of myocardial relaxation when compared to the control heart. The inotropic responses to dibutyryl-adenosine 3′,5′-cyclic-monophosphate (DBcAMP) and forskolin were also prominently reduced in the type 1 diabetic heart compared to control [73,80] but were not evident in the type 2 diabetic heart [34]. Therefore, β-adrenergic sensitivity seems to be affected both in the STZ-induced type 1 and type 2 diabetic hearts.

Competitive binding studies have also reported differences in β-adrenergic density and/or number in diabetic tissue [75]. A number of reports suggest a significant decrease in myocardial membrane β-adrenoceptor density in STZ-induced type 1 diabetic hearts [80–82], while other workers report either an increase [83] or no change [75] in the density of β-adrenergic binding sites in STZ-induced type 1 diabetic membranes [83]. Moreover, receptor number seems to be unaltered in type 2 diabetic hearts [34] although it appears that their affinity for agonists did not seem to be consolidated [81] in both type 1 and type 2 diabetic hearts [84].

Competitive binding studies have shown [80] that the interaction between β-adrenoceptor and Gs-protein is not altered in type 1 diabetic hearts. This observation may imply that the dysfunctional responsiveness associated with type 1 diabetic hearts may not necessarily caused by a alteration in either the cAMP or changes in G-proteins but is more likely to be caused by a defect distal to the adenylate cyclase (AC) system.

INTRACELLULAR CALCIUM AND ITS ROLE IN CONTRACTILE FUNCTION AND FLUX BALANCE IN THE DIABETIC HEART

Resting calcium

Resting cell $[Ca^{2+}]_i$ levels are determined mainly by Ca^{2+} leaking out of the cell. This is counterbalanced by the sarcolemmal Ca-ATPase pump and the sarcolemmal Na^+/Ca^{2+} exchanger [85]. The Na/Ca exchanger provides the predominant mechanism for Ca^{2+} efflux during cardiac diastole [86].

Some reports suggest that diastolic $[Ca^{2+}]_i$ is reduced [87–89] while others [73,90] have reported no significant changes between type 1 diabetic and control cardiomyocytes. These discrepancies may be due to differences in the time treatment of STZ and the type of fluorescent probe used to measure the $[Ca^{2+}]_i$.

In the STZ-induced neonatal model of type 2 diabetes elevated levels of basal $[Ca^{2+}]_i$ have been reported [34]. Moreover, Allo et al. [91] observed that the relative fluorescence of fura-2 at 502 nm was higher in cells from type 2 diabetic hearts suggesting an increase in basal $[Ca^{2+}]_i$ compared to control.

Sodium/calcium exchanger and resting calcium

Any changes associated with the Na^+/Ca^{2+} are likely to be associated with changes in resting Ca^{2+}. The Na^+/Ca^{2+} exchanger is partly regulated by intracellular sodium concentration ($[Na^+]_i$). It has been shown that intracellular $[Na^+]_i$ is reduced in

STZ-induced type 1 diabetic myocytes [92], and this may be due to a reduction in the Na^+/H^+ exchanger which has been reported [93]. Reduced $[Na^+]_i$ would result in the reversed operation of the Na^+/Ca^{2+} exchanger, resulting in a decrease in cytoplasmic Ca^{2+} [93].

Conversely, Allo et al. [91] have suggested that a significant decrease in the ability of the Na^+/K^+-ATPase activity would lead to increased levels of $[Na^+]_i$. Moreover, significant reduction in Na^+/K^+-ATPase activity has been reported type 1 [94] and type 2 [5] diabetic induced hearts. Decreased Na^+/K^+-ATPase activity is be matched by a increase in $[Na^+]_i$ resulting in increased in Na^+/Ca^{2+} exchanger activity and a rise in basal $[Ca^{2+}]_i$, which has been reported in type 2 diabetes [91].

Systolic calcium

The transient rise of $[Ca^{2+}]_i$ released from the SR is thought to be graded and dependent upon the amount of trigger Ca^{2+} entering the cardiac cell via the single L-type channel and possibly through the Na^+/Ca^{2+} exchanger operating in reverse mode [38,39]. The effects of diabetes on systolic $[Ca^{2+}]_i$ in ventricular myocytes obtained from type 1 diabetic hearts are still unclear. Lagadic-Gossmann et al. [87] demonstrated that the peak systolic Ca^{2+} transient was reduced in type 1 STZ-induced rat cardiomyocytes by 43% compared to control. A slower decay of Ca^{2+} transient was reported in type 1 STZ-induced ventricular myocytes [61,87], while other reports have observed either little or no significant differences in the characteristics of the Ca^{2+} transient from diabetic hearts [73]. Yu et al. [95] reported that depolarisation of the sarcolemmal membrane with potassium chloride (KCl) produced a dose dependent, and rapid increase in $[Ca^{2+}]_i$ that was enhanced in the diabetic cells, while other workers have shown that β-adrenoceptor stimulation with isoprenaline (1×10^{-8} and 1×10^{-7} M) [96] and ociprenaline (1×10^{-7} and 1×10^{-6} M) [74] increased the amplitude of $[Ca^{2+}]_i$ transient, but the extent of potentiation in the diabetic cells was less. Little data are available to suggest any alteration in systolic Ca^{2+} in type 2 diabetic cells.

Defects in the mechanisms, which are involved in Ca^{2+} transport including sarcolemmal Ca^{2+}-ATPase, L-type Ca^{2+} channels, Na^+/Ca^{2+} exchanger or SR Ca^{2+} uptake or release mechanisms, may be responsible for changes in Ca^{2+} mobilisation within the diabetic cardiac myocyte.

SARCOLEMMAL CALCIUM-ATPASE PUMP

In the STZ-induced type 1 diabetic heart, the sarcolemmal Ca^{2+}-ATPase pump has been reported to be significantly depressed in 18 and 24 days [97] and 8 week [98,99] diabetic preparations. There is some evidence to suggest that the sarcolemmal Ca^{2+}-ATPase pump activity in the type 2 diabetic heart is decreased slightly compared to control [91] although the degree of impairment reported is not enough to adversely effect Ca^{2+} homeostasis. Any alteration in the sarcolemmal [98] Ca^{2+}-ATPase pump could contribute to a defect in the transport of Ca^{2+} across the myocardial membrane in the diabetic heart.

L-TYPE CALCIUM CHANNELS AND CALCIUM CURRENT

Initial depolarisation, usually by an action potential leads to the voltage-gated opening of L-type Ca^{2+} channels [50]. In type 1 diabetic myocytes a few reports have suggested that L-type Ca^{2+} channel opening is impaired. Bergh et al. [100] have reported that Ca^{2+} influx was significantly reduced in both acute and chronic diabetes compared to age-matched controls, while, Yu et al. [95] proposed that the L-type Ca^{2+} channel in type 1 diabetes showed enhanced activity and was qualitatively and quantitatively altered. Moreover, the density of L-type I_{Ca} was also significantly reduced by diabetes and the fast time constant of I_{Ca} inactivation, which represents mainly the SR Ca^{2+} release-induced inactivation, was significantly higher in diabetic than in normal myocytes. Moreover, a decrease in I_{Ca} was also observed in chronic (24–30 week old) diabetic myocytes [101]. The decrease in I_{Ca}, which is the main source of trigger Ca^{2+} for SR Ca^{2+} release, may explain the significantly lowered peak systolic $[Ca^{2+}]_i$ previously shown in diabetic myocytes [102]. Other reports suggest that the current density-voltage relationships and steady-state inactivation curves of I_{Ca} are not significantly altered in type 1 STZ-diabetic ventricular cells [73,103,104]. While, Tamada et al. [73] showed no significant difference in the stimulating effects either of isoproterenol, forskolin, or DBcAMP on the I_{Ca} between control and type 1 diabetic myocytes. It is speculated that the response of the L-type Ca^{2+} channel to its activation and opening, is dependent on its phosphorylated state [105], which in turn regulates the length of time it is opened for, and consequently the regulation of I_{Ca}. Phosphoprotein phosphatases 1, 2A, 2B and 2C, within the sarcolemma regulate the life span of the opening time of the L-type Ca^{2+} channel, which in the normal heart is likely to be around a few seconds [106]. In type 2 diabetic hearts the activity of phosphatase 1 has been found to be decreased, thus augmenting the time the L-type channel is open [107]. One possibility is that the time span of opening is deranged in the diabetic heart.

Na^+/Ca^{2+} EXCHANGER

The Na^+/Ca^{2+} exchanger has a pivotal role in the extrusion of Ca^{2+} from the cytosol following a Ca^{2+} transient. Although the relative activity of decreasing $[Ca^{2+}]_i$ is only 7% in the rat [108], it is the predominant mechanism of removing Ca^{2+} out of the cell. Any compositional change within the sarcolemmal membrane or protein change of the exchanger may lead to an abnormal accumulation of Ca^{2+} within the cell following systole and consequent rise of Ca^{2+} within SR. Of the three cloned isoforms of the Na^+/Ca^{2+} exchanger, NCX1 is expressed at highest levels in the heart [109]. Many studies have reported diminished Na^+/Ca^{2+} exchanger activity in sarcolemmal samples taken from STZ-induced [93,97,99] and alloxan treated type 1 diabetic hearts [110]. Other studies using STZ-induced type 2 diabetic hearts have also reported a reduction in sarcolemmal Na^+/Ca^{2+} exchanger activity [91].

Hattori et al. [109] have demonstrated a 30% reduction in the protein and mRNA levels of the NCX 1. Moreover, a reduction in the Na^+/Ca^{2+} exchange machinery may contribute decreased Na^+/Ca^{2+} exchanger function in the diabetic heart. However, Teshima et al. [111] reported no reduction in mRNA Na^+/Ca^{2+} exchanger expression followuing 3 and 12 weeks STZ treatment. In contrast, Schaffer et al. [112] showed that mRNA levels were unchanged in 12–14 month STZ-induced type 2 diabetic hearts.

The Na^+/Ca^{2+} current ($I_{Na\text{-}Ca}$) has been reported to be significantly decreased in the 3–4 [102] and 8 [109] week-treated STZ-induced type 1 diabetic myocytes. Moreover, it was shown that the decreased density of $I_{Na\text{-}Ca}$ was prevented by insulin intervention [109]. It has also been reported that insulin evokes a dose dependent rise in Na^+/Ca^{2+} exchanger activity, which is significantly decreased (63%) in the diabetic heart [112]. In addition, the Na^+/Ca^{2+} exchanger activity in cultured type 2 cardiomyocytes is decreased when they are incubated in a media containing high glucose. In contrast, insulin was found to reverse the effect. Taken together, these observations indicate that the determinants of diabetes i.e. hyperglycaemia and insuliopenia may possibly contribute to a reduced activity observed in the Na^+/Ca^{2+} exchanger and Ca^{2+} flux in diabetic heart cells. It is known that hyperglycaemia plays a role in glycolation of specific key proteins and/or activation of protein kinase C [113] and insulin is closely linked to changes in membrane phospholipid bilayers [114].

SARCOPLASMIC RETICULUM Ca^{2+} CONTENT

Ryanodine is a neutral plant alkaloid, which is a specific and selective ligand for the CaRyR within the SR [60]. It produces a progressive decline in cardiac muscle contraction [60]. At low concentrations (1–30 nM), ryanodine is thought to bind to high affinity sites resulting in the release of Ca^{2+} from the SR. [^{3}H] ryanodine has been employed previously to show that the number of binding sites in type 1 diabetic heart is reduced compared to control [60]. Ca^{2+} influx accumulates around the CaRyR at the SR where it binds to CaRyR receptors to trigger the SR Ca^{2+} release. Reduced density of CaRyR might lead to an impairment of Ca^{2+} release from the SR, depressed shortening and rate of shortening, although it has yet to be reported if the decrease in numbers of CaRyR (reported in type 1 diabetic hearts) is indicative of the sensitivity of Ca^{2+} release from the SR. Total protein CaRyR [115] and expression of mRNA [111] CaRyR have been reported to be significantly depressed in the STZ-induced diabetic heart.

Caffeine increases SR Ca^{2+} channel opening, thus promoting Ca^{2+} leakage into the cytoplasm. The permanent opening of Ca^{2+} channels prevents re-introduction and accumulation of Ca^{2+} into the SR [116]. The peak $[Ca^{2+}]_i$ induced by caffeine can be used as a measurement of an index of releasable Ca^{2+} from the SR, although it should be noted that caffeine also affects myofilaments sensitisation as well as inhibiting phosphodiesterase (which can increase cAMP and in turn activate of cAMP dependent protein Kinase) [95]. Exogenous Ca^{2+} in the presence of caffeine has been shown to be extruded out of the SR into the cytoplasm. Several studies have demonstrated that the amplitude of the caffeine-induced Ca^{2+} transient is depressed in type 1 diabetic cardiomyocytes [73,87,117]. Yu et al. [60] reported that caffeine-induced contracture and

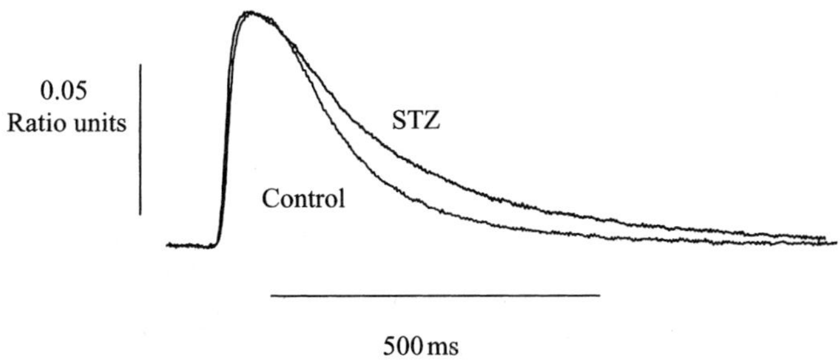

Figure 4. Representative fast time-base recordings of Ca^{2+} transients in electrically stimulated (1 Hz) ventricular myocytes, superfused with normal Tyrode at 35–37°C, from STZ-induced diabetic compared to control rats.

subsequent Ca^{2+} transient in diabetic myocytes to be 75% that of control cells. Rapid cooling contractures (RCC) is another established method of assessing SR Ca^{2+} release in the contracted cell. Rapid cooling (from 30°C–1°C) of the SR (in situ) results in the rapid release of Ca^{2+} from the SR, this is followed by a contracture. Experimental data using type 1 diabetic cells have demonstrated, depressed RCC [117]. Bouchard and Bose [118] showed a 50% reduction of RCC in type 1-diabetic cells, while Yu et al. [60] observed a reduction in the amplitude of RCC in the diabetic heart that was 68% that of control cells. This evidence suggests that a reduction in caffeine and rapid cooling induced contracture seen in type 1 diabetic cardiac cells is indicative of a diminished Ca^{2+} storage mechanism in the SR. However, little or no experimental evidence exists to establish altered Ca^{2+} content within the SR of type 2 diabetic hearts.

SARCOPLASMIC RETICULUM ATPase PUMP

The SR possesses a pump (SERCA) which is distinct from the sarcolemmal Ca^{2+}-ATPase pump. The decay of the Ca^{2+} transient is initiated by the re-uptake of Ca^{2+} into the SR by SERCA [50,51] and the extrusion of Ca^{2+} from the cell by the Na^+/Ca^{2+} exchanger [37,52,53]. Ventricular myocytes re-uptake of Ca^{2+} into the SR accounts for 92% of the total removal of Ca^{2+} from the cytosol, while the Na^+/Ca^{2+} exchanger accounts for approximately 7% in the rat [108]. In type 1 induced-diabetic hearts, it has been shown that contractile dysfunction is associated with a longer phase of systolic $[Ca^{2+}]_i$ which contributes a prolonged $[Ca^{2+}]_i$ transient duration [87]. Similarly, unpublished data from our laboratory using 8–12 week-STZ-treated rats have also shown a prolongation of the $[Ca^{2+}]_i$ transient duration (Fig. 4). Some workers have reported that the prolonged $[Ca^{2+}]_i$ transient duration is associated with a slower uptake of Ca^{2+} back into the SR. It has also been reported that altered SR Ca^{2+}-uptake activities in diabetic animals were accompanied by a significant decrease in the level of the Ca^{2+}-pump ATPase [115]. Several other studies have observed a decreased activity of the SERCA pump on the SR in STZ-induced type 1 diabetic cells [119].

Some workers have reported a significant reduction in mRNA expression [111,120,121] and protein activity [115] of the SERCA pump in type 1 induced diabetic hearts [97,122,123]. However, in 3 and 5 week old STZ-induced diabetic rats there was no reduction in the relative level of ventricular SERCA2 mRNA expression in neither diabetic nor insulin treated rats [124]. In type 2 diabetic hearts Misra et al. [123] reported that SR isolated from the JCR:LA-cp model of type 2 diabetic hearts showed unaltered activities compared to control. On the other hand, Schaffer et al. [5] using isolated SR from STZ-induced type 2 diabetic hearts showed that a small but significant depression of SERCA activity. Although the SERCA pump is important in decreasing the beat-to-beat $[Ca^{2+}]_i$ levels, it is incapable of extruding Ca^{2+} from the cell. Therefore, steady-state increases of $[Ca^{2+}]_i$ in diabetic myocytes cannot be explained by a defective SR Ca transport system alone [5].

PHOSPHOLAMBAN

A PKA-dependent protein, phospholamban, regulates the activity of the SERCA pump. In its unphosphorylated form, phospholamban acts as an inhibitory mechanism on the SERCA pump, but when it becomes phosphorylated, it accelerates the uptake of Ca^{2+} from the cytoplasm into the SR [72]. The decrease in Ca^{2+} uptake into the SR, reported in diabetic hearts [125] could be attributable to an alteration in the level of phospholamban or its phosphorylated state. Gando et al. [77] showed that stimulation with isoprenaline resulted in a 3-fold increase in phospholamban phosphorylation using ^{32}P incorporation in control myocytes, however, no significant increase was observed in diabetic cells. Moreover, Gando et al. [77] also showed that forskolin activation of phospholamban phosphorylation was depressed in diabetic hearts compared to control, respectively. An increase in protein phosphatase activity in diabetic compared with control hearts may contribute in minimising the effects of c-AMP mediators like isoprenaline [77]. Total protein content of phospholamban using Western blot technique has been shown to be either significantly increased [126] or decreased [115] in 6 week old myocytes taken from STZ treated type 1 diabetic hearts. Northern blot analysis has also shown that the expression of mRNA encoding phospholamban in the diabetic heart is significantly increased [120] after 6 weeks of treatment but there was no change [111] in 3 and 12 week treated STZ-induced type 1 diabetic hearts compared to control. These studies suggest that an alteration in phospholamban level or expression and/or protein phosphatase level in the diabetic heart may play a role in decreased Ca^{2+} uptake that has reported in the type 1 diabetic heart.

CONCLUSION

Current evidence suggests that an altered process that underpins the mechanism of E-C coupling is responsible for the contractile dysfunction seen in diabetic heart cells. In particular, it has been suggested that abnormal Ca^{2+} movement is responsible for the impairment seen in diabetic hearts. Human studies have shown that diabetes can induce a state of cardiomyopathy, which is characterised by abnormal systolic and diastolic compliance [5,16,19,20]. Studies using experimentally induced diabetes have reported depressed SV, AO, positive (+dP/dt) and negative (−dP/dt) left ventricular developed in whole heart [54] decreased speed of contraction, a prolongation in the contraction, and a delay in relaxation in papillary muscles [21] and alterations in the kinetics of contractile properties of isolated ventricular myocytes from experimentally induced type 1 diabetes. Moreover, reductions in aortic output (AO), ventricular pressure, and cardiac work in whole hearts from type 2 induced models of diabetes have been reported. Although β-adrenergic receptor affinity seems unaltered by diabetes, impaired responsiveness to β-agonists have been reported in type 1 [76] [73,77–79] and type 2 induced diabetic hearts [34]. Basal $[Ca^{2+}]_i$ levels have been shown to be either, high [87] or unchanged [73] in type 1 diabetic cells and elevated in type 2 diabetic myocytes [34]. Resting $[Na^+]_{i,}$ which could be attributable to Ca^{2+} imbalance through the Na^+/Ca^{2+} exchanger has been reported to be lowered in type 1 diabetic cells [92], which may be due to a reduction in the Na^+/H^+ exchanger [93] and higher in type 2 cells through a consequence of reduced Na^+/K^+-ATPase activity [91]. Changes in L-type Ca^{2+} channel activity have been reported in type 1 diabetics hearts [100]. Moreover, a decrease in I_{Ca} was also observed in chronic (24–30 week old) diabetic myocytes [101]. The decrease in I_{Ca}, which is the main source of trigger Ca^{2+} for SR Ca^{2+} release, may explain the significantly lowered peak systolic $[Ca^{2+}]_i$ previously shown in diabetic myocytes [102]. Other reports suggest that the current density-voltage relationships and steady-state inactivation curves of I_{Ca} are not significantly altered in type 1 STZ-diabetic ventricular cells [73,103,104]. Caffeine and RCC studies used in type 1 diabetic cardiomyocytes have shown that the amplitude of the caffeine-induced Ca^{2+} transient is depressed in type 1 diabetic cardiomyocytes [73,87,117] suggesting a dysfunction in the Ca^{2+} storage mechanism within the SR. This may be brought about by a reduction in the activity of the SERCA pump, which has been reported in type 1 [115,119] and small alterations in type 2 diabetes [5]. The Na^+/Ca^{2+} exchanger has been shown to be dramatically reduced in type 1 induced [97] and type 2 [91] diabetic hearts leading to a rise in $[Ca^{2+}]_i$. Moreover change in Na^+/Ca^{2+} exchanger protein, mRNA expression [109] and $I_{Na\text{-}Ca}$ [102,109] have all been reported in type 1 hearts although mRNA levels were unchanged in 12–14 month STZ-induced type 2 diabetic hearts [112]. Figure 5a. represents a schematic model of Ca^{2+} homeostasis in a typical STZ-induced type 1 cardiomyocyte. In this model it is shown that all major transporter mechanisms within the myocyte may contribute synergistically to alter $[Ca^{2+}]_i$ homeostasis. Figure 5b. represents a schematic model in a typical STZ-induced type 2 cardiomyocyte, in which Na^+/Ca^{2+} exchanger activity is significantly reduced, the SR appears slightly altered and Ca^{2+} pumps and CaRyR channels appear normal. This results in altered Ca^{2+} equilibrium, which is shifted towards the SR (due to reduced Ca^{2+} efflux), resulting in Ca^{2+} overload.

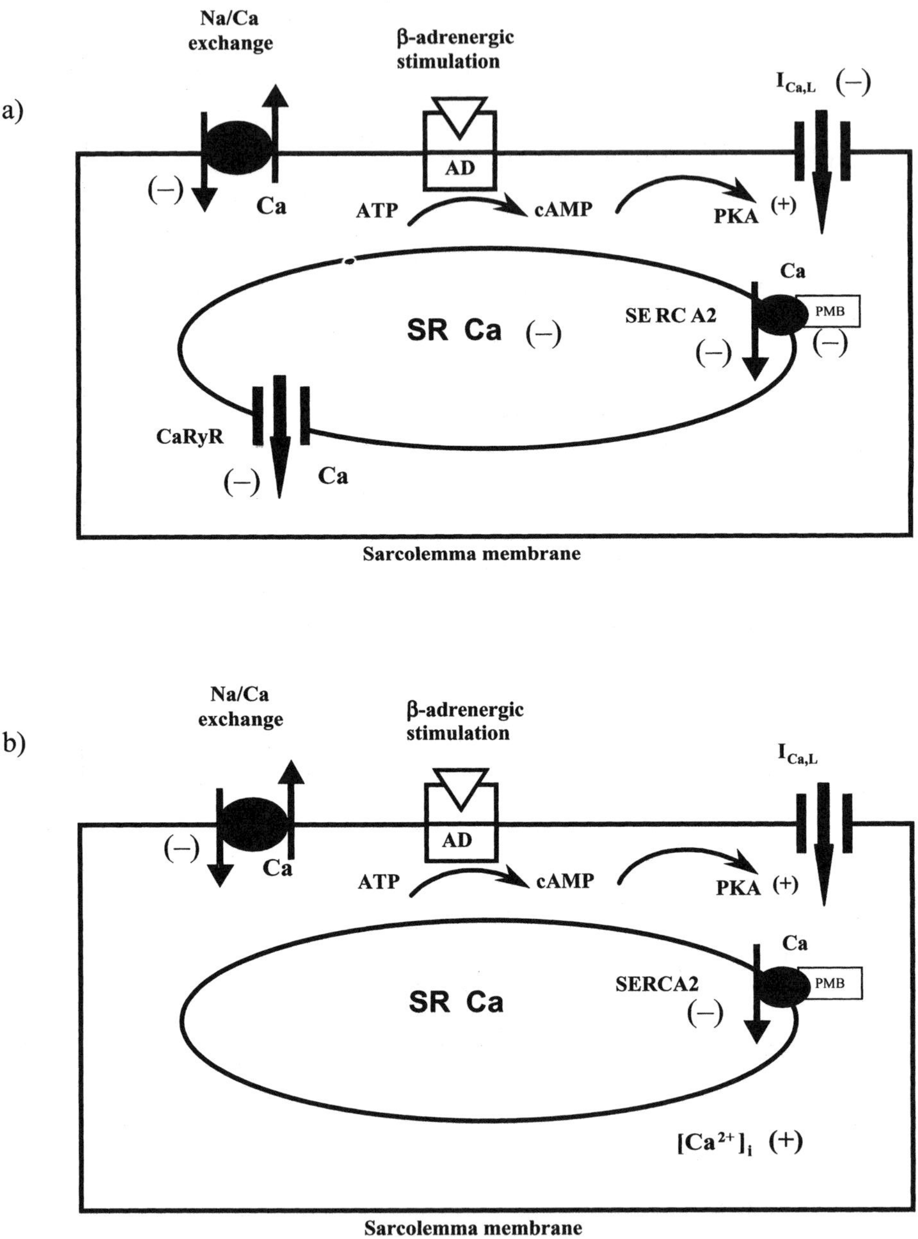

Figure 5. Schematic model of E-C coupling and Ca^{2+} homeostasis in cardiomyocytes of STZ-induced (a) type 1 diabetes and (b) type 2 diabetes. In model (a) it is suggested that a derangement in Ca^{2+} mobilisation is associated with a dysfunction of the different Ca^{2+} transporters. In model (b) it is postulated that the Na^+/Ca^{2+} exchanger is deranges resulting in the elevation of $[Ca^{2+}]_i$.

In conclusion, it is suggested that contractile dysfunction of the diabetic heart is associated with a derangement in the cellular Ca^{2+} homeostasis, possibly through mechanisms of uptake of Ca^{2+} into the SR or its extrusion from the cell (e.g. in type 1 diabetes) and through an impaired activity of the Na^+/Ca^{2+} exchanger (e.g. type 2 diabetes).

ACKNOWLEDGEMENTS

Supported by the British Heart Foundation.

REFERENCES

1. Williams G, Pickup JC. 1999. Handbook of Diabetes London: Blackwell Science Ltd.
2. Harris M, Zimmet P. 1997. Classification of diabetes mellitus and other categories of glucose intolerance. In International Textbook of Diabetes Mellitus, ed. AK Zimmet, R DeFronzo, and H Keen, pp. 9–23. Chichester: Wiley.
3. Amos AF, Mccarty DJ, Zimmet P. 1997. The rising global burden of diabetes and its complications: estimates and projections to the year 2010. Diabet Med 14 Suppl 5:S1–S85.
4. King H, Aubert RE, Herman WH. 1998. Global burden of diabetes, 1995–2025: prevalence, numerical estimates, and projections. Diabetes Care 21:1414–1431.
5. Schaffer SW. 1991. Cardiomyopathy associated with noninsulin-dependent diabetes. Mol Cell Biochem 107:1–20.
6. Thorsby P, Undlien DE, Berg JP, Thorsby E, Birkeland KI. 1998. Diabetes mellitus—a complex interaction between heredity and environment Tidsskr. Nor Laegeforen. 118:2519–2524.
7. Dhalla NS, Pierce GN, Innes IR, Beamish RE. 1985. Pathogenesis of cardiac dysfunction in diabetes mellitus. Can J Cardiol 1:263–281.
8. Julien J. 1997. Cardiac complications in non-insulin-dependent diabetes mellitus. Journal Of Diabetes And Its Complications 11:123–130.
9. Schernthaner G. 1996. Cardiovascular mortality and morbidity in type-2 diabetes mellitus. Diabetes Res Clin Pract 31 Suppl:S3–13.
10. Mahgoub MA, Abd-Elfattah AS. 1998. Diabetes mellitus and cardiac function. Mol Cell Biochem 180:59–64.
11. Raman M, Nesto RW. 1996. Heart disease in diabetes mellitus. Endocrinol Metab Clin North Am 25:425–438.
12. Laakso M. 1999. Hyperglycemia and cardiovascular disease in type 2 diabetes. Diabetes 48:937–942.
13. Albanna II, Eichelberger SM, Khoury PR, Witt SA, Standiford DA, Dolan LM, Daniels SR, Kimball TR. 1998. Diastolic dysfunction in young patients with insulin-dependent diabetes mellitus as determined by automated border detection. Journal of The American Society of Echocardiography 11:349–355.
14. Kiss A, Kertesz T, Koltai MZ, Cserhalmi L, Jermendy G, Kammerer L, Zrinyi T, Pogatsa G. 1988. Left ventricular diastolic function in diabetics. Acta Physiol Hung 71:227–232.
15. Litwin SE, Raya TE, Anderson PG, Daugherty S, Goldman S. 1990. Abnormal cardiac function in the streptozotocin-diabetic rat. Changes in active and passive properties of the left ventricle. J Clin Invest 86:481–488.
16. Astorri E, Fiorina P, Gavaruzzi G, Astorri A, Magnati G. 1997. Left ventricular function in insulin-dependent and in non-insulin-dependent diabetic patients: Radionuclide assessment. Cardiology 88:152–155.
17. Nicolino A, Longobardi G, Furgi G, Rossi M, Zoccolillo N, Ferrara N, Rengo F. 1995. Left-ventricular diastolic filling in diabetes-mellitus with and without hypertension. Am J Hypertens 8:382–389.
18. Akella AB, Sonnenblick EH, Gulati J. 1996. Alterations in myocardial contractile proteins in diabetes-mellitus. Coronary Artery Disease 7:124–132.
19. Vanninen E, Mustonen J, Vainio P, Lansimies E, Uusitupa M. 1992. Left ventricular function and dimensions in newly diagnosed non-insulin-dependent diabetes mellitus. Am J Cardiol 70:371–378.

20. Astorri E, Fiorina P, Contini CA, Albertini D, Magnati G, Astorri A, Lanfredini M. 1997. Isolated and preclinical impairment of left ventricular filling in insulin-dependent and non-insulin-dependent diabetic patients. Clin Cardiol 20:536–540.
21. Fein FS, Kornstein LB, Strobeck JE, Capasso JM, Sonnenblick EH. 1980. Altered myocardial mechanics in diabetic rats. Circ Res 47:922–933.
22. Tahiliani AG, Vadlamudi RV, Mcneill JH. 1983. Prevention and reversal of altered myocardial function in diabetic rats by insulin treatment. Can J Physiol Pharmacol 61:516–523.
23. Collins JF, Pawloski-Dahm C, Davis MG, Ball N, Dorn GW, Walsh RA. 1996. The role of the cytoskeleton in left ventricular pressure overload hypertrophy and failure. J Mol Cell Cardiol 28: 1435–1443.
24. Howarth FC, Singh J. 1999. Altered handling of calcium during the process of excitation-contraction coupling in the streptozotocin-induced diabetic rat heart—A short review. International Journal Diabetes 7:52–64.
25. Goto Y, Kakizaki M, Masaki N. 1975. Spontaneous diabetes produced by selective breeding of normal Wistar rats. Proc JPN Acad 51:80–85.
26. Surwit RS, Feinglos MN, Livingston EG, Kuhn CM, McCubbin JA. 1984. Behavioral manipulation of the diabetic phenotype in ob/ob mice. Diabetes 33:616–618.
27. Bray GA. 1977. The Zucker-fatty rat: a review. Fed Proc 36:148–153.
28. Kawano K, Hirashima T, Mori S, Saitoh Y, Kurosumi M, Natori T. 1992. Spontaneous long-term hyperglycemic rat with diabetic complications. Otsuka Long-Evans Tokushima Fatty (OLETF) strain. Diabetes 41:1422–1428.
29. Ren J, Bode AM. 2000. Altered cardiac excitation-contraction coupling in ventricular myocytes from spontaneously diabetic BB rats. Am J Physiol 279:H238–H244.
30. Berdanier CD. 1991. The BHE rat: an animal model for the study of non-insulin-dependent diabetes mellitus. FASEB J 5:2139–2144.
31. Kalderon B, Gutman A, Levy E, Shafrir E, Adler JH. 1986. Characterization of stages in development of obesity-diabetes syndrome in sand rat (Psammomys obesus). Diabetes 35:717–724.
32. Portha B, Blondel O, Serradas P, McEvoy R, Giroix MH, Kergoat M, Bailbe D. 1989. The rat models of non-insulin dependent diabetes induced by neonatal streptozotocin. Diabete Metab 15:61–75.
33. Weir GC, Clore ET, Zmachinski CJ, Bonner-Weir S. 1981. Islet secretion in a new experimental model for non-insulin-dependent diabetes. Diabetes 30:590–595.
34. Schaffer SW, Allo S, Punna S, White T. 1991. Defective response to cAMP-dependent protein kinase in non-insulin-dependent diabetic heart. Am J Physiol 261:E369–E376.
35. Ward WK, Beard JC, Halter JB, Pfeifer MA, Porte DJ. 1984. Pathophysiology of insulin secretion in non-insulin-dependent diabetes mellitus. Diabetes Care 7:491–502.
36. Schaffer SW, Wilson GL. 1993. Insulin resistance and mechanical dysfunction in hearts of Wistar rats with streptozotocin-induced non-insulin-dependent diabetes mellitus. Diabetologia 36:195–199.
37. Barry WH, Bridge JHB. 1993. Intracellular calcium homeostasis in cardiac myocytes. Circulation 87(6):1806–1815.
38. Lipp P, Niggli E. 1994. Sodium current-induced calcium signals in isolated guinea-pig ventricular myocytes. J Physiol 474:439–446.
39. Leblanc N, Hume JR. 1990. Sodium current-induced release of calcium from cardiac sarcoplasmic reticulum. Science 248:372–376.
40. Sipido KR, Carmeliet E, Pappano A. 1995. Na^+ current and Ca^{2+} release from the sarcoplasmic reticulum during action potentials in guinea-pig ventricular myocytes. J Physiol 489:1–17.
41. Sham JSK, Cleemann L, Morad M. 1992. Gating of the cardiac Ca^{2+} release channel: The role of Na^+ current and Na^+—Ca^+ exchange. Science 255:850–853.
42. Beuckelmann DJ, Wier WG. 1988. Mechanism of release of calcium from sarcoplasmic reticulum of guinea-pig cardiac cells J Physiol 405:233–255.
43. Cannell MB, Berlin JR, Lederer WJ. 1987. Effect of membrane potential changes on the calcium transient in single rat cardiac muscle cells. Science 238:1419–1423.
44. Eisner DA, Trafford AW. 2000. No Role for the Ryanodine Receptor in Regulating Cardiac Contraction? News Physiol Sci 15:275–279.
45. Fabiato A. 1983. Calcium-induced release of calcium from the cardiac sarcoplasmic reticulum. Am J Physiol 14:C1–C14.
46. Litwin SE, Li J, Bridge JH. 1998. Na^+/Ca^{2+} exchanger ge and the trigger for sarcoplasmic reticulum Ca release: studies in adult rabbit ventricular myocytes. Biophys J 75:359–371.

47. Muller P. 1965. Ouabain effects on cardiac contraction, action potential and cellular potassium. Circ Res 17:46–56.
48. Levi AJ, Ferrier GR. 1997. Biophys J 72 (2):A161-Tu-Pos130 (Abstr.).
49. Lipp P, Laine M, Tovey SC, Burrell KM, Berridge MJ, Li W, Bootman MD. 2000. Functional InsP3 receptors that may modulate excitation-contraction coupling in the heart. Curr Biol 10:939–942.
50. Bers DM. 1991. Excitation-contraction coupling and cardiac contractile force. Dordrecht, The Netherlands: Kluwer Academic Publishers.
51. Balke CW, Egan TM, Wier WG. 1994. Processes that remove calcium from the cytoplasm during excitation-contraction coupling in intact rat heart cells J Physiol 474:447–462.
52. Barcenas-Ruiz L, Beuckelmann DJ, Weir WG. 1987. Sodium-calcium exchange in the heart: Membrane currents and changes in $[Ca^{2+}]_i$. Science 238(4834), 1720–1722.
53. Jorgensen AO, Shen ACY, Daly P, MacLennan DH. 1982. Localization of Ca^{2+} Mg^{2+}-ATPase of the sarcoplasmic reticulum in adult rat papillary muscle. J Cell Biol 93:883–892.
54. Regan TJ, Ettinger PO, Khan MI, Jesrani MU, Lyons MM, Oldewurtel HA, Weber M. 1974. Altered myocardial function and metabolism in chronic diabetes mellitus without ischemia in dogs. Circ Res 35:222–237.
55. Fein FS, Sonnenblick EH. 1994. Diabetic cardiomyopathy. Cardiovasc Drugs Ther 8:65–73.
56. Lagadic-Gossman D, Jourdon P, Feuvray D. 1994. Cardiac contractile activity and action-potential in spontaneously diabetic bb rats. Sciences Et Techniques De L Animal De Laboratoire 19:207–212.
57. Cameron NE, Cotter MA, Robertson S. 1989. Contractile properties of cardiac papillary muscle in streptozotocin-diabetic rats and the effects of aldose reductase inhibition. Diabetologia 32: 365–370.
58. Cotter MA, Cameron NE, Robertson S. 1992. Polyol pathway-mediated changes in cardiac muscle contractile properties: studies in streptozotocin-diabetic and galactose-fed rats. Exp Physiol 77: 829–838.
59. Ren J, Walsh MF, Hamaty M, Sowers JR, Brown RA. 1999. Augmentation of the inotropic response to insulin in diabetic rat hearts. Life Sci 65:369–380.
60. Yu Z, Tibbits GF, Mcneill JH. 1994. Cellular functions of diabetic cardiomyocytes: contractility, rapid-cooling contracture, and ryanodine binding. Am J Physiol 266:H2082–H2089.
61. Ren J, Davidoff AJ. 1997. Diabetes rapidly induces contractile dysfunctions in isolated ventricular myocytes. Am J Physiol 41:H148–H158.
62. Okayama H, Hamada M, Hiwada K. 1994. Contractile dysfunction in the diabetic-rat heart is an intrinsic abnormality of the cardiac myocyte. Clin Sci (Colch.) 86:257–262.
63. Howarth FC, Qureshi MA, Bracken NK, Winlow W, Singh J. 2001. Time-dependent effects of strptozotocin-induced diabetes on contraction of ventricular myocytes from rat heart. Emirates Medical Journal 19:35–41.
64. Wold LE, Relling DP, Colligan PB, Scott GI, Hintz KK, Ren BH, Epstein PN, Ren J. 2001. Characterization of contractile function in diabetic hypertensive cardiomyopathy in adult rat ventricular myocytes. J Mol Cell Cardiol 33:1719–1726.
65. Ren J. 2000. Attenuated cardiac contractile responsiveness to insulin-like growth factor I in ventricular myocytes from biobreeding spontaneous diabetic rats. Cardiovasc Res 46:162–171.
66. Ishitani T, Hattori Y, Sakuraya F, Onozuka H, Makino T, Matsuda N, Gando S, Kemmotsu O. 2001. Effects of Ca^{2+} sensitizers on contraction, $[Ca^{2+}]_i$ transient and myofilament Ca^{2+} sensitivity in diabetic rat myocardium: potential usefulness as inotropic agents. J Pharmacol Exp Ther 298:613–622.
67. Schaffer SW, Tan BH, Wilson GL. 1985. Development of a cardiomyopathy in a model of noninsulin-dependent diabetes. Am J Physiol 248:H179–H185.
68. Schaffer SW, Mozaffari MS, Artman M, Wilson GL. 1989. Basis for myocardial mechanical defects associated with non-insulin-dependent diabetes. Am J Physiol 256:E25–E30.
69. Howarth FC, Qureshi MA. 2002. Characteristics of ventricular myocyte shortening after administration of streptozotocin to neonatal rats. Archives of physiology and biochemistry (in press).
70. Trautwein W, Hescheler J. 1990. Regulation of cardiac L-type calcium current by phosphorylation and G proteins. Ann Rev Physiol 52:257–274.
71. Kranias EG, Solaro RJ. 1982. Phosphorylation of Troponin I and phospholamban during catecholamin stimulation of rabbit heart. Nature 298(5870):182–184.
72. Tada M, Katz AM. 1982. Phosphorylation of the sarcoplasmic reticulum and sarcolemma. Annual Review of Physiology 44:401–423.

73. Tamada A, Hattori Y, Houzen H, Yamada Y, Sakuma I, Kitabatake A, Kanno M. 1998. Effects of beta-adrenoceptor stimulation on contractility, $[Ca^{2+}]_i$ and Ca^{2+} current in diabetic rat cardiomyocytes. Am J Physiol 43:H1849–H1857.
74. Ha T, Kotsanas G, Wendt I. 1999. Intracellular Ca^{2+} and adrenergic responsiveness of cardiac myocytes in streptozotocin-induced diabetes. Clin Exp Pharmacol Physiol 26:347–353.
75. Sellers DJ, Chess-Williams R. 2001. The effect of streptozotocin-induced diabetes on cardiac beta-adrenoceptor subtypes in the rat. J Auton Pharmacol 21:15–21.
76. Atkins FL, Dowell RT, Love S. 1985. beta-Adrenergic receptors, adenylate cyclase activity, and cardiac dysfunction in the diabetic rat. J Cardiovasc Pharmacol 7:66–70.
77. Gando S, Hattori Y, Akaishi Y, Nishihira J, Kanno M. 1997. Impaired contractile response to beta adrenoceptor stimulation in diabetic rat hearts: Alterations in beta adrenoceptors-G protein adenylate-cyclase system and phospholamban phosphorylation. J Pharmacol Exp Ther 282(1): 475–484.
78. Heyliger CE, Pierce GN, Singal PK, Beamish RE, Dhalla NS. 1982. Cardiac alpha- and beta-adrenergic receptor alterations in diabetic cardiomyopathy. Basic Res Cardiol 77:610–618.
79. Horackova M, Murphy MG. 1988. Effects of chronic diabetes mellitus on the electrical and contractile activities, $45Ca^{2+}$ transport, fatty acid profiles and ultrastructure of isolated rat ventricular myocytes. Pflugers Arch 411:564–572.
80. Gando S. 1994. Pharmacological studies on alterations in myocardial beta-adrenoceptors and their intracellular signal transduction in experimental diabetic rats. Hokkaido Igaku Zasshi 69:1140–1153.
81. Nishio Y, Kashiwagi A, Kida Y, Kodama M, Abe N, Saeki Y, Shigeta Y. 1988. Deficiency of cardiac beta-adrenergic receptor in streptozocin-induced diabetic rats. Diabetes 37:1181–1187.
82. Menotti A, Blackburn H, Seccareccia F, Kromhout D, Nissinen A, Aravanis C, Giampaoli S, Mohacek I, Nedeljkovic S, Toshima H. 1997. The relation of chronic diseases to all-cause mortality risk—the Seven Countries Study. Ann Med 29:135–141.
83. Austin CE, Chess-Williams R. 1991. Diabetes-induced changes in cardiac beta-adrenoceptor responsiveness: effects of aldose reductase inhibition with ponalrestat. Br J Pharmacol 102:478–482.
84. Ramanadham S, Tenner TEJ. 1987. Alterations in the myocardial beta-adrenoceptor system of streptozotocin-diabetic rats. Eur J Pharmacol 136:377–389.
85. Schaffer SW, Mozaffari M. 1996. Abnormal mechanical function in diabetes: relation to myocardial calcium handling. Coron Artery Dis 7:109–115.
86. Golden KL, Ren J, O'Connor J, Dean A, DiCarlo SE, Marsh JD. 2001. In vivo regulation of Na/Ca exchanger expression by adrenergic effectors. Am J Physiol Heart Circ Physiol 280: H1376–H1382.
87. Lagadic-Gossmann D, Buckler KJ, Le Prigent K, Feuvray D. 1996. Altered Ca^{2+} handling in ventricular myocytes isolated from diabetic rats. Am J Physiol 270:H1529–H1537.
88. Hayashi H, Noda N. 1997. Cytosolic Ca^{2+} concentration decreases in diabetic rat myocytes. Cardiovasc Res 34:99–103.
89. Noda N, Hayashi H, Miyata H, Suzuki S, Kobayashi A, Yamazaki N. 1992. Cytosolic Ca^{2+} concentration and pH of diabetic rat myocytes during metabolic inhibition. J Mol Cell Cardiol 24: 435–446.
90. Yu Z, Quamme GA, Mcneill JH. 1994. Depressed $[Ca^{2+}]_i$ responses to isoproterenol and cAMP in isolated cardiomyocytes from experimental diabetic rats. Am J Physiol 266:H2334–H2342.
91. Allo SN, Lincoln TM, Wilson GL, Green FJ, Watanabe AM, Schaffer SW. 1991. Non-insulin-dependent diabetes-induced defects in cardiac cellular calcium regulation. Am J Physiol 260: C1165–C1171.
92. Katoh H, Noda N, Hayashi H, Satoh H, Terada H, Ohno R, Yamazaki N. 1995. Intracellular sodium concentration in diabetic rat ventricular myocytes. Jpn Heart J 36:647–656.
93. Pierce GN, Ramjiawan B, Dhalla NS, Ferrari R. 1990. Na^+/H^+ exchange in cardiac sarcolemmal vesicles isolated from diabetic rats. Am J Physiol 258:H255–H261.
94. kato K, Chapman DC, Rupp H, Lukas A, Dhalla NS. 1999. Alterations of heart function and Na^+/K^+-ATPase activity by etomoxir in diabetic rats. J Appl Physiol 86:812–818.
95. Yu JZ, Quamme GA, Mcneill JH. 1995. Altered $[Ca^{2+}]_i$ Mobilization in diabetic cardiomyocytes—responses to caffeine, KCl, ouabain, and ATP. Diabetes Research and Clinical Practice 30:9–20.
96. Noda N, Hayashi H, Satoh H, Terada H, Hirano M, Kobayashi A, Yamazaki N. 1993. Ca^{2+} transients and cell shortening in diabetic rat ventricular myocytes. Jpn Circ J 57:449–457.

97. Takeda N, Dixon IC, Hata T, Elimban V, Shah KR, Dhalla NS. 1996. Sequence of alterations in subcellular organelles during the development of heart dysfunction in diabetes. Diabetes Research and Clinical Practice 30:S–S.
98. Heyliger CE, Prakash A, Mcneill JH. 1987. Alterations in cardiac sarcolemmal Ca^{2+} pump activity during diabetes mellitus. Am J Physiol 252:H540–H544.
99. Makino N, Dhalla KS, Elimban V, Dhalla NS. 1987. Sarcolemmal Ca^{2+} transport in streptozotocin-induced diabetic cardiomyopathy in rats. Am J Physiol 253:E202–E207.
100. Bergh CH, Hjalmarson A, Sjogren KG, Jacobsson B. 1988. The effect of diabetes on phosphatidylinositol turnover and calcium influx in myocardium. Horm Metab Res 20:381–386.
101. Wang DW, Kiyosue T, Shigematsu S, Arita M. 1995. Abnormalities of K^+ and Ca^{2+} currents in ventricular myocytes from rats with chronic diabetes. Am J Physiol 269:H1288–H1296.
102. Chattou S, Diacono J, Feuvray D. 1999. Decrease in sodium-calcium exchange and calcium currents in diabetic rat ventricular myocytes. Acta Physiol Scand 166:137–144.
103. Schneider JA, Sperelakis N. 1975. Slow Ca^{2+} and Na^+ responses induced by isoproterenol and methylxanthines in isolated perfused guinea-pig hearts exposed to elevated K. J Mol Cell Cardiol 7:249–273.
104. Jourdon P, Feuvray D. 1993. Calcium and potassium currents in ventricular myocytes isolated from diabetic rats. J Physiol (Lond.) 470:411–429.
105. Sperelakis N. 1988. Regulation of calcium slow channels of cardiac muscle by cyclic nucleotides and phosphorylation. J Mol Cell Cardiol 20(Suppl)2:75–105.
106. Hescheler J, Kameyama M, Trautwein W, Mieskes G, Soling HD. 1987. Regulation of the cardiac calcium channel by protein phosphatases. Eur J Biochem 165:261–266.
107. Allo SN, Schaffer SW. 1990. Defective sarcolemmal phosphorylation associated with noninsulin-dependent diabetes. Biochim Biophys Acta 1023:206–212.
108. Bers DM. 2002. Cardiac excitaion-contraction coupling. Nature 415:198–205.
109. Hattori Y, Matsuda N, Kimura J, Ishitani T, Tamada A, Gando S, Kemmotsu O, Kanno M. 2000. Diminished function and expression of the cardiac Na^+/Ca^{2+} exchanger in diabetic rats: implication in Ca^{2+} overload. J Physiol 527 Pt 1:85–94.
110. Kato M, Kako KJ. 1988. Na^+/Ca^{2+} exchange of isolated sarcolemmal membrane: effects of insulin, oxidants and insulin deficiency. Mol Cell Biochem 83:15–25.
111. Teshima Y, Takahashi N, Saikawa T, Hara M, Yasunaga S, Hidaka S, Sakata T. 2000. Diminished expression of sarcoplasmic reticulum Ca^{2+}-ATPase and ryanodine sensitive Ca^{2+} Channel mRNA in streptozotocin-induced diabetic rat heart. J Mol Cell Cardiol 32:655–664.
112. Schaffer SW, Ballard-Croft C, Boerth S, Allo SN. 1997. Mechanisms underlying depressed Na^+/Ca^{2+} exchanger activity in the diabetic heart. Cardiovasc Res 34:129–136.
113. Giles TD, Ouyang J, Kerut EK, Given MB, Allen GE, McIlwain EF, Greenberg SS. 1998. Changes in protein kinase C in early cardiomyopathy and in gracilis muscle in the BB/Wor diabetic rat. Am J Physiol 274:H295–H307.
114. Saltiel AR. 1994. The paradoxical regulation of protein phosphorylation in insulin action. FASEB J 8:1034–1040.
115. Netticadan T, Temsah RM, Kent A, Elimban V, Dhalla NS. 2001. Depressed levels of Ca^{2+} cycling proteins may underlie sarcoplasmic reticulum dysfunction in the diabetic heart. Diabetes 50:2133–2138.
116. Rousseau E, Meissner G. 1987. Single cardiac sarcoplasmic reticulum Ca^{2+}-release channel: activation by caffeine. Am J Physiol 256:H328–H333.
117. Woodbury LA, Hecht HH. 1952. Effects of cardiac glycosides upon the electrical activity of single ventricular fibres of the frog heart, and their relation to the digitalis effect of the electrocardiogram. Circulation 6:172–182.
118. Bouchard RA, Bose D. 1991. Influence of experimental diabetes on sarcoplasmic reticulum function in rat ventricular muscle. Am J Physiol 260:H341–H354.
119. Ganguly PK, Pierce GN, Dhalla KS, Dhalla NS. 1983. Defective sarcoplasmic reticular calcium transport in diabetic cardiomyopathy. Am J Physiol 244:E528–E535.
120. Kim HW, Ch YS, Lee HR, Park SY, Kim YH. 2001. Diabetic alterations in cardiac sarcoplasmic reticulum Ca^{2+}-ATPase and phospholamban protein expression. Life Sci 70:367–379.
121. Russ M, Reinauer H, Eckel J. 1991. Diabetes-induced decrease in the mRNA coding for sarcoplasmic reticulum Ca^{2+}-ATPase in adult rat cardiomyocytes. Biochem Biophys Res Commun 178:906–912.

122. Lopaschuk GD, Tahiliani AG, Vadlamudi RV, Katz S, Mcneill JH. 1983. Cardiac sarcoplasmic reticulum function in insulin- or carnitine-treated diabetic rats. Am J Physiol 245:H969–H976.
123. Misra T, Gilchrist JS, Russell JC, Pierce GN. 1999. Cardiac myofibrillar and sarcoplasmic reticulum function are not depressed in insulin-resistant JCR:LA-cp rats. Am J Physiol 276:H1811–H1817.
124. Zarain-Herzberg A, Yano K, Elimban V, Dhalla NS. 1994. Cardiac sarcoplasmic reticulum Ca^{2+}-ATPase expression in streptozotocin-induced diabetic rat heart. Biochem Biophys Res Commun 203:113–120.
125. Satoh N, Sato T, Shimada M, Yamada K, Kitada Y. 2001. Lusitropic effect of MCC-135 is associated with improvement of sarcoplasmic reticulum function in ventricular muscles of rats with diabetic cardiomyopathy. J Pharmacol Exp Ther 298:1161–1166.
126. Zhong Y, Ahmed S, Grupp IL, Matlib MA. 2001. Altered SR protein expression associated with contractile dysfunction in diabetic rat hearts. Am J Physiol 281:H1137–H1147.

G.N. Pierce, M. Nagano, P. Zahradka, and N.S. Dhalla (eds.).
ATHEROSCLEROSIS, HYPERTENSION AND DIABETES.
Kluwer Academic Publishers. Boston.

PROTEIN KINASE C SIGNALING AND EXPRESSION OF THE DIABETIC CARDIAC PHENOTYPE

BARINDER PAL SINGH KANG, BABATUNDE FASIPE, KAMEELAH BROADWAY, MARJAN CHEGOUNCHI, LEONARD G. MEGGS, and ASHWANI MALHOTRA

Department of Medicine, Division of Nephrology, UMDNJ-New Jersey Medical School, 185 South Orange Avenue, Newark, New Jersey—07103, USA

Summary. The focus of this review will be recent advances in the molecular biology of protein kinase C (PKC) signaling in cardiac myocytes and the application of these novel techniques to study the pathobiology of diabetic cardiac myopathy. The PKC family of serine/threonine kinases have been implicated in a diverse array of biologic responses in health and disease. Compelling evidence has linked PKC signaling to hyperglycemia mediated cell injury. Although the cardiac myocyte has not been traditionally considered a major target cell for insulin, high ambient concentration of glucose promotes the activation of cardiac PKC isozymes, that target physiologically relevant intracellular substrates. The availability of genetically engineered mice, with targeted activation of distinct PKC isozyme (PKCε) in cardiac muscle cells and the development of selective peptide PKC modulators, provides an approach to examine PKC signaling events in the diabetic heart, and to explore the in vivo and in vitro consequences of this signaling cascade. The rapid growth of knowledge in this area is critical to the development of therapeutic strategies with the potential to arrest or reverse the progression of diabetic cardiomyopathy.

Key words: Protein Kinase C (PKC), Hyperglycemia, Diabetes Mellitus, Cardiac Myocytes, PKC Isozymes

Address for Correspondence: Ashwani Malhotra, PhD, Associate Professor, Division of Nephrology and Hypertension, Department of Medicine, MSB C-521, UMDNJ-New Jersey Medical School, 185 South Orange Avenue, Newark, New Jersey—07103. Phone: 973-972-1922; Fax: 973-972-3578; e-mail: malhotas@umdnj.edu

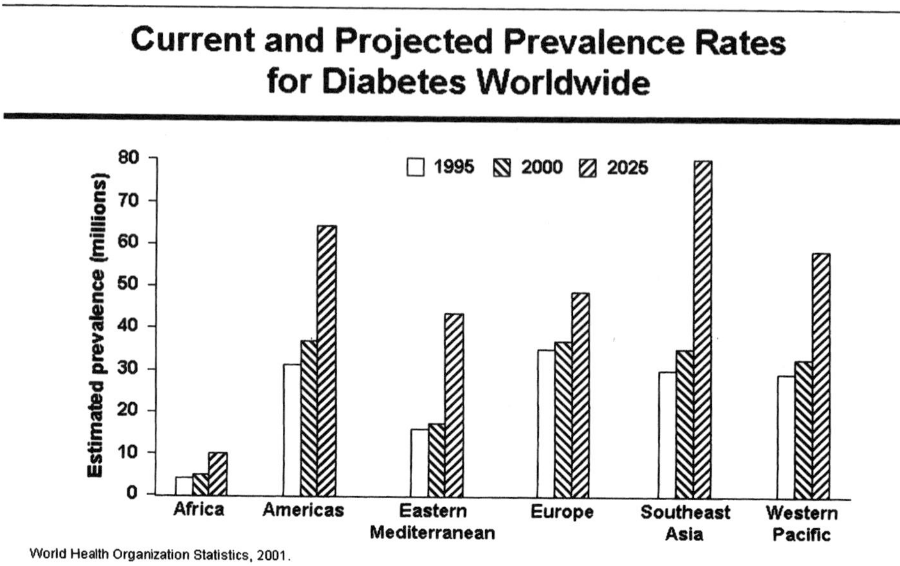

Figure 1. Data from the World Health Organization show that during the next 25 years, the diabetes epidemic is expected to grow in all regions, most markedly in the Americas, the Eastern Mediterranean, and Southeast Asia. The risk is greatest in areas where there is a high prevalence of low-birth-weight babies combined with dietary habits in later life that result in obesity and high body mass index.

INTRODUCTION

The term diabetes mellitus (DM) refers to a spectrum of syndromes ultimately leading to hyperglycemia. Each point along the line is associated with either an absolute or relative deficiency of insulin coupled with varying degree of peripheral resistance to the actions of insulin. In the United States it is estimated that more than 15.4 million persons are afflicted with DM of which only 60% have been diagnosed [1]. If the current worldwide trend (Fig. 1) continues it is estimated that more than 250 million will have the disorder by 2010. In 1998, the cost of DM to the medical care system in the United State was $104 billion, with projected increases of 10–12% per annum [1].

DM is classified as Type 1 or Type 2 based on age of onset and the presence or absence of insulin. Type 1 DM results from cell mediated destruction of the beta cells of pancreatic islets. Circulatory markers of destruction are autoantibodies to insulin, islet cells, glutamic acid decarboxylase (GAD) and several tyrosine phosphatases [2]. This disorder is strongly associated with the HLA system and influenced by linkages to the DQA, DQB and DRB [3]. Non-genetic factors also play a role since the rate of concordance of type 1 diabetes in monozygotic twins is less than 50%. Type 2 DM is a heterogeneous disorder that is characterized by a degree in insulin resistance and a defective beta cell secreting function. In the United States, 95% of patients have Type 2 DM. This disorder has a strong genetic basis, with a concordance among monozygotic twins approaching 100% [4].

Until recently, the existence of a distinct diabetic cardiomyopathy has been a matter of debate. However, the Framingham Heart Study documented significant correlation between DM and left ventricular mass and thickness in women [5,6]. Subsequent studies [7] have shown that DM also alters the mechanical performance of the heart, as evidenced by the presence of diastolic dysfunction and early modification of left ventricular structure and function. Carefully performed studies indicate the prevalence of diastolic dysfunction in patients with well-controlled Type 2 DM to be approximately 65% [8]. More recently, apoptosis or programmed cell death has also been reported in the diabetic heart [9,10]. Apoptosis, which is frequently not detected by routine morphological evaluation, is characterized by nuclear condensation, membrane blebbing and the formation of apoptotic bodies. Cell death by apoptosis is a tightly orchestrated event, under the control of genetic programs, which have been highly conserved during the evolutionary process. The molecular events that direct expression of the death signal and diastolic dysfunction in the diabetic heart have been the subject of intense investigation. Activation of the protein kinase C (PKC) family of serine/threonine kinases is a well-known intracellular signaling response following exposure to high ambient glucose concentration [11]. Before reviewing evidence of PKC signaling and the expression of the diabetic cardiac phenotype, it appropriates to highlight recent changes in the classification of PKC family members.

CLASSIFICATION OF PKC ISOZYMES

Currently, at least 12 PKC isozymes have been cloned [12], and individual isozymes have been implicated in such diverse cellular responses as proliferation, contractility, hypertrophy and apoptosis [13–21]. Expression of this family of serine/threonine kinases in myocardial tissue has been reported to be species dependent and developmentally regulated [22–24]. Adult rat ventricular myocytes (ARVM) co-express multiple PKC isozymes (α, β_1, β_2, δ, ε, and ζ), with PKCδ and ε, the major isozymes detected by immunoblotting [25]. Until recently, PKC isozymes were categorized under 3 categories, conventional (α, β_1/β_2 and γ), novel (δ, ε, η, and θ) and atypical (ζ and λ). A fourth subfamily, composed of two closely related isozymes (μ, ν), has recently been identified by cloning and sequence analysis [12]. PKC isozymes (Fig. 2) are characterized by the presence of highly conserved COOH-terminal kinase domains (C3/C4) while differing at NH_2-terminal regulatory regions (C1) [12,23]. Members of the conventional subfamily possess two NH_2-terminal regulatory domains (C1/C2), and require Ca^{2+}, phospholipids, diacylglycerol (DAG) or phorbol ester for activation [23]. The C1 domain binds DAG and phorbol esters, while the C2 domain binds anionic phospholipids in a Ca^{2+} dependent manner [12]. The novel PKC isozymes are structurally related to the conventional subfamily, differing by the absence of the Ca^{2+} binding domain. The atypical PKC isozymes are distinguished by deletion of the Ca^{2+} binding domain and resistance to activa-

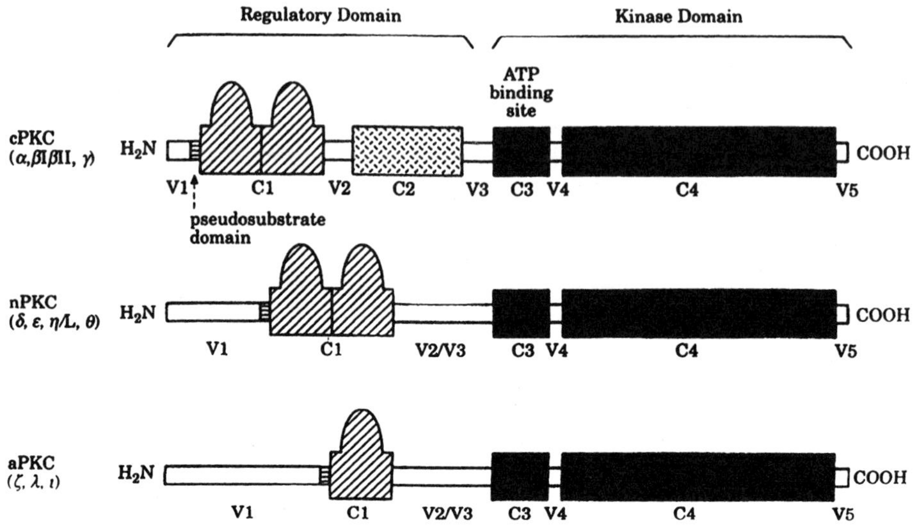

Figure 2. Schematic representation of the domain structure of PKC isoforms. Four conserved domains (C1–C4) and five variable domains (V1–V5) are identified. The C1 domain is divided into two parts corresponding to the two cysteine-rich zinc finger-like sequences. PKCμ, an additional member of the atypical PKC family with phorbol ester-independent kinase activity is not included in this schematic. PKCμ differs from other aPKCs in that it contains two cysteine-rich zinc finger-like domains which are unusually widely spaced. "Reproduced with permission from Molecular and Cellular Biochemistry, 225:97–107, 2001".

tion by DAG or phorbol esters [23,24,26]. Activating molecules for this subfamily include phosphatidylserine (PS) [27], phosphatidylinositol triphosphate (3,4,5-IP_3) [28] and the octapeptide angiotensin II [24]. The latter peptide has been reported to promote translocation of PKCζ in vascular smooth muscle cells [29] and cardiac myocytes [24]. A fourth subfamily has recently been established with the cloning of PKCν, which along with PKCμ, comprise the new grouping [12]. The cDNA of PKCν was isolated with the assistance of a search of the human expressed sequence tag database. Sequence analysis of the predicted gene product indicated a protein composed of 890 amino acid residues, and 77.3% homology with PKCμ [12]. At the COOH-terminus, the PKCν protein contains a pleckstrin homology (PH) sequence of amino acids (417–542), inserted between the cysteine-rich domain and catalytic domain. PH domains are present in a number of proteins involved in cell signaling events [30–33] and these regions of shared homology may serve to promote intra and intermolecular interactions [34]. Tissue expression of PKCν has been detected by Northern blot analysis in all adult tissues, including myocardium [12]. The ubiquitous expression of PKCν, suggest it may serve a basic house keeping function in cells.

HYPERGLYCEMIA ACTIVATES CARDIAC PKC ISOZYMES

Although in vivo models of human disease have served as a paradigm to study pathophysiology, limitations exist with respect to establishing cause and effect. ARVM co-express multiple PKC isozymes [23,35], increasing the complexity of determining the in vivo functional implications of PKC activation. As discussed above, DM is characterized by the development of a progressive cardiomyopathy that is independent of the vasculopathy [36–38]. However, the intracellular signaling events that promote expression of the diabetic cardiac phenotype have remained elusivc. Employing an in vitro system, in which ARVM are enzymatically dissociated from myocardial tissue, our laboratory [39; Fig. 3] has shown that 25 mM glucose is a potent stimulus for translocation and activation of cardiac PKC isozymes (β_1, β_2, δ, ε and ζ). Glucose induced PKC translocation was characterized by a delayed onset, requiring more than 1 hour of exposure to 25 mM glucose (Fig. 4). The latter property may serve to protect cardiac myocytes from transient glucose elevations, or reflect the time required for glucose-induced activation of signaling pathways involved in PKC translocation. Surprisingly, delayed onset of PKC translocation was followed by an impressive increase in the membrane immunoreactivity of several PKC isozymes. Importantly, translocation of PKCβ_1/β_2 and PKCε was sustained at 24 hours, suggesting these isozymes may be preferentially expressed in response to high ambient glucose concentration.

Although hyperglycemia dominates the pathophysiology of diabetes mellitus, the application of an in vitro system, to study the effects of high ambient glucose on isolated cardiac muscle cells has obvious limitations. However, the above findings provide the basis for an interesting comparison with those reported following in vivo exposure to hyperglycemia. Our findings [39] differ somewhat from those reported in whole heart tissue from STZ diabetic rats, in which an increase in the membrane association of one or several of the following isozymes, PKCα, β_2, δ, and ε, has been reported [40–43]. Differences between our results and those reported in whole heart tissue from STZ diabetic rats may reflect physiological changes associated with the in vivo diabetic state, such as increased PKCα expression in the non-myocyte compartment of the myocardium [43]. It must also be acknowledged that chronic exposure to high glucose concentration may result in downregulation in the expression of some, but not all PKC isozymes. As a case in point, Malhotra and colleagues [41] employing the STZ model reported that only cardiac PKCε exhibited evidence of sustained translocation and activation. However, this study was limited to PKCδ and ε, and did not attempt to characterize the response of cardiac PKC isozymes to high glucose, or the signaling events by which glucose promotes PKC translocation. Moreover, compelling evidence has also been presented for the activation of PKCβ_2 as a determinant of cardiac phenotype in diabetic rats [44]. The pathogenic role of PKCβ_2 was confirmed by demonstrating prevention of the histological and functional lesions, in mice treated with a selective PKCβ isoform inhibitor [44]. Moreover, transgenic mice with targeted overexpression of the PKCβ_2

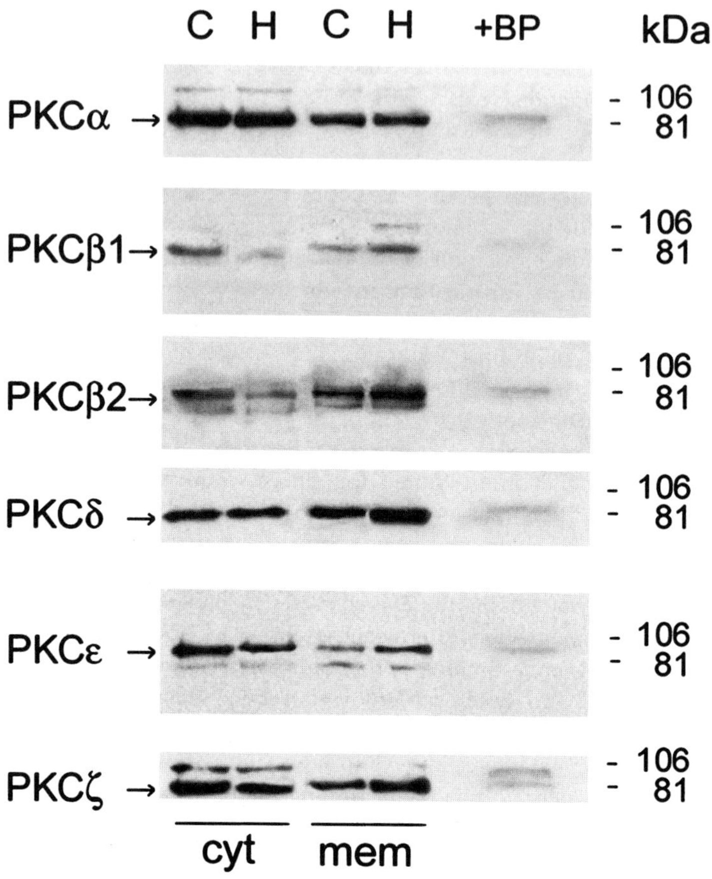

Figure 3. Representative Western Blot analysis of PKCα, β_1, β_2, δ, ε and ζ showing translocation from cytosolic (cyt) to membrane (mem) fraction. These fractions were extracted from cardiac myocytes exposed to 5 mM (C) and 25 mM (H) glucose for 12 hours. The quantity of protein loaded was 25 μg (cytosolic) and 50 μg (membrane). Blocking peptides (+BP) for each of the isozymes are also shown. "Copyright© 2001 American Diabetes Association From Diabetes, Vol 50, 2001; 1918–1926; Reprinted with permission from *The American Diabetes Association*".

isozyme in cardiac myocytes, exhibit a cardiac phenotype characterized by left ventricular hypertrophy, myocyte necrosis, multifocal fibrosis and impaired left ventricular performance [15]. Taken together, the available evidence indicates that high ambient glucose concentration is a potent stimulus for the redistribution of cardiac PKC isozymes, and suggests a role for multiple isozymes in the signaling events that result in the expression of the diabetic cardiac phenotype.

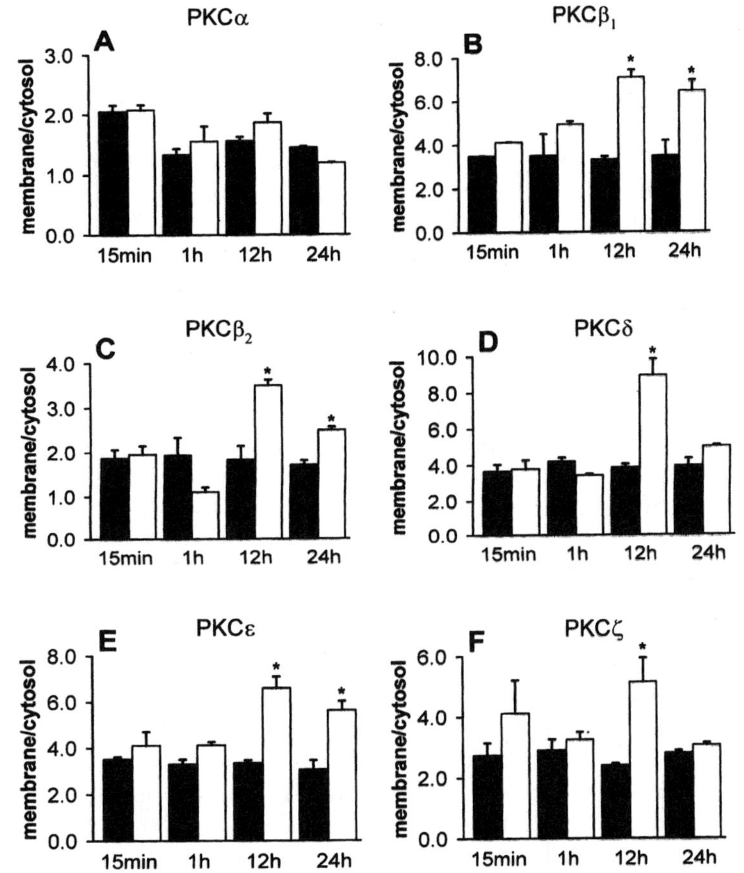

Figure 4. Time course for translocation of PKC isozymes (Fig. 4:A–F) in adult rat ventricular myocytes exposed to 5 mM glucose (■) and 25 mM glucose (□). Membrane immunoreactivity for PKCβ_1, β_2, δ, ε and ζ was increased following exposure to 25 mM glucose for 12 hours. The response was sustained for PKCβ_1, β_2 and ε at 24 hours. Data points represent 2–4 independent observations. Group comparisons: ⋆ represents 5 mM glucose *vs* 25 mM glucose; ⋆ = $p \leq 0.05$. "Copyright© 2001 American Diabetes Association From Diabetes, Vol 50, 2001; 1918–1926; Reprinted with permission from *The American Diabetes Association*".

MECHANISM(S) OF GLUCOSE INDUCED PKC ACTIVATION

Multiple lines of evidence have implicated activation of the phospholipase C, and the generation of the phospholipid DAG, as the mechanism of PKC translocation in response to hyperglycemia [45–48]. Our laboratory [41] and others [47,49–52], have reported that pathologic stimuli such as hyperglycemia, hypoxia and oxidative stress, may promote PKC translocation via alternate pathways or by direct activation. We have recently demonstrated that in vitro exposure of ARVM to 25 mM glucose, in the presence of the phospholipase C inhibitor, D609, did not prevent subcellular redistribution of PKCβ_1 and PKCε (Fig. 5). This result was somewhat unexpected since DAG is a phospholipid activator of PKCβ_1 and ε, and suggests that 25 mM glucose recruits these isozymes through alternate signaling pathways. In contrast, D609 blocked the translocation of PKCβ_2, δ, and ζ (Fig. 5). These findings indicate that 25 mM glucose redistributes these isozymes through a pathway involving phospholipase C. It should be noted that at concentrations less than 100 μM, D609 failed to inhibit translocation of PKCβ_2, δ, and ζ. The dose of D609 required to demonstrate a partial inhibitory effect on glucose induced redistribution of PKC isozymes, may reflect initial activation of phospholipase C in the presence of 25 mM glucose. Alternatively, D609 has been reported to exhibit a higher affinity for phosphatidylcholine-specific phospholipase C than phosphatidylinositol-specific phospholipase C [50]. However, the selectivity of D609 for the latter enzyme has been documented in vitro, under conditions of agonist and stretch dependent activation of phospholipase C [53,54]. It must also be recognized that higher doses of inhibitors may be required to block translocation of PKC isozymes in response to noxious external stimuli. For example, 100 μM of D609 was required to inhibit cardiac PKC translocation in response to ANG II and hypoxia, but failed to attenuate PKC redistribution in response to oxidative stress [35]. Interestingly, a cause and effect relationship between hyperglycemia induced generation of reactive oxygen species (ROS), and activation of PKC has recently been documented [55]. Two main sites for the generation of ROS have been identified at the inner mitochondria membrane: the NADH dehydrogenase at complex I, and the interface between ubiquinone and complex III. The tricarboxylic acid cycle provides the substrate for glucose induced ROS generation. The overproduction of ROS in response to hyperglycemia was inhibited by interventions that block transport of electrons at complex I or uncouple oxidative phosphorylation. Normalizing levels of mitochondrial ROS has been shown to prevent glucose-induced activation of PKC [56], implicating altered redox status as a trigger for PKC signaling under hyperglycemic conditions.

In a recent communication [39], our laboratory (Fig. 6) has reported that exposure of ARVM to 25 mM glucose provokes the release of angiotensin II (ANG II), coupled with angiotensin II type-1 receptor (AT-1R)-dependent redistribution of PKC isozymes. The application of physical forces, such as mechanical stretch, to in vitro cultures of cardiac myocytes, has been reported to be a stimulus for the release of ANG II [57]. Our finding that 25 mM glucose provokes the release of ANG II, implies that these discordant external stimuli may activate a common pathway. Alternatively, release of ANG II from cardiac myocytes may be coupled with increased intracellular generation of this peptide. To determine if glucose induced release of ANG II is coupled with the activation of ANG II signal transduction pathways that promote PKC translocation, the selective AT-1R antagonist, losartan, was added to cultures of freshly isolated ARVM maintained at 25 mM glucose concentration. Losartan completely reversed translocation of PKC-β_1, β_2, δ and ε (Fig. 7). Conversely, the selective angiotensin II type-2 receptor (AT-2R) antagonist, PD 123,319,

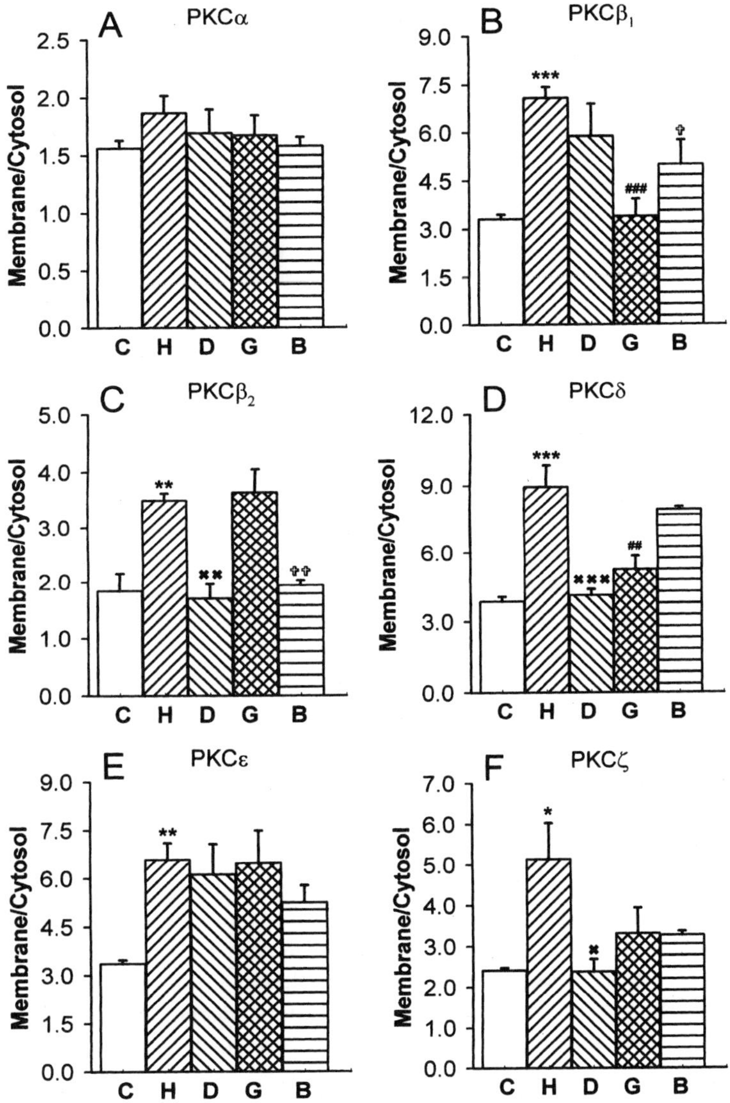

Figure 5. Effect of D609, genistein and BAPTA/AM on translocation of PKC isozymes (Fig. 5:A–F) in adult rat ventricular myocytes exposed to 25 mM glucose for 12 hours. Note that none of the inhibitors had a uniform inhibitory effect on PKC translocation. D609 completely reversed PKCβ_2, δ and ζ. Genistein blocked translocation of PKCβ_1 and δ. BAPTA/AM inhibited translocation of PKCβ_1 and β_2. C = 5 mM glucose; H = 25 mM glucose; D = 25 mM glucose + D609 (100 μM); G = 25 mM glucose + Genistein (100 μM) and B = 25 mM glucose + BAPTA/AM (25 μM). Data points represent 3–5 independent observations. * represents C *vs* H; × represents H *vs* D; # represents H *vs* G and + represents H *vs* B. * *or* × *or* ✞ = $p \leq 0.05$; ** *or* ×× *or* ## *or* ✞✞ = $p \leq 0.01$; *** *or* ××× *or* ### = $p \leq 0.001$. "Copyright© 2001 American Diabetes Association From Diabetes, Vol 50, 2001; 1918–1926; Reprinted with permission from *The American Diabetes Association*".

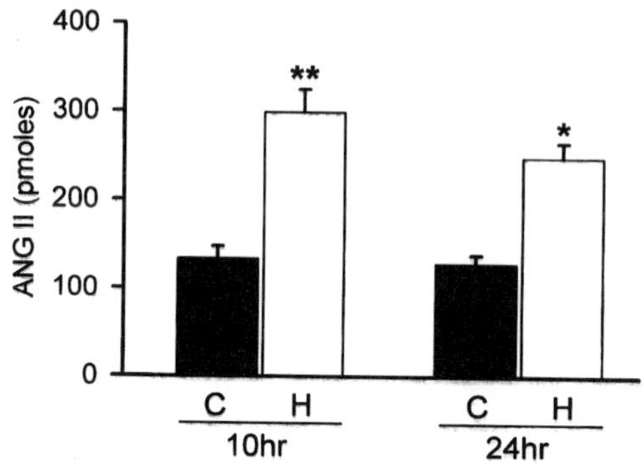

Figure 6. Effect of 5 mM (■) and 25 mM (□) glucose on ANG II release from adult rat ventricular myocytes at 10 and 24 hours. Data represent 6–10 independent observations. C = 5 mM glucose and H = 25 mM glucose. Group comparisons: * represents C *vs* H. * = $p \leq 0.05$; ** = $p \leq 0.001$. "Copyright© 2001 American Diabetes Association From Diabetes, Vol 50, 2001; 1918–1926; Reprinted with permission from *The American Diabetes Association*".

did not alter the redistribution of PKC isozymes in response to 25 mM glucose (Fig. 8).

COMPARTMENTALIZATION FACILITATES PKC: SUBSTRATE INTERACTION

In the presence of an activating signal, PKC isozymes bind to specific anchoring proteins, collectively known as receptors for activated C kinases (RACKS) [58,59]. The molecular weight of RACKS purified from rat heart and brain are in the range of 30–36kDa [58,59]. RACKS engage their respective PKC isozymes at a site distinct from the substrate-binding domain (Fig. 9). This interaction facilitates the compartmentalization of PKC isozymes at locations within the cell, such as the nucleus, cytoplasm and cytoskeleton that are in close proximity to target substrates. The identification of evolutionary conserved sequences within the interacting domain of PKC isozymes, and detection of autoregulatory sites at the regulatory domain, have provided the background to explore conformational adaptations of the PKC molecule, in the active and quiescent state [34]. The initial description of autoregulatory sites [60] was instrumental in the identification of the pseudo-substrate sequence. The latter motifs mediate intramolecular interactions by linking the regulatory and catalytic domains, maintaining kinases in an inactive state [60]. Mochly-Rosen and co-workers [52,53,61], have capitalized on the above observation to develop synthetic peptides corresponding to the pseudo-substrate sequence that may induce or inhibit endogenous PKC activity. Peptides that stabilize the interaction between pseudo-substrate and RACK binding sites of PKC isozymes, promote the inactive conformational alignment, in which the catalytic domain is concealed [34,60]. The unique binding interactions of individual PKC isozymes with their respective RACKS [58,59] has made it possible to design peptide modulators with a high degree of selectivity and specificity [52,53]. Thus far, the most compelling

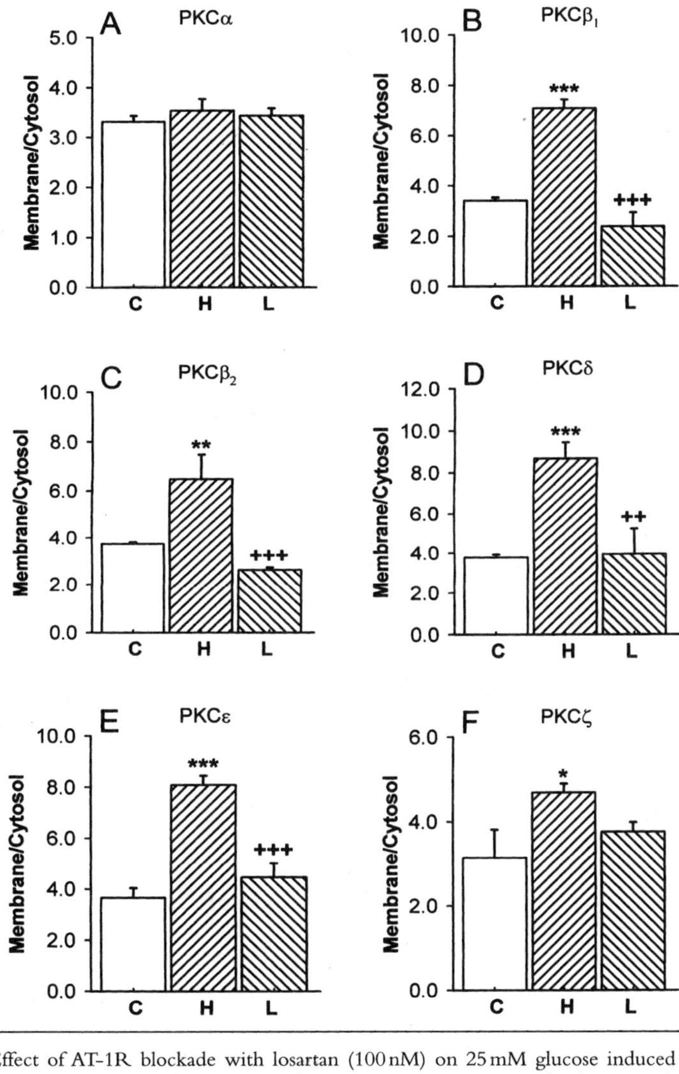

Figure 7. Effect of AT-1R blockade with losartan (100 nM) on 25 mM glucose induced PKC translocation (Fig. 7:A–F) in adult rat ventricular myocytes. Losartan completely reversed translocation of PKCβ_1, β_2 and ε. C = 5 mM glucose; H = 25 mM glucose; L = 25 mM glucose + losartan (100 nM). Data represent 3–6 independent observations. Group comparisons: * represents C *vs* H and + represents H *vs* L. * = $p \le 0.05$; ** *or* ++ = $p \le 0.01$; *** *or* +++ = $p \le 0.001$. "Copyright© 2001 American Diabetes Association From Diabetes, Vol 50, 2001; 1918–1926; Reprinted with permission from *The American Diabetes Association*".

evidence demonstrating the efficacy of this approach has been the application of synthetic peptides to modulate PKCε translocation, in cardiac myocytes [52,61]. For example, the octapeptide antagonist εV1, is derived from the first unique region (V1) of PKCε, which is comprised of 142 amino acids [34]. A recombinant εV1

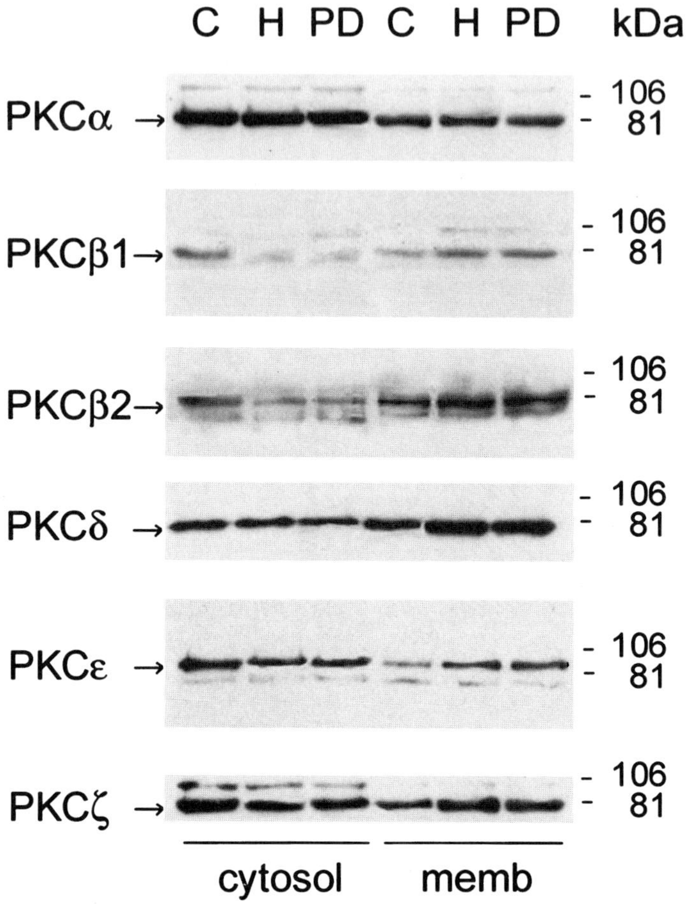

Figure 8. Representative Western Blot analysis of PKCα, β_1, β_2, δ, ε and ζ showing translocation from cytosolic (cytosol) to membrane (memb) fraction. These fractions were extracted from cardiac myocytes exposed to 5 mM (C), 25 mM (H) glucose and 25 mM glucose + 100 nM AT-2R blocker, PD123,319 (PD), for 12 hours. AT-2R blocker did not inhibit the translocation of PKCβ_1, β_2, δ, ε and ζ. The quantity of protein loaded was 25 μg (cytosolic) and 50 μg (membrane).

fragment was shown to selectively inhibit agonist and phorbol ester induced PKCε translocation [52] whereas, activation of other cardiac PKC isozymes was not affected by this peptide. A similar strategy has been utilized to identify short sequences of homology between PKC isozymes and their respective RACKS [61], to interfere with intra-molecular interactions, and promote the active PKC conformation [34]. A decided advantage of this approach is the selective modification of PKC activity, in an isozyme specific manner [62]. The peptide ζε-RACK, was devel-

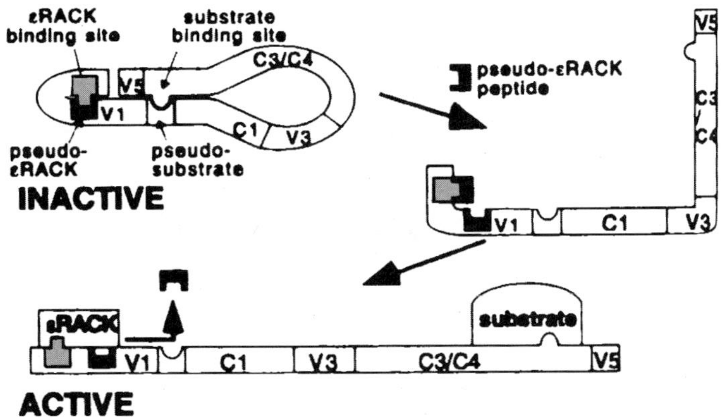

Figure 9. Model of the pseudo-εRACK site in the inactive and active forms of PKCε and the putative mode of action of the pseudo-εRACK peptide as agonist. An intramolecular association is shown between inactive PKCε and the pseudo-εRACK site at the V1 domain of PKCε. In addition, an intramolecular interaction is depicted between the substrate binding site of PKCε and the pseudo-substrate site, and between the V1 and V5 domains. In the presence of the pseudo-εRACK peptide, spontaneous dissociation of the pseudo-εRACK site is postulated to occur, promoting transition to the active form of PKCε. Replacing the pseudo-εRACK peptide with εRACK, completes the transition to active PKCε. "Reproduced with permission from Molecular and Cellular Biochemistry, 225:97–107, 2001".

oped as the first isozyme-selective PKC agonist [59,63]. ζε-RACK promotes translocation of PKCε, by displacing the pseudo-εRACK sequence, facilitating the interaction of PKCε with its corresponding RACK. This approach has also been employed to generate PKCε transgenic mice [52].

GLUCOSE INDUCED PHOSPHORYLATION OF TROPONIN I IS PKC DEPENDENT

An important limitation of previous studies concerning the physiologic effects and phenotypic expression of PKC signals has been the identification of target substrates. Translocation and activation of PKC isozymes may not be concurrent events, and the extent and duration of PKC redistribution may not be an index of PKC activity [64]. To determine whether exposure of ARVM to 25 mM glucose promotes both translocation and activation of PKC isozymes, our laboratory [39] examined the phosphorylation status of troponin I (TnI). Although this sarcomeric protein is known to be a substrate for several PKC isozymes, PKC-β_2 and ε, have been reported to preferentially target TnI in the diabetic myocardium [65]. *In vitro* studies performed with TnI mutants [66], have identified several phosphorylation sites for PKC isozymes and indicate that the critical residues responsible for reduced Ca^{2+} sensitivity and ATPase activity, are located at ser-43/ser-45. Our results clearly indicate an upregulation of TnI phosphorylation, when ARVM are exposed to 25 mM glucose for 12–24 hours. Stoichiometrically, the TnI protein was found to exhibit a comparatively greater increase in the phosphorylation of serine than thre-

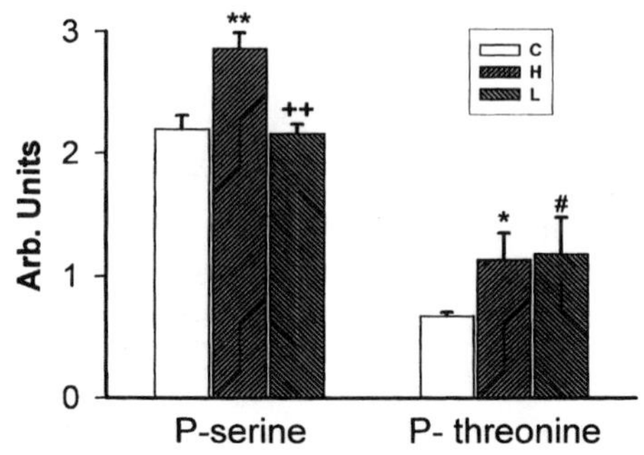

Figure 10. Effect of losartan (100 nM) on 25 mM glucose induced phosphorylation of TnI. Losartan selectively blocked phosphorylation of TnI serine residues, but did not inhibit threonine phosphorylation. C = 5 mM glucose; H = 25 mM glucose; L = 25 mM glucose + losartan (100 nM). Data represent 5–8 independent observations. Group comparisons: * represents C *vs* H; + represents H *vs* L and # represents C *vs* L. * *or* # = $p \leq 0.05$ and ** *or* ++ = $p \leq 0.01$.

onine residues. Interestingly, losartan completely reversed serine phosphorylation, but had no detectable effect on the phosphorylation of threonine residues (Fig. 10). The latter observation implies that activated PKC isozymes differentially target serine/threonine residues on TnI, with the AT-1R dependent isozymes, PKC-β_1, β_2, δ and ε, exclusively phosphorylating TnI serine residues. Although our laboratory has focused on the interaction between PKC and the TnI protein, high ambient concentrations of glucose promote the redistribution of several PKC isozymes, potentially affecting multiple biological functions of the diabetic myocardium. For example, PKC-ε has been reported to confer protection against cell death by hypoxia [53], and to promote ischemic preconditioning of cardiac myocytes [67]. The latter properties may prove to be extremely valuable in determining the balance between cell death and cell survival in the diabetic heart.

PKC ISOZYMES AND CELL SURVIVAL

Recently, evidence has emerged documenting specific signaling from PKC isozymes to mitogen activated protein kinase (MAPK) cascades [68,69]. Constitutively active mutants of PKC δ and ε, were introduced into myocytes, by infection with replication deficient adenoviral vectors [69], to determine if these isozymes differentially activate distinct members of the MAPK family (ERK, JNK, p38^{MAPK}), and whether overexpression of PKCδ or ε was sufficient to induce apoptosis. The results provide evidence in support of the notion that PKC dependent signals target distinct subfamilies of MAPK. For example, PKCε overexpression was found to be coupled with activation of ERK, whereas infection with PKCδ induced activation of JNK p38 sub-families of MAPK. Interestingly, overexpression of PKCδ, was found to induce apoptosis, whereas, PKCε was cytoprotective. The mechanism of PKCε

cyto-protection was not specifically addressed, although overexpression of PKCδ was noted to result in a time dependent decrease in endogenous PKCε levels. Alternatively, ERK dependent signals have been reported to protect against apoptosis in a number of cell lines [70–72], and PKCε recruitment of the ERK module may activate a survival program in cardiac myocytes [69]. ERK dependent signals have been reported to target serine residues of the anti-apoptotic Bcl-2 protein, providing a molecular basis for transmission of survival signals by this pathway [73,74]. Conversely, activation of the JNK and p38 subfamilies has been reported to induce cell death by apoptosis [75,76]. An important limitation of previous work demonstrating the cardiotrophic and survival phenotypes induced by PKCε dependent signals [52,53,58,59] concerns the identity of downstream effectors targeted by the activated isozyme.

Finally, the mitochondria are key determinants of cell death and cell survival [77]. Cytochrome c release by mitochondria and depolarization of the mitochondria membrane potential are crucial events in triggering oxidant induced myocyte apoptosis [78]. In contrast, pharmacologic activation of the mitoK^{+}_{ATP} channel has recently been reported to precondition myocytes to ROS [79], and more specifically, inhibit apoptosis induced by oxidative stress. Since PKC is an important component of the signaling cascade that confers ischemic preconditioning-induced cardio-protection [52], and directly linked to the survival pathway coupled with the activation of mitoK^{+}_{ATP}, it seem reasonable to suggest that PKC isozymes may protect against glucose induced ROS death signals by this mechanism. Future investigations to test this hypothesis should provide yet another dimension to the multiple biologic events modulated by the PKC family of isozymes.

ACKNOWLEDGEMENTS

This work was partially supported by research grant from "Foundation of UMDNJ Annual Grants Program (A.M)" and the support from Summit Area Public Foundation through the generosity of Mrs. Elaine B. Burnett Fund.

REFERENCES

1. Report of the expert committee on the diagnosis and classification of diabetes mellitus. 2000. Diabetes Care 23(Suppl 1):S4–S19.
2. Garcia MJ, McNamara PM, Gordon T, Kannel WB. 1974. Morbidity and mortality in the Framingham population sixteen-year follow-up study. Diabetes 23:105–111.
3. Kannel WB, McGee DL. 1979. Diabetes and Cardiovascular diseases. The Framingham Heart Study. JAMA 241:2035–2038.
4. Galderisi M, Anderson KM, Wilson PWF, Levy D. 1991. Echocardiographic Evidence for the Existence of a Distinct Diabetic Cardiomyopathy. (The Framingham Heart Study) Am J Cardiol 68:85–89.
5. Ruderman NB, Haudenschild C. 1974. Diabetes as an artherogenic factor. Prog Cardiovasc Dis 26:272–412.
6. Geiss LS, Herman WH, Smith PJ. 1995. In Diabetes in America. National Diabetes Data Group Report. NIDDK, Bethesda, MD, 233–257.
7. Liu JE, Palmieri V, Roman MJ, Bella JN, Fabsitz R, Howard BV, Welty TK, Lee ET, Devereux RB. 2001. The impact of diabetes on left ventricular filling pattern in normotensive and hypertensive adults: the Strong Heart Study. J Am Coll Cardiol 37:1943–1949.

8. Zabalgoitia M, Ismaeil MF, Anderson L, Maklady FA. 2001. Prevalence of diastolic dysfunction in normotensive, asymptomatic patients with well-controlled type 2 diabetes mellitus. Am J Cardiol 87:320–323.
9. Fiordaliso F, Li B, Latini R, Sonnenblick EH, Anversa P, Leri A, Kajstura J. 2000. Myocyte death in streptozotocin-induced diabetes in rats is angiotensin II dependent. Lab Invest 80:513–527.
10. Fiordaliso F, Leri A, Cesselli D, Limana F, Safai B, Nadal-Ginard B, Anversa P, Kajstura J. 2001. Hyperglycemia activates p53 and p53-regulated genes leading to myocyte cell death. Diabetes 50:2363–2375.
11. Williams B. 1995. Glucose-induced vascular smooth muscle dysfunction: the role of protein kinase C. J Hypertens 13:477–486.
12. Hayashi A, Seki N, Hattori A, Kozuma S, Saito T. 1999. PKCν a new member of the protein kinase C family, composes a fourth subfamily with PKCμ. Biochim Biophys Acta 1450:99–106.
13. Wikman-Coffelt J, Wu ST, Parmley WW, Mason DT. 1991. Angiotensin II and phorbol esters depress cardiac performance and decrease diastolic and systolic Ca^{2+} in isolated perfused rat hearts. Am Heart J 122:786–794.
14. Bowling N, Walsh RA, Song G, Estridge T, Sandusky GE, Fouts RL, Mintze K, Pickard T, Roden R, Bristow MR, Sabbah HN, Mizrahi JL, Gromo G, King GL, Vlahos CJ. 1999. Increased protein kinase C activity and expression of Ca^{2+}-sensitive isoforms in the failing human heart. Circulation 99:384–391.
15. Wakasaki H, Koya D, Schoen FJ, Jirousek MR, Ways DK, Hoit BD, Walsh RA, King GL. 1997. Targeted overexpression of protein kinase C β_2 isoform in myocardium causes cardiomyopathy. Proc Natl Acad Sci U S A 94:9320–9325.
16. Barr LF, Campbell SE, Baylin SB. 1997. Protein kinase C-β_2 inhibits cycling and decreases c-myc-induced apoptosis in small cell lung cancer cells. Cell Growth Differ 8:381–392.
17. Berra E, Municio MM, Sanz L, Frutos S, Diaz-Meco MT, Moscat J. 1997. Positioning atypical protein kinase C isoforms in the UV-induced apoptotic signaling cascade. Mol Cell Biol 17:4346–4354.
18. Emoto Y, Kisaki H, Manome Y, Kharbanda S, Kufe D. 1996. Activation of protein kinase Cδ in human myeloid leukemia cells treated with 1-beta-D-arabinofuranosylcytosine. Blood 87:1990–1996.
19. Murray NR, Fields AP. 1997. Atypical protein kinase C_ι protects human leukemia cells against drug-induced apoptosis. J Biol Chem 272:27521–27524.
20. Kajstura J, Cigola E, Malhotra A, Li P, Cheng W, Meggs LG, Anversa P. 1997. Angiotensin II induces apoptosis of adult ventricular myocytes in vitro. J Mol Cell Cardiol 29:859–870.
21. Ron D, Mochly-Rosen D. 1995. An autoregulatory region in protein kinase C: the pseudoanchoring site. Proc Natl Acad Sci USA 92:492–496.
22. Rybin VO, Steinberg SF. 1994. Protein kinase C isoform expression and regulation in the developing rat heart. Circ Res 74:299–309.
23. Steinberg SF, Goldberg M, Rybin VO. 1995. Protein kinase C isoform diversity in the heart. J Mol Cell Cardiol 27:141–153.
24. Takeishi Y, Jalili T, Ball NA, Walsh RA. 1999. PKC translocation without changes in Galphaq and PLC-beta protein abundance in cardiac hypertrophy and failure. Am J Physiol 277:H2298–H2304.
25. Naruse K, King GL. 2000. Protein kinase C and myocardial biology and function. Circ Res 86:1104–1106.
26. Dutil EM, Toker A, Newton AC. 1998. Regulation of conventional protein kinase C isozymes by phosphoinositide-dependent kinase 1 (PDK-1). Curr Biol 8:1366–1375.
27. Gschwendt M, Leibersperger H, Kittstein W, Marks F. 1992. Protein kinase Cζ and ε in murine epidermis. TPA induces down-regulation of PKC ε but not PKC ζ. FEBS Lett 307:151–155.
28. Nakanishi H, Brewer KA, Exton JH. 1993. Activation of the ζ isozyme of protein kinase C by phosphatidylinositol 3,4,5-trisphosphate. J Biol Chem 268:13–16.
29. Liao DF, Monia B, Dean N, Berk BC. 1997. Protein kinase C-ζ mediates angiotensin II activation of ERK1/2 in vascular smooth muscle cells. J Biol Chem 272:6146–6150.
30. Haslam RJ, Koide HB, Hemmings BA. 1993. Pleckstrin domain homology. Nature 363:309–310.
31. Mayer BJ, Ren R, Clark KL, Baltimore D. 1993. A putative modular domain present in diverse signaling proteins. Cell 73:629–630.
32. Gibson TJ, Hyvonen M, Musacchio A, Saraste M, Birney E. 1994. PH domain: the first anniversary. Trends Biochem Sci 19:349–353.
33. Lemmon MA, Ferguson KM, Schlessinger J. 1996. PH domains: diverse sequences with a common fold recruit signaling molecules to the cell surface. Cell 85:621–624.
34. Souroujon MC, Mochly-Rosen D. 1998. Peptide modulators of protein-protein interactions in intracellular signaling. Nat Biotechnol 16:919–924.

35. Takeishi Y, Jalili T, Ball NA, Walsh RA. 1999. Responses of cardiac protein kinase C isoforms to distinct pathological stimuli are differentially regulated. Circ Res 85:264–271.
36. Rodrigues B, Cam MC, McNeill JH. 1998. Metabolic disturbances in diabetic cardiomyopathy. Mol Cell Biochem 180:53–57.
37. Rodrigues B, McNeill JH. 1992. The diabetic heart: Metabolic causes for the development of a cardiomyopathy. Cardiovasc Res 26:913–922.
38. Bell DSH. 1995. Diabetic cardiomyopathy: A unique entity or a complication of coronary artery disease? Diabetes Care 18:708–714.
39. Malhotra A, Kang BPS, Cheung S, Opawumi D, Meggs LG. 2001. Angiotensin II promotes glucose-induced activation of cardiac protein kinase C isozymes and phosphorylation of troponin I. Diabetes 50:1918–1926.
40. Inoguchi T, Battan R. Handler E, Sportsman JR, Heath W, King GL. 1992. Preferential elevation of protein kinase C isoform beta II and diacylglycerol levels in the aorta and heart of diabetic rats: Differentail reversiblity to glycemic control by islet cell transplantation. Proc Natl Acad Sci USA 89:11059–11063.
41. Malhotra A, Reich D, Nakouzi A, Sanghi V, Geenen DL, Buttrrick PM. 1997. Experimental diabetes is associated with functional activation of protein kinase Cε and phosphorylation of troponin I in the heart, which are prevented by angiotensin II receptor blockade. Circ Res 81:1027–1033.
42. Giles TD, Ouyang J, Kerut EK, Given MB, Allen GE, McIlwain EF, Greenberg SS. 1998. Changes in protein kinase C in early cardiomyopathy and in gracilis muscle in the BB/Wor diabetic rat. Am J Physiol 274:H295–H307.
43. Kang N, Alexander G, Park JK, Maasch C, Buchwalow I, Luft FC, Haller H. 1999. Differential expression of protein kinase C isoforms in streptozotocin-induced diabetic rats. Kidney Int 56:1737–1750.
44. Ishii H, Jirousek MR, Koya D, Takagi C, Xia P, Clermont A, Bursell SE, Kern TS, Ballas LM, Heat WF, Stramm LE, Feener EP, King GL. 1996. Amelioration of vascular dysfunction in diabetic rats by an oral PKCβ inhibitor. Science 272:728–731.
45. Haller H, Baur E, Quass P, Behrend M, Lindschau C, Distler A, Luft FC. 1995. High glucose concentrations and protein kinase C isoforms in vascular smooth muscle cells. Kidney Int 47:1057–1067.
46. Shiba T, Inoguchi T, Sportsman JR, Heath WF, Bursell S, King GL. 1993. Correlation of diacylglycerol level and protein kinase C activity in rat retinal circulation. Am J Physiol 265:E783–E793.
47. Xia P, Inoguchi T, Kern TS, Engerman RL, Oates PJ, King GL. 1994. Characterization of the mechanism for the chronic activation of diacylglycerol-protein kinase C pathway in diabetes and hypergalactocemia. Diabetes, 43:1122–1129.
48. Ayo SH, Radnik R, Garoni JA, Troyer DA, Kreisberg JI. 1991. High glucose increases diacylglycerol mass and activates protein kinase C in mesangial cell cultures. Am J Physiol 261:F571–F577.
49. Gu X, Bishop SP. 1994. Increased protein kinase C and isozyme redistribution in pressure-overload cardiac hypertrophy in the rat. Circ Res 75:926–931.
50. Goldberg M, Zhang HL, Steinberg SF. 1997. Hypoxia alters the subcellular distribution of protein kinase C isoforms in neonatal rat ventricular myocytes. J Clin Invest 99:55–61.
51. Mochly-Rosen D, Wu G, Hahn H, Osinska H, Liron T, Lorenz JN, Yatani A, Robbins J, Dorn GW II. 2000. Cardiotrophic effects of protein kinase C epsilon: analysis by in vivo modulation of PKC epsilon translocation. Circ Res 86:1173–1179.
52. Gray MO, Karliner JS, Mochly-Rosen D. 1997. A selective ε-protein kinase C antagonist inhibits protection of cardiac myocytes from hypoxia-induced cell death. J Biol Chem 272:30945–30951.
53. Jiang T, Kuznetsov V, Pak E, Zhang H, Robinson RB, Steinberg SF. 1996. Thrombin receptor actions in neonatal rat ventricular myocytes. Circ Res 78:553–563.
54. Sadoshima J, Izumo S. 1993. Mechanical stretch rapidly activates multiple signal transduction pathways in cardiac myocytes: potential involvement of an autocrine/paracrine mechanism. EMBO J 12:1681–1692.
55. Nishikawa T, Edelstein D, Du XL, Yamagishi S, Matsumura T, Kaneda Y, Yorek MA, Beebe D, Oates PJ, Hammes HP, Giardino I, Brownlee M. 2000. Normalizing mitochondrial superoxide overproduction blocks three pathways of hyperglycemic damage. Nature 404:787–790.
56. Lando D, Pongratz I, Whitelaw ML. 2000. A redox mechanism controls differential DNA binding activities of hypoxia-inducible factor [HIF] 1δ abd the HIF-like factor. J Biol Chem 275:4618–4627.
57. Leri A, Claudio PP, Li Q, Wang X, Reiss K, Wang S, Malhotra A, Kajstura J, Anversa P. 1998. Stretch-mediated release of angiotensin II induces myocyte apoptosis by activating p53 that enhances the local renin angiotensin system and decreases the Bcl-2-to-Bax ratio in the cell. J Clin Invest 101:1326–1342.

58. Mochly-Rosen D, Gordon AS. 1998. Anchoring proteins for protein kinase C: a means for isozyme selectivity. FASEB J 12:35–42.
59. Mochly-Rosen D. 1995. Localization of protein kinases by anchoring proteins: a theme in signal transduction. Science 268:247–251.
60. Kobe B, Heirerhorst J, Kemp BE. 1997. Intrasteric regulation of protein kinases. Adv Sec Mess Phosphoprot Res 31:29–40.
61. Johnson JA, Gray MO, Chen CH, Mochly-Rosen D. 1996. A protein kinase C translocation inhibitor as an isozyme-selective antagonsit of cardiac function. J Biol Chem 271:24962–24966.
62. Malhotra A, Kang BPS, Opawumi D, Belizaire W, Meggs LG. 2001. Molecular biology of protein kinase C signaling in cardiac myocytes. Mol Cell Biochem 225:97–107.
63. Dorn GW 2nd, Souroujon MC, Liron T, Chen CH, Gray MO, Zhou HZ, Csukai M, Wu G, Lorenz JN, Mochly-Rosen D. 1999. Sustained in vivo cardiac protection by a rationally designed peptide that causes ε protein kinase C translocation. Proc Natl Acad Sci USA 96:12798–12803.
64. Trilivas I, McDonough PM, Brown JH. 1991. Dissociation of protein kinase C redistribution from the phosphorylation of its substrates. J Biol Chem 266:8431–8438.
65. Takeishi Y, Chu G, Kirkpatrick DM, Li Z, Wakasaki H, Kranias EG, King GL, Walsh RA. 1998. In vivo phosphorylation of cardiac troponin I by protein kinase Cβ2 decreases cardiomyocyte calcium responsiveness and contractility in transgenic mouse hearts. J Clin Invest 102:72–78.
66. Jideama NM, Noland TA Jr, Raynor RL, Blobe GC, Fabbro D, Kazanietz MG, Blumberg PM, Hannun YA, Kuo JF. 1996. Phosphorylation specificities of protein kinase C isozymes for bovine cardiac troponin I and troponin T and sites within these proteins and regulation of myofilament properties. J Biol Chem 271:23277–23283.
67. Goto M, Cohen MV, Downey JM. 1996. The role of protein kinase C in ischemic preconditioning. Ann N Y Acad Sci 793:177–190.
68. Clerk A, Sugden PH. 2001.Untangling the web: Specific signaling form PKC isoforms to MAPK cascades. Circ Res. 89:847–849.
69. Heidkamp MC, Bayer AL, Martin JL, Samarel AM. 2001.Differential activation of mitogen-activated protein kinase cascades and apoptosis by protein kinase C ε and δ in neonatal rat ventricular myocytes. Circ Res 89:882–890.
70. Peruzzi F, Prisco M, Dews M, Salomoni P, Grassille E, Romano G, Calabretts B, Baserga R. 1999. Multiple signaling pathways of the insulin-like growth factor in protection form apoptosis. Mol Cell Biol 19:7203–7215.
71. Ruderman JV. 1993. MAP kinase and the activation of quiescent cells. Curr Opin Cell Biol 5:207–213.
72. Zhengui X, Dickens M, Raingeaud J, Davis RJ, Greenberg ME. 1995. Opposing effects of ERK and JNK-p38 MAP kinases. Science 24:1326–1331.
73. Ito T, Deng X, Carr B, May WS. 1997. Bcl-2 phosphorylation required for anti-apoptosis function. J Biol Chem 272:11671–11673.
74. Horiuchi M, Hayashida W, Kambe T, Yamada T, Dzau VJ. 1997. Angiotensin type 2 receptor dephosphorylates Bcl-2 by activating MAP kinase phosphatse-1 and induces apoptosis. J Biol Chem 272:19022–19026.
75. Wang Y, Hyang S, Sah VP, Ross J, Brown JH, Han H, Chien K. 1998. Cardiac muscle cell hypertrophy and apoptosis induced by distinct members of the p39 MAP kinse family. J Biol Chem 273:2161–2168.
76. Kummer JL, Pravin KR, Heidenreich KA. 1997. Apoptosis induced by withdrawral of trophic factors is mediated by p38 MAP kinase. J Biol Chem 272:20490–20494.
77. Akao M, Ohler A, O'Rourke B, Marban E. 2001. Mitochondrial ATP sensitive potassium channels inhibit apoptosis induced by oxidative stress in cardiac cells. Circ Res 88:1267–1275.
78. Wang Y, Kyoji H, Ashraf M. 1999. Activation of mitochondrial ATP-sensitive K^+ channel for cardiac protection against ischemic injury is dependent on protein kinase C activity. Circ Res 85:731–741.
79. Takashi E, Wang Y, Ashraf M. 1999. Activation of mitochondrial K_{ATP} channel elicits late preconditioning against myocardial infarction via protein kinase C signaling pathway. Circ Res 85:1146–1153.

G.N. Pierce, M. Nagano, P. Zahradka, and N.S. Dhalla (eds.).
ATHEROSCLEROSIS, HYPERTENSION AND DIABETES.

OXIDATIVE STRESS IN CARDIOVASCULAR COMPLICATIONS OF DIABETES

FIROOZEH FARAHMAND, HUIQUAN LOU, and PAWAN K. SINGAL

Summary. The burden of cardiovascular disease related to diabetes will increase substantially in the coming decades. Diabetes, formerly thought as a problem of glucose metabolism, produces most of its harm by effects on the cardiovascular system. Atherosclerosis and other cardiovascular complications account for most of the deaths due to diabetes. Diabetics with cardiovascular complications fare worse than their counterparts. There is convincing experimental and clinical evidence that in diabetics the oxidative stress is increased. There are various mechanisms that contribute to the formation of free radicals and cause oxidative stress. Less certain however, is whether oxidative stress causes the development of long-term complications of diabetes or merely reflects one of the associated processes that are affected by diabetes. The precise mechanisms by which oxidative stress accelerates complications of diabetes are only partly known. There is, however, evidence for the role of protein kinase C, advanced glycation end products and activation of certain transcription factors.

***Key words*:** Antioxidants, Free Radicals, Diabetes Mellitus, Cardiac Pathologies, Vasculopathy

INTRODUCTION

Diabetes mellitus with its associated complications is one of the major health disorders worldwide. The number of diabetics is on the rise and it is projected that by the year 2010 there will be 300 million diabetic patients. The incidence of ischemic

Address for Correspondence: Dr. Pawan K. Singal, Institute of Cardiovascular Sciences, St. Boniface General Hospital Research Centre, Room R3022, 351 Taché Avenue, Winnipeg, MB R2H 2A6, Canada. Tel: (204) 235-3416; Fax: (204) 233-6723; e-mail: psingal@sbrc.ca

heart disease (IHD) is higher and the risk of mortality from IHD is also two to four times higher in people with non-insulin dependent diabetes mellitus (NIDDM) than in general population, accounting for approximately 40% deaths in NIDDM. Hyperglycemia is clearly recognized as the primary culprit in the pathogenesis of diabetic complications. Glycation, the nonenzymatic adduction of glucose to protein, represents one possible mechanism by which excessive levels of glucose in the plasma, in the interstitial fluid and within the cells, could lead to pathophysiologic damage. However, diabetologists have also reported patients, who despite prolonged periods of poor glycemic control, have escaped the worst vascular complication, and others who quickly develop complications even when glycemic control is good. Thus, there are other, yet not understood factors which may link hyperglycemia to tissue damage. More recently, an increase in oxidative stress and a decrease in antioxidants has been suggested to play a role [1,2,3,4]. The present review focusses on the hypothesis that increased oxidative stress may play a role in the poor cardiovascular outlook in diabetic patients.

There is convincing experimental as well as clinical evidence that the generation of free radicals is increased in both NIDDM and IDDM. Furthermore, the onset of diabetes is closely associated with increased oxidative stress which may contribute to the progression of diabetes as well as its cardiovascular complications (Fig. 1). There are various mechanisms that contribute to the formation of free radicals. The precise mechanism by which oxidative stress may accelerate the development of complications in diabetes are only partly known. There is, however, evidence for the role of protein kinase C, advanced glycation end products (AGE) and activation of transcription factors. The exact signalling pathways and the interactions with free radicals remain a matter of discussion. Additionally, results of recent studies suggest a role of free radicals in the development of insulin resistance. This new concept of oxidative stress, being an important trigger in the onset and progression of diabetes and its complications, may offer a unique therapeutic option for the treatment of diabetes and its complications.

OXIDATIVE STRESS

In physiologic conditions, about 95% of the oxygen consumed is tetravalently reduced, through cytochrome oxidase enzyme system, resulting in the formation of water and production of adenosinetriphosphate to perform vital metabolic functions. Less than 5% of the oxygen is reduced through univalent pathway where also four electrons are added, but one at a time. In this process, a variety of highly reactive oxygen species (ROS) are produced, which have a very short half life and react with unsaturated sites in subcellular structures as well as macromolecules. The term oxidative stress, refers to a condition when there is a serious imbalance between the production of free radicals and antioxidant defence in favour of free radicals [5,6]. A free radical can be defined as any atom or molecule that contains an unpaired electron in its outermost electron shell and the examples are superoxide anion (O_2^-), hydroxyl radical (OH), and peroxyradical (ROO). Free radicals can be pro-

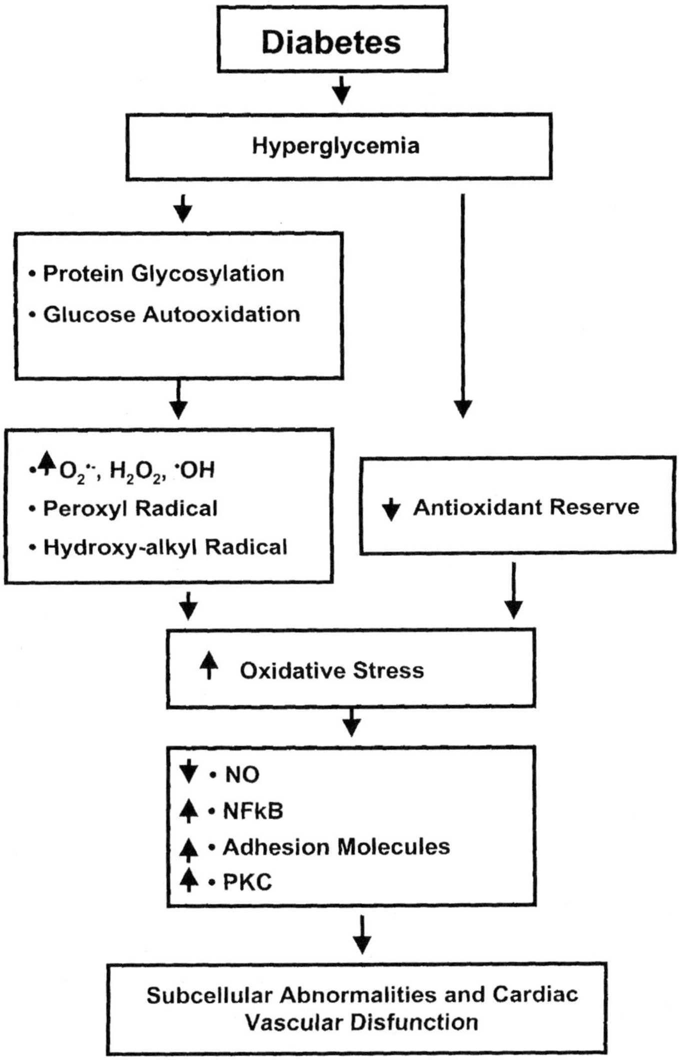

Figure 1. Oxidative Stress in Diabetes—induced Cardiovascular Complications.

duced by several different biological and biochemical processes within the body such as autooxidation of catecholamines and activation of polymorphs, arachidonic acid cascade and different oxidation-reduction reactions. In addition, free radicals can be produced during an exposure to radiation, such as gamma rays which can split water to produce OH in vascular endothelium and other cells.

THE EVIDENCE FOR INCREASED OXIDATIVE STRESS IN DIABETES

Patient studies

There seems to be general agreement that the production of free radicals is increased in diabetic patients. Free radical damage to DNA has been well demonstrated, and several DNA damage products including 8-hydroxydeoxyguanosine (8-OH dG), 8-hydroxyadenine and 7-methyl-8-hydroxyguanine, have been identified in human urine of diabetics [7]. Lipid peroxidation is important in vivo for several reasons, in particular it is suggested to contribute to the development of atherosclerosis by the modifications of low-density lipoprotein [5,8,9]. Elevated levels of reactive oxygen species (ROS) and insufficient antioxidant protection lead to enhanced LDL oxidation in diabetes. Supplementation with the antioxidant, RRR-α tocopherol, offers significant protection against LDL oxidation in diabetic patients [10,11,12,13].

Several clinical studies have reported increased levels of oxidative stress markers, e.g., lipid hydroperoxides, 8-epi-PGF2a 8-OH dG and ox-LDL in both type 1 and type 2 Diabetes when compared to healthy age matched subjects [14,15]. Four fold higher median concentration of 8-OH dG in mononuclear cells of diabetic patients was observed as compared to controls [14]. The study showed for the first time greater oxidative damage to DNA in diabetic patients as compared to control. An approximately two-fold increase in the plasma oxidative stress, as indicated by 8-epi-PGF2a and ROOH, was observed in diabetic patients when compared to healthy subjects [16]. A relationship between increase in oxidative stress as indicated by hydroperoxides and antioxidant decrease in tocopherol has also been noted. A decrease in antioxidant capacity has also been observed in the plasma of diabetic patients [16,17,18].

Animal studies

In rats, made diabetic with a single injection of streptozotocin (STZ, 65 mg/kg), there was reduced myocardial function, increased oxidative stress and reduced myocardial antioxidant reserve [3]. Treatment with probucol (10 mg/kg/day), an antioxidant, did not reverse the weight loss induced by diabetes but serum glucose levels of diabetic rats were significantly reduced from 603.7 ± 40 mg/dl to 422.6 ± 33. STZ administration induced about an 80% decrease in insulin levels, whereas in the diabetic group that received the probucol this reduction was about 62%. Probucol also improved cardiac function in diabetic rats .

SOD activity was reduced by about 50% in diabetic rats as compared to control. The group treated only with probucol had significantly more SOD than control. In diabetic group, probucol caused small but significant increase in SOD activity. Diabetic rats showed lower levels of GSHPx than control and probucol improved this enzymatic activity. LPO was about 100% higher in diabetic group than in control. Probucol reduced these levels but they were still higher than control. Clearly reduced cardiac function in diabetics is associated with reduced antioxidant reserve as well as increased oxidative stress and antioxidant treatment using probucol modulated these changes [3].

POSSIBLE SOURCES OF OXIDATIVE STRESS IN DIABETES

The evidence for an increased oxidative stress has been convincingly demonstrated; however, less is known about the sources and the mechanism by which these reactive oxygen radicals are generated in diabetes. A proposed chronology of events in the pathogenesis of oxidative stress due to hyperglycemia, including intermediary steps to tissue damage, has been shown in Fig. 1. Oxidative stress may result from an overproduction of precursors to reactive oxygen radicals and/or decreased efficiency of inhibitory scavenger systems. The stress may be amplified by an autocatalytic cycle of metabolic stress, tissue damage and cell death, [19,20]. Two mechanisms, non-enzymatic glycosylation and autooxidative glycosylation, have been proposed that may explain how hyperglycemia can cause increased ROS formation [21,22,23].

The term of autooxidative glycosylation was introduced to describe the proposed role of reducing sugar as a catalyst of oxidative chemical modification and cross linking of proteins [20,22,24]. In fact, advanced glycation end (AGE) products can be produced by aerobic, non-enzymatic glycation of protein, in the presence of even a small concentration of transitional metals [25]. The reduced oxygen products formed in the autooxidation of protein bound Amadori products include superoxide and hydrogen peroxide [26]. In addition, AGE products can stimulate the release of ROS in endothelium by a receptor-mediated (RAGE) process. It is likely that all the proteins in the body can undergo glycation, if exposed to high glucose or glucose α-phosphate. Intracellular proteins in insulin requiring tissues of diabetics may be partially protected from glycation despite extracellular hyperglycemia because glucose is not entering the cell due to deficiency of or resistance to insulin [27]. Nevertheless, analysis of tissue samples from diabetic subjects exhibits a generalized increase in glycation [20].

The polyol pathway may also contribute to non-enzymatic glycation of proteins, because fructose can bind non-enzymatically to protein (so called fructation), and fluorescence of collagen from diabetic animals, is decreased by inhibitors of aldol reduction [19].

It has been shown that glucose under physiological conditions, produces oxidants that possess reactivity similar to the hydroxy free radicals [20]. The process of glucose oxidation results in dicarbonyl compound formation which is accompanied by O_2^- production. That high glucose stimulates the generation of O_2^- in human umbilical vein endothelial cells has been demonstrated [28]. These data and the observation that the production of O_2^- are not prevented by inhibitors of nitric oxide synthases, P-450-dependent oxygenase and lipo and cyclooxygenase suggest that the autooxidation of glucose may be one of the major sources of ROS in diabetes. That hyperglycemia and oxidative stress are related very closely is also supported by in vivo studies [28–30].

There is much evidence from experimental studies that the formation of ROS is a direct consequence of hyperglycemia. Incubation of endothelial and smooth muscle cells with increasing concentrations of glucose initiates formation of ROS

[28,31]. A significant increase was observed at glucose concentrations as high as 10 mM [28]. In addition, AGE products have been shown to simulate the formation of ROS by a receptor mediated process [32]. Recently, it has shown that the intracellular formation of AGE and lipid peroxidation are closely linked processes. Inhibition of lipid peroxidation also prevented the formation of AGE products [33]. Thus there are various mechanisms known by which ROS may be generated in diabetes, and much experimental evidence has accumulated to show that various types of vascular cells are able to produce ROS under hyperglycemic condition.

Altered antioxidant enzyme defences

It has been shown that non-enzymatic glycosylation (glycation) of human CuZn superoxide dismutase leads to a gradual inactivation of the enzyme in vitro as well as in vivo and the level of glycated CuZnSod is increased in the erythrocyte of patients with diabetes mellitus [20]. Furthermore, the generation of glutathione is delayed in the presence of high glucose causing an impairment of antioxidant defence [29]. Antioxidant reserve has also been shown to be reduced in the myocardium of rats made diabetic using streptozotocin [3].

CARDIOVASCULAR COMPLICATIONS OF DIABETES

Observations that oxidative stress impairs endothelium-dependent vasodialtion [34,35], triggers the expansion of mesangial cells and is related to the incidence of type 2 diabetes [36], suggest that oxidative stress may play an important role in the initiation of the pathophysiological cascade of events leading to vascular and other diabetic complications. Conversely, evidence has also been presented that oxidative stress may not occur early in the disease process of diabetes, but may be rather an underlying pathogenic factor in the progression of the disease [37]. One of the major problems in assessing the issue of when oxidative stress occurs in the disease process and whether there is an accumulation of free radicals derived tissue damage during the disease is the stability of oxidation products (37).

Patients with both insulin-dependent (IDDM) and non-insulin-dependent (NIDDM) diabetes mellitus suffer from an increased incidence of cardiovascular disease when compared with control population (38). These vascular complications take the form of premature and accelerated atherosclerosis of large arteries (macrovascular disease) or increased permeability of capillaries associated with thickening of the basement membrane (microvascular disease). That invivo hyperglycemia and oxidative stress are closely linked is supported by the determination of the total radical trapping antioxidant parameter (TRAP) in control subjects and in diabetic patients (39). Activation of membrane bound, macrophage like NADH oxidase in endothelial cells and smooth muscle cells has been reported in hypertension and hypercholesterolemia. Agiotensin (II) is a strong activator of this enzyme in vascular cells (40). Alternatively, it has been suggested that the electron flux in endothelial NO synthase (NOS III) becomes uncoupled in hyperglycemia. In such an uncoupled state the electrons flowing from the reductase domain to the oxygenase domain in the NOS complex, are diverted to the molecular oxygen rather than to L-arginine. In this regard, not only the production of ROS but also the activation of NFkB and the induction of apoptosis was prevented in human and rat endothelial cells in the presence of inhibitors of NOS [41].

In bovine aortic endothelial cells, it has been shown that the mitochondrial electron flux becomes uncoupled from ATP synthesis in hyperglycemic conditions [42]. The production of ROS could be prevented by various couplers of the mitochondrial electron chain. Furthermore, activation of PKC, the polyol pathway, the transcription factor NFkB and the increased formation of AGE products were influenced by ROS (42). An accelerated conversion of glucose to fructose by the sorbitol pathway has a significant impact on the redox state of the cell. The conversion of glucose by this pathway consumes NADPH and leads to an increased NADH flux in mitochondria.

That hyperglycemia leads to an activation of protein kinase C in all cells and tissues, which take up glucose independently from insulin, might therefore not only be mediated by an increase in diacylglycerol (DAG) which is a strong activator of protein kinase C (PKC), but also by the enhanced formation of ROS [43,44]. Thus several lines of reasoning suggest AGE and ROS are able to activate PKC and that activation of PKC is the common downstream mechanism to which multiple cellular and functional abnormalities in the diabetic vascular tissue can be attributed, including changes in vascular flow, vascular permeability , extracellular matrix components and cell growth. Clearly ROS play an important role in the activation of biochemical pathways involved in the pathogenesis of vascular complications (Fig. 1).

Activation of redox-sensitive transcription factors by AGE and hyperglycemia

AGE products accumulate during the course of diabetes and are believed to induce endothelial dysfunction characterized by an impaired regulation of blood flow by highly thrombogenic and pro-coagulant state of vascular wall [45]. These vascular alterations are thought to be relavant to the progression of diabetic complications. Recent studies have shown that interactions of AGE-modified proteins with specific AGE receptors result in the degradation of AGE proteins and induce signal transduction pathway causing impairment of endothelium dependent vasodilation, an increase in procoagulant activity, induction of cell adhesion molecules, increased vasoconstriction and other vascular dysfunctions [45].

As a result of activation of these signal transduction pathways-binding of AGE to RAGE (receptor for AGE), vascular cells (smooth muscle cells, macrophages, endothelial cells) generate ROS [26,46], which may also result in the depletion of cellular antioxidant reserve (eg, glutathione, ascorbate), and the activation of redox sensitive transcription factors, such as NFkB [26]. In experiments using vascular cells, the generation of ROS and the activation of NfkB, is not only caused by AGE, but also by high concentrations of glucose, might indicate a link between elevated post-prandial glucose levels and the development of vascular complications [28]. Taken together, these experimental and clinical data suggest that activation of the oxidative stress and sensitive transcription factors such as NFkB and AP-1 represents an important pathogenic link between hyperglycemia and the remodelling of the vessel wall in diabetics [47,48].

Abnormalities in vascular tone and blood flow have been found in many organs of diabetic animals and patients, including heart, kidney, retina, peripheral arteries and microvessels. There is considerable evidence that nitric oxide reacts in a diffusion-controlled way with superoxide anions to produce peroxynitrate [49]. Thus, a simultaneous formation of ROS would consequently reduce the amount of biologically active nitric-oxide and lead to the impairment of vasodilation. Such thinking is supported by the fact that the impaired endothelium-dependent relaxation was restored by the addition of superoxide dismutase (SOD), an enzyme which inactivates the O_2^- very effectively as well as with pretreatment of diabetic animals with alpha-tocopherol [35]. In addition to superoxide anions, AGE products have been shown to quench NO and may therefore be important modulator of endothelial dependent vasodilation [50]. Recent clinical studies have shown that antioxidants are able to restore or at least improve the disturbed endothelium dependent vasodilation in diabetic patients and in patients with coronary artery disease [51]. ROS and PKC activation regulates vascular cell permeability and vascular cell proliferation which are two important events in the pathogenic cascade of endothelial dysfunction and whose abnormalities can lead to microvascular and macrovascular complications [52,53].

Oxidative stress directly induced by hyperglycemia, or indirectly by endothelin 1 (ET-1) may lead to activation of redox-sensitive transcription factors. It has been shown that antioxidants as well as inhibition of PKC activity by selective inhibitors decrease cell proliferation and permeability in aortic smooth muscle and mesangial cells, thus supporting a close relationship between oxidative stress and PKC activation [47,48].

CHANGES IN EXTRACELLULAR MATRIX

Thickening of capillary basement membrane is one of the early structural abnormalities observed in the vascular system in diabetes [54]. Histologically, increases in type IV and VI collagen, fibronectin and laminin, in addition to decreases in proteoglycan are observed in the heart [30,55], as well as in vascular beds of diabetic patients. Experimental studies have shown that these alterations in vascular bed can be prevented by high doses of antioxidants such as tocopherol and inhibition of PKC.

In conclusion, there is strong evidence that a relative increase in free radicals and thus, oxidative stress play a role in the development of cardiovascular complications of diabetes. Research over the past ten years suggests that oxidative stress plays a role in this pathway as a link between hyperglycemia and the typically observed pathophysiological features including cardiovascular complications of diabetes.

ACKNOWLEDGEMENTS

The research reviewed herein was supported by a grant from the Canadian Institutes of Health Research. Firoozeh Farahmand was supported by a Fellowship from the Faculty of Graduate Studies, University of Manitoba.

REFERENCES

1. Kaul N, Siveski-Iliskovic N, Hill M, Slezak J, Singal PK. 1993. Free radicals and the heart. Pharmacol Toxicol Methods 30:55–67.
2. Kaul N, Siveski-Iliskovic N, Thomas TP, Hill M, Khaper N, Singal PK. 1995. Probucol improves antioxidant activity and modulates development of diabetic cardiomyopathy. Nutrition 11: 551–554.
3. Kaul N, Siveski-Iliskovic N, Hill M, Khaper ••, Seneviratne C, Singal PK. 1996. Probucol treatment reverses antioxidant and functional deficit in diabetic cardiomyopathy. Mol Cell Biochem 160–161:283–288.
4. Godin DV, Wohaieb SA, Garnett ME, Goumeniouk AD. 1988. Antioxidant enzyme alterations in experimental and clinical diabetes. Mol Cell Biochem 84:223–231.
5. Halliwell B, Cross CE, Gutteridge JMC. 1992. Free radicals, antioxidants and human disease: Where we are now? J Lab Clin Med 119:598–620.
6. Singal PK, Petkau A, Gerrard JM, Hrushovetz S, Foerster J. 1988. Free radicals in health and disease. Mol Cell Biochem 84:121–122.
7. Whiteman M, Jenner A, Halliwell B. 1997. Hypochlorous acid-induced base modification in isolated calf thymus DNA. Chem Res Toxicol 10:1240–1246.
8. Steinberg D, Parthasarathy S, Carew TE. 1989. Beyond cholesterol. Modifications of low-density lipoprotein that increases its atherogenicity. New Engl J Med 320:915–924.
9. Carew TE, Schwenke DC, Steinberg D. 1987. Antiatherognic effect of probucol unrelated to it hypocholeteolemic effect: evidence that antioxidants invivo can selectively inhibit low density lipoprotein degradation in macrophage-rich fatty streaks and slow the progression of altherosclersis in the Watanable heritable hyperlipemic rabbit. Proc Natl Acad Sci USA 84:7725–7729.
10. Jha P, Flather M, Lonn E, FarKouh M, Yusuf S. 1995. The antioxidant vitamins and cardiovascular disease. A critical review of epidemiologic and clinical data. Ann Intern Med 123:860–872.
11. Rudich A, Kozlovsky N, Potashnik R, Bashan N. 1998. Oxidant stress reduces insulin responsiveness in 3T3-L1 adipocyte and skeletal muscle insulin resistance. Diabetolgia 41(Suppl. 1):A34.
12. Stephens NG, Parsons A, Schofield PM, et al. 1996. A randomized controlled trial of vitamin E in patients with coronary diseases: The Cambridge heart antioxidant study (CHAOS). Lancet 347: 781–786.
13. Rimm EB, Stampfer MJ, Ascherio A. 1993. Vitamin E consumption and coronary heart disease in men. N Engl J Med 328:1450–1456.
14. Dandona P, Thusu K. 1996. Oxidative damage DNA in diabetes mellitus. Lancet 347:444–445.
15. Greisbacher A, Kinderhauser M, Andet ••. 1995. Enhanced serum levels of TBARS in diabetes mellitus. Am J Med 98:469–475.
16. Nourouz-Zadeh J, Tajaddini-Sarmadi J. 1995. Elevated levels of authentic plasma hydroperoxides in NIDDM. Diabetes 44:1054–1058.
17. Tsai EC, Hirch IB, Brunzell JD, Chait A. 1994. Reduced plasma peroxyl radical; trapping capacity and increased susceptibility of LDL to oxidation in poorly controlled IDDM. Diabetes 43:1010–1014.
18. Chari SN, Nath N, Rathi AB. 1984. Glutathione and its redox system in diabetic polymorphonuclear leukocytes. Am J Med Sci 287:14–15.
19. Suarez G, Rajaram R, Oronsky AL, Gawinowicz MA. 1989. Nonenzymatic glycation of bovine serum albumin by fructose (fructation). Comparison with the Maillard reaction initiated by glucose. J Biol Chem 264:3674–3679.
20. Arai K, Maguchi S, Fuji S, Ishibashi H, Oikawa K, Taniguchi N. 1987. Glycation and inactivation of human Cu-Zn-superoxide dismutase. Identification of the in vitro glycated sites. J Biol Chem 262: 16969–16972.
21. Wolff SP, Dean RT. 1987. Glucose auto-oxidation and protein modification. The potential role of "autoxidative glycosylation" in diabetes. Biochem J 245:243–250.
22. Bunn HF. 1981. Nonenzymatic glycosylation of protein: relevance to diabetes. Am J Med 70:325–330.
23. Thornalley PJ, Wolff SP, Crabbe MJ, Stern A. 1984. The oxidation of oxyhaemoglobin by glyceraldehyde and other simple monosaccharides. Biochem J 217:615–622.

24. Ahmed MU, Thorpe SR, Baynes JW. 1986. Identification of N epsilon-carboxymethyllysine as a degradation product of fructoselysine in glycated protein. J Biol Chem 261:4889–4894.
25. Sakurai T, Tsuchiya S. 1988. Superoxide production from nonenzymatically glycated protein. FEBS Lett 236:406–410.
26. Yan SD, Schmidt AM, Anderson GM, Zhang J, Brett J, Zou YS, Pinsky D, Stern D. 1994. Enhanced cellular oxidant stress by the interaction of advanced glycation end products with their receptors/binding proteins. J Biol Chem 269:9889–9897.
27. Higgins PJ, Garlick RL, Bunn HF. 1982. Glycosylated hemoglobin in human and animal red cells. Role of glucose permeability. Diabetes 31:743–748.
28. Du XL, Stockklauser-Farber K, Rosen P. 1999. Generation of reactive oxygen intermediates, activation of NfkappaB, and induction of apoptosis in human endothelial cells by Glucose: Role of nitric oxide synthase? Free Radic Med Biol 27:752–763.
29. Kashiwagi A, Asahina T, Ikebuchi M, et al. 1994. Abnormal glutathione metabolism and increased cytotoxicity caused by H2O2 in human umbilical vein endothelial cells, cultured in high glucose medium. Diabetollogia 37:264–269.
30. Ceriello A. 1997. Acute hyperglycemia and oxidative stress generation. Diabet Med 14:S45–S49.
31. Wascher TC, Toplak H, Krejs GJ, Simecek S, Kukovetz WR, Graier WF. 1994. Intracellular mechanisms involved in D-glucose mediated amplification of agonist-induced Ca response and EDRF formation in vascular endothelial cells. Diabetes 43:984–991.
32. Mullarkey C, Edestein D, Brownlee M. 1990. Free radical generation by early glycation products: a mechanism for accelerated arteriogenesis in diabetes. Biochem Biophys Res Commun 173:932–939.
33. Giardino I, Fard AK, Hatchell DL, Brownlee M. 1998. Aminoguanidine inhibits reactive oxygen species formation, lipid peroxidation, and oxidant-induced apoptosis. Diabetes 47:1114–1120.
34. Diedrich D, Skopec J, Diedrich A, Dai FX. 1994. Endothelial dysfunction in mesentric resistance arteries of diabetics rats: role of free radicals. Am J Physiol 266: H1153–H1161.
35. Rosen P, Ballhausen T, Bloch W, Addics K. 1995. Endothelial relaxation is disturbed by oxidative stress in diabetic heart: The influences of tocopherol as antioxidant. Diabetolgia 38:1157–1168.
36. Sundaram RK, Bhaskar A, Vijayalingam S, Viswanatthan M, Mohan R, Shanmugasundaram KR. 1996. Antioxidant status and lipid peroxidation in type II diabetes with and without complications. Clin Sci 90:255–260.
37. Baynes JW. 1991. Role of oxidative stress in development of complications in diabetes. Diabetes 40:405–411.
38. Jarrett RJ, McCartney P, Keen H. 1982. The Bedford survey: ten year mortality rates in newly diagnosed diabetics, borderline diabetics and normoglycaemic controls and risk indices for coronary heart disease in borderline diabetics. Diabetologia 22:79–84.
39. Wolff SP. 1993. Diabetes mellitus and free radicals. Br Med Bull 49:642–652.
40. Warnholz A, Nickenig G, Schulz E, et al. 1999. Increased NADH-oxidase-mediated superoxide production in the early stages of atheroscleros evidence for involvement of the renin-angiotensin system. Circulation 99:2027–2033.
41. Rosen P, Bartels H, Berkels R, Kirrmizugul I, Rosen R. 2000. Short term glucose stimulates the generation of reactive oxygen species, but eliminates free nitric oxide. Diabetes 49:134–135.
42. Nishikawa T, Edelstein D, Du XL, et al. 2000. Normalizing mithochondrial superoxide production blocks three pathways of hyperglycemic damage. Nature 404:787–790.
43. Nishizuka Y. 1992. Intracellular signaling by hydrolysis of phospholipids and activation of protein kinase C. Science 258:607–614.
44. King GI, Ishii H, Koya D. 1997. Diabetic vascular dysfunctions: a model of excessive activation of protein kinase C. Kidney Int 52:S77–S85.
45. Bierhaus A, Chevion S, Chevion M, et al. 1997. Advanced glycation end-products (AGEs) induced activation of NF-kB is suppressed by alpha-lipoic acid in cultured endothelial cells. Diabetes 1 46: 1481–1490.
46. Schmidt A-M, Zhang JH, et al. 1994. Interaction of advanced glycation end-products with their endothelial cells receptor leads to enhanced expression of VCAM-1: A mechanism for augmented monocyte-vessel wall interactions in diabetes. FASEB J 8:3841–3842.
47. Bursell SE, Cletmont AC, Aiello LP, et al. 1999. High-dose Vitamine E supplementation normalize retinal blood flow and creatinine clearance in patients with type I diabetes. Diabetes care 22: 1245–1251.
48. Kunisaki M, Bursell S-E, Clermont AC, et al. 1995. Vitamin E prevents diabetes-induced abnormal retinal blood flow via the diacyl-glycerol-protein kinase C pathway. Am J Physio 269:E239–E246.

49. Ohara Y, Peterson TE, Harrison DG. 1997. Hypercholesterolemia increases endothelial superoxide anion production. Hypertension 30:934–941.
50. Bucala R, Tracy KJ, Ceramin A. 1991. Advanced glycation products quench nitric oxide and mediate defective endothelim dependent vasodilation in experimental diabetes. J Clinical Invest 97:22–28.
51. Ting HH, Timimi FK, Haley EA, et al. 1997. Vitamin C improves endothelium dependent vasodilation in forearm resistance vessels of humans with hypercholesterolemia. Circulation 95:2617–2622.
52. Park IS, Kiyomoto H, Abboud SL, Abboud HE. 1997. Expression of transforming growth factor-beta and type IV collagen in early streptozotocin-induced diabetes. Diabetes 46:473–480.
53. Oliver JA, Adenylate cyclase and protein kinase C. 1990. Mediate opposite actions on endothelial junctions. J Cell Physiol 145:536–542.
54. Scheinman JL, Fish AJ, Matas AJ, Michael AF. 1987. The immunohistopathology of glomerular antigens. II. The glomerular basement membrane, actomyosin, and fibroblast surface antigens in normal, diseased and transplanted human kidneys, Am J Pathol 90:71–88.
55. Walker JD, Viberti GC. 1994. Pathophysiology of microvascular disease: an overview. In Chronic Complications of Diabetes, Pickup JC, Williams G (eds). Blackwell Scientific: Oxford, UK 11–19.

G.N. Pierce, M. Nagano, P. Zahradka, and N.S. Dhalla (eds.).
ATHEROSCLEROSIS, HYPERTENSION AND DIABETES.
Kluwer Academic Publishers. Boston.

AUGMENTED ENERGY TRANSFER IN RAT HEART MITOCHONDRIA: COMPENSATORY RESPONSE TO ABNORMAL HOUSEHOLD OF ENERGY IN ACUTE DIABETES

ATTILA ZIEGELHÖFFER,[1] IVETA WACZULÍKOVÁ,[2]
TANYA RAVINGEROVÁ,[1]
BARBARA ZIEGELHÖFFER-MIHALOVIČOVÁ,[3]
JAN NECKÁŘ,[4] and JÁN STYK[1]

[1] *Institute for Heart Research, Slovak Academy of Sciences, Bratislava, Slovak Republic;* [2] *Department of Biophysics and Chemical Physics, Faculty of Mathematics, Physics and Informatics, Comenius University, Bratislava, Slovak Republic;* [3] *Carl-Ludwig-Institute of Physiology, University of Leipzig, Leipzig, Germany;* [4] *Institute of Physiology, Academy of Sciences of the Czech Republic and Centre of Cardiovascular Research, Prague, Czech Republic*

Summary. Objectives: Hearts of rats with diabetes mellitus are generally characterized by energy demands exceeding their energy production. Nevertheless, although working permanently in energy deficiency, the diabetic hearts may also exhibit decreased vulnerability to ischemia and calcium overload. This points to presence of adaptation changes in cardiac energetics, in which at least that limited amount of energy which the diabetic heart mitochondria can produce, may be transported through the mitochondrial membrane to sites of its utilization at a non-limiting rate.
Aim: Study of diabetes-induced adaptation in cardiac energetics from molecular mechanisms to functional significance by means of: i) Identification and elucidation of biochemical and biophysical changes that may be linked to augmentation of energy transfer in diabetic cardiomyocytes and thus, associated with adaptation of the myocardium to diabetes. ii) Disclosing the functional significance of the diabetes-induced adaptation in cardiac energetics, by investigating mitochondrial membrane fluidity, ATPase activities and formation of

Address of the Corresponding Author: Attila Ziegelhöffer, PhD, DSc, Institute for Heart Research, Slovak Academy of Sciences, Dúbravská cesta 9, SK 842 33 Bratislava, Slovak Republic. Phone: (004212) 5477 4406; Fax: (004212) 5477 6637; e-mail: usrdzigy@savba.sk

mitochondrial contact sites (MiCS), facilitating the Ca-dependent, high capacity of energy transfer from mitochondria, in conjunction with testing the ischemic tolerance of heart.
Methods: Hearts of diabetic and age-matched adult male control rats were investigated on the 8th day after streptozotocin administration ($55\,mg \cdot kg^{-1}$ i.v.). Metabolic status of animals was monitored estimating the levels of glucose, glycohemoglobin, triacylglycerol, cholesterol in the blood or serum, respectively. After excision, the hearts were Langendorff-perfused with either 1.6 or $2.2\,mmol \cdot l^{-1}$ $CaCl_2$, subjected to calcium paradox or to cardiac arrest by replacing calcium for cadmium ions. MiCS formation was assessed by cytochemical detection of the mitochondrial isoform of creatine phosphokinase (mCPK) octameres and was quantified stereologically as MiCS to mitochondrial surface ratio (S_S). Mg-dependent and 2,4-dinitrophenol-stimulated ATPase activities as well as fluorescence anisotropy of diphenylhexatriene and membrane fluidity were estimated as indicators of functional and biophysical status in isolated preparation of cardiac mitochondria. For comparison, the same biophysical variables were also tested in a fraction of sarcolemmal membranes isolated from diabetic hearts. Ischemic tolerance (IT) of hearts was evaluated in anesthetized open-chest animals subjected to 30 min occlusion of LAD coronary artery followed by 4 h reperfusion, monitoring ischemic arrhythmias and by measuring the size of infarcted area (tetrazolium double staining).
Results: In control hearts, increasing Ca^{2+} induced both, positive inotropic response (dP/dt increase from 2270 ± 220 to 2955 ± 229, $p < 0.01$) and elevated MiCs formation (S_S increase from 0.070 ± 0.011 to 0.123 ± 0.012, $p < 0.01$). In diabetic hearts, basic MiCS formation was already comparable with that induced by elevated Ca^{2+} in control hearts and could not be further stimulated by Ca^{2+}. High MiCS formation (high capacity energy transfer from mitochondria) in diabetic hearts was also associated with significantly ($p < 0.01$) increased membrane fluidity and slightly elevated ATPase activities of cardiac mitochondria. This finding was in contrast to that in diabetic heart sarcolemma and it could be attributed to different roles of both membrane systems. In control hearts, ventricular tachycardia represented 55.4% of total arrhythmias and occurred in 90% of the animals. In diabetic hearts, arrhythmia profile was similar to that in controls, and the incidence of tachyarrhythmias and their severity were not enhanced (arrhythmia score: 3.18 ± 0.4 vs. 3.30 ± 0.3 in controls). The infarct size normalized to the size of area at risk in controls exceeded that in the diabetic hearts (69.2 ± 2.2% vs. 52.3 ± 5.8%, $p < 0.05$).
Conclusions: Ca-signaling represents the link between the energy delivery from mitochondria (via MiCS) and energy requirements of the heart. In contrast to cardiac sarcolemma, the mitochondria of diabetic hearts exhibit increased membrane fluidity and ATPase activities. These changes seem to belong to endogenous mechanisms of myocardial protection, they are associated with top stimulation of MiCS formation i.e., of energy transport from mitochondria via MiCS, and contribute to increased resistance of diabetic hearts to irreversible cell damage.

Key words: Adaptation of heart to diabetes, Tolerance to ischemia, Endogenous protective mechanisms in heart, Mitochondrial contact sites, Mitochondrial membrane fluidity

INTRODUCTION

It was convincingly demonstrated that metabolic disorganization resulting from diabetes induces myocardial remodeling [1,2] as well as irregularities in function of cardiac subcellular membrane systems [3,4], associated with abnormalities in function of receptors [5], ion transport [6,7] and calcium handling [2,5,6]. In some cases, particularly in type 2 diabetes, these alterations may even lead to an increase in the level of free Ca^{2+} in the cytoplasm ($[Ca^{2+}]_i$). Nevertheless, whether $[Ca^{2+}]_i$ increases or not, the diabetic heart always exhibits amplified and prolonged calcium transients [8]. Diabetes-induced abnormalities also concern cardiac energetics. The latter is characterized by decreased, nevertheless predominating utilization of endogenous glycogen prior to exogenous glucose, for energy production [9]. However, neither thc glycolysis, which is believed to be the main energy supplier of the subcellular membrane systems [10,11], nor the oxidative phosphorylation, expected to supply all other energy consuming systems, produce in diabetes adequate amounts of energy. This is manifested in energy demands that exceed the energy production in cardiac cells [9,12,13]. However, in spite of the overall metabolic deterioration and permanent energy deficiency, diabetic hearts do not stop to beat but, particularly in the acute phase of the disease, they may even exhibit increased tolerance to ischemia [14,15,16,17] and calcium overload [2,6,13,18], as well as decreased sensitivity to reperfusion-induced ventricular arrhythmias [15,19,20]. This points to a diabetes-induced adaptation of the myocardium at least in dealing with energy.

As concerns the mitochondria from chronic diabetic hearts, they were shown to have decreased F1 ATPase activity, impaired function of the citric acid cycle and oxidative production of ATP [3,21]. In acute phase of the disease, these alterations seemed to be, at least in part, compensated by significantly increased formation of mitochondrial contact sites (MiCS) enabling high capacity energy transport through the mitochondrial membrane [8]. The outcome of all these alterations are proportionally lowered myocardial contents of adenosine triphosphate (ATP) and adenosine diphosphate (ADP), as well as of creatine phosphate (CP) in acute and also in chronic diabetes [9,13]. Proportionality in ATP, ADP, and CP decrease is manifested by ATP/ADP and ATP/CVP ratios not differing considerably from those in tissue of the normal heats [12]. This indicates that, in contrary to some expectations, at least the intracellular energy transfer may be not limiting in the diabetic hearts [8]. The latter assumption is strongly supported by our earlier results [22]: diabetic hearts which were always shown to have amplified Ca^{2+} transients [18], exhibited an MiCS formation identical with the maximal MiCS formation which could be achieved in healthy hearts by increased offer of calcium [8,22] and was coupled with a positive inotropic response [22,23].

The present paper is devoted to elucidation of functional significance of the diabetes-induced adaptation in cardiac energetics. This goal was followed by investigating alterations in fluidity of the mitochondrial membranes, characterized by stationary fluorescence anisotropy of diphenylhexatriene and the related changes in mitochondrial Mg^{2+}-ATPase activities, coupled with formation of MiCS, which facilitate the Ca^{2+}-dependent high capacity energy transfer from the mitochondria in conjunction with testing the ischemic tolerance of the diabetic heart.

MATERIALS AND METHODS

All experiments were performed in accordance with the Guide for the Care and Use of Laboratory Animals published by the US National Institute of Health (NIH publication No. 85–23, revised 1985).

Induction of diabetes and assessment of metabolic status of the animals

Experiments were performed on adult male Wistar rats. Animals were kept on standard pellet diet with free access to water. Diabetes mellitus was induced by a single dose of streptozotocin (Sigma-Aldrich, Germany, $55\,mg \cdot kg^{-1}$ i.v.). Full manifestation of the disease was confirmed by estimation of glucose [24] and glycohemoglobin [25] in the blood as well as cholesterol [26] and triacylglycerols [27] in serum. In addition, diabetic animals were also daily tested for glucose content in urine, by means of test stripes (DIABUR – 5000, Glucose, Urine, Roche, Mannheim, Germany). Experiments were performed on the 8th day after streptozotocin administration. Parallel to the group of acute diabetic animals (initial body weight 232 ± 10 g) a group of age- and weight-matched healthy animals (initial body weight 230 ± 13 g) served as control.

Isolated heart preparation

Animals were killed by cervical dislocation. Hearts were quickly excised and Langendorff-perfused at 37°C (perfusion pressure 75 mm Hg; 15 min perfusion following 15 min stabilization perfusion without recirculation of perfusate) with Krebs-Henseleit solution (K-H) containing (in $mmol \cdot l^{-1}$): 118.5 NaCl, 25.0 $NaHCO_3$, 1.2 $MgSO_4$, 1.2 Na_2HPO_4, 3.0 KCl, 11.1 glucose and either 1.6 or 2.2 $CaCl_2$, gassed with 95% O_2 and 5% CO_2, pH 7.4. *Hearts with calcium paradox*: 15 min stabilized perfusion with K-H containing $1.6\,mmol \cdot l^{-1}$ $CaCl_2$ followed by 3 min Ca^{2+} depletion with calcium free K-H containing $0.1\,mmol \cdot l^{-1}$ EDTA, and finally by 12 min Ca^{2+} repletion again with K-H containing $1.6\,mmol \cdot l^{-1}$ $CaCl_2$. The function of perfused hearts was monitored estimating dP/dt (for more details see 2,13,22). *Inhibition of the Ca^{2+} signal for MiCS formation:* Heart arrest induced by replacement of Ca^{2+} for Cd^{2+} ions administered intracoronarily (5 ml of $5\,mmol \cdot l^{-1}$ $CdCl_2$ applied in a bolus) immediately at the end of perfusion similar to that in the control hearts (for more details see 8). These groups of diabetic and control hearts were further processed for cytochemical determination of MiCS.

Cytochemical detection of MiCS formation

MiCS were assessed by cytochemical detection of octameric form of the mitochondrial creatine phosphokinase [28]. The method is based on reduction of thiocarbamyl nitro blue tetrazolium chloride salt in the presence of lactate and glucose-6-phosphate dehydrogenase. Thin sections of embedded tissue slices were examined in electron microscope. MiCS formation was quantified stereologically [29] as the ratio of MiCS surface to mitochondria surface (S_S). The testing grid was superimposed over the electronmicrographs and the ratio of intersections of cycloids with MiCS and intersections of cycloids with mitochondrial membranes was counted (for more details see 8,29).

Assessment of ischemic tolerance of the hearts

Ischemic tolerance was evaluated in pentobarbital-anesthetized, artificially ventilated (Ugo Basile, Italy), open chest diabetic as well as age- and weight-matched control animals. Rats were subjected to 30 min occlusion of the LAD coronary artery followed by 4 h reperfusion of the ischemic area. Evaluation involved the monitoring of ischemic arrhythmias (Hellige Servomed, Switzerland) and measuring the size of infarction by means of the tetrazolium staining technique [30]. Arrhythmias were evaluated in accordance with The Lambeth Convention [15,20,31].

Measurement of infarct size

After 4 h of reperfusion, the hearts were arrested in diastole with 0.25 mg verapamil (Isoptin, Knoll, Germany) injected into the right jugular vein. The hearts were excised and washed with 20 ml saline through the cannulated aorta. The LAD coronary artery was then reoccluded and the ischemic zone was delineated by staining the non-ischemic tissue with 5% potassium permanganate (Lachema, Czech Republic) dissolved in 2 ml of water, through the aorta. After washing out the solution thoroughly with saline and releasing the occlusion, the hearts were perfused with 1% 2,3,5-triphenyltetrasolium chloride (TTC, Sigma-Aldrich, Germany) dissolved in 0.1 $mol \cdot l^{-1}$ phosphate buffer (pH 7.4) to stain surviving mocardium of the area at risk. The hearts were than incubated in the effluent of TTC for 20 min. Than, hearts were cut perpendicularly to the long axis of the ventricle into slices 1 mm thick and stored overnight in 10% neutral formaldehyde solution. The day after the infarct-size staining, the right ventricular free wall was separated and both sides of the slices were photographed. The infarct size (IS), size of the area at risk (AR) and the size of the left ventricle (LV) were determined by planimetry. The IS was normalized to the to AR and to LV (IS/AR and IS/LV, respectively); the size of AR was normalized to LV (AR/LV) [30].

Isolated preparations of cardiac sarcolemma and mitochondria

Sarcolemmal membranes: isolated sarcolemmal membranes from diabetic and control rat hearts were prepared from 10% (weight/volume) homogenates of the myocardium, by the method of hypotonic shock, followed by treatment with 0.6 $mol \cdot l^{-1}$ sodium iodide (NaI). The resulting membrane fraction was highly enriched in sarcolemma and contained less than 3% of sarcoplasmic reticulum and/or mitochondrial membranes (estimated by measuring the activities of marker enzymes of the sarcoplasmic reticulum and mitochondria). For more details see Vrbjar et al. [32]. *Mitochondria*: Excised hearts were cooled down to 0°C, washed free of blood, cleaned from pericardium, vessels, valves and fat and minced fine with pair of scissors. For isolation of mitochondria the differential centrifugation procedure of Lehninger et al. [33] was applied. *Briefly*: Mitochodria were liberated from the fine cut tissue by gentle homogenization (teflon homogenizer) in a medium containing in mmol·l^{-1}: 20 Tris.HCl, 4 EDTA, 180 KCl. After repeated spuning down and washing, the final mitochondrial fraction was resuspended in 50 mmol·l^{-1} Tris-HCl buffer (pH 7.4), adjusted to a final protein concentration of 75 μg/50 μl and used for further investigations. The resulting mitochondrial fraction was contaminated to less than 3% by membranes of sarcoplasmic reticulum and/or sarcolemma (estimated by measuring the activities of the respective marker enzymes). For more details see [34].

Estimation of mitochondrial ATPase activities

Activities of the oligomycin-sensitive Mg^{2+}-dependent ATPase of isolated mitochondria were estimated in 1 ml of incubation medium containing in mmol·l^{-1}: 250 imidazol buffer, pH 7.4; 40 $MgCl_2$, 40 ATP.Tris and 75 μg of mitochondrial protein. When estimating the total Mg^{2+}-dependent and dinitrophenol stimulated activity of the enzyme, the incubation medium contained in addition also 0.1 mmol·l^{-1} 2,4-dinitrophenol. After 10 min preincubation at 37°C, the reaction was started with addition of ATP and terminated (after 20 min) by an equal volume (1 ml) of ice-cold 12% trichloroacetic acid (TCA). Enzyme activities were measured by estimating the amounts of orthophosphate liberated by ATP splitting and expressed in mmol P_i·g^{-1} of mit. prot·h^{-1}. Protein was estimated according to Lowry et al. [35] using bovine serum albumin as a standard. Inorganic phosphorus was determined using the method of Taussky and Schorr [36].

Measurement of membrane fluidity

Fluidity of the mitochondrial and sarcolemmal membranes was determined by means of 1,6-diphenyl-1,3,5-hexatriene (DPH, Sigma-Aldrich, Germany)—a fluorescent probe commonly used for monitoring of structural ordering of membranes. Isolated mitochondrial or sarcolemmal membranes (diluted 40 times) were stained in 50 mmol·l^{-1} Tris·HCl buffer containing 1 μmol·l^{-1} DPH. Subsequently the steady-state anisotropy of DPH was measured at room temperature with the SPECORD M-40 (Germany) spectrophotometer. The measured steady-state fluorescence of DPH characterizes the state of stiffness of phospholipid acyl chains in the lipid bilayer of membranes and is in a reversal proportion to fluidity of membrane lipids. Incorporation of DPH into the membranes was characterized by fluorescence anisotropy decay in the 1–60 min range. Experimental data were fitted to an exponential curve using the least square method. The rate constant of DPH incorporation (k) was calculated according to the equation:

$$r(t) = R_S + (R_0 - R_S)\exp(-kt)$$

where t is the time measured from the addition of DPH; R_0 and R_S represent minimalized values of the fit at the beginning and at the completion of DPH passage

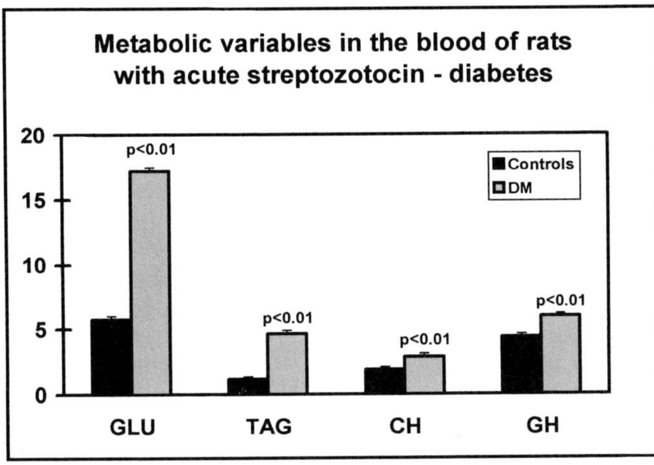

Figure 1. Glu—glucose; TAG—triacylglycerols; CH—cholesterol; GH—glycohemoglobin. Data for GLU and TAG are given in mmol/l, for CH in g/l, and for GH in % of the total hemoglogin content; Data represent means ± SEM; n = 51.

through the membrane into the hydrophobic core. Fore more details see Šikurová et al. [37].

Statistics

Results were evaluated as means ± S.E.M. One-way analysis of variance ANOVA followed by Tukey method were applied to test for any significant differences in normally distributed variables among the groups. Non-Gaussian distributed variables, such as incidences of ventricular tachycardia and fibrillations were compared using the Fisher's exact test. Differences between groups with $p < 0.05$ or less were considered as significant.

RESULTS AND DISCUSSION

Metabolic status of the animals

The levels of glucose and contents of glycohemoglobin in blood and of triacylglycerols and cholesterol in serum (Fig. 1), monitored to characterize the metabolic status of healthy control animals, were fully comparable with normal metabolic values reported earlier [5,6,38]. In contrast, the group of diabetic animals exhibited a significant ($p < 0.01$) elevation in the values of glucose, triacylglycerols, cholesterol, and glycohemoglobin amounting to 199.7, 394.9, 52.2, and 36.5%, respectively. Forty eight hours after streptozotocin administration and later on, the animals exhibited positive glucosuria. In addition, the latter findings were also accompanied by enhanced Amadori product formation manifested in a 31% ($p < 0.01$) increase

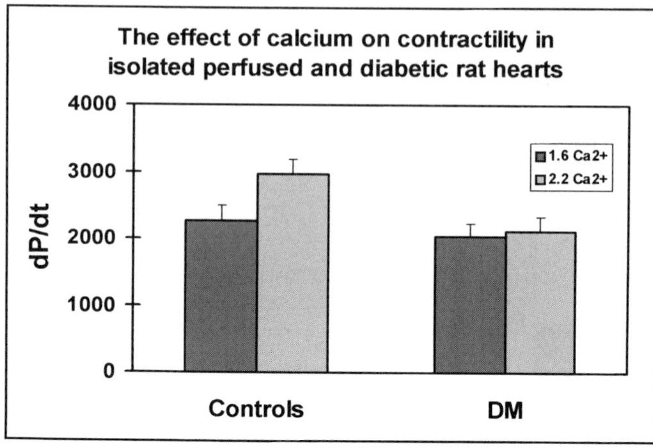

Figure 2. Abbreviations: C 1.6 Ca^{2+}, C 2.2 Ca^{2+}, DM 1.6 Ca^{2+}, DM 2.2 Ca^{2+}—control and diabetic hearts perfused with either 1.6 or 2.2 Ca^{2+}, mmol/l. Data represent means ± SEM; n = 10 – 12. Significances for dP/dt: C 2.2 Ca^{2+} vs. C 1.6 Ca^{2+}, DM 1.6 Ca^{2+} as well as DM 2.2 Ca^{2+}—$p < 0.05$.

in fructosamine content of the heart sarcolemma (from 2.68 ± 0.14 to 3.51 ± 0.45 mg^{-1}·prot.) and confirmed the presence of completely developed diabetes. For details concerning fructosamine estimation see [18]. All these values are in agreement with the biochemical findings presented in our earlier studies [5,6,18,38].

Heart Inotropy and MiCS formation

In healthy control hearts, elevation of Ca^{2+} concentration in perfusate expectantly led to an enhanced calcium influx into the heart cells and augmented, consequently, the intracellular Ca^{2+} transients that, in turn, propagated a signal for both: i) an increase of heart contractility, manifested in an increase of dP/dt (Fig. 2), that is always coupled with increased utilization of ATP (not shown), and ii) an increase in MiCS formation (Fig. 3). It is believed, that increase in MiCS formation reflects an activation of the energy delivery pathway, particularly of transfer of the high-energy phosphate bonds from the mitochondria to the cytoplasm [39,40]. In cardiac cells, this occurs to meet the increased energy demands of the heart [8,23]. In our experiments, this assumption was proved by Ca^{2+}-induced positive inotropic response, manifested in an increase of dP/dt amounting 30.2%, $p < 0.01$ (Fig. 2), and also in elevated MiCS formation, represented by an S_S increase amounting 75.7%, $p < 0.01$ (Fig. 3). On the other hand, replacement of Ca^{2+} by Cd^{2+} ions led to a weakening of Ca^{2+} signal and caused a fast and significant ($p < 0.01$) depression in MiCS formation (Fig. 3). That again proved the key role of the Ca^{2+} signal in mechanism of coupling between MiCS formation and the energy demands of the myocardium. In diabetic hearts, already the basic MiCS formation was identi-

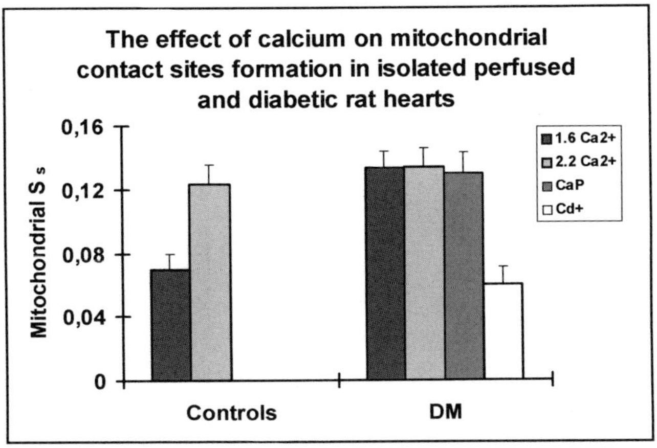

Figure 3. Abbreviations: C 1.6 Ca^{2+}, C 2.2 Ca^{2+}, DM 1.6 Ca^{2+}, DM 2.2 Ca^{2+}—control and diabetic hearts perfused with either 1.6 or 2.2 Ca^{2+}, mmol/l; DM CaP—diabetic hearts with calcium paradox; DM Cd—diabetic hearts with Ca^{2+} replaced by Cd^{2+}. Data represent means ± SEM; n = 10 – 12. Significances for S_s: C 1.6 Ca^{2+} and DM Cd vs. C 2.2 Ca^{2+}, DM 1.6 Ca^{2+}, DM 2.2 Ca^{2+} as well as DM CaP—$p < 0.05$.

cal with that which could be maximally achieved in healthy control hearts, upon perfusion with elevated calcium. Nevertheless, neither the elevated Ca^{2+} in perfusion medium, nor the induction of calcium paradox proved to be potent enough to induce any considerable stimulation in MiCS formation in diabetic hearts (Fig. 3). This indicated, that in acute diabetic hearts, the Ca^{2+} signal for augmentation of energy delivery through the mitochondrial membrane is already permanently present and its regulatory effect is maximally developed.

Biophysical properties of mitochondria and sarcolemma: role of the membrane fluidity

Mitochondrial contact sites are dynamic structures formed by molecular conglomerates consisting of molecules of ATP/ADP-phosphotransferase (ATP/ADP-translocase) in the inner-, porine in the outer mitochondrial membrane, and of the octameric isoform of mitochondrial creatine phosphokinase in the intermembrane space. In electrone microscope MiCS appear as points of contacts between the inner- and outer mitochondrial membranes. But, in fact, each molecular conglomerate (MiCS) crosses mitochondrial membrane in a single span that also serves as an energy transport channel [8,23,28,39,40]. MiCS are ephemeral structures, formed more abundantly when energy demands of the cells are high and again disintegrated when the need for their function is declining [8,22.23]. It may be assumed, that active formation and/or disintegration of MiCS may be associated with considerable changes in membrane fluidity, particularly in cardiac mitochondria. But, in spite of that, little exact data were available in this respect since yet. Our present exper-

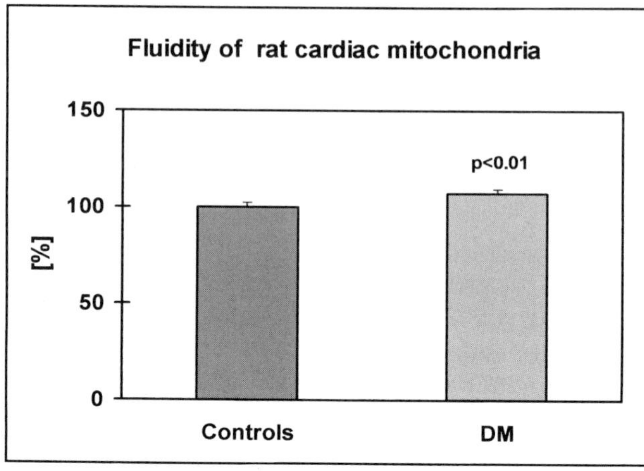

Figure 4. Abbreviations: r—steady-state fluorescence anisotropy of diphenylhexatriene; DM—diabetic hearts. Data represent means ± SEM, expressed in per cent of the control value. Actual value of r for the controls amounts to 0.347. n = 9 for controls, and 8 for DM.

imental data revealed that in acute, but fully developed diabetes (8 days), when the hearts are not yet failing, and the intracellular Ca^{2+} signaling and MiCS formation are augmented, the fluidity of mitochondrial membranes becomes significantly ($p < 0.01$) increased (Fig. 4). It may be assumed that the mechanism of MiCS formation requires free movements of numerous molecules in the membrane. The sequence of these movements starts with entry of Ca^{2+} and acceptance of the Ca^{2+} signal somewhere in the membrane. It is followed by octamerising mCPK (still unknown mechanism). The series of consequent steps is finished by pulling of both mitochondrial membranes together, an event associated with formation of the molecular triplet (of MiCS) in the place where the membranes are closest approaching themselves. Hence, a concomitant increase in membrane fluidity seems to be the proper condition that might secure the whole process. But, on the other hand, free radicals are believed to play an important role in pathogenesis of diabetes [41,42]. When attacked by reactive oxygen species, subcellular membranes usually exhibit decreased fluidity and increased lipoperoxidation [18,38,43,44]. In order to check whether the increased fluidity may be a response specific only for cardiac mitochondria in acute diabetes, the fluidity of isolated heart sarcolemmal membranes was also investigated in this stage of the disease (Fig. 5). Results revealed that in contrast to mitochondria, sarcolemmal membranes from acute diabetic hearts exhibited significantly ($p < 0.001$) decreased membrane fluidity. It is little probable, that our findings of increased membrane fluidity in mitochondria of acute diabetic hearts are really questioning the free radical-paradigm. It sounds more likely, that during the acute phase of diabetes, when the endogenous mechanisms of protection, leading to adaptation of the myocardium, are strongly activated, mitochondrial functions become also activated.

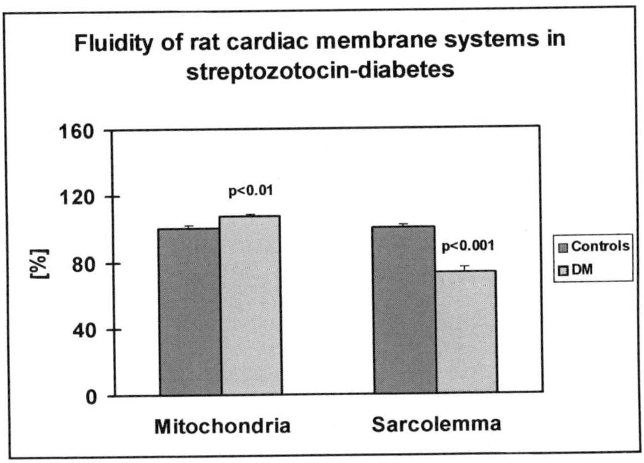

Figure 5. Abbreviations: r—steady-state fluorescence anisotropy of diphenylhexatriene; DM—diabetic hearts. Data represent means ± SEM, expressed in per cent of the control values. Actual values of r for the controls amount to 0.347 for mitochondria (n = 9 for control, and 8 for DM) and 0.185 for sarcolemma.

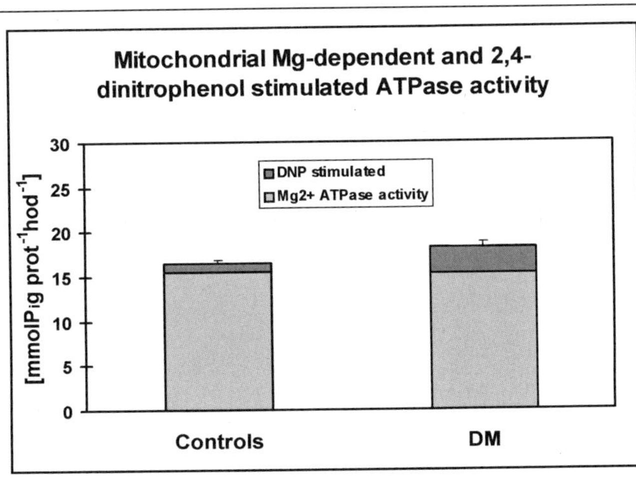

Figure 6. Abbreviations: DNP—2,4-dinitrophenol; DM—diabetic hearts. Data represent means ± SEM; n = 9, and 8 respectively. Mg^{2+}-stimulated plus DNP-stimulated portions represent the total Mg^{2+}-ATPase activity. Significance of the total activity in controls vs. DM was $p < 0.05$.

A 10.6% increase in total mitochondrial ATPase activity (the Mg^{2+}-activated + DNP-stimulated portions of activity), which accompanied the observed increase in membrane fluidity, is also testifying for some enhancement in metabolic activity of the mitochondria (Fig. 6). All these variables indicate that in acute phase of strep-

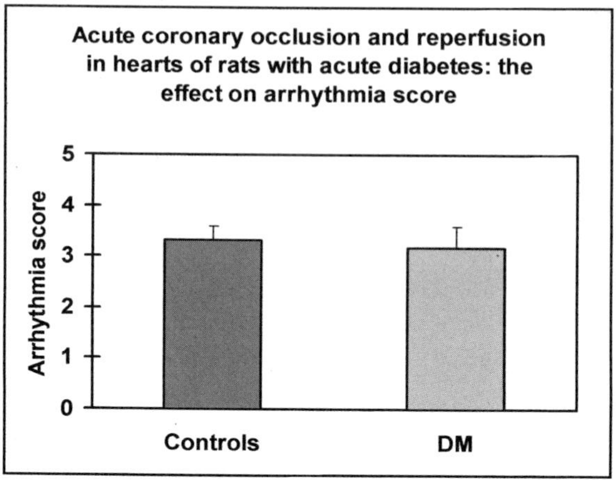

Figure 7. Abbreviation: DM—hearts from diabetic animals. Data represent means ± SEM; n = 12. Non-significant.

tozotocin-diabetes, mitochondria may substantially participate in energy household of the diabetic heart.

Ischemic tolerance

In order to evaluate the significance of augmented energy transfer from mitochondria for function and particularly for ischemia tolerance of the myocardium, adapted to work in conditions of acute diabetes, hearts of diabetic rats were subjected to acute coronary occlusion and reperfusion of the occluded area. In healthy control hearts, ventricular tachycardia after LAD coronary artery ligation represented 55.4% of the total arrhythmias and occurred in 90 % of the animals. In diabetic rats, arrhythmia profile was similar to that in the control group, and the incidence of tachyarrhythmias and their severity were not enhanced (arrhythmia score 3.18 ± 0.4 vs. 3.3 ± 0.3 in the controls, $p > 0.05$). The results in Fig. 7 indicate that in comparison with control hearts, the diabetic hearts are not more susceptible to ventricular arrhythmias induced by acute myocardial ischemia. On the other hand, the infarct size normalized to the size of area at risk (Fig. 8) was by 16.9% ($p < 0.05$) smaller in the diabetic hearts than in control hearts.

General conclusions

1) Hearts of rats with acute but fully developed streptozotocin-diabetes exhibit activated mechamisms of endogenous protection, which allows them to adapt to work at unfavorable conditions of diabetes.
2) Cardiac mitochondria from rats with acute diabetes exhibit increased membrane fluidity and elevated mitochondrial ATPase activities. These changes seem to belong either to endogenous protection or to adaptation mechanisms.

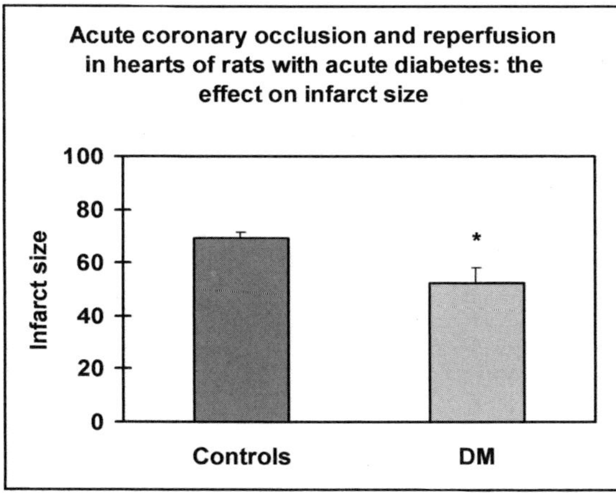

Figure 8. Abbreviation: DM—hearts from diabetic animals. Data represent means ± SEM; n = 12. Significance:—*p < 0.05.

3) Ca^{2+}-signaling represents the link between the energy delivery from mitochondria (via MiCS) and the energy requirements of the heart.
4) In diabetic hearts, which are performing permanently in energy deficiency, the augmented (to maximum) energy transport via MiCS seems to be a part of adaptation changes. This contributes to increased resistance of diabetic hearts to various forms of damage.
5) In the acute phase of diabetes, rat hearts are more resistant to irreversible cell injury.

ACKNOWLEDGMENTS

Authors are indebted to D. Pancza who spare no effort in performing the experiments with perfused hearts and monitoring the arrhythmias as well as to Kristina Nagyová, Juraj Rievaj, and Jozef Tánczos, pregraduate students of biophysics and physiology, who also participated in the study. The excellent technical assistance of A. Brichtová, A. Macsáliová, I. Blažíčková, M. Hýbelová, Z. Hradecká and E. Havránková is also gratefully appreciated. Supported in part with VEGA grants 2/7157/22, 2/2063/22, 2/7155/21 and 1/7673/20.

REFERENCES

1. Dhalla NS, Liu X, Panagia V, Takeda N. 1998. Subcellular remodeling and heart dysfunction in chronic diabetes. Cardiovasc Res 40:239–247.
2. Ziegelhöffer A, Ravingerová T, Styk J, Džurba A, Volkovová K, Čársky J, Waczulíková I. 1998. Hearts with diabetic cardiomyopathy: Adaptation to calcium overload. Exp Clin Cardiol 3:158–161.
3. Pierce GN, Dhalla NS. 1984. Heart mitochondrial function in chronic experimental diabetes in rats. Can J Cardiol 1:48–54.

4. Pierce GN, Ramjiwan B, Meng H-P. 1991. Cardiac sarcolemma membrane alterations during the diabetic cardiomyopathy. In: The Diabetic Heart. Ed. M Nagano and NS Dhalla, 229–236. New York: Raven Press.
5. Gøtzshe O. 1991. Myocardial calcium uptake and catecholamine sensitivity in experimental diabetes. In: The Diabetic Heart. Ed. M Nagano and NS Dhalla, 199–208. New York: Raven Press.
6. Ziegelhöffer A, Ravingerová T, Styk J, Tribulová N, Volkovová K, Šeboková J, Breier A. 1996. Diabetic cardiomyopathy in rats: biochemical mechanisms of elevated tolerance to calcium overload. Diabetes Res Clin Pract 31:S93–S103.
7. Ziegelhöffer A, Kjeldsen K, Bundgaard H, Breier A, Vrbjar N, Džurba A. 2000. Na,K-ATPase in the myocardium: Molecular principles, functional and clinical aspects. Gen Physiol Biophys 19:9–47.
8. Ziegelhöffer-Mihalovičová B, Okruhlicová L', Tribulová N, Ravingerová T, Volkovová K, Šeboková J, Ziegelhöffer A. 1997. Mitochondrial contact sites detected by creatine phosphokinase activity in the hearts of normal and diabetic rats. Is mitochondrial contact site formation a calcium dependent process? Gen Physiol Biophys 16:329–338.
9. Strödter D, Willmann P, Willmann J, Federlin K, Schaper W. 1991. In: The Diabetic Heart. Ed. M Nagano and NS Dhalla, 383–393. New York: Raven Press.
10. Fedelešová M, Dhalla NS, Balasubramanian V, Ziegelhöffer A. 1972. Energy dependent stimulation of membrane bound Mg^{2+} and Na^{+}-K^{+}-ATPase by glucose. In: Les Surcharges Cardiaques (Heart Overloading), Colloque INSERM. Ed. P Hatt, 217–221. Paris: INSERM.
11. Askenasy N. 2001. Glycolysis protects sarcolemmal membrane integrity during total ischemia in the rat heart. Basic Res Cardiol 96:612–622.
12. Seymour A-M, Brosnan MJ. 1991. Nuclear magnetic resonance investigations of energy metabolism in diabetic cardiomyopathy. In: The Diabetic Heart. Ed. M Nagano and NS Dhalla, 371–382. New York: Raven Press.
13. Ravingerová T, Styk J, Pancza D, Tribulová N, Šeboková J, Volkovová K, Ziegelhöffer A, Slezák J. 1996. Diabetic cardiomyopathy in rats: alleviation of myocardial dysfunction caused by Ca^{2+} overload. Diabetes Res Clin Pract 31:S105–S112.
14. Tani M, Neely JR. 1988. Hearts from diabetic rats are more resistant to in vitro ischemia: possible role of altered Ca^{2+} metabolism. Circ Res 62:931–940.
15. Ravingerová T, Kolář F, Neckář J, Štetka R, Volkovová K, Ziegelhöffer A, Styk J. 2001. Ventricular arrhythmias following coronary artery occlusion in rats: is the diabetic heart less or more sensitive to ischemia? Basic Res Cardiol 96:160–168.
16. Ravingerová T, Štetka R, Barančík M, Volkovová K, Pancza D, Ziegelhöffer A, Styk J. 2001. Response to ischemia and endogenous myocardial protection in the diabetic heart. In: Diabetes and Cardiovascular Disease. Ed. A Angel, N Dhalla, G Pierce and P Singal, 285–293. New York: Kluwer Academic/Plenum Publishers.
17. Strnisková M, Neckář J, Barančík M, Kolář F, Ravingerová T. 2001. Rats with acute diabetes mellitus are more resistant to ischemic injury. J Mol Cell Cardiol 33:A114
18. Ziegelhöffer A, Ravingerová T, Styk J, Šeboková J, Waczulíková I, Breier A, Džurba A, Volkovová K, Čársky J, Turecký L. 1997. Mechanisms that may be involved in calcium tolerance of the diabetic heart. Mol Cell Biochem 176:191–198.
19. Kusama Y, Hearse DL, Avkiran M. 1992. Diabetes and susceptibility of reperfusion-induced vetricular arrhythmias. J Mol Cell Cardiol 24:411–421.
20. Ravingerová T, Štetka R, Pancza D, Uličná O, Ziegelhöffer A, Styk J. 2000. Susceptibility to ischemia-induced arrhythmias and the effect of preconditioning in the diabetc rat heart. Physiol Res 49:607–616.
21. Kuo HT, Moore KH, Giomelli F, Wiener J. 1983. Defective oxidative metabolism of heart mitochondria from genetically diabetic mice. Diabetes 32:181–187.
22. Bakker A, Bernaert I, De Bie M, Ravingerová T, Ziegelhöffer A. 1994. The effect of calcium on mitochondrial contact sites: a study on isolated rat hearts. Biochim Biophys Acta 1224:583–588.
23. Ziegelhöffer-Mihalovičová B, Ziegelhöffer A, Ravingerová T, Kolář F, Jacob W, Tribulová N. 2002. Regulation of mitochondrial contact sites in neonatal, juvenile, and diabetic hearts. 2002 Mol Cell Biochem 236:37–44.
24. Tinder P. 1969. Determination of blood glucose using 4-amino phenazon as oxygen acceptor. J Clin Path 22:246–253.
25. Burrin JM, Worth R, Ashworth AA, Alberti KGMM. 1980. Automated colorimetric estimation of glycosylated hemoglobin. Clin Chim Acta 106:45–50.

26. Watson D. 1960. A simple method for determination of serum cholesterol. Clin Chim Acta 5:613–615.
27. Fossati P, Prencipe L. 1982. Serum triglycerides determined colorimetrically with an enzyme that produces hydrogen peroxide. Clin Chem 28:2077–2080.
28. Biermans W, Bernaert I, De Bie M, Nijs B, Jacob W. 1989. Ultrastructural localisation of creatine kinase activity in the contact sites between inner and outer mitochondrial membranes in rat myocardium. Biochim Biophys Acta 974:74–80.
29. Baddeley AJ, Gundersen HJG, Cruz-Olive RM. 1986. Estimation of surface area of vertical sections. J Microsc (Oxford) 142:259–276.
30. Neckář J, Papoušek F, Nováková O, Ošt'ádal B, Kolář F. 2002. Cardioprotective effects of chronic hypoxia and ischaemic preconditioning are not additive. Basic Res Cardiol 97:161–167.
31. Walker MJA, Curtis MJ, Hearse DJ, Campbell RWS, Jansen MJ, Yellon DM, Cobbe SM, Coker SM, Harness JB, Harron WG, Higgins AJ, Julian DG, Lab MJ, Manning AS, Northover BJ, Parratt JR, Riemersma RA, Riva E, Russell DC, Sheridan DJ, Winslow E, Woodward B. 1988. The Lambeth Conwentions: guide-lines for study of arrhythmias in ischaemia, infarction and reperfusion. Cardiovasc Res 22:447–455.
32. Vrbjar N, Soos J, Ziegelhöffer A. 1984. Secondary structure of heart sarcolemmal proteins during interaction with metallic cofactors of (Na,K)-ATPase. Gen Physiol Biophys 3:317–325.
33. Lehninger AL, Carafoli E, Rossi CS. 1967. Energy linked ion movements in mitochondrial systems. Advanced Enzymology 29:259–320.
34. Ziegelhöffer A, Monošíková R, Džurba A, Vrbjar N. 1982. Influence of ischemia on the activities of mitochondrial creatine phosphokinase in the myocardium. Bratisl Lek Listy (Bratislava Medical Letters) 77:566–575.
35. Lowry OH, Rosebrough NJ, Farr AR, Randall RJ. 1953. Protein measurement with the folin phenol reagent. J Biol Chem 193:265–275.
36. Taussky AA, Shorr EE. 1953. A microcolorimetric method for determination of inorganic phosphorus. J Biol Chem 202:575–583.
37. Šikurová L, Nemcová P, Kvasnička P, Hianik T. 1997. Fluorescence anisotropy studies of ACTH interaction with lecithin bilayers. J Fluorescence 7:151S–153S.
38. Ziegelhöffer A, Styk J, Ravingerová T, Šeboková J, Volkovová K, Waczulíková I, Čársky J, Džurba A, Dočolomanský P. 1999. Prevention of processes coupled with free radical formation prevents also the development of calcium resistance in the diabetic heart. Life Sci 65:1999–2001.
39. Wyss M, Smeiting J, Wevers RA, Wallimann T. 1992. Mitochondrial creatine kinase: A key enzyme of aerobic energy metabolism. Biochim Biophys Acta 1102:119–166.
40. Knoll G, Brdiczka D. 1993. Changes in freeze fractured mitochondrial membranes correlated to their energy state—dynamic interactions of the boundary membranes. Biochim Biophys Acta 773:102–110.
41. Oberley LW. 1988. Free radicals and diabetes. Free Rad Biol Med 5:113–124.
42. Baynes JW. 1991. Role of oxidative stress in development of complications in diabetes. Diabetes 40:405–412.
43. Waczulíková I, Šikurová L, Čársky J. 2002. Fluidity gradient of erythrocyte membranes in diabetics: the effect of resorcylidene aminoguanidine. Bioelectrochemistry 55:53–55.
44. Watala C, Winocour P. 1992. The relationship of chemical modification of membrane proteins and plasma lipoproteins to reduced membrane fluidity of erythrocytes of diabetic subjects. Clin Chem Clin Biochem 30:513–519.

G.N. Pierce, M. Nagano, P. Zahradka, and N.S. Dhalla (eds.).
ATHEROSCLEROSIS, HYPERTENSION AND DIABETES.

KETOSIS, TUMOR NECROSIS FACTOR-α AND CARDIOVASCULAR DISEASE IN TYPE-1 DIABETIC PATIENTS

SUSHIL K. JAIN, ROBERT MCVIE, and JOSEPH A. BOCCHINI, JR.

Department of Padiatrics, Louisiana State University Health Sciences Center, Shreveport, LA 71130, USA

Summary. The molecular mechanisms by which ketosis promotes the vascular disease, morbidity and mortality in type-1 diabetic patients are unclear. Elevated blood level of TNF-α, a pro-inflammatory cytokine, is a risk factor in the development of vascular inflammation and cardiovascular disease. This chapter has focused on the following points: (1) Hyperketonemic diabetic patients have significantly higher levels of TNF-α compared with normoketonemic diabetic patients and normal controls. There is a significant correlation between ketosis and oxidative stress as well as between the oxidative stress and TNF-α levels in the blood of diabetic patients. (2) Ketone body acetoacetate (AA) treatment increases TNF-α secretion and increases oxygen radicals production in U937 monocyte cells. However, β-hydroxybutyrate did not have any effect on TNF-α secretion or oxygen radicals production in U937 cells. (3) Exogenous addition of antioxidant N-acetylcysteine prevents stimulation of TNF-α secretion caused by AA alone or with high glucose (HG). The effect of AA or HG on TNF-α secretion was inhibited by specific inhibitors of protein kinase A, p38-MAPK and NFkB. Thus, ketosis increases circulating TNF-α levels, which can promote the development of cardiovascular disease in diabetic patients.

***Key words*:** TNF-α, Oxygen redicals, Diabetes, Ketosis

ABBREVIATIONS

TNF-α: Tumor Necrosis Factor-alpha; AA: acetoacetate; BHB: β-hydroxybutyrate; NKD:normoketonemic diabetics; HKD: hyperketonemic diabetics; HG: High-

Address for Correspondence: Dr. Sushil K. Jain, Department of Pediatrics, LSU Health Sciences Center, 1501 Kings Highway, Shreveport, LA 71130. Tel: 1-318-675-6086; Fax: 1-318-675-6059; e-mail: sjain@lsuhsc.edu

glucose; PMA:phorbol 12-myristate 13-acetate; AKB: α-ketobutyrate; NAC: N-acetylcysteine; ROS: reactive oxygen species; ERK: extracellular signal–regulated kinase; MAPK: mitogen-activated protein kinase; JNK: c-jun N-terminal kinase; NFkB: Nuclear transcription factor.

INTRODUCTION

Diabetes mellitus is a chronic disease affecting 6–8% of the total population, with nearly 600,000 new cases diagnosed each year. The total cost of patient care is more than 100 billion dollars per year. Vascular inflammation and complications are the leading cause of morbidity and mortality in the diabetic population and remain a major public health issue [1,2]. The risk factors include hyperglycemia, hyperosmolarity, free fatty acids, ketosis, dehydration, and change in pH, altered insulin-glucagon ratio, pro-inflammatory cytokines (such as TNF-α, IL-6 and IL-1β), and several other unknown factors [2]. Hyperglycemia is one of the major risk factors in the development of vascular complications [3]. Many of the biochemical pathways by which hyperglycemia may cause cellular damage include: increased polyol pathway and associated changes in the intracellular redox state, increased diacylglycerol synthesis with consequent activation of specific protein kinase C isoforms, increased nonenzymatic glycation of both intra- and extracellular proteins, and increased oxidative stress [1–5].

In addition to hyperglycemia, type-1 diabetic patients frequently experience ketosis from excessive fat breakdown because body fuel is derived mainly from fat when the body is in a state of insulin deficiency [6]. In general, diabetic patients receiving regular health care have better controlled ketosis. Yet, during routine check-ups they frequently are found to have 1 to 2 mM concentrations of ketones in their blood, which is much higher than the normal level. Over the long term, diabetic patients with frequent episodes of ketosis have higher incidences of vascular disease, general pain and discomfort, loss of productivity and shortened life spans. The molecular mechanisms of altered protein function and gene expression in ketosis induced tissue injury are not known.

TNF-α AND VASCULAR INFLAMMATION IN DIABETES

Tumor Necrosis Factor-alpha (TNF-α) is produced by macrophages and other cell types and can stimulate the release of interleukins, prostaglandin and chemokines [7]. It has been suggested that increased TNF-α production and decreased insulin sensitivity are causally linked in vivo [7–11]. Elevated circulating levels of TNF-α can cause induction of interleukins and adhesion molecules and thereby increase monocyte-endothelial cell adhesion, which is now recognized as an early and rate-limiting step in the development of vascular disease and arteriosclerosis [12,13]. Several pro-inflammatory cytokines including TNF-α, IL-6 and IL-1β play a significant role in the advancement of vascular complications in many models of inflammation including diabetes [2].

OXIDATIVE STRESS, KETOSIS AND DIABETES

The levels of lipid peroxidation products in the blood are higher in diabetic patients in general [14–19] and much higher in diabetic patients with poor glycemic control and vascular disease [19–21]. Recent studies have demonstrated that the ketone body AA can generate oxygen radicals, cause glutathione (GSH) depletion, and increase lipid peroxidation and apoptosis in human endothelial cells and monocytes [22,23]. Oxidative stress levels are higher in the RBC and plasma of hyperketonemic (HKD) compared with normoketonemic type-1 diabetic (NKD) patients [24,25]. Oxidative stress in diabetes may arise from a variety of mechanisms, such as excessive oxygen radical production as a result of the auto-oxidation of glucose [26], the activation of P-450-like activity by the glucose metabolite NADPH [27], glycated proteins [28] and the ketone body AA [22,24], and the depletion of NADH by the activation of aldose reductase [29] and glycation of antioxidative enzymes, which limits their capacity to detoxify oxygen radicals [30,31]. The proposed mechanism by which AA could generate oxygen radicals and cause cellular lipid peroxidation may involve its auto-oxidation, or some unknown metabolite of AA may also generate ROS. Ketosis can increase extra-mitochondrial oxidation of fatty acids and generation of hydrogen peroxide and thereby increase oxidative stress in HKD patients. The normalization of superoxide radical generation prevents glucose-induced activation of protein kinase C, formation of advanced glycation end products, sorbitol accumulation, and NFkB activation in cultured endothelial cells [29].

KETOSIS AND TNF-α SECRETION

Figures 1 illustrate significantly higher levels of TNF-α in diabetic patients (D) compared with age-matched normal subjects (N). However, when D was divided into NKD and HKD groups, HKD patients had significantly higher levels of TNF-α compared with those of NKD patients ($p < 0.01$). There was no difference in the levels of TNF-α in NKD patients compared with those of age-matched normal subjects. We used blood concentrations of AA as an index of ketosis. Diabetic patients whose blood level of AA was =>>0.3 μM were considered HKD and those with <0.3 μM were considered NKD. There was no difference in duration of diabetes (5.1 ± 1 vs. 5.8 ± 1 yrs) and ages (12 ± 1 vs. 13 ± 1 yrs) between NKD and HKD, and in ages between N (12 ± 1) and D (13 ± 1) groups. HbA_{1c} levels between NKD (10.3 ± 1.5%) and HKD (11 ± 1.3%) were not significantly different. This suggests that ketosis increases the production of TNF-α in diabetic patients. This study also found a significant relationship ($r = 0.36$, $p < 0.05$, $n = 34$) between the ketosis (as determined by AA level) and oxidative stress (as assessed by protein oxidation level, as well as between the protein oxidation and TNF-α levels ($r = 0.47$, $p < 0.02$, $n = 34$) in the blood of type-1 diabetic patients.

In order to examine the biochemical mechanisms leading to elevate TNF-α levels in HKD patients, we studied the TNF-α secretion by a U937 monocytic cell line cultured with elevated levels of AA or BHB with and without high-glucose (HG) levels in the culture medium. Figure 2 shows that AA; BHB or AKB alone does

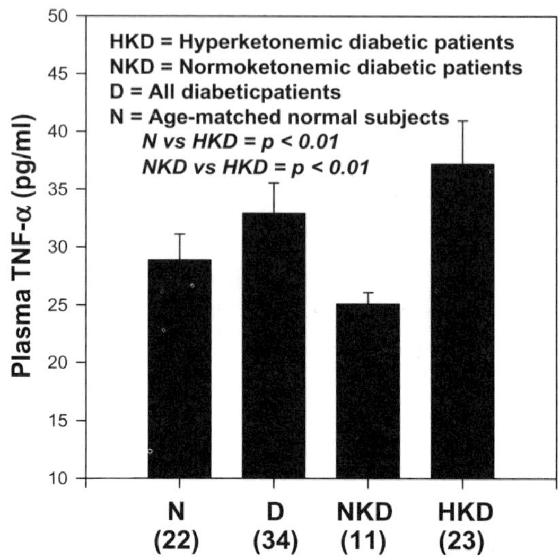

Figure 1. Plasma TNF-α levels in normo- and hyper-ketonemic diabetic patients and age-matched normal subjects.

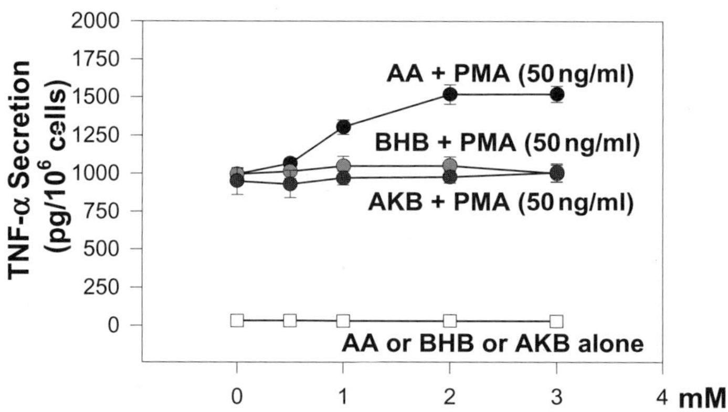

Figure 2. Effect of acetoacetate (AA) or β-hydroxybutyrate (BHB) or α-ketobutyrate (AKB) on TNFα secretion by cultured U937 monocytes.

not have any effect on TNF-α secretion in unstimulated monocytes. However, in PMA-activated monocytes, AA caused a concentration-dependent increase in TNF-α secretion.

Figure 3 shows that AA at levels similar to those frequently encountered in diabetic patients can cause ROS production in monocytes. Neither BHB nor AKB had

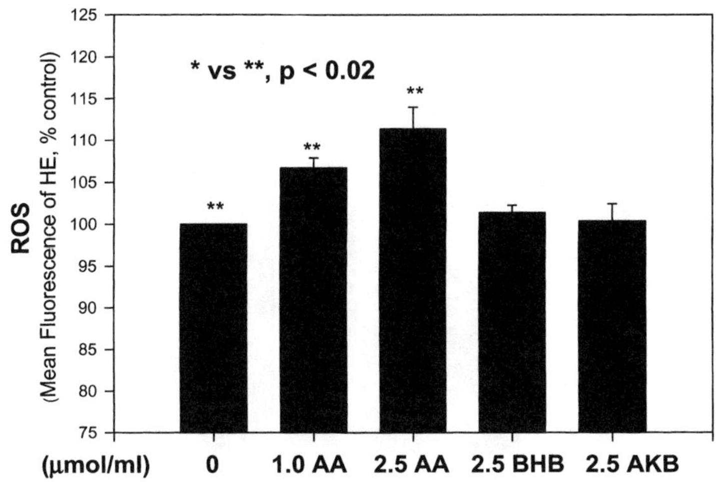

Figure 3. Effect of AA, BHB and α-ketobutyrate (AKB) on ROS production in U937 cells (24 hrs).

any effect on ROS production. There is an increase in TNF-α production caused by the peroxide in activated monocytes [32]. HG also resulted in a modest increase in TNF-α secretion in PMA-activated monocytes (Fig. 4). The effect of AA on TNF-α secretion was observed even in the presence of HG. However, treatment with elevated levels of BHB alone or in the presence of HG, or AKB or mannitol did not have any change on TNF-α secretion compared with basal levels (Fig. 4). Thus, elevated AA levels can promote TNF-α secretion in both *in vitro* cell cultures model and *in vivo* in type-1 diabetic patients. This also suggest a role of oxidative stress in the enhanced TNF-α secretion in AA-treated U937 monocytes.

Figure 5 illustrates that exogenous addition of dibutyryl cAMP lowered the production of TNF-α in AA, HG or AA + HG treated monocytes. Similarly, forsokolin, which stimulates the endogenous production of cAMP, caused a significant inhibition of TNF-α secretion by AA, HG and AA + HG. AA and AA + HG treatment significantly lowered cAMP levels in monocytes (data not given). This suggests that elevated TNF-α production is mediated by cAMP depletion.

H89 (an inhibitor of protein kinase) and SB203580 (an inhibitor of p38-MAPK) as well as a cell permeable NFkB inhibitor (NFkB-SN50) completely inhibited the TNF-α secretion in both AA and HG-treated monocytes (data not given). These studies suggest a role of protein kinase and p38-MAPK in the signal transduction pathways and possible up regulation of NFkB and TNF-α synthesis and secretion by cells treated with AA and HG.

The oxidative stress caused by excessive ROS generation or hyperglycemia has been shown to affect a variety of signal transduction pathways involving mitogen-activated protein kinase (MAPK) such as extracellular signal–regulated kinases

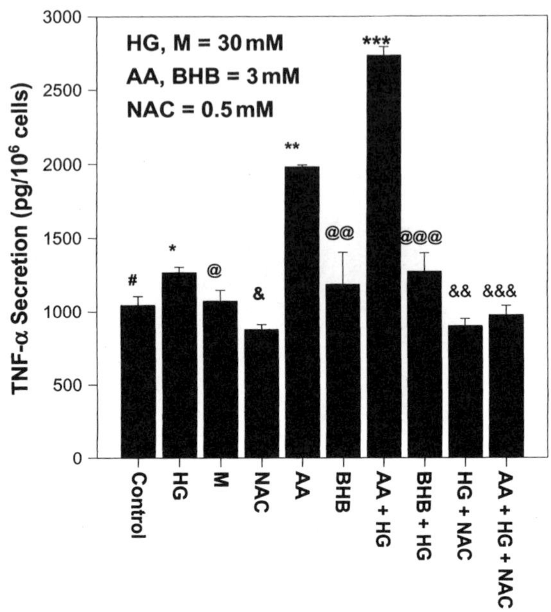

Figure 4. Effect of high glucose (HG), mannitol (M), AA, HG and NAC on TNF-α secretion by activated monocytes. Differences between values marked #vs*, #vs**, #vs***, and *vs&&, ***vs&&& are significant ($p < 0.02$).

(ERK-2), p38 and c-jun N-terminal kinase (JNK) [33]. HG can up-regulate expression of transcription factors NFkB and activating protein-1 and the TNF-α gene in monocytes. This expression of the TNF-α gene is mediated by the protein kinases p38 and JNK-1, which are dependent and independent of oxidative stress pathways [33,34]. Several studies advocate the importance of the p38 pathway in diabetes [35]. cAMP-dependent protein kinases (PKA) can activate phosphorylation of substrate proteins and cross talk with MAPKs pathways and proteins that are involved in signal transduction pathways leading to altered gene expression and modulation of physiological processes [34]. cAMP is known to modulate cytokine production in a number of cell types [36]. Whether ketosis affects expression of proteins associated with cytokine signal transduction pathways or has similar effects on endothelial cells TNF-α secretion is not known.

The vascular complications in diabetes could be a multifactorial event involving several cells types, inflammatory cytokines, chemokines, adhesion molecules and other unknown etiological factors. In diabetic patients, monocytes are exposed to ketone bodies for a prolonged period of time, thus becoming targets of an oxidized environment similar to that of the endothelial cells of the blood vessels. It is therefore plausible to suggest that ketosis may initiate some of these pathological events.

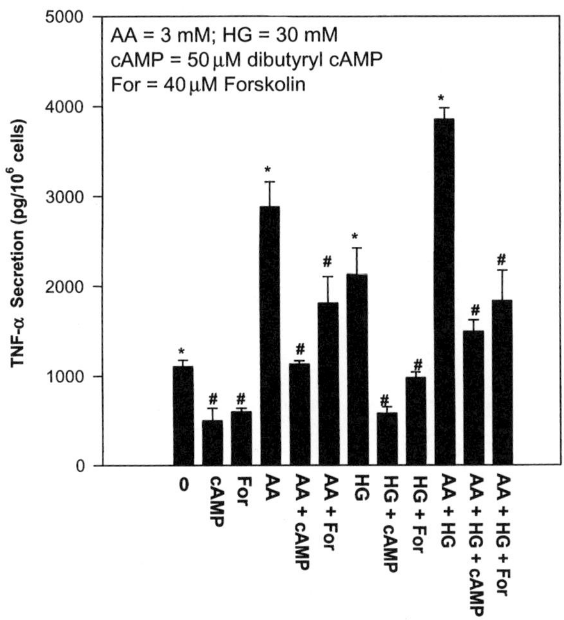

Figure 5. Effect of cAMP and Forsokollin on TFN-α Secretion by AA and HG-treated Cultured Monocytes. Differences in values marked *vs# are significant ($p < 0.01$).

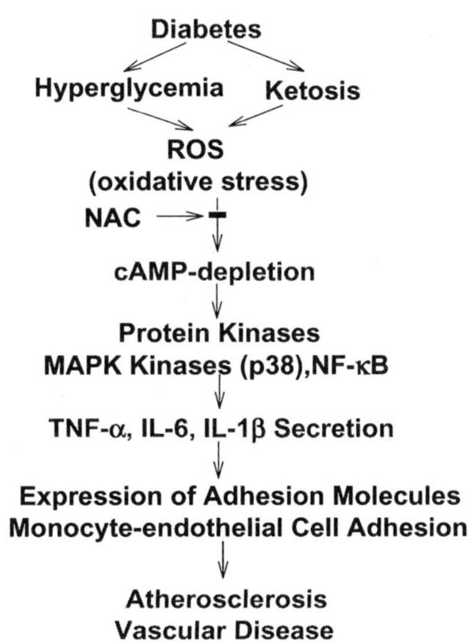

Figure 6. Proposed mechanism for the role of ketosis and cytokines in vascular disease of diabetes Diabetes

CONCLUSION

Ketosis can increase TNF-α secretion in a U937 monocyte cell culture model and in type-1 diabetic patients. Figure 6 illustrates the proposed mechanism by which ketosis and hyperglycemia can increase blood levels of pro-inflammatory cytokines, monocyte-endothelial cells adhesion and vascular disease. The effect of the ketone body AA on TNF-α secretion is apparently mediated by cAMP deficiency and the activation of protein kinase A, along with p38-MAPK and NFkB. The evidence that the antioxidant NAC can prevent the secretion of TNF-α in AA-treated cultured monocytes needs to be explored at the clinical level to see whether its supplementation can prevent or delay the excess vascular disease observed among diabetic patient population.

ACKNOWLEDGEMENTS

Authors are thankful to Georgia First for editing this manuscript. This study was supported by a Stiles Grant Award by the LSUHSC at Shreveport.

REFERENCES

1. DCCT Research Group. 1996. The absence of a glycemic threshold for the development of long-term complications: The perspective of the diabetes control and complications trial. Diabetes 45:1289–1298.
2. Rader DJ. 2000. Inflammatory markers of coronary risk. New Engl J Med 343:1179–1182.
3 Strowig SM, Raskin P. 1995. Glycemic control and the complications of diabetes. Diab rev 3:237–257.
4 Baynes, JW. 1991. Role of oxidative stress in development of complications in diabetes. Diabetes 40:405–411.
5. Ruderman NB, Williamson JR, Brownlee M. 1992. Glucose and diabetic vascular disease. FASEB J 6:2905–2914.
6. Champe PC, Harvey RA. 1994. In Lippincott's illustrated reviews: Biochemistry. J. B. Lippincott Co. 171–190.
7. Kern PA, Ranganathan S, Li C, Wood L, Ranganathan G. 2001. Adipose tissue tumor necrosis factor and interleukin-6 expression in human obesity and insulin resistance. Amer J Physiol 280:E745–5.
8. Halse R, Pearson SL, McCormack JG, Yeaman SJ, Taylor R. 2001. Effects of tumor necrosis factor-a on insulin action in cultured human muscle cells. Diabetes 50:1102–1109.
9. Hotamisligil GS, Budavari A, Murray D, Spiegleman BM. 1994. Reduced tyrosine kinase activity of the insulin receptor in obesity-diabetes: central role of tumor necrosis factor-á. J Clin Invest 94:1543–1549.
10. Saghizadeh M, Ong JM, Garvey WT, Henry RR, Kern PA. 1996. Th expression of TNF alpha by human muscle. Relationship to insulin resistance. J Clin Invest 97:1111–1116.
11. Solomon SS. 1975. Effect of insulin and lipolytic hormones on cyclic AMP phosphodieterase activity in normal and diabetic rat adipose tissue. Endocrinology 96:1366–1373.
12. Jialal I, Devaraj S. 1996. The role of oxidized low density lipoprotein in atherogenesis. J Nutr 126: 1053S–1057S.
13. Devaraj S, Jialal I. 2000. Alpha-tocopherol supplementation decreases serum C-reactive protein and monocyte interleukin-6 levels in normal volunteers in type-2 diabetic patients. Free Rad Biol Med 29:790–792.
14. Rajeswari P, Natarajan R, Nadler JL, Kumar D. 1991. Glucose induces lipid peroxidation and inactivation of membrane associated iron transport enzymes in human erythrocytes in vivo and in vitro. J. Cell Physiol 149:100–109.
15. Jain SK, Krueger SK, McVie R, Jaramillo JJ, Palmer M, Smith T. 1998. Relationship of blood thromboxane-B_2 with lipid peroxides and effect of vitamin E and placebo supplementation on TxB_2 and lipid peroxide levels in Type-1 diabetic patients. Diab Care 21:1511–1516.

16. Zoppini G, Targher G, Monauni T, Faccini G, Pasqualini E, Martinelli C, Zenalri ML, Muggeo M. 1996. Increase in circulating products of lipid peroxidation in smokers with IDDM.Diab Care 19:1233–1236.
17. Dominguez C, Rutz E, Gussinye M, Carrascosa A. 1998. Oxidative stress at onset and in early stages of type-1 diabetes in children and adolescents. Diab Care 21:1736–1742.
18. Santini SA, Marra G, Giardina B, Cotroneo P, Mordente A, Martorana GE, Manto A, Ghirlanda G. 1997. Defective plasma antioxidant defenses and enhanced susceptibility to lipid peroxidation in uncomplicated IDDM. Diabetes 46:1853–1858.
19. Ozben T, Nacitarhan S, Tuncer N. 1995. Plasma and urine malondialdehyde levels in non-insulin dependent diabetic patients with and without microalbuminuria. Int J Clin & Lab Res 25:162–164.
20. Jain SK, McVie R, Duett J, Herbst JJ. 1989. Erythrocyte membrane lipid peroxidation and glycosylated hemoglobin in diabetes. Diabetes 38:1539–1543.
21. Nishikawa T, Edelstein D, Du XL, Yamagishi S, Matsumura T, Kaneda Y, Yorek MA, Beebe D, Oates PJ, Hammes HP, Giardino I, Brownlee M. 2000. Normalizing mitochondrial superoxide production blocks three pathways of hyperglycemic damage. Nature 404:787–790.
22. Jain SK, Kannan K, Lim G. 1998. Ketosis (acetoacetate) can generate oxygen radicals and cause increased lipid peroxidation and growth inhibition in human endothelial cells. Free Rad Biol Med 25:1083–1088.
23. Jain SK, Kannan K, McVie R. 1999. Effect of hyperketonemia on blood monocytes in type 1 diabetic patients and apoptosis in cultured U937 monocytes. Antioxidants Redox Signal 1:211–220.
24. Jain SK, McVie R. 1999. Hyperketonemia can increase lipid peroxidation and lower glutathione levels in human erythrocytes in vitro and in type 1 diabetic patients. Diabetes 48:1850–555.
25. Jain SK, McVie R, Jackson R, Levine SN, Lim G. 1999. Effect of hyperketonemia on lipid peroxidation levels of plasma in diabetic patients. Diabetes Care 22:171–175.
26. Wolff S, Jiang ZY, Hunt JV. 1991. Protein glycation and oxidative stress in diabetes mellitus and aging. Free Rad Biol Med 10:339–352.
27. Jain SK. 1989. Hyperglycemia can cause membrane lipid peroxidation and osmotic fragility in human red blood cells. J Biol Chem 264:21340–21345.
28. Mullarkey CJ, Edelstein D, Brownlee M. 1990. Free radical generation by early glycation products: A mechanism for accelerated atherogenesis in diabetes. Biochem Biophys Res Commun 173: 932–939.
29. Nishikawa T, Edelstein D, Du XL, Yamagishi S, Matsumura T, Kaneda Y, Yorek MA, Beebe D, Oates PJ, Hammes HP, Giardino I, Brownlee M. 2000. Normalizing mitochondrial superoxide production blocks three pathways of hyperglycemic damage. Nature 404:787–790.
30. Arai K, Maguchi S, Fujii S, Ishibash H, Oikawa K, Taniguchi N. 1987. Glycation and inactivation of human Cu-Zn-superoxide dismutase. Identification of the in vitro glycated sites. J Biol Chem 262: 16969–16972.
31. Rajeswari P, Natarajan R, Nadler JL, Kumar D. 1991. Glucose induces lipid peroxidation and inactivation of membrane associated iron transport enzymes in human erythrocytes in vivo and in vitro. J Cell Physiol 149:100–109.
32. Jain SK, Kannan K. 2001. Chromium chloride inhibits oxidative stress and TNF- secretion caused by exposure to high glucose in cultured monocytes. Biochem Biophys Res Commun 289:687–691.
33. Guha M, Bai W, Nadler JL, Natarajan R. 2000. Molecular mechanisms of tumor necrosis factor a gene expression in monocytic cells via hyperglycemia-induced oxidant stress-depemdent and independent pathways. J Biol Chem 275:17728–17739.
34. Jain SK, Kannan K, Lim G, McVie R, Bocchini JA. Hyperketonemia increases TNF-α secretion in cultured U937 monocytes and type-1 diabetic patients. Diabetes 51:2287–2293 (2002).
35. Igarashi M, Wakasaki H, Takahara N, Ishii H, Jiang Z-Y, Yamauchi T, Kuboki K, Meier M, Rhodes CJ, King GL. 1999. Glucose or diabetes activates p38 mitogen-activated protein kinase via different pathways. J Clin Invest 103:185–195.
36. Kannan K, Jain SK. 2000. Oxidative stress and apoptosis. Pathophysiology 7:153–163.

G.N. Pierce, M. Nagano, P. Zahradka, and N.S. Dhalla (eds.).
ATHEROSCLEROSIS, HYPERTENSION AND DIABETES.
Kluwer Academic Publishers. Boston.

EPIGENETIC ALTERATIONS IN DIABETIC CARDIOMYOPATHY

PATRICK K. UMEDA,[1] REGINA P. SHIAU,[1] MAKESHA MIGGINS,[1] and JAMES B. CAULFIELD[2]

Departments of [1] Medicine and [2] Pathology, University of Alabama at Birmingham, Birmingham, Alabama, USA

Summary. DNA methylation of the β-myosin heavy chain (HC) promoter plays a primary role in altering the structure and function of the failing heart. The modification of specific promoter sequences induces a cardiomyopathy in a transgenic mouse model and *de novo* DNA methylation occurs in the myocytes of failing but not of nonfailing human hearts. To determine if comparable epigenetic alterations of the β-myosin HC promoter are involved in diabetic cardiomyopathy, we used the bisulfite mapping technique to examine DNA methylation of the human β-myosin HC promoter in left ventricular tissue of non-insulin-dependent diabetic patients obtained at autopsy. Genomic DNA was treated with bisulfite, a 320-bp region of the β-myosin HC promoter containing 7 CpG methylation sites was amplified by PCR and cloned in a plasmid vector, and cytosine methylation was assessed by DNA sequencing of >20 clones. Of the 7 CpG sites, three are methylated *de novo* in failing human hearts. In DNA from the type 2 diabetic hearts (n = 12), only one of the latter 3 CpG sites is methylated to a substantial extent. The same change in DNA methylation occurs in solid-organ transplants (n = 3) with steroid-induced diabetes as well as in type 1 diabetics (n = 2). These data indicate that unique alterations in DNA methylation are associated with diabetes. As in the failing heart, such epigenetic modifications of the β-myosin HC promoter may play a primary role in altering the phenotype of the diabetic heart.

Key words: DNA methylation, Diabetic cardiomyopathy, Heart failure, Myosin heavy chain gene, Epigenetic mechanisms

Corresponding Author: Patrick K. Umeda, PhD, Division of Cardiovascular Diseases, University of Alabama at Birmingham, Zeigler Research Building, Rm 302, 703 19th Street South, Birmingham, Alabama 35294. Phone: 205-934-7569; Fax: 205-975-5150; e-mail: Pumeda@cardio.dom.uab.edu

INTRODUCTION

A high incidence of heart failure in diabetics is not surprising considering that hypertension, hyperlipidemia, obesity, atherosclerosis and coronary disease, and kidney disease are frequently associated with diabetes. However, even in the absence of coronary disease, diabetic patients exhibit a 4–6 fold increase in the incidence of congestive heart failure [1]. The epidemiologic data and the presence of cardiomegaly and congestive heart failure that is not due to coronary disease in some diabetics [2] suggest a distinct form of "cardiomyopathy" associated with diabetes. Clinical studies identifying alterations in heart function in diabetic patients in the preclinical stages [3,4] further suggest a cardiomyopathy that is not solely due to other pathologies associated with diabetes.

Studies in various animal models of diabetes have identified functional, biochemical, and molecular changes in the diabetic ventricle [5,6]. Abnormalities in diastolic and systolic function have been correlated with intrinsic alterations in calcium homeostasis [5–7], sarcolemmal and sarcoplasmic ion transporters [8–10], metabolism [11], mitochondrial function [12], contractile function [13,14], contractile protein [6,15] and isomyosin [16–18] expression, and the extracellular matrix [19,20]. On the other hand, diabetes has also been associated with microvascular changes [21], which in the setting of hypertension may accentuate ischemic damage and the progression to heart failure. Since many of the cardiac alterations associated with diabetes are similar to those found in end-stage heart failure, it is difficult to distinguish the primary effects of diabetes on the heart from subsequent changes in heart function due to complications of the disease.

While there is considerable interest in the role of transcription factors [22] and signal transduction pathways [23–25] in cardiac hypertrophy and failure, we have identified a transgenic mouse model that suggests novel mechanisms for modulating the heart phenotype. In transgenic mice, the presence of heterologous β-myosin HC promoter sequences is sufficient to produce the structural and functional changes of the heart that are associated with moderate heart failure [26]. These changes include RV and LV dilatation, myofibrillar disarray, excess mitochondria, depressed contractile function *in vivo* and in isolated papillary fibers, altered calcium homeostasis, and blunted coronary vasomotor responses. These phenotypic effects are intrinsic to the heart, since the altered heart function in the transgenic model occurs in the absence of cardiovascular disease, hypertension, or any overt developmental defects. Furthermore, the cardiomyopathy is not due to insertional mutagenesis, since it occurs in all transgenic mouse lines that contain the relevant sequences. In this transgenic mouse model, specific sequences of the β-myosin HC promoter modulate the heart phenotype.

The cardiomyopathic alterations in our transgenic mouse model are not only due to the presence of specific gene sequences but also due to the methylation of those sequences [27]. In one transgenic mouse line where genomic imprinting modulates the DNA methylation of the transgene locus, the cardiomyopathy is only observed in animals with a methylated transgene. In other lines, the transgene is methylated regardless of its parental origin and all transgenic animals exhibit cardiac alterations. Thus, in this model, DNA methylation appears to be a regulatory switch that initiates the effects of the β-myosin HC promoter sequences.

Our transgenic mouse model suggests that specific alterations in DNA methylation are associated with clinical heart failure. In human hearts, the selective methylation of endogenous β-myosin HC promoter sequences is correlated with congestive heart failure (see Results). To determine if selective alterations in DNA methylation also occur in diabetes, we have compared the DNA methylation of the β-myosin HC gene promoter in diabetic hearts with that in nonfailing and in failing human hearts. Here we show that specific sites within the human β-myosin HC promoter are methylated *de novo* in diabetic hearts. Moreover, we show that the modification observed in diabetes is distinct from those that occur in end-stage heart failure.

MATERIALS AND METHODS

Human heart specimens

Specimens were obtained from the left ventricle (LV) of explanted hearts following heart transplantation and from the LV of hearts at the time of autopsy. Portions of the LV (200–400 mg) were frozen in liquid nitrogen and stored at –80°C. Autopsy specimens were generally obtained within 12–24 hours of death. The procurement and analysis of human tissues were reviewed and approved by the Institutional Review Board.

DNA extraction

Approximately 200 mg of frozen LV tissue was suspended in 0.5 ml of a solution containing 400 mM NaCl, 10 mM Tris-HCl, pH 7.5, 0.5% SDS, 5 mM EDTA, 200 μg/ml Proteinase K (Boehringer-Mannheim), dispersed with a Teflon pestle, and incubated at 55°C overnight. The residual tissue mass was dispersed by vortexing, and 135 μL of saturated NaCl solution was added to the lysate. The mixture was chilled on ice for 5–10 minutes and then centrifuged at 16,000 × g for 10 minutes. Genomic DNA was precipitated from the supernatant by adding 0.4 volumes of isopropanol. The solution was centrifuged at 16,000 × g for 5 minutes, and the precipitate washed with 30% isopropanol, then with 70% ethanol, and dried. The precipitate was then dissolved in 150 μL of 10 mM Tris-HCl, pH 7.5, 1 mM EDTA.

To remove the residual RNA, the DNA solution was made 10 mM in EDTA and 0.5% in SDS. Thirty micrograms of heat-treated RNase was added and the mixture incubated at 37°C for 30 minutes. Proteinase K (Boehringer-Mannheim) was added to a final concentration of 100 μg/ml and the solution incubated at 55°C for 2 hours. The sample was extracted once with an equal volume of phenol : chloroform (1 : 1) and twice with chloroform alone. One-tenth volume of 2 M NaOAc, pH 5.4 and 2 volumes of ethanol were added to the final aqueous phase and the DNA precipitated at –20°C overnight. The DNA precipitate was recovered by centrifugation, washed with 70% ethanol, dried, and dissolved in 100–200 μL of 10 mM Tris-HCl, pH 7.5, 1 mM EDTA. The yield of genomic DNA ranged from 50 to 100 μg.

Bisulfite genomic sequencing

The genomic DNA (1.5 μg) was treated with sodium bisulfite essentially as described by Clark *et al.* [28]. Free bisulfite was removed by gel filtration on a 1-ml tuberculin-syringe spin column of Sephadex G-50 fine (equilibrated with 10 mM Tris-HCl, pH 7.5, 1 mM EDTA). Sodium hydroxide was added to the sample to a final concentration of 0.3 M and the sample incubated at 37°C for 15 minutes. The solution was then brought to 0.3 M in either NaOAc (pH 5.4) or KOAc (pH 5), 2 μg of linear acrylamide (Ambion) added as carrier, and the DNA precipitated with 3 volumes of ethanol at −80°C. The DNA precipitate was recovered by centrifugation, washed with 70% ethanol, dried, and then dissolved in 25 μL of 10 mM Tris-HCl, pH 7.5, 1 mM EDTA.

A 391-bp portion of the "sense" strand of the human β-myosin HC promoter (−95 to −485) was initially amplified with the following primers: A) 5′-TTG GATATAGGATTTGGG-3′, B) 5′-AACTATTATCACTAAAAACATTTCCCC-CAA-3′. Amplifications were performed in a 20-μL reaction mixture containing: 67 mM Tris-HCl, pH 8.85, 6.7 mM $MgCl_2$, 16.6 mM $(NH4)_2SO_4$ 150 μm dNTe, 160 μg/ml BSA, 0.2 μM of each primer, 1.6% formamide (deionized), 0.5 units AmpliTaq (Applied Biosystems), and 1 μL of bisulfite-modified DNA. The reaction mixture was overlaid with mineral oil and the PCR amplification carried out on an MJ Research thermocycler under the following conditions: 94°C/4 min × 1 cycle; 94°C/1 min, 53°C/2 min, 72°C/3 min, × 5 cycles; 94°C/30 sec, 53°C/ 2 min, 72°C/1 min, × 35 cycles; and 72°C/5 min × 1 cycle.

Nested PCR was performed with the following primers: C) 5′-GGATGTAG GTTTTAGGTTAGGAAAGTAGGG-3′, D) 5′-ACATTTCCCCCAAACTCC-3′. The second amplification was performed in a 20-μL reaction mixture containing: Pfu Buffer 3 (Stratagene), 200 μM dNTP, 0.2 μM primers, 0.5 units Pfu or TurboPfu (Stratagene) and 1 μL of a 1:10 dilution of the initial (Taq) PCR reaction. The cycling conditions were: 96°C/1 min, 50°C/2 min, 72°C/2 min, × 1 cycle; 94°C/ 1 min, 50°C/2 min, 72°C/2 min, × 30 cycles; 72°C/5 min × 1 cycle.

The nested PCR reaction was fractionated on a 1.5% agarose gel in Tris-borate-EDTA buffer. The 365-bp human β-myosin HC promoter fragment was recovered by running the DNA fragment onto DEAE-nitrocellulose (Schleicher & Schuell). The DNA fragment was eluted from the filter with 100 μL of 1.5 M NaCl, 20 mM Tris-HCl, pH 7.5, 2 mM EDTA at 70°C for 15 minutes. The elution was repeated with a second aliquot of the high salt solution. The DNA fragment was precipitated at −80°C following the addition of 1/20 volume of 2 M NaOAc, pH 5.4 and 2.5 volumes of ethanol. The DNA precipitate was recovered by centrifugation, washed with 70% ethanol, dried, and dissolved in 10 mM Tris-HCl, pH 7.5, 1 mM EDTA.

The 365-bp fragment was ligated into pBluescript KS(-) (Stratagene) that had been linearized with EcoRV, and the ligated DNA was transformed into supercompetent E. coli DH5α (Invitrogen) or DH10B (Invitrogen) according to the manufacturer's protocol. Plasmid DNAs were sequenced using Sequenase version 2.0 DNA sequencing kit (USB) and analyzed on a 5% Long Ranger (BioWhittaker)-urea sequencing gel. DNA sequencing was also performed by Center for AIDs Research Sequencing Core at UAB on an ABI Prism Model 3100.

The frequency of methylcytosine at specific sites was determined by sequencing more than 20 clones for each patient specimen. The distribution of DNA methylation for each experimental group was then obtained by averaging the frequency distributions for the corresponding patients.

The PCR primers B and C actually correspond to the rabbit β-myosin HC promoter sequences. The rabbit primers consistently produced the appropriate PCR fragments even though they contained 1–3 nucleotide mismatches with the corresponding human β-myosin HC promoter sequences.

RESULTS

Table 1 shows age and pathology associated with the patients in this study. Non-failing control hearts were from patients with minimal indications of heart disease or hypertrophy. These patients also had no prior history of type 2 diabetes. Failing hearts consisted of explanted hearts obtained at the time of heart transplantation. The LV ejection fraction (when available) shows the diminished heart function in these patients. The diabetic hearts were obtained primarily from type 2 diabetics. These patients suffered from other clinical conditions that included hypertension, athersclerosis, ischemic heart disease and cardiac failure. Only one exhibited cardiomegaly with no coronary artery disease and could be diagnosed with diabetic cardiomyopathy.

To assess DNA methylation of the endogenous β-myosin HC promoter in human hearts, we used the bisulfite mapping technique [28,29]. In this method, cytosine (but not methylcytosine) residues are converted to uracil with sodium bisulfite. Individual DNA strands for a region of interest are then amplified by PCR and subcloned, and the residual cytosines (*i.e.*, methylcytosines) identified by DNA sequencing of individual clones. In this method, DNA methylation can be resolved at the sequence level. The extent to which specific cytosine residues are modified in the original DNA is estimated by sequencing a number of clones (molecules).

In our transgenic mouse model, sequences extending from −130 to −670 of the rabbit β-myosin HC promoter mediate changes in the heart phenotype. The corresponding region of the human β-myosin HC promoter is highly conserved in nucleotide sequence [30] and contains a cluster of 7 CpG methylation sites located between −130 and −450. The latter region also contains binding sites for a number of transcription factors and has been shown to encode both negative and positive cis-regulatory elements of the β-myosin HC gene [30–32]. To determine if the human β-myosin HC promoter is differentially methylated in cardiac failure and diabetes, we focused on the CpG methylation sites between −130 and −450.

Table 1. Experimental Groups

Non-Failing Hearts

Patient	Sex	Age	Pathology/cause of death
1	M	10 m	Drowning
2	M	57	Stroke
3	F	19	Primary pulmonary hypertension
4	F	8 m	Biliary atresia

Failing Hearts

Patient	Sex	Age	LVEF	Pathology
5	M	49	0.10	Ischemic heart disease
6	F	10	—	Transposition of great vessels
7	M	24	0.10	Idiopathic dilated cardiomyopathy
8	M	42	0.12	Idiopathic dilated cardiomyopathy
9	F	51	0.10	Idiopathic dilated cardiomyopathy
10	F	16	unavail.	Idiopathic dilated cardiomyopathy
11	F	20	unavail.	Idiopathic dilated cardiomyopathy
12	F	59	unavail.	Idiopathic dilated cardiomyopathy
13	F	14 m	unavail.	Myocarditis
14	M	54	0.15	Ischemic heart disease
15	F	50	unavail.	Idiopathic dilated cardiomyopathy
16	M	54	unavail.	Dilated cardiomyopathy
17	F	46	0.10	Dilated cardiomyopathy
18	M	59	unavail.	Ischemic heart disease
19	M	61	0.20	Idiopathic dilated cardiomyopathy

Diabetic Hearts

Patient	Sex	Age	Type	Pathology/cause of death
20	M	63	2	CAD, pulmonary thromboemboli
21	F	45	2	Congestive heart failure
22	M	74	2	Bronchopneumonia
23	M	68	2	Ruptured aortic aneurysm
24	F	46	2	Heart failure, arrhythmia
25	M	72	2, post-transplant	Pneumonia (heart transplant-9 yr)
26	F	87	2	CAD, MI, heart failure
27	M	59	2	Heart failure, pulmonary edema
28	F	68	2	Acute promyelocytic leukemia
29	M	61	2	Idiopathic pulmonary fibrosis
30	M	81	2	CAD
31	F	66	2, post-transplant	Disseminated aspergillosis (heart transplant-2 yr)
32	M	47	2	Bronchopneumonia
33	F	43	2	Extensive *Pseudomonas* infection, myocarditis
34	F	68	2	Severe CAD, heart failure
35	M	76	2	Squamous cell carcinoma of the lungs
36	M	42	2	Pulmonary thromboemboli
37	M	48	2, post-transplant	Hemorrhagic diathesis (heart transplant-1 yr)
38	F	36	1	Superior vena cava syndrome
39	F	33	1	Cerebral vascular accident

Type 2 diabetic patients 21, 24, 26, 27, 33 and 34 were in heart failure. The post-transplantation survival for patients 25, 31 and 37 is indicated along with the pathology or cause of death. LVEF, left ventricular ejection fraction; m, months; MI, myocardial infarction; CAD, coronary artery disease.

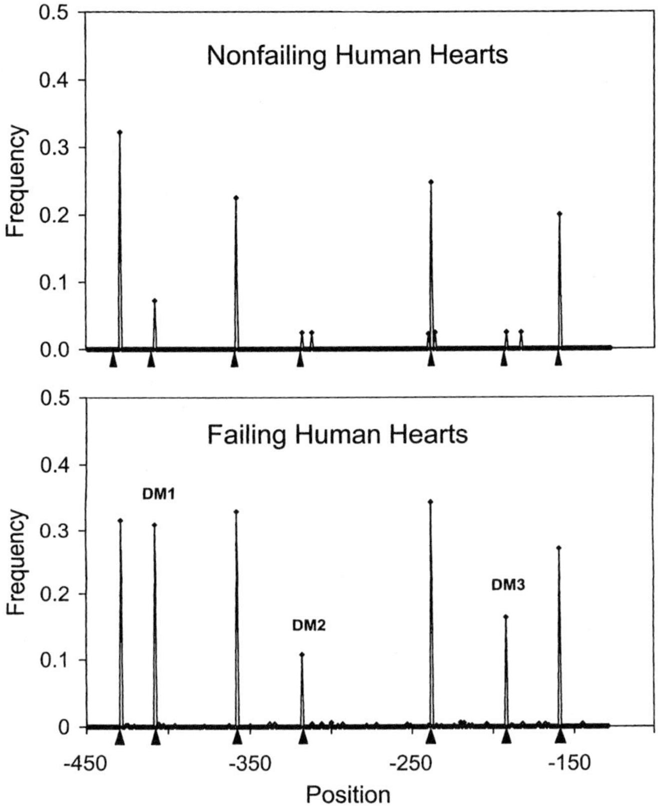

Figure 1. DNA Methylation of the Human β-Myosin HC Promoter in Nonfailing and Failing Human Hearts. The upper panel shows the relative proportion (frequency) of methylcytosine residues over a 320-bp region of the promoter in nonfailing human ventricles (n = 4). The lower panel shows the distribution observed in genomic DNA from explanted, failing hearts (n = 15). The location of this region in the human β myosin HC gene is indicated on the abscissa. The solid triangles at the bottom indicate the location of the CpG methylation sites. DM1, DM2, and DM3 designate the sites that are methylated differentially or *de novo* in failing hearts.

Specific sites of the β-myosin HC promoter are methylated in failing human hearts

To determine if the endogenous β-myosin HC promoter is differentially methylated in human heart failure, we compared methylation patterns in DNA from LV tissue of nonfailing and explanted failing hearts. Figure 1 shows the distribution of methylcytosines in the 320-bp region of the endogenous β-myosin HC promoter. The frequency of methylcytosines corresponds to the proportion of DNA molecules that are methylated at a particular site. Only data for the "sense" strand are shown. As seen in Fig. 1, DNA methylation occurs primarily at CpG dinucleotides.

Methylcytosine residues at other locations generally correspond to the modification of CpNpG sites (33). In ventricular DNA from nonfailing hearts (top panel), only 4 of the 7 CpG sites are methylated at the frequency of 0.2–0.4. Modifications at the other CpG sites are substantially less frequent. By contrast, in ventricular DNA from failing hearts, all 7 sites are methylated (bottom panel). Four CpG sites are modified to the same extent as in nonfailing hearts; the other three sites (designated as DM1, DM2 and DM3) are differentially methylated in failing human hearts. These data indicate that specific sites in the promoter are modified *de novo* in failing human hearts.

The relevance of the differential methylation of the β-myosin HC promoter to cardiac failure is indicated by other studies. First, in failing human hearts, alterations in DNA methylation are not observed in other regions of the genome (data not shown). Second, the analyses of nuclei isolated by laser-assisted microdissection indicate that the methylation of DM1, DM2 and DM3 occurs predominantly in myocytes, but not in nonmyocytes, of failing human hearts (data not shown). Third, the level (frequency) of methylation in DNA from myocyte nuclei is 2–3 fold higher than that in DNA from whole LV tissue. Finally, in animal models of hypertrophy and failure, altered methylation of the endogenous β-myosin HC promoter is observed in cardiac hypertrophy but becomes more extensive in overt heart failure (data not shown). The selective methylation of the β-myosin HC promoter in myocytes of the heart and the progression of such changes in experimental models of hypertrophy and failure are consistent with a role for the methylation of the endogenous β-myosin HC promoter in mediating the phenotypic changes that occur in cardiac failure.

Methylation of the β-myosin HC promoter is altered in non-insulin-dependent diabetic hearts

To determine if alterations in DNA methylation are associated with the cardiomyopathic changes in diabetes, we examined the methylation profiles in type 2 diabetic hearts obtained at autopsy. Most of the patients had other clinical conditions (Table 1) that could potentially affect DNA methylation. Based on the data in Fig. 1, diabetic patients with cardiac failure were likely to show extensive changes in DNA methylation in the promoter sequences. As for the other type 2 diabetic patients, we postulated that, by analyzing many patients, any change common to diabetes would be evident while modifications resulting from other clinical conditions would be averaged into the background.

As shown in Fig. 2, specific alterations in the DNA methylation of the β-myosin HC promoter were evident in hearts of type 2 diabetics. In type 2 diabetics who were not in heart failure (top panel), the DNA methylation profile is slightly different from that of nonfailing control hearts. One of the differentially methylated sites (DM1) is modified to a substantial level while DNA methylation at the other sites, including DM2 and DM3, is similar to that in nonfailing control hearts. In type 2 diabetics who were in cardiac failure (bottom panel), the pattern of methylation is similar to that observed in explanted failing human hearts (Fig. 1). All three differentially methylated sites are modified with the level of modification at DM1

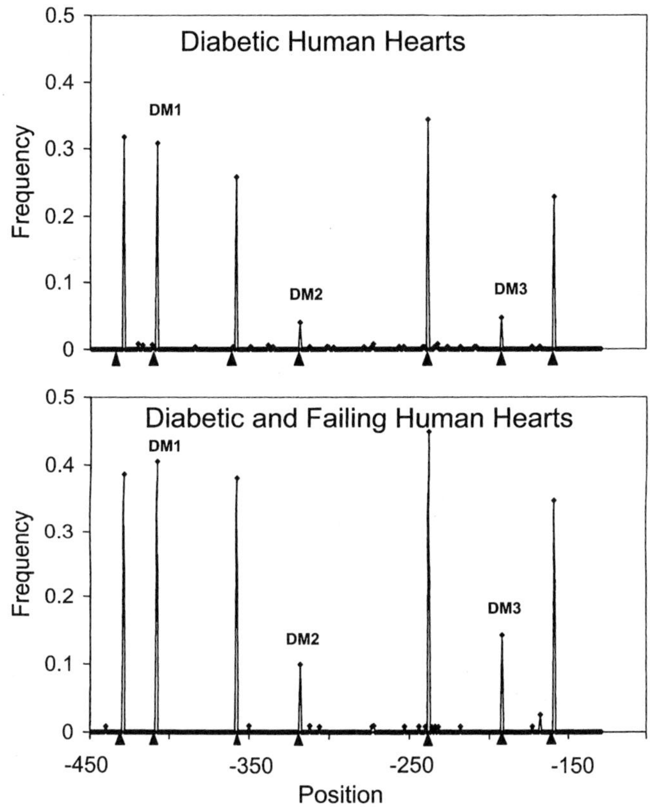

Figure 2. DNA Methylation of the Human β-Myosin HC Promoter in Diabetic Human Hearts. The figure shows the relative proportion (frequency) of methylcytosine residues over a 320-bp region of the promoter in type 2 diabetic LV tissues obtained at autopsy. The distribution in type 2 diabetics who were not in heart failure (n = 12) is shown in the top panel. The data for type 2 diabetics who were in heart failure (n = 6) are shown in the bottom panel. The location of this region in the human β myosin HC gene is indicated on the abscissa. The solid triangles at the bottom indicate the location of the CpG methylation sites. DM1, DM2, and DM3 designate the sites that are methylated differentially or *de novo* in failing hearts.

(but not DM2 and DM3) being slightly higher than that in explanted failing human hearts. The selective methylation of DM1 in type 2 diabetic hearts suggests that the human β-myosin HC promoter is methylated *de novo* in diabetes. Furthermore, the data show that the alteration in methylation that is associated with diabetes is distinct from those in heart failure.

The β-Myosin HC promoter is methylated de novo in steroid-induced diabetes

Since many of the diabetic patients had long standing disease (Table 1), it is possible that the selective change in DNA methylation could be due to other

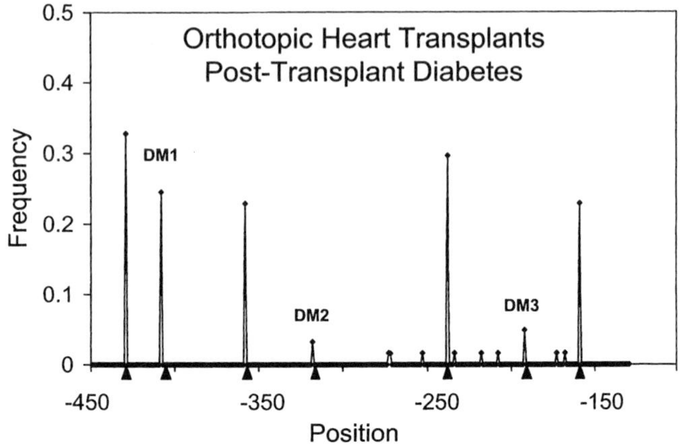

Figure 3. DNA Methylation of the Human β-Myosin HC Promoter in Steroid-Induced Diabetes. The figure shows the distribution of methylcytosine residues in a 320-bp region of the human β-myosin HC promoter in steroid-induced diabetic hearts. The LV specimens were from patients who developed type 2 diabetes following heart transplantation (n = 3). The diabetes probably resulted from the steroids used in the immunosuppression therapy. The solid triangles at the bottom indicate the location of the CpG methylation sites. DM1, DM2, and DM3 designate the sites that are methylated differentially or *de novo* in failing hearts.

complications of the disease. To obtain some insight into temporal change in DNA methylation, we were able to analyze LV specimens from three patients who developed type 2 diabetes following heart transplantation. In these patients, the diabetes resulted from the use of steroids in immunosuppression therapy. The post-transplantation survival for two patients was 1–2 years; for the other patient, it was 9 years. As shown in Fig. 3, the distribution of methylcytosines in the steroid-induced diabetic hearts was similar to that of spontaneous type 2 diabetics. Only one differentially methylated site (DM1) is modified to a significant extent. Since this change in DNA methylation occurred in donor hearts that presumably exhibited the DNA methylation profile of nonfailing hearts, the data indicate that the modification associated with type 2 diabetics is inducible, probably occurs early in diabetes, and is unlikely to be due to other complications of the disease.

The β-myosin HC promoter is selectively methylated in type 1 diabetic hearts

We have also examined the pattern of DNA methylation of the β-myosin HC promoter in a limited number of type 1 diabetic hearts. As shown in Fig. 4, type 1 diabetic hearts exhibit the specific methylation of DM1 found in type 2 diabetes. However, DM3 also is methylated, but at a slightly lower level than in failing hearts (Figs. 1 and 2). The modification of DM3 may be related to the severity of the diabetes. These data show that specific changes in the methylation of the β-myosin HC promoter are observed in insulin-dependent diabetes.

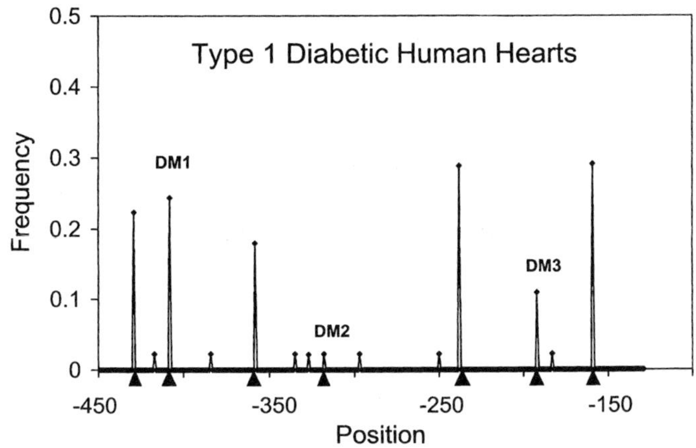

Figure 4. DNA Methylation of the Human β-Myosin HC Promoter in Type 1 Diabetic Hearts. The figure shows the distribution of methylcytosine residues in a 320-bp region of the promoter in type 1 diabetic hearts (n = 2). The solid triangles at the bottom indicate the location of the CpG methylation sites. DM1, DM2, and DM3 designate the sites that are methylated differentially or *de novo* in failing hearts.

DISCUSSION

Our studies show that alterations in DNA methylation occur in diabetic hearts. Using the bisulfite mapping technique to analyze a region of the human β-myosin HC promoter, we find that a specific site is methylated *de novo* in the hearts of type 2 diabetics. The modification at this site appears to be selective, as other sites in the promoter either remain unmodified or are methylated to the same level as in nonfailing control hearts. This alteration in methylation is present in orthotopic heart transplants with steroid-induced diabetes. Thus, this alteration is inducible and may occur early in diabetes. Furthermore, the specific alteration in DNA methylation occurs in both type 2 diabetes and in type 1 diabetic hearts. Overall, the data suggests that a specific change in DNA methylation of the β-myosin HC promoter is associated with diabetes.

The alteration in methylation in diabetic hearts occurs in a region of the genome that apparently can affect the structure and function of the heart. In transgenic mice, the methylation of this region of the β-myosin HC promoter is sufficient to produce the phenotypic changes that are associated with cardiac failure. In this transgenic mouse model, DNA methylation serves as a switch initiating the cardiomyopathic effects. In human failing hearts and animal models of heart failure, the methylation of this region of the endogenous β-myosin HC promoter is enhanced and is consistent with having a role in modulating the phenotype of the heart. Thus, the change in methylation observed in diabetic hearts may be related to the change in heart structure and function associated with diabetes.

The pattern of DNA methylation associated with diabetes is distinct from that observed in heart failure. In diabetics with heart failure, however, the unique pattern observed in diabetes changes to the pattern seen in failing human hearts. It is possible that the alteration observed in diabetes reflects an early event in the progression to cardiac failure. Alternatively, the dynamic changes in the methylation of the promoter could suggest that different mechanisms are involved in modifying the DNA in diabetes and in cardiac failure. The further increase in the level of methylation at DM1 (but not DM2 and DM3) in failing hearts of diabetics would favor the latter possibility. Thus, the analysis of DNA methylation suggests a mechanism by which diabetes may directly induce the changes in the heart that are associated with heart failure.

The mechanism by which alterations in DNA methylation mediate changes in the heart is not known. DNA methylation has long been associated with inactive genes and the repression of gene expression [34]. Methylated DNA is often associated with heterochromatin [35] or inactive regions of the genome. This correlation of DNA methylation and gene silencing may result from alterations in chromatin mediated by modified histones [36], the recruitment of histone deacetylase to methylation sites [37], or altering the binding sites of specific transcription factors [38]. In some instances, however, DNA methylation also mediates positive effects on gene expression [39,40]. For example, in the imprinted insulin-like growth factor-2 receptor gene, expression of the maternal allele is dependent on the methylation of an imprinting control region in the second intron of the gene [39]. Thus, DNA methylation may be instrumental in initiating a pattern of gene expression as well as in suppressing an existing regulatory scheme.

DNA methylation generally is not recognized as a mechanism for modulating gene expression in the adult heart. Early studies assessing global DNA methylation failed to identify any significant change in the heart other than an overall decrease with age [41]. One recent report examined the methylation of the β-myosin HC promoter in the right atrium of hypertrophied human hearts [42]. In that study, DNA methylation of three sites in the β-myosin HC promoter was inversely related to the transcription of the gene. It is possible that the alterations in methylation in LV tissue detected in our analyses may also affect transcription of the β-myosin HC gene. One of the differentially methylated sites (DM3) is located near a positive cis-element of the promoter [31,32,43]. The other two differentially modified sites are in regions of the promoter that appear to mediate negative effects of promoter function in the heart [30,44]. Thus, it is not clear what the net effect of the differential methylation might be on transcription of the β-myosin HC gene. The cardiomyopathy in transgenic mice containing only heterologous β-myosin HC promoter sequences, however, would suggest that the primary effect of DNA methylation on the heart phenotype is independent of any change in the expression of the β-myosin HC gene.

In one sense, the regulatory processes that we are dealing with here may be considered to be epigenetic. Epigenetics refers to mitotically and/or meiotically heritable changes in gene function that do not result from a change in the DNA sequence. As shown in transgenic mice, cardiomyopathic alterations can be inherited through a discrete segment of the genome and these effects are mediated through the modification of that gene segment by DNA methylation. Epigenetic mechanisms play major roles in either maintaining or altering cellular fates during development [45]. Such mechanisms are responsible for a number of cellular processes (e.g., X-inactivation and various forms of gene silencing) and are essential for development [46]. Epigenetic effects mediated by DNA methylation can control the spatial and temporal expression of genes during muscle development [47,48] and also are important in genomic "imprinting" [39,40,49]. Thus, the "epigenetic" effect of the β-myosin HC promoter on the heart is consistent with this developmental theme of modulating or altering the fate of cells or tissues.

The concept of "epigenetic" modulation of gene expression in the adult heart is novel. Such a concept predicts that various mechanisms acting through the methylation of the β-myosin HC promoter could mediate the development or progression of cardiomyopathic alterations in the heart. The *de novo* methylation of specific promoter sequences in diabetes may exemplify such a paradigm for altering the structure and function of the heart.

ACKNOWLEDGEMENTS

This work was supported by grants from the National Institutes of Health (HL66911) and the American Heart Association (9950381).

REFERENCES

1. Kannel WB, Hjortland M, Castelli WP. 1974. Role of diabetes in congestive heart failure: the Framingham Study. Am J Cardiol 34:29–34.
2. Rubler S, Dlugash J, Yuceoglu YZ, Kumral T, Branwood AW, Grishman A. 1972. New type of cardiomyopathy associated with diabetic glomerulosclerosis. Am J Cardiol 30:595–602.
3. Ahmed SS, Jaferi GA, Narang RM, Regan TJ. 1975. Preclinical abnormality in left ventricular function in diabetes mellitus. Am Heart J 89:153–158.
4. Regan TJ, Lyons MM, Ahmed SS, Levinson GE, Oldewurtel HA, Ahmad MR, Haider B. 1977. Evidence for cardiomyopathy in familial diabetes mellitus. J Clin Invest 60:884–899.
5. Schaffer SW. 1991. Cardiomyopathy associated with noninsulin-dependent diabetes. Mol Cell Biochem 107:1–20.
6. Dhalla NS, Liu X, Panagia V, Takeda N. 1998. Subcellular remodeling and heart dysfunction in chronic diabetes. Cardiovas Res 40:239–247.
7. Yu JZ, Rodrigues B, McNeill JH. 1997. Intracellular calcium levels are unchanged in the diabetic heart. Cardiovas Res 34:91–98.
8. Ganguly PK, Pierce GN, Dhalla KS, Dhalla NS. 1983. Defective sarcoplasmic reticular calcium transport in diabetic cardiomyopathy. Am J Physiol 244:E528–E535.
9. Heyliger CE, Prakash A, McNeill JH. 1987. Alterations in cardiac sarcolemmal Ca^{2+} pump activity during diabetes mellitus. Am J Physiol 525:H540–H544.
10. Pierce GN, Dhalla NS. 1983. Sarcolemmal Na^+-K^+ ATPase activity in diabetic rat heart. Am J Physiol 245:C241–C247.
11. Stanley WC, Lopaschuk GD, McCormack JG. 1997. Regulation of energy substrate metabolism in the diabetic heart. Cardiovas Res 34:25–33.
12. Flarsheim CE, Grupp IL, Matlib MA. 1996. Mitochondrial dysfunction accompanies diastolic dysfunction in diabetic rat heart. Am J Physiol 271:H192–H202.
13. Fein FS, Kornstein LB, Strobeck JE, Capasso JM, Sonnenblick EH. 1980. Altered myocardial mechanics in diabetic rats. Circ Res 47:922–933.

14. Garber DW, Neely JR. 1983. Decreased myocardial function and myosin ATPase in hearts from diabetic rats. Am J Physiol 244:H586–H591.
15. Malholtra A, Lopez MC, Nakouzi A. 1995. Troponin subunits contribute to altered myosin ATPase activity in diabetic cariomyopathy. Mol Cell Biochem 151:165–172.
16. Dillman WH. 1980. Diabetes mellitus induces changes in cardiac myosin of the rat. Diabetes 29:579–582.
17. Pierce GN, Dhalla NS. 1981. Cardiac myofibrillar ATPase activity in diabetic rats. J Mol Cell Cardiol 13:1063–1069.
18. Malhotra A, Penpargkul S, Fein FS, Sonnenblick EH, Scheuer J. 1981. The effect of streptozotocin-induced diabetes in rats on cardiac contractile proteins. Circ Res 49:1243–1250.
19. Thompson EW. 1988. Structural manifestations of diabetic cardiomyopathy in the rat and its reversal by insulin treatment. Am J Anat 182:270–282.
20. Sima A, Popov D, Starodub O, Stancu C, Cristea C, Stern D, Simionescu M. 1997. Pathobiology of the heart in experimental diabetes: immunolocalization of lipoproteins, immunoglobulin G, and advanced glycation endproducts proteins in diabetic and/or hyperlipidemic hamster. Lab Invest 77:3–18.
21. Factor SM, Minase T, Cho S, Fein F, Capasso JM, Sonnenblick EH. 1984. Coronary microvascular abnormalities in the hypertensive-diabetic rat. A primary cause of cardiomyopathy? Am J Pathol 116:9–20.
22. Molkentin JD, Lu J-R, Antos CL, Markham B, Richardson J, Robbins J, Grant SR, Olson EN. 1998. A calcineurin-dependent transcriptional pathway for cardiac hypertrophy. Cell 93:215–228.
23. Arber S, Hunter JJ, Ross J Jr, Hongo M, Sansig G, Borg J, Perriard J-C, Chien KR, Caroni P. 1997. MLP-deficient mice exhibit a disruption of cardiac cytoarchitectural organization, dilated cardiomyopathy, and heart failure. Cell 88:393–403.
24. D'Angelo DD, Sakata Y, Lorenz JN, Boivin GP, Walsh RA, Liggett SB, Dorn GW II. 1997. Transgenic GαQ overexpression induces cardiac contractile failure in mice. Proc Natl Acad Sci USA 94:8121–8126.
25. Akhter SA, Luttrell LM, Rockman HA, Iaccarino G, Lefkowitz RJ, Koch WJ. 1998. Targeting the receptor-Gq interface to inhibit *in vivo* pressure overload myocardial hypertrophy. Science 280:574–577.
26. Umeda PK, Norton P, Shiau RP, Perry GJ, Urthaler F, Caulfield JB. 1996. Sequences of the rabbit β myosin heavy chain promter produce a condition of chronic heart failure in transgenic mice. Circulation 94:I–408.
27. Umeda PK, Norton P, Shiau RP, Caulfield JB. 1997. Cardiomyopathy in rabbit β myosin heavy chain promoter mice involves the methylation of the transgene. Circulation 96:I–181.
28. Clark SJ, Harrison J, Paul CL, Frommer M. 1994. High sensitivity mapping of methylated cytosines. Nucl Acid Res 22:2990–2997.
29. Frommer M, McDonald LE, Millar DS, Collis CM, Watt F, Grigg GW, Molloy PL, Paul CL. 1992. A genomic sequencing protocol that yields a positive display of 5-methylcytosine residues in individual DNA strands. Proc Natl Acad Sci USA 89:1827–1831.
30. Vyas DR, McCarthy JJ, Tsika RW. 1999. Nuclear protein binding at the β-myosin heavy chain A/T-rich element is enriched following increased skeletal muscle activity. J Biol Chem 274:30832–30842.
31. Edwards JG, Bahl JJ, Flink IL, Cheng SY, Morkin E. 1994. Thyroid hormone influences β myosin heavy chain (β MHC) expression. Biochem Biophys Res Comm 199:1482–1488.
32. Cribbs LL, Shimizu N, Yockey CE, Levin JE, Jakovcic S, Zak R, Umeda PK. 1989. Muscle specific regulation of a transfected rabbit myosin heavy chain β gene promoter. J Biol Chem 264:10672–10678.
33. Clark SJ, Harrison J, Frommer M. 1995. CpNpG methylation in mammalian cells. Nature Genetics 10:20–27.
34. Razin A, Cedar H. 1991. DNA methylation and gene expression. Microbiol Rev 55:451–458.
35. Bestor TH. 1990. DNA methylation: evolution of a bacterial immune function into a regulator of gene expression and genome structure in higher eukaryotes. Phil Trans Royal Soc London (Series B) 326:179–187.
36. Tamaru H, Selker EU. 2001. A histone H3 methyltransferase controls DNA methylation in *Neurospora crassa*. Nature 414:277–283.
37. Nan X, Ng H-H, Johnson CA, Laherty CD, Turner BM, Eisenman RN, Bird A. 1998. Transcriptional repression by the methyl CpG-binding protein MeCP2 involves a histone deacetylase complex. Nature 393:386–389.

38. Hark AT, Schoenherr CJ, Katz KJ, Ingram RS, Levorse JM, Tilghman SM. 2000. CTCF mediates methylation-sensitive enhancer-blocking activity at the *H19/Igf2* locus. Nature 405:486–489.
39. Wutz A, Smrzka OW, Schweifer N, Schellander K, Wagner EF, Barlow DP. 1997. Imprinted expression of the *Igf2r* gene depends on an intronic CpG island. Nature 389:745–749.
40. Murrell A, Heeson S, Bowden L, Constancia M, Dean W, Kelsey G, Reik W. 2001. An intragenic methylated region in the imprinted *Igf2* gene augments transcription. EMBO Reports 2:1101-1106.
41. Romanov GA, Zin'kovskaia GG, Berbyshev GD, Vaniushin BF. 1979. Age- and tissue-specific differences in intragenome distribution of 5′-methylcytosine in cow's DNA. Biokhimiia 44:1576–1581.
42. Clifford CP, Nunez DJ. 1998. Human beta-myosin heavy chain mRNA prevalence is inversely related to the degree of methylation of regulatory elements. Cardiovas Res 38:736–743.
43. Shimizu N, Prior G, Umeda PK, Zak R. 1992. *Cis*-acting elements responsible for muscle-specific expression of the myosin heavy chain β gene. Nucl Acids Res 20:1793–1799.
44. Umeda PK, Carter RL, Hall RS, Welborn JM, Bugaisky LB. 1990. Regulation of the myosin heavy chain β promoter in skeletal and cardiac muscles. In: The Dynamic State of Muscle Fibers. Ed. D Pette, 61–74, New York, Walter de Gruyter.
45. Holliday R, Pugh JE. 1975. DNA modification mechanisms and gene activity during development. Science 187:226–232.
46. Riggs AD, Porter TN. 1996. Overview of epigenetic mechanisms. In: Epigenetic Mechanisms of Gene Regulation. Ed. VEA Russo, RA Martienssen, AD Riggs, 29–45, New York, Cold Spring Harbor Laboratory Press.
47. Grieshammer U, McGrew MJ, Rosenthal N. 1995. Role of methylation in maintenance of positionally restricted transgene expression in developing muscle. Development 121:2245–2253.
48. Brunk BP, Goldhamer DJ, Emerson CP Jr. 1996. Regulated demethylation of the myoD distal enhancer during skeletal myogenesis. Develop Biol 177:490–503.
49. Reik W, Howlett SK, Surani MA. 1990. Imprinting by DNA methylation:from transgenes to endogenous gene sequences. Development 108:99–106.

INDEX